Elsevier's Integrated

Anatomy and Embryology

Elsevier's Integrated
Anatomy and
Embryology

Bruce Ian Bogart PhD

Module Director
Morphological and Developmental Basis of Medicine
Anatomy Unit Director
Department of Cell Biology
New York University
School of Medicine
New York, New York

Victoria H. Ort PhD

Embryology Unit Co-Director
Department of Cell Biology
New York University
School of Medicine
New York, New York

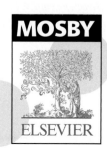

MOSBY
ELSEVIER

1600 John F. Kennedy Blvd
Suite 1800
Philadelphia, PA 19103-2899

ELSEVIER'S INTEGRATED ANATOMY & EMBRYOLOGY   ISBN-13: 978-1-4160-3165-9

Copyright © 2007 by Mosby, Inc., an affiliate of Elsevier Inc.

All rights reserved. No part of this publication may be reproduced or transmitted in any form or by any means, electronic or mechanical, including photocopying, recording, or any information storage and retrieval system, without permission in writing from the publisher. Permissions may be sought directly from Elsevier's Health Sciences Rights Department in Philadelphia, PA, USA: phone: (+1) 215 239 3804, fax: (+1) 215 239 3805, e-mail: healthpermissions@elsevier.com. You may also complete your request on-line via the Elsevier homepage (http://www.elsevier.com), by selecting 'Customer Support' and then 'Obtaining Permissions.'

Notice

Knowledge and best practice in this field are constantly changing. As new research and experience broaden our knowledge, changes in practice, treatment, and drug therapy may become necessary or appropriate. Readers are advised to check the most current information provided (i) on procedures featured or (ii) by the manufacturer of each product to be administered, to verify the recommended dose or formula, the method and duration of administration, and contraindications. It is the responsibility of the practitioner, relying on their own experience and knowledge of the patient, to make diagnoses, to determine dosages and the best treatment for each individual patient, and to take all appropriate safety precautions. To the fullest extent of the law, neither the Publisher nor the Authors assume any liability for any injury and/or damage to persons or property arising out or related to any use of the material contained in this book.

The Publisher

Library of Congress Cataloging-in-Publication Data

Bogart, Bruce Ian.
  Elsevier's integrated anatomy & embryology / Bruce Ian Bogart, Victoria H. Ort.
    p. ; cm.—(Elsevier's integrated series)
  Includes index.
  ISBN 978-1-4160-3165-9
  1. Human anatomy. 2. Embryology. 3. Human anatomy. 4. Embryology. I. Ort, Victoria H. II. Title.
III. Title: Elsevier's integrated anatomy and embryology. IV. Title: Integrated anatomy & embryology.
V. Series.
  [DNLM: 1. Anatomy. QS 4 B674e 2007]
  QM23.2.B64 2007
  611—dc22

                                                                    2007002640

Acquisitions Editor: Kate Dimock
Developmental Editor: Andrew Hall

Working together to grow
libraries in developing countries

www.elsevier.com | www.bookaid.org | www.sabre.org

ELSEVIER   BOOK AID International   Sabre Foundation

Printed in China

Last digit is the print number: 9 8 7 6 5 4 3 2 1

We dedicate this book to our families and colleagues who have been wonderfully supportive throughout the years and especially during this endeavor, and to the memory of our dear friend Dr. Lawrence Prutkin, who would have greatly enjoyed a New York University School of Medicine anatomy textbook.

Preface

Many medical schools have changed their curriculum from anatomic radiology to molecular biology and translational research due to the enormous growth in biomedical science. Given this situation, we set out to develop a hybrid anatomy text that could be used as a primary source in students' first year and again as a review book for the boards, clerkships, and electives. We hope to add a significant amount of anatomic information, such as the peripheral distribution of the cranial nerves, to our Web page to enrich the anatomy information available to the interested student. We sincerely hope that you find this text valuable as a first year student, and again when you return to anatomy in your third and fourth years, and even after you graduate.

Bruce Ian Bogart, PhD
Victoria H. Ort, PhD

Editorial Review Board

Chief Series Advisor
J. Hurley Myers, PhD
Professor Emeritus of Physiology and Medicine
Southern Illinois University School of Medicine
and
President and CEO
DxR Development Group, Inc.
Carbondale, Illinois

Anatomy and Embryology
Thomas R. Gest, PhD
University of Michigan Medical School
Division of Anatomical Sciences
Office of Medical Education
Ann Arbor, Michigan

Biochemistry
John W. Baynes, MS, PhD
Graduate Science Research Center
University of South Carolina
Columbia, South Carolina

Marek Dominiczak, MD, PhD, FRCPath, FRCP(Glas)
Clinical Biochemistry Service
NHS Greater Glasgow and Clyde
Gartnavel General Hospital
Glasgow, United Kingdom

Clinical Medicine
Ted O'Connell, MD
Clinical Instructor
David Geffen School of Medicine
UCLA
Program Director
Woodland Hills Family Medicine Residency Program
Woodland Hills, California

Genetics
Neil E. Lamb, PhD
Director of Educational Outreach
Hudson Alpha Institute for Biotechnology
Huntsville, Alabama
Adjunct Professor
Department of Human Genetics
Emory University
Atlanta, Georgia

Histology
Leslie P. Gartner, PhD
Professor of Anatomy
Department of Biomedical Sciences
Baltimore College of Dental Surgery
Dental School
University of Maryland at Baltimore
Baltimore, Maryland

James L. Hiatt, PhD
Professor Emeritus
Department of Biomedical Sciences
Baltimore College of Dental Surgery
Dental School
University of Maryland at Baltimore
Baltimore, Maryland

Immunology
Darren G. Woodside, PhD
Principal Scientist
Drug Discovery
Encysive Pharmaceuticals Inc.
Houston, Texas

Microbiology
Richard C. Hunt, MA, PhD
Professor of Pathology, Microbiology, and Immunology
Director of the Biomedical Sciences Graduate Program
Department of Pathology and Microbiology
University of South Carolina School of Medicine
Columbia, South Carolina

Neuroscience
Cristian Stefan, MD
Associate Professor
Department of Cell Biology
University of Massachusetts Medical School
Worcester, Massachusetts

Pharmacology
Michael M. White, PhD
Professor
Department of Pharmacology and Physiology
Drexel University College of Medicine
Philadelphia, Pennsylvania

Physiology
Joel Michael, PhD
Department of Molecular Biophysics and Physiology
Rush Medical College
Chicago, Illinois

Pathology
Peter G. Anderson, DVM, PhD
Professor and Director of Pathology Undergraduate Education
Department of Pathology
University of Alabama at Birmingham
Birmingham, Alabama

Contents

Chapter 1 Introduction to Anatomical Terminology, Basic Anatomical Concepts, and Early

Embryonic Stages *1*

Chapter 2 Introduction to the Peripheral Nervous System *11*

Chapter 3 The Back *23*

Chapter 4 The Thorax *35*

Chapter 5 The Abdomen *77*

Chapter 6 Posterior Abdominal Wall *127*

Chapter 7 Pelvis and Perineum *141*

Chapter 8 Lower Limb *195*

Chapter 9 Upper Limb *241*

Chapter 10 Head and Neck *291*

Case Studies *397*

Case Study Answers *401*

Index *405*

Series Preface

How to Use This Book

The idea for Elsevier's Integrated Series came about at a seminar on the USMLE Step 1 exam at an American Medical Student Association (AMSA) meeting. We noticed that the discussion between faculty and students focused on how the exams were becoming increasingly integrated—with case scenarios and questions often combining two or three science disciplines. The students were clearly concerned about how they could best integrate their basic science knowledge.

One faculty member gave some interesting advice: "read through your textbook in, say, biochemistry, and every time you come across a section that mentions a concept or piece of information relating to another basic science—for example, immunology—highlight that section in the book. Then go to your immunology textbook and look up this information, and make sure you have a good understanding of it. When you have, go back to your biochemistry textbook and carry on reading."

This was a great suggestion—if only students had the time, and all of the books necessary at hand, to do it! At Elsevier we thought long and hard about a way of simplifying this process, and eventually the idea for Elsevier's Integrated Series was born.

The series centers on the concept of the *integration box*. These boxes occur throughout the text whenever a link to another basic science is relevant. They're easy to spot in the text—with their color-coded headings and logos. Each box contains a title for the integration topic and then a brief summary of the topic. The information is complete in itself—you probably won't have to go to any other sources—and you have the basic knowledge to use as a foundation if you want to expand your knowledge of the topic.

You can use this book in two ways. First, as a review book . . .
When you are using the book for review, the integration boxes will jog your memory on topics you have already covered. You'll be able to reassure yourself that you can identify the link, and you can quickly compare your knowledge of the topic with the summary in the box. The integration boxes might highlight gaps in your knowledge, and then you can use them to determine what topics you need to cover in more detail.

Second, the book can be used as a short text to have at hand while you are taking your course . . .
You may come across an integration box that deals with a topic you haven't covered yet, and this will ensure that you're one step ahead in identifying the links to other subjects (especially useful if you're working on a PBL exercise). On a simpler level, the links in the boxes to other sciences and to clinical medicine will help you see clearly the relevance of the basic science topic you are studying. You may already be confident in the subject matter of many of the integration boxes, so they will serve as helpful reminders.

At the back of the book we have included case study questions relating to each chapter so that you can test yourself as you work your way through the book.

Online Version

An online version of the book is available on our Student Consult site. Use of this site is free to anyone who has bought the printed book. Please see the inside front cover for full details on the Student Consult and how to access the electronic version of this book.

In addition to containing USMLE test questions, fully searchable text, and an image bank, the Student Consult site offers additional integration links, both to the other books in Elsevier's Integrated Series and to other key Elsevier textbooks.

Books in Elsevier's Integrated Series

The nine books in the series cover all of the basic sciences. The more books you buy in the series, the more links that are made accessible across the series, both in print and online.

 Anatomy and Embryology

 Histology

 Neuroscience

 Biochemistry

 Physiology

 Pathology

 Immunology and Microbiology

 Pharmacology

 Genetics

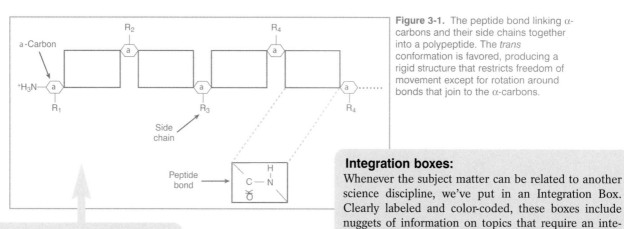

Figure 3-1. The peptide bond linking α-carbons and their side chains together into a polypeptide. The *trans* conformation is favored, producing a rigid structure that restricts freedom of movement except for rotation around bonds that join to the α-carbons.

Artwork:
The books are packed with 4-color illustrations and photographs. When a concept can be better explained with a picture, we've drawn one. Where possible, the pictures tell a dynamic story that will help you remember the information far more effectively than a paragraph of text.

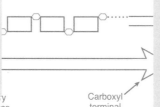

Integration boxes:
Whenever the subject matter can be related to another science discipline, we've put in an Integration Box. Clearly labeled and color-coded, these boxes include nuggets of information on topics that require an integrated knowledge of the sciences to be fully understood. The material in these boxes is complete in itself, and you can use them as a way of reminding yourself of information you already know and reinforcing key links between the sciences. Or the boxes may contain information you have not come across before, in which case you can use them as a springboard for further research or simply to appreciate the relevance of the subject matter of the book to the study of medicine.

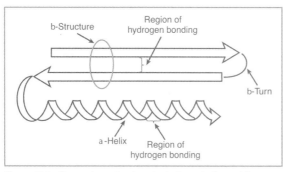

Figure 3-3. Secondary structure includes α-helix and β-pleated sheet (β-sheet).

MICROBIOLOGY

Prion Diseases

Prions (PrPSc) are formed from otherwise normal neurologic proteins (PrP) and are responsible for encephalopathies in humans (Creutzfeldt-Jakob disease, kuru), scrapie in sheep, and bovine spongiform encephalopathy. Contact between the normal PrP and PrPSc results in conversion of the secondary structure of PrP from predominantly α-helical to predominantly β-pleated sheet. The altered structure of the protein forms long, filamentous aggregates that gradually damage neuronal tissue. The harmful PrPSc form is highly resistant to heat, UV irradiation, and protease enzymes.

Since proline has no free hydrogen to contribute to helix stability, it is referred to as a "helix breaker." The α-helix is found in most globular proteins and in some fibrous proteins (e.g., α-keratin).

Text:
Succinct, clearly written text, focusing on the core information you need to know and no more. It's the same level as a carefully prepared course syllabus or lecture notes.

*-structure) consists of
tabilized by hydrogen
f adjacent sequences.
(parallel) or opposite (antiparallel) direction. β-Structures are found in 80% of all globular proteins and in silk fibroin.

Supersecondary Structure and Domains

Supersecondary structures, or *motifs*, are characteristic combinations of secondary structure 10–40 residues in length that recur in different proteins. They bridge the gap between the less specific regularity of secondary structure and the highly specific folding of tertiary structure. The same motif can perform similar functions in different proteins.

- The four-helix bundle motif provides a cavity for enzymes to bind prosthetic groups or cofactors.
- The β-barrel motif can bind hydrophobic molecules such as retinol in the interior of the barrel.
- Motifs may also be mixtures of both α and β conformations.

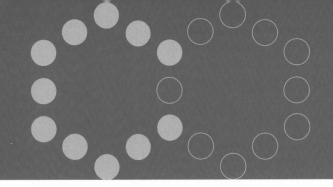

Introduction to Anatomic Terminology, Basic Anatomic Concepts, and Early Embryonic Stages

1

CONTENTS

TERMINOLOGY AND ANATOMIC POSITION
Planes and Sections
Basic Components in the Study of Anatomy

ORGANIZATIONAL PLAN OF THE TRUNK WALL
Skin
Fascia
Skeleton
Muscle
Joints

EMBRYONIC EARLY STAGES: BILAMINAR AND TRILAMINAR EMBRYO
Gastrulation: The Process That Produces the Trilaminar Embryo
Para-axial (Somitic) Mesoderm

INTERMEDIATE MESODERM DEVELOPMENT

●●● TERMINOLOGY AND ANATOMIC POSITION

Terms such as "up" and "down" or "to the side" only have meaning if everyone starts with a universal standard. In anatomy this standard is the anatomic position, which is a standing or erect position with the palms of the hands facing forward (Fig. 1-1). In this position, a structure located toward the front of the human body is referred to as *anterior*, while a structure located toward the back is referred to as *posterior*. "Dorsal" (back) is also used to describe the back, while "ventral" (belly) is used to describe the front of the body.

A structure can be "superior to" (above) or "inferior to" (below) another structure in any part of the body. Terms with similar meaning are *cranial*, which refers to the region of the head, and *caudal*, which refers to the region of the tail. The term *medial* pertains to structures located toward the middle or median longitudinal axis of the human body, while *lateral* structures are situated more toward the side (see Figs. 1-1A and 1-1B). *Superficial* means closer to the surface, or skin, and *deep* refers to farther away from the surface of the body (Table 1-1).

An eponym is the use of an individual's name for a structure or disease. Since eponyms convey little structural information, they are omitted from many anatomy texts. However, some clinicians still use these terms, so the more commonly encountered eponyms are included in this text.

Planes and Sections

The human body can be dissected with reference to three planes—sagittal, transverse, and coronal—either by means of imaging technologies such as computer axial tomography (CAT scanning), magnetic resonance imaging (MRI) or by dissection.

A plane is two dimensional, such as superior/inferior or anterior/posterior. A section is a cut through a structure and therefore has a third dimension, e.g., an anterior/posterior section through the body (cross-section).

The *sagittal plane*, separates the body vertically into right and left portions. Such a section in the middle (median) is called a *midsagittal plane*, while one alongside the midline is a *parasagittal plane*. A cross-section, or horizontal section, divides the body into "superior" and "inferior" portions (see Fig. 1-1C).

The *transverse plane* is a plane at right angles to the long axis of a structure or the sagittal plane. Thus, we can discuss a cross-section of an artery, vein, or nerve as well as one through the entire body.

Finally, the *coronal* (frontal) *plane* is the plane that separates the "anterior" portion of the body from the "posterior" portion. Coronal refers to a crown-like structure,

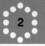

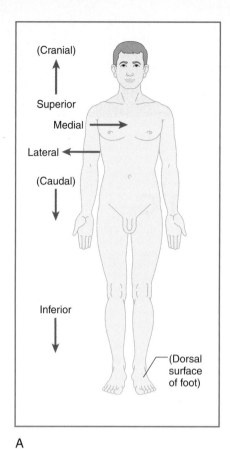

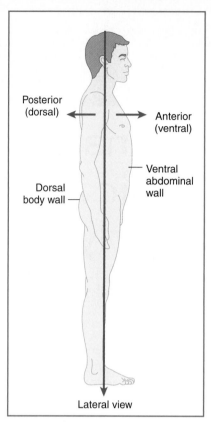

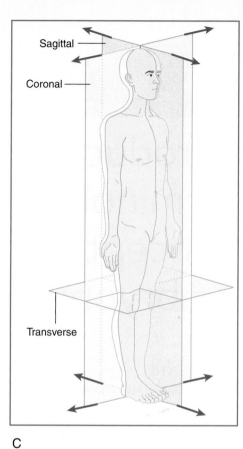

A   B   C

Figure 1-1. A, Anatomic position of the human body. **B,** Lateral view of the anatomic position of the human body. **C,** Planes through the human body.

and a coronal plane divides the body in the same manner as the coronal suture of the skull (see Figs. 1-1B, 1-1C, and Table 1-2).

Basic Components in the Study of Anatomy

The basic components in the study of structure are morphology, relationships, arterial supply, venous drainage, lymphatic drainage, and innervation.

Morphology can be defined as form and structure or what it looks like. Often, but not always, a structure's name tells you

TABLE 1-1. Summary of Terms

Term	Definition	Similar Term	Opposite Term
Anterior	Closer to front	Ventral	Posterior
Posterior	Closer to back	Dorsal	Anterior
Superior	Located above	Cranial	Inferior
Inferior	Located below	Caudal	Superior
Rostral	Located toward the beak	Embryo term for superior	Caudal
Medial	Toward the middle	—	Lateral
Lateral	Toward the side	—	Medial
Median	In the midline	—	—
Superficial	Near the skin or body surface	—	Deep
Deep	Away from the skin or body surface	—	Superficial

TABLE 1-2. Summary of Planes and Sections

Plane	Definition	Similar Term
Sagittal	Separates the body vertically	—
Parasagittal	Separates the body vertically but parallel to the midline	—
Horizontal	Separates the body into upper (superior) and lower (inferior) portions	Cross-section, transverse
Coronal	Separates the body into anterior and posterior portions	—

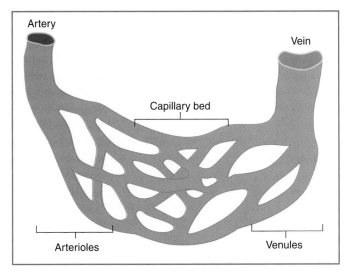

Figure 1-2. Circulation.

something about its appearance. Morphology includes size, shape, weight, and sex dimorphism (male/female differences). *Relationship* pertains to a structure's location or association relative to other structures in the body. Relationships given in terms of the body wall and its bony landmarks are referred to as surface anatomy. The relationships of the organs typically start with bony landmarks, since these are the most stable points in the human body. Relationships are also described in terms of other organs.

The blood supply of a structure consists of both its *arterial supply* and *venous drainage*. Arteries are vessels that carry blood away from the heart, while veins carry blood toward the heart regardless of the level of oxygenated or deoxygenated blood. Arteries branch into arterioles that form arterial capillaries leading to venous capillaries, which collect into venules and finally join to form veins (Fig. 1-2).

Capillaries

Capillaries are thin-walled vessels, devoid of smooth muscle, formed by endothelial cells and their basement membranes (see Fig. 1-2). This network, or "bed," of fine vessels allows almost all elements of blood except red cells to leave the circulatory system to find extravascular spaces and become the interstitial fluid within tissue or organ spaces external to the cells. It is at the level of the capillary bed that exchange of gases and metabolites actually takes place.

Collateral Circulation

Collateral circulation occurs when more than one artery brings blood to a specific organ or part of an organ. For example, the thoracic wall receives blood from both the anterior and posterior intercostal arteries. The area where a secondary (collateral) artery joins a primary artery is referred to as an *anastomosis* (communication) between the two vessels. This arrangement also characterizes the venous drainage. It is obvious that two vessels are better than one in providing nourishment to an organ. However, there are several instances

in the human body where only one artery provides blood to a specific organ or part of an organ. Such an artery is called an *end artery*. Blockage (occlusion) of an end artery results in cell death or necrosis. For example, occlusion of the central artery of the retina produces loss of vision.

Lymphatics

Lymphatics are the drainage system of the interstitial fluid in the tissue spaces. Lymphatic capillaries carry all components of blood except red blood cells. Afferent vessels end just under the capsule of a lymph node, while efferent vessels arise from the medulla (center) of a lymph node. The lymphatic efferent capillaries form larger vessels that eventually empty into the venous circulation close to the heart (approximately where the subclavian vein joins the internal jugular vein). On the left side these large lymphatic vessels enter the venous circulation as the thoracic duct and on the right side as the right main lymphatic duct. *The key point is that lymph is always returned to the venous circulation.*

The lymphatic drainage of a structure is extremely important in clinical medicine. The skin and superficial fascia superior to the umbilicus (navel) drain toward the axillary (arm

PHYSIOLOGY & PATHOLOGY

Fluid Movement

Fluid movement across the walls of capillaries is determined by capillary hydrostatic pressure, which usually forces fluid out; interstitial fluid hydrostatic pressure, which can vary; plasma colloidal osmotic pressure, which is produced by the higher concentration of protein in capillary blood that exerts a strong inward osmotic pressure; and the interstitial fluid osmotic pressure that causes a strong outward osmotic pressure into the interstitial spaces.

Edema (an abnormal accumulation of fluid in the interstitial space) can be produced by an abnormal leakage of fluid from capillaries. A diminished lymphatic drainage of the interstitial spaces can also cause fluid accumulation in the interstitial spaces.

PATHOLOGY

Conditions of the Arterial Wall

Arteriosclerosis is a thickening of the arterial wall due to calcium (Ca^{++}) deposits, whereas atherosclerosis is a subintimal thickening (plaque) formed by the accumulation of mostly smooth muscle cells and a mixture of intracellular and extracellular lipids, connective tissue, and glycosaminoglycans in the tunica intima, or innermost arterial layer. Both conditions can narrow or occlude medium and large arteries. Clot formation on the plaque presents a risk of thrombosis. The clot within the artery may cause infarct at a distal site in the vessel with diminished oxygen (O_2) supply. With extended time, collateral branches, if present, sometimes open as the lumen of a collateral artery narrows.

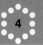

pit) nodes, while inferior to the umbilicus these same layers drain toward the superficial inguinal (groin) nodes. For most other structures, lymphatic drainage follows arteries (in reverse direction) and veins back to the larger lymphatic vessels. It is important to understand lymphatic drainage, since disease often spreads from the tissue spaces via the lymphatic vessels. This is especially true of metastatic carcinoma and infection, whereby cancer cells or microorganisms can travel from a primary lesion to the lymph nodes that drain the diseased structure—and beyond.

Innervation

Innervation, the nerve supply of a structure, is covered in depth in the next section. Nerves, arteries, veins, and lymphatic vessels usually enter an organ together as a neurovascular bundle. The point where they enter an organ is usually indented and referred to as the hilum (or hilus) of the organ. As a rule, neurovascular bundles also enter the deep surfaces of muscles.

●●● ORGANIZATIONAL PLAN OF THE TRUNK WALL

The organizational plan of the trunk wall begins with the skin, or epidermis plus dermis, and works inward (Fig. 1-3). These structures are derived from the embryonic germ layers, ectoderm, and mesoderm (somites and the somatic portion of the lateral mesoderm).

Skin

Skin consists of an epithelial layer, or epidermis, and a connective tissue layer, or dermis. The skin has hair whose distribution patterns and amounts vary greatly. Hair distribution over some parts of the body is sex-dependent (for example, the groin). The skin also contains sweat glands, many of which are under direct control of the sympathetic nervous system, and numerous sensory nerve endings as well as cutaneous (from Latin *cutis*, "skin") blood vessels and lymphatics.

Fascia

Just under the skin is the fascia. This is a layer of connective tissue that wraps, or envelops, part of the body. There are three types of fascia: superficial, deep, and subserous (extraserous).

Superficial Fascia

Superficial (subcutaneous) fascia is also referred to as the hypodermis. It is found just internal to, and intimately adherent to, dermis throughout the body (see Fig. 1-3).

The superficial fascia is composed of two layers: an outer fatty layer and an inner membranous layer. The outer fatty layer varies from place to place on the body and from person to person. This layer is always somewhat thicker in the lower abdominal wall and is virtually absent in the eyelids. It responds to estrogens and is therefore relatively thicker in women. In both sexes it is a layer where fat can accumulate. The inner

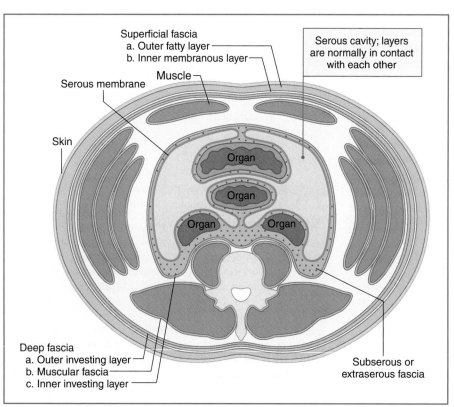

Figure 1-3. The typical layers of the body; the serous cavity is actually a potential cavity between the layers of the serous membrane.

membranous layer of superficial fascia, constant throughout the body, is an elastic membrane adherent to the fatty layer.

In general, the superficial fascia is very loosely applied to the deeper layers of the body. The student can demonstrate this by gently pinching his or her own forearm or abdomen. However, superficial fascia adheres to the deeper layers in several places. One example is the region just inferior to the inguinal region, where the inner (membranous) layer of superficial fascia actually fuses with the outer layer of deep fascia.

Deep Fascia

Deep fascia (see Fig. 1-3), the principal fascia of the body, functions to hold muscles and other structures in their proper relative positions. This type of fascia is devoid of fat; it surrounds each skeletal muscle, fills in gaps between muscles, stretches between muscles and bones, and forms broad fascial sheets that separate the musculoskeletal system from (1) the superficial fascia and (2) the various body cavities.

Different parts of the deep fascia have additional names. The fascia that surrounds each skeletal muscle is the muscular deep fascia, or epimysium. The fascia that externally envelops the overall musculoskeletal system is the outer investing layer of deep fascia; this grayish, sheet-like fascial layer is very well developed over the extremities and in the neck. The inner investing layer of deep fascia separates the musculoskeletal system from the body cavities (thorax, abdomen, pelvis). This layer is also named according to the specific cavity it surrounds, but instead of using the term "inner," use the Latin prefix endo-. Thus, the inner investing layer of deep fascia in the thorax is called the *endothoracic fascia*, in the abdomen the *endoabdominal fascia*, and in the pelvis the *endopelvic fascia*.

The inner investing layer of deep fascia can also be named according to its related skeletal muscle. Thus, endoabdominal fascia that lines the inner surface of the transversus abdominis muscle is referred to as transversalis fascia, and endopelvic fascia deep to the obturator internus muscle is called obturator internus fascia. It should be remembered that these examples are all just parts of the continuous inner investing layer.

Subserous (Extraserous) Fascia

The last major category of fascia is the subserous (extraserous) fascia. This layer abuts the external surfaces of the serous membranes and may include a substantial amount of fatty connective tissue. When this connective tissue appears around an organ without an overlying serous membrane, it is referred to as the *adventitia* of that organ. In the abdomen, the subserous fascia expands to help hold certain organs in proper position. The subserous fasciae of the abdomen and pelvis can also be referred to collectively as extraperitoneal fascia.

The serous membranes (see Fig. 1-3) are sheets of flat mesothelial cells that line the body cavities. Serous is derived from the Latin word for "watery-like," and the serous membranes secrete a watery fluid as a lubricant. The serous membranes of the thorax are the two pleural membranes and the pericardium, while the serous membrane of the abdomen and pelvis is the peritoneum. Additionally, in males, there are two serous membranes associated with the testes, the tunicae vaginalis testis.

The serous cavity (see Fig. 1-3) is a potential cavity or space between the layers of the serous membrane. Typically, the serous cavity contains only serous fluid. Illustrations such as Figure 1-3 are often misleading because they show the serous membranes artificially separated into a cavity when in the healthy individual it is only a potential cavity. This is artistic license, but not true in the living.

Skeleton

The skeletal system consists of bones and cartilage that are articulated (connected together) by joints. Bone consists of a specialized connective tissue. Bones have compact layers and a core, or *marrow*, cavity. Externally, the bone is covered by the periosteum, which is continuous with muscle tendon and provides both the bone and periosteum with its arterial supply. The periosteum also has osteogenic cells. Bones form levers, which can be moved by skeletal muscles. In addition, they are protective of the central nervous system and many organs, and some have bone marrow that is hemopoietic (capable of blood cell formation).

Classification of Bones

The skeletal system is subdivided into an axial and an appendicular skeletal system. The axial skeletal system consists of the skull, vertebral column, and ribs. The appendicular skeletal system consists of the bones of the upper limb starting with the clavicle and of the lower limb starting with the hip bone or os coxae.

Bones have different shapes. Flat bones have a thin, flattened morphology. Long bones form long levers of the limbs. Short bones typically have diameters equal in size to each other and are also associated with the hands and feet, while irregular bones make up a group having irregular or complex shapes such as the vertebrae, wrist bones, and ankle bones. Compact bone is the dense, hard outer layer of long and irregular bones. The inner trabecular portion of a bone is called spongy, or cancellous, bone and is filled by bone marrow.

Muscle

There are three types of muscle: skeletal, smooth, and cardiac. Skeletal muscle contracts to move levers (bones) and joints. They are under voluntary control. Smooth muscle is considered to be involuntary and is associated with many organs.

HISTOLOGY

Formation of Bone

Bones develop by one of two different processes. Membrane bone formation takes place in the vascularized mesenchyme, whereas endochondral bone formation is the replacement of a cartilage model by bone matrix.

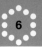

Cardiac muscle is also considered to be involuntary and is associated with the heart.

Skeletal Muscle

Skeletal muscle is typically attached by means of tendons to bone, cartilage, or ligaments. In a few rare cases, muscles can be attached to an organ (eye) or skin (muscles of facial expression). The stable point is the "origin." In the limbs, it is usually the proximal (closer to the trunk or midline) point, while the insertion is the attachment point that moves. In the limbs, the insertion is usually the distal (away from the trunk or midline) point.

Skeletal muscle is dependent on its neurovascular bundle, which consists of nerves, blood vessels, and lymphatics.

Joints

There are three types of joints: fibrous, cartilaginous, and synovial. Additionally, joints can be classified as *diarthrodial*, which allow for the greatest freedom of movement; *amphiarthrodial*, which are slightly moveable; and *synarthrodial*, which do not allow for movement (Table 1-3).

●●● EMBRYONIC EARLY STAGES: BILAMINAR AND TRILAMINAR EMBRYO

Starting after implantation with the bilaminar embryonic disc stage of development (Fig. 1-4), the cells facing the primordial amnionic cavity are referred to as the epiblast, while the cells facing the yolk sac are referred to as the hypoblast (see Figs. 1-4A to 1-4C). The epiblast cells will form the lining of the amnionic cavity (amnion), while hypoblast cells produce the lining of most of the yolk sac. At this point, the bilaminar embryo is a flat disc between the amnionic cavity and the yolk sac (see Fig. 1-4D).

TABLE 1-3. Classification of Joints*

Joint Name	Description
Fibrous joints	Consist of union of two bones by fibrous tissue
Syndesmosis	Bones that are separated but joined by ligaments
Suture	Union of two bones by fibrous tissue with almost no motion possible
Gomphosis	A socket that receives a process that sits in the socket, such as the root of a tooth that fits into an alveolus in the jaw
Cartilaginous joints	Have apposing bony surfaces united by cartilage
Synchondrosis	Has cartilage connecting the apposed surfaces, which typically are converted to bone, such as the epiphyses and diaphyses of long bones
Symphysis	Joint between two bones connected by fibrocartilage usually found in the midline
Synovial (diarthrodial) joints	Occur between opposing bony surfaces covered with a layer of hyaline cartilage or fibrocartilage
	Has a joint cavity lined by a synovial membrane that secretes synovial fluid and a fibrous capsule reinforced by ligaments

*Synarthrodial joints consist of a union of two bones that does not allow for movement.

Gastrulation: The Process That Produces the Trilaminar Embryo

Epiblast Cells

Early in this process, the rostral (cephalic or cranial in the adult) portion of the hypoblast thickens to interact with the epiblast cells to become the future oropharyngeal membrane.

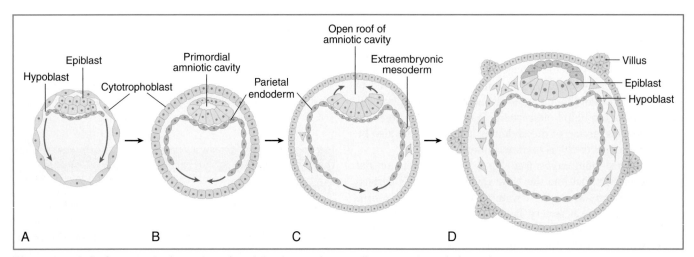

Figure 1-4. A–D, Steps in the formation of the bilaminar embryo, yolk sac, and amniotic cavity.

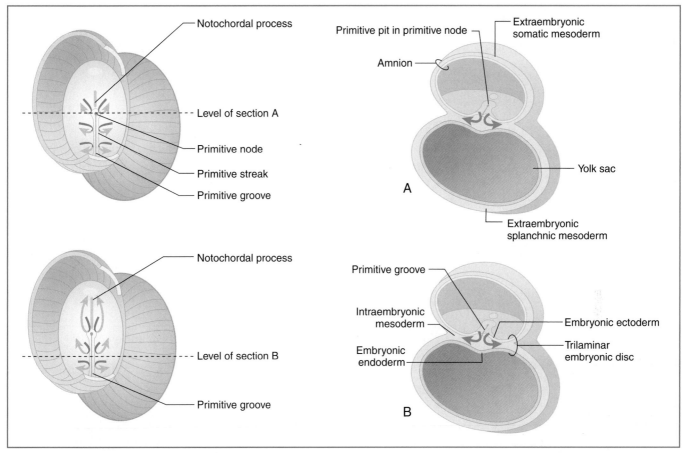

Figure 1-5. Craniocaudal and transverse sections through embryo demonstrating epiblast cells producing the notochord by invaginating through the primitive node and producing the embryonic mesoderm by invaginating through the primitive streak.

A similar region develops at the caudal portion of the embryo, and is called the cloacal plate or membrane.

Epiblast cells migrate to the midline to form a furrow called the *primitive streak*, which is located at the caudal end of the embryo. At the rostral (cephalic) end of the streak, there is a slight elevation called the *primitive node* surrounded by a depression called the *primitive pit*. The appearance of the primitive streak establishes the anterior-posterior, left-right, and dorsal-ventral axes (Fig. 1-5).

Once the streak is established, epiblast cells migrate toward the primitive streak, invaginate into it, and displace the hypoblast cells of the bilaminar disc to form the definitive endoderm layer (Figs. 1-5 to 1-7). The next wave of cells from the epiblast forms an intermediate layer between the endoderm and epiblast layers to become mesoderm (see Figs. 1-6 and 1-7). As the cells populate the middle mesodermal layer, they migrate laterally and rostrally (see Fig. 1-7). The rostrally migrating cells pass around the oropharyngeal membrane from each side and meet at the cranial end of the embryo to form the cardiogenic plate (the future heart; see Figs. 1-7 and 1-8).

Some epiblast cells migrate to the primitive pit and pass rostrally in the midline (see Fig. 1-7) until they reach the buccopharyngeal membrane, beyond which they cannot pass because of the fusion of the epiblast layer with the endodermal layer. These epiblast cells form the axial mesoderm. The cells closest to the buccopharyngeal membrane form the mesoderm of the prechordal plate that will be important in the formation of the face and forebrain. The remaining column of cells will form the notochord (see Fig. 1-7). The

CLINICAL MEDICINE

Sacrococcygeal Teratoma

Occasionally the primitive streak fails to regress at the appropriate time and persists as a tumor at the base of the spine, a sacrococcygeal teratoma. Sacrococcygeal teratomas often contain various types of tissues, since they are derived from the pluripotent cells of the primitive streak. These tumors are most often found in females and usually are malignant and therefore must be removed neonatally. The tumor has a morbidity of 10% neonatally that increases to greater than 50% by 6 months of age.

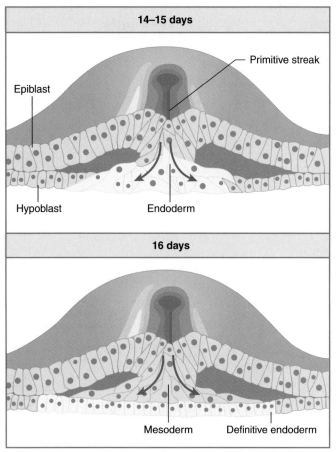

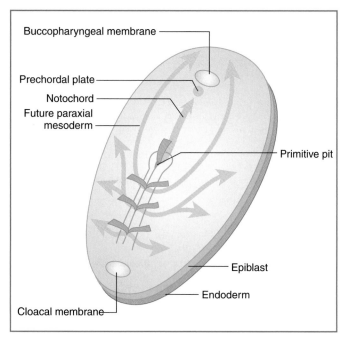

Figure 1-7. Formation of notochord and embryonic mesoderm.

Figure 1-6. Transverse sections through embryo at the level of the primitive streak demonstrating epiblast migration in the formation of the embryonic endoderm and mesoderm.

cells that do not migrate out of the epiblast become the ecto-derm. The primitive streak degenerates by the fourth week, and the embryo is now a trilaminar embryo (see Fig. 1-8).

Neurulation

The next step is the formation of the neural tube, which is the precursor to the brain and spinal cord, a process called *neurulation* (Fig. 1-9). The ectodermal cells just dorsal to the notochord increase in height to form a thickened neural plate (see Fig. 1-9A). The neural plate folds inward (invaginates) to form the neural groove, while the elevations at the groove's

open end are called the neural folds (see Fig. 1-9B). As the groove deepens, the elevations fuse with each other to form the neural tube, which separates from the overlying surface ectoderm and appears to sink into the underlying mesoderm. The future neural crest cells migrate out of the neural folds as they fuse to become the neural crest cells, which now lie between the ectoderm and the neural tube.

Paraxial (Somitic) Mesoderm

The axial mesoderm is found in the midline as notochord and prechordal plate mesoderm. Mesoderm peripheral to the notochord develops into three paired components: paraxial, intermediate, and lateral mesoderm.

The paraxial, or somitic, mesoderm forms paired segments, or *somitomeres*, starting in the cephalic region of the embryo, which then continue to form in a craniocaudal fashion. This initially results in 42 to 44 pairs of somites, but with the loss of one occipital somite and several coccygeal somites, there

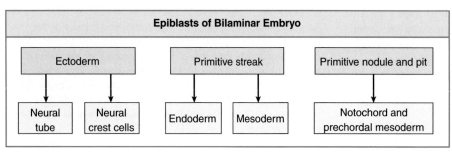

Figure 1-8. Formation of the endoderm, mesoderm, and ectoderm from epiblast during gastrulation.

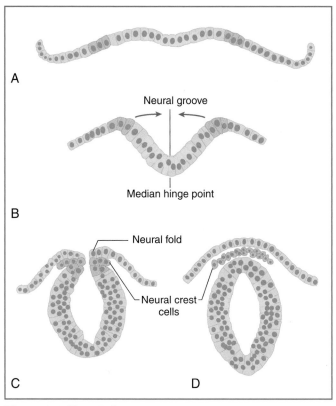

Figure 1-9. Neurulation.

are approximately 36 remaining somites (Fig. 1-10A). Each somite initially divides into two components (Fig. 1-10B): the ventral medial portion that interfaces with the notochord produces the sclerotome and the remainder forms the dermomyotome, whose intermediate cells subsequently form the myotome (Figs. 1-10C, D). The remaining laterally located dermatome cells spread out beneath the ectoderm to form the dermis. The sclerotome forms the vertebral column. The myotome produces the skeletal muscle of the trunk and limbs. A key fact in understanding the innervation pattern of the trunk and limbs is that a myotome and dermatome develop from a single somite, which will be innervated by the same spinal nerve.

●●● INTERMEDIATE MESODERM DEVELOPMENT

Lateral plate mesoderm divides into somatic (parietal) mesoderm and visceral (splanchnic) mesoderm. The somatic lateral mesoderm forms the parietal serous membranes of the body cavities and the limb mesoderm that forms the skeleton of the limbs. The visceral lateral mesoderm forms the smooth muscle and connective tissue components of the cardiovascular, lymphatic, and gastrointestinal systems and the respiratory tract.

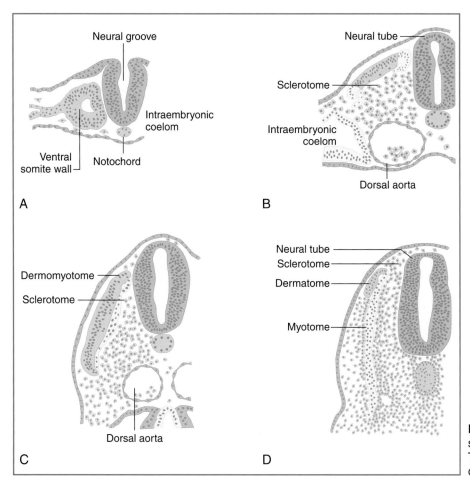

Figure 1-10. Somite develops into a sclerotome and a dermomyotome. The dermomyotome divides into a dermatome and myotome.

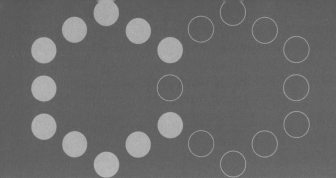

Introduction to the Peripheral Nervous System

2

CONTENTS

INTRODUCTION

PERIPHERAL NERVOUS SYSTEM

SPINAL CORD (CENTRAL NERVOUS SYSTEM)

OVERVIEW OF THE AUTONOMIC NERVOUS SYSTEM
Sympathetic Nervous System
Parasympathetic Nervous System
Visceral Afferent Neurons

REFERRED PAIN

CLASSIFICATION OF NEURONAL FIBERS

DEVELOPMENT OF THE SPINAL CORD AND PERIPHERAL NERVOUS SYSTEM

●●● INTRODUCTION

The nervous system comprises the central nervous system (CNS) and the peripheral nervous system (PNS). The CNS is surrounded and protected by the skull (neurocranium) and vertebral column and consists of the brain and the spinal cord. The PNS exists primarily outside these bony structures.

The entire nervous system is composed of neurons, which are characterized by their ability to conduct information in the form of impulses (action potentials), and their supporting cells plus some connective tissue. A neuron has a cell body (perikaryon) with its nucleus and organelles that support the functions of the cell and its processes. Dendrites are the numerous short processes that carry an action potential toward the neuron's cell body, and an axon is the long process that carries the action potential away from the cell body. Some neurons appear to have only a single process extending from only one pole (a differentiated region of the cell body) that divides into two parts (Fig. 2-1). This type of neuron is called a pseudounipolar neuron because embryonically it develops from a bipolar neuroblast in which the two axons fuse. Multipolar neurons (Fig. 2-2) have multiple dendrites and typically a single axon arising from an enlarged portion of the cell body called the axon hillock. These processes extend from different poles of the cell body.

One neuron communicates with other neurons or glands or muscle cells across a junction between cells called a synapse. Typically, communication is transmitted across a synapse by means of specific neurotransmitters, such as acetylcholine, epinephrine, and norepinephrine, but in some cases in the CNS by means of electric current passing from cell to cell.

Many axons are ensheathed with a substance called myelin, which acts as an insulator. Myelinated axons transmit impulses much faster than nonmyelinated axons. Myelin consists of concentric layers of lipid-rich material formed by the plasma membrane of a myelinating cell. In the CNS, the myelinating cell is the oligodendrocyte, and in the PNS it is the Schwann cell. The myelinated sheath is periodically interrupted by segments lacking myelin, called the *nodes of Ranvier*.

The CNS regions that contain myelinated axons are termed *white matter* because myelinated processes appear white in color, whereas the portions of the CNS composed mostly of nerve cell bodies are called *gray matter*.

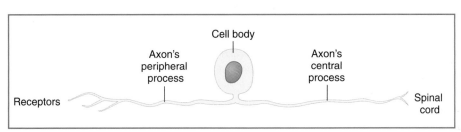

Figure 2-1. An afferent (sensory) neuron. Note the cell body and the peripheral and central processes, which form an axon. For a spinal nerve, the cell body is located in the dorsal root ganglion of the dorsal root.

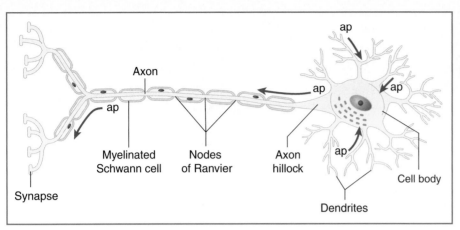

Figure 2-2. A myelinated efferent (motor) neuron. Note the direction of the action potential (ap) toward the synapse with another neuron or with skeletal muscle.

PHYSIOLOGY

Action Potential in the Nodes of Ranvier

The exposed portions of the axon at the nodes of Ranvier have a high density of voltage-dependent Na^+ channels while the voltage-dependent K^+ channels are located in the myelinated portions of the axon. This arrangement allows the action potential to "jump" from one node to another in a rapid saltatory, or leaping, conduction. Thus, the conduction velocity of myelinated axons is higher than the conduction velocity of nonmyelinated axons of the same size.

CLINICAL MEDICINE

Multiple Sclerosis

Multiple sclerosis (MS) is an autoimmune demyelinating disease of the central nervous system. Extensive loss of myelin, which occurs predominantly in the white matter, produces axonal degeneration and even loss of the cell bodies. In some cases, remyelination occurs, resulting in partial or complete recovery periods. This relapsing-remitting form of MS is the most common form of MS at the time of initial diagnosis.

(involuntary movements). These divisions can be traced back to the embryonic origins of the structures that they innervate, starting at the level of the trilaminar embryo. The somatic nervous system innervates structures derived from ectoderm, paraxial mesoderm, and lateral plate somatic mesoderm. The autonomic nervous system supplies structures derived from endoderm, intermediate mesoderm, and lateral plate visceral mesoderm.

In both the somatic system and autonomic system, neurons and their nerves are classified according to function. Individual neurons that carry impulses away from the CNS are called *efferent*, or *motor* neurons. The axons of these multipolar neurons are also referred to as efferent fibers and they synapse on muscles or glands. Neurons that carry impulses to the CNS are called *afferent*, or *sensory*, neurons. In the somatic system, these neurons carry impulses that originate from receptors for external stimuli (pain, touch, and temperature), referred to as *exteroceptors*. In addition, receptors located in tendons, joint capsules, and muscles convey position sense that is known as *proprioception*. Afferent neurons that run with the autonomic system carry impulses from interoceptors located within visceral organs that convey stretch as well as pressure, chemoreception, and pain.

●●● PERIPHERAL NERVOUS SYSTEM

The PNS encompasses the nervous system external to the brain and spinal cord. In the PNS, axons (fibers) are collected into bundles supported by connective tissue to form a nerve.

The PNS consists of 31 pairs of spinal nerves (Fig. 2-3), which arise from the spinal cord, and 12 pairs of cranial nerves, which originate from the brainstem. In addition, the nervous system contains both the somatic system and the autonomic system, each with portions within the CNS and PNS. The somatic system mediates information between the CNS and the skin, skeletal muscles (voluntary movements), bones, and joints. The autonomic system, in contrast, mediates information between the CNS and visceral organs

HISTOLOGY

Nerve Tissue

The epineurium, perineurium, and endoneurium organize the nerve into smaller and smaller bundles. The epineurium is continuous with the dura mater at or just distal to the intervertebral foramen; the arachnoid mater follows the ventral and dorsal roots to join the pia mater. Laterally the layers of arachnoid that follow the nerve roots fuse with each other, sealing the subarachnoid space and joining the perineurium. The pia mater is closely associated with the CNS, but the pia mater is reflected off the CNS to cover the arteries, which are now described as lying in a subpial space that is continuous with the perivascular spaces.

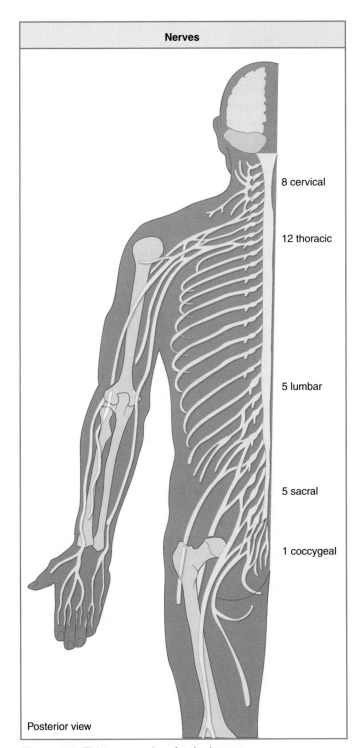

Nerves

8 cervical

12 thoracic

5 lumbar

5 sacral

1 coccygeal

Posterior view

Figure 2-3. Thirty-one pairs of spinal nerves.

●●● SPINAL CORD (CENTRAL NERVOUS SYSTEM)

The spinal cord is a long tubular structure that is divided into a peripheral white matter (composed of myelinated axons) and a central gray matter (cell bodies and their connecting fibers). When viewed in cross section, the gray matter has pairs of horn-like projections into the surrounding white matter. These horns are called ventral horns, dorsal horns, and lateral horns, but in three dimensions they represent columns that run the length of the spinal cord.

The ventral horns contain the cell bodies of motor neurons and their axons (Fig. 2-4). A collection of neuronal cell bodies in the CNS is a nucleus. Axons of the ventral horn nuclei leave the spinal cord in bundles called ventral roots. These motor fibers innervate skeletal muscles.

The lateral (intermediolateral) horns contain the cell bodies for the sympathetic nervous system at spinal cord levels T1–L2 and for the parasympathetic nervous system at spinal cord levels S2–S4. The axons from these neurons also leave the spinal cord through the ventral root and will synapse in various peripheral ganglia. A collection of neuronal cell bodies in the PNS is a ganglion. It is important to note that synapses occur within ganglia of the autonomic nervous system but not within the sensory ganglia of the somatic nervous system.

The dorsal horns receive the sensory fibers originating in the peripheral nervous system. Sensory fibers reach the dorsal horn by means of a bundle called the dorsal root (see Fig. 2-4). The dorsal root ganglion is part of the dorsal root. The sensory fibers have their cell bodies located in swellings called the *dorsal root ganglia*. The dorsal root contains sensory fibers (axons), while the dorsal root ganglia contain sensory cell bodies (and their axons). The central axons of the sensory neuron enter the dorsal horn of the gray matter. Some of these fibers will run in tracts (a bundle of fibers in the CNS) of the white matter to reach other parts of the CNS. Other axons will synapse with intercalated neurons (interneurons), which in turn synapse with motor neurons in the ventral horn to form a reflex arc.

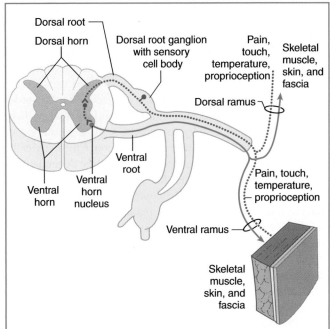

Dorsal root

Dorsal horn

Dorsal root ganglion with sensory cell body

Pain, touch, temperature, proprioception

Skeletal muscle, skin, and fascia

Dorsal ramus

Ventral root

Ventral horn

Ventral horn nucleus

Pain, touch, temperature, proprioception

Ventral ramus

Skeletal muscle, skin, and fascia

Figure 2-4. A typical cross-section of the spinal cord demonstrates the central location of the gray matter and the peripheral location of the white matter.

Although the dorsal root is essentially sensory and the ventral root is motor, the two roots come together within the bony intervertebral foramen to form a mixed spinal nerve (i.e., it contains both sensory and motor fibers). The spinal cord is defined as part of the CNS, but the ventral and dorsal roots are considered parts of the PNS. Outside the intervertebral foramen, the mixed nerve divides into a ventral ramus (from the Latin for "branch") and a dorsal ramus (see Fig. 2-4). The larger ventral ramus supplies the ventrolateral body wall and the limbs; the smaller dorsal ramus supplies the back. Since the ventral and dorsal rami are branches of the mixed nerve, they both carry sensory and motor fibers.

A spinal cord segment is the portion of the spinal cord that gives rise to a pair of spinal nerves. Thus, the spinal cord gives rise to 8 pairs of cervical nerves (C1–C8), 12 pairs of thoracic nerves (T1–T12), 5 pairs of lumbar nerves (L1–L5), 5 pairs of sacral nerves (S1–S5), and 1 pair of coccygeal nerves (Co1) (see Fig. 2-3). The spinal cord segments are numbered in the same manner as these nerves.

●●● OVERVIEW OF THE AUTONOMIC NERVOUS SYSTEM

The autonomic nervous system differs structurally and physiologically from the somatic nervous system. The autonomic nervous system is often defined as a motor neuronal system, generally concerned with involuntary body functions, in contrast to the somatic nervous system, which has both motor and sensory neurons responsible for voluntary muscle function and general sensation. The autonomic nervous system innervates smooth muscle, cardiac muscle, and glands. Again, there are sensory fibers from the viscera that run with the autonomic nerves but are historically not considered part of it.

Anatomically, the motor component of the somatic nervous system consists of a single neuron: an efferent neuron with its cell body located in the ventral horn of the spinal cord and whose axon runs to innervate skeletal muscle. However, the autonomic nervous system consists of a chain of two efferent neurons to innervate smooth muscle or glands. The first-order neuronal cell body is located in a CNS nucleus, and its fiber (axon) travels peripherally to synapse with a second-order neuron, which is located in a PNS ganglion. Physiologically, smooth and cardiac muscles are not completely dependent on autonomic motor neurons for contraction. In contrast, skeletal muscle is completely dependent on somatic motor innervation to contract and to remain viable. Indeed, first paralysis, followed by atrophy, results when skeletal muscle loses its innervation.

The first-order autonomic neurons have their cell bodies located in the CNS, either in the lateral (intermediolateral) horn of the spinal cord or in the brain stem. The cell bodies of first-order neurons give rise to myelinated axons that run from the CNS to synapse on second-order neurons in a ganglion, located completely outside the CNS. These cell bodies give rise to unmyelinated axons that innervate smooth muscle, cardiac muscle, and glands.

The first-order neurons and their fibers are referred to as *preganglionic* (presynaptic), and the second-order neurons and their fibers are *postganglionic* (postsynaptic). Each autonomic preganglionic fiber synapses with several postganglionic neurons. This arrangement allows preganglionic neurons to stimulate multiple postganglionic neurons whose postganglionic fibers reach smooth muscle and glands by means of several different pathways.

The autonomic nervous system is subdivided into the sympathetic and parasympathetic nervous systems. These terms refer to the specific locations of preganglionic and postganglionic cell bodies, as well as neurohumoral transmitters and function.

Sympathetic Nervous System

The sympathetic nervous system supplies visceral structures throughout the entire body. It supplies visceral structures associated with the skin (sweat glands, blood vessels, and arrector pili muscles) and deeper visceral structures of the body (blood vessels, smooth muscle in the walls of organs, and various glands).

The sympathetic preganglionic cell bodies are located in the lateral horns of thoracic spinal cord segments 1 through 12 plus lumbar segments 1 and 2 (Fig. 2-5). The axons of these preganglionic cells leave the spinal cord along with the somatic motor axons by means of the ventral horn and root at each of these levels (T1–L2) to join the mixed spinal nerve (Fig. 2-6). This outflow is referred to as the *thoracolumbar outflow*. The preganglionic sympathetic fibers follow the spinal nerve's ventral ramus and then leave the ventral ramus to enter the sympathetic ganglia of the sympathetic trunk. The sympathetic trunk is one of the paired elongated nerve strands characterized by ganglia and interganglionic (interconnecting) segments that parallel the vertebral column. The paired sympathetic trunks are lateral to the vertebral column starting at the level of the first cervical vertebra, and they run anterolaterally onto the vertebral column in the lumbar and sacral regions. The myelinated bundle of preganglionic fibers from the ventral ramus to the sympathetic trunk is called a *white ramus communicans* (white communicating branch; plural, *rami communicantes*) (see Figs. 2-6 and 2-7).

Thus, there are 14 pairs of white rami communicantes, arising from the 12 pairs of thoracic spinal nerves and the first two pairs of lumbar spinal nerves. Therefore, only 14 spinal cord segments (T1–L2) contain preganglionic sympathetic cell bodies, and only 14 pairs of white rami communicantes enter the sympathetic trunk carrying preganglionic fibers to synapse with the postganglionic nerve cells in all 22–23 sympathetic chain ganglia. *The preganglionic fibers can synapse in the thoracic and upper lumbar ganglia or run either up or down the chain, but not both, to synapse in cervical, lumbar, or sacral ganglia.* Postganglionic sympathetic fibers leave the sympathetic chain to enter all 31 pairs of spinal ventral rami by means of the 31 pairs of gray rami communicantes.

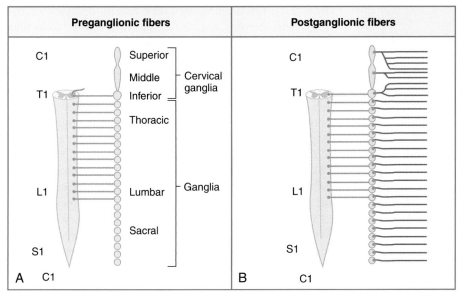

Figure 2-5. Preganglionic sympathetic fibers leave the ventral rami of mixed spinal nerves (T1–L2) to enter the sympathetic chain ganglia by means of 14 pairs of white rami communicantes (**A**), while 31 pairs of gray rami communicantes leave the sympathetic chain ganglia (**B**). (Only the left half of the thoracolumbar outflow is illustrated.)

Once the preganglionic sympathetic fibers enter the sympathetic chain ganglion, there are three possibilities to synapse with postganglionic neurons. They can (1) synapse in a chain ganglion as soon as they enter the sympathetic chain, (2) synapse in a chain ganglion after traveling up or down the chain (see Fig. 2-6), or (3) pass through the sympathetic chain ganglion without synapsing and form a specific splanchnic nerve (containing preganglionic fibers) and then synapse in a ganglion closer to the organ that it innervates (see Fig. 2-7).

This last possibility is as if a specific sympathetic chain ganglion for an organ had migrated out of the chain and moved closer to the organ, lengthening the preganglionic fibers but sometimes shortening the postganglionic ones (see Fig. 2-7). The route that a particular sympathetic neuron takes depends on its ultimate destination. The neurons that supply

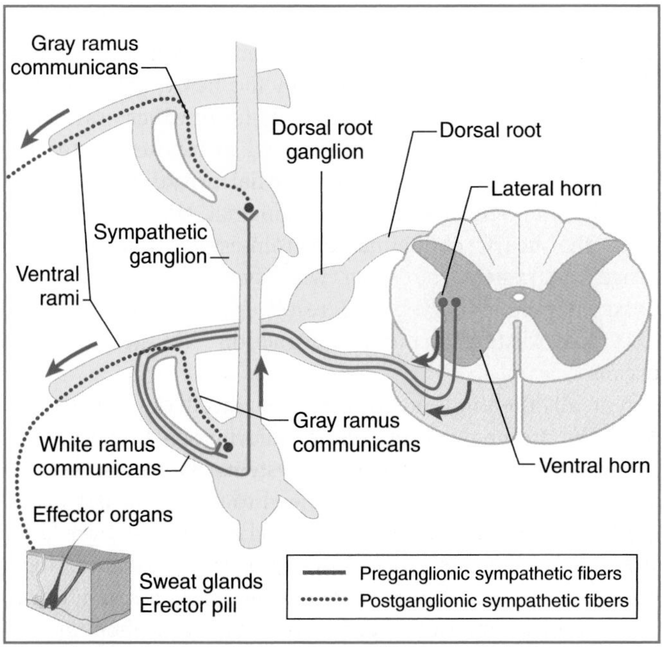

Figure 2-6. Sympathetic pathway to sweat glands, arrector pili muscles, and the smooth muscle of blood vessels in the body wall.

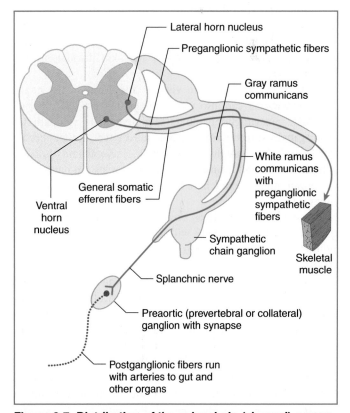

Figure 2-7. Distribution of the splanchnic (visceral) nerves. Preganglionic sympathetic fibers pass through the sympathetic ganglia to form greater, lesser, least, and lumbar splanchnic nerves that supply visceral structures in the abdomen and pelvis.

TABLE 2-1. Location of Preganglionic and Postganglionic Neuronal Cell Bodies for Splanchnic Nerves Arising from Spinal Cord Levels T5–T12; L1, L2, (L3)

Name of Nerve	Spinal Cord Level of Origin	Preaortic Ganglia Where Synapse Occurs
Greater splanchnic nerve	T5–T9	Celiac and to a lesser extent superior mesenteric ganglia
Lesser splanchnic nerve	T10–T11	Aorticorenal and superior mesenteric ganglia
Least splanchnic nerve	T12	Renal plexus
Lumbar splanchnic nerve	L1, L2, (L3)	Inferior mesenteric ganglion and minute intermesenteric and hypogastric ganglia

blood vessels, arrector pili muscles, and sweat glands in the skin can use either option one or option two and then leave the sympathetic chain at every level by means of grey rami communicantes (unmyelinated communicating branches) to rejoin all 31 pairs of spinal ventral rami (see Fig. 2-5). These postganglionic sympathetic fibers then run in both ventral and dorsal rami to supply the skin throughout the body.

Fibers that will innervate visceral structures in the head, neck, and thorax can also use either of the first two options, but their postganglionic fibers then leave the sympathetic chain ganglia directly as splanchnic nerves that are named for the organs they supply. For example, cervical and thoracic cardiac nerves and thoracic pulmonary nerves are part of the cardiopulmonary splanchnic nerves that supply the heart and lungs.

The neurons that pass *through* the sympathetic chain ganglia without synapsing will innervate visceral structures in the abdomen and pelvis (see Fig. 2-7). These are the so-called named splanchnics: greater, lesser, least, and lumbar splanchnic nerves (Table 2-1). These nerves travel to autonomic ganglia, which are generically referred to as *preaortic (prevertebral) ganglia.* The postganglionic fibers from these preaortic ganglia run with various arteries to reach the viscera of the abdomen and pelvis. The postganglionic fibers from these preaortic ganglia follow the arteries that have the same names as the ganglia (i.e., the postganglionic fibers of the superior mesenteric ganglion follow the branches of the superior mesenteric artery.)

The term splanchnic is derived from the Greek and means "visceral." Reminder: not all sympathetic nerves with the designation "splanchnic" are bundles of preganglionic fibers (Table 2-2). There are many other visceral branches of the sympathetic nervous system that are also called "splanchnic nerves" that contain postganglionic fibers. These splanchnic nerves arise from cervical and upper thoracic sympathetic ganglia and as postganglionic nerves run directly to organs in the head, neck, and thorax that they innervate (see parasympathetic nervous system). Postganglionic sympathetic fibers in branches of the upper thoracic sympathetic ganglia also supply the thoracic aorta. *None of the splanchnic nerves run in gray rami communicantes.*

For the thoracoabdominal outflow to provide preganglionic sympathetic neurons to synapse in the 22–23 chain ganglia, one preganglionic fiber must synapse with approximately 33 postganglionic neurons at different levels of the sympathetic chain. Thus, a preganglionic axon synapses with many postganglionic neuronal cell bodies. In addition, one postganglionic cell body receives many synapses from other preganglionic axons. This may account for the wide dissemination and possibly amplification of sympathetic innervation.

Parasympathetic Nervous System

The parasympathetic portion of the autonomic nervous system is called the *craniosacral outflow* because it has its preganglionic cell bodies in the brainstem and in the sacral portion of the spinal cord. Parasympathetic fibers run in cranial nerves III, VII, IX, and X. The sacral parasympathetic outflow arises from the intermediolateral horn of sacral spinal cord segments 2, 3, 4, and its fibers are called *pelvic splanchnics* (Fig. 2-8 and Table 2-3).

Visceral Afferent Neurons

Visceral sensory fibers also run with the autonomic nerves. These neurons carry specific information from the viscera. The sensory impulses arising from the heart, great vessels, respiratory and gastrointestinal system, which run with parasympathetic neurons, are involved in reflexes controlling blood pressure, respiration rate, partial pressures of carbon dioxide, etc. Sensory fibers for pain that arise in receptors from the heart, abdominal gastrointestinal tract, rectum, urogenital system, etc., run with sympathetic and sacral parasympathetic nerves and result from inflammation or excessive distention and contraction of the involved organs.

Not all afferent functions are perceived on a conscious level. We are unaware of sensory information that regulates the respiratory and circulatory systems. However, we are aware of hunger, thirst, and the need to urinate or defecate.

Pain from the viscera is perceived differently from pain from the somatic structures. Visceral pain is typically diffuse. Often visceral pain is *perceived* as arising from a region of the body wall distant from the involved organ, a phenomenon called referred pain. Understanding the mechanism of referred pain helps identify the organ that may be involved and thus aids in the diagnosis of the underlying disease.

TABLE 2-2. Location of Preganglionic and Postganglionic Neuronal Cell Bodies for Segmental Sympathetic Supply

Spinal Cord Segment Containing Cell Bodies of Preganglionic Fibers	Location of Postganglionic Cell Bodies in Sympathetic Ganglia/Mode of Exit of Postganglionic Fibers	Region and/or Effector Organ Supplied
T1–T5	Superior and middle cervical chain ganglia fibers exit by means of gray rami communicantes to ventral rami spinal nerves C1–C5	Sweat glands, arrector pili muscles, and blood vessels of neck and face
T3–T6	Inferior cervical and upper thoracic chain ganglia fibers exit by means of gray rami communicantes to ventral rami of spinal nerves C6–C8, T1–T5	Sweat glands, arrector pili muscles, and blood vessels of upper limb and thoracic wall
T1–T6	Superior, middle, and inferior cervical and upper thoracic chain ganglia 1–6 fibers exit directly as visceral branches; **they do not use gray rami communicantes**	Cardiopulmonary nerves to heart, trachea, lungs, and lower esophagus
T2–L1	Thoracic chain ganglia 1–12 and lumbar ganglia 1, 2 postganglionic fibers exit through gray rami communicantes to ventral rami of spinal nerves T1–L1	Sweat glands, arrector pili muscles, and blood vessels of trunk body wall
T5–L2 Some preganglionic fibers pass through splanchnic chainganglia without synapsing to form sympathetic nerves (greater, lesser, least and lumbar splanchnic nerves) without synapsing to supply:	Preaortic (celiac, superior mesenteric, inferior mesenteric, aorticorenal) ganglia Postganglionic sympathetic fibers from these ganglia supply	Gastrointestinal and urogenital organs of the abdominopelvic cavity
T9–L2	Lumbosacral chain ganglia fibers exit through gray rami communicantes to ventral rami of spinal nerves T9–L2	Sweat glands, arrector pili muscles, and blood vessels of lower limb

●●● REFERRED PAIN

Referred pain can be defined as pain from deep organs perceived as arising from a dermatome or dermatomes of the body wall distant or remote from the actual diseased organ. The visceral sensory fibers for pain run with sympathetic and parasympathetic splanchnic nerves. The key to understanding referred pain is that both the cutaneous region where the pain is perceived and the involved organ are innervated by fibers associated with the same spinal cord segment or segments.

The general somatic sensory fibers for somatic pain run in spinal nerves. Many visceral sensory pain fibers run in the sympathetic nerves and join the spinal nerves by means of their white rami communicantes (see Table 2-2). Thus, both somatic pain fibers and visceral pain fibers have cell bodies that are in the same dorsal root ganglia and enter the dorsal horn together *to synapse on the same second-order neurons.* The CNS mistakenly recognizes visceral pain as arising from a portion of the body wall, which does not have a direct relationship to the involved organ.

HISTOLOGY

Morphology of Motor and Sensory Cells

Not only do motor and sensory cells have specific locations, they also have specific morphologies. Motor cells are typically multipolar with numerous dendrites, whereas sensory neurons typically have round cell bodies with one or two axons.

CLINICAL MEDICINE

Sensing Pain

A myocardial infarction (heart attack) typically produces deep pain on the left side of the chest and radiating pain into the medial side of the left arm, forearm, and even the little finger. Somatic sensory fibers from these regions of the body wall and upper left limb synapse in the same spinal cord segments, T1–T4 or T5, as the visceral sensory fibers from the heart. The CNS does not clearly distinguish the origin of this pain, and it perceives the pain as coming from the body wall and upper left limb.

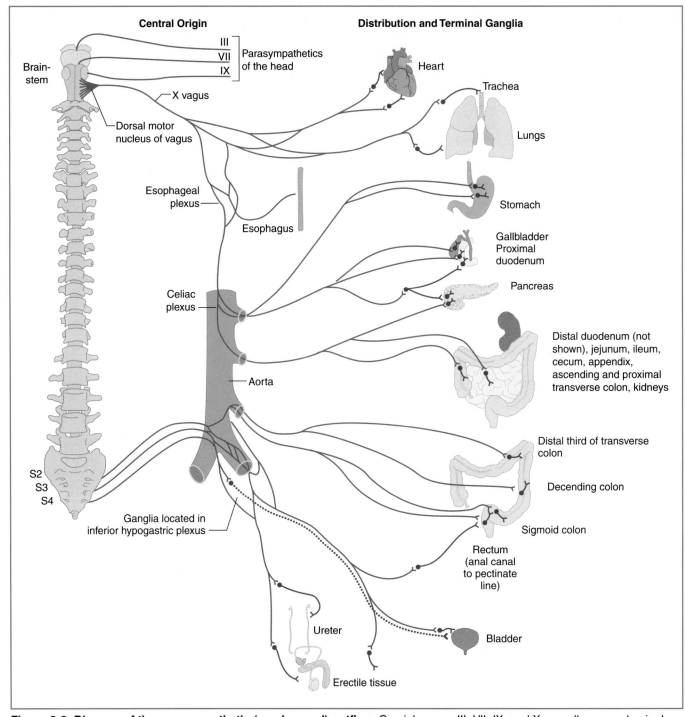

Figure 2-8. Diagram of the parasympathetic (craniosacral) outflow. Cranial nerves III, VII, IX, and X as well as sacral spinal cord segments S2, S3, and S4 have relatively long preganglionic fibers (blue) that synapse in ganglia either in or close to the effector organs. Short postganglionic fibers (red) then innervate specific structures in these organs.

Both the autonomic and visceral sensory innervation to many of the organs of the trunk are well known, whereas this is less clear for other organs. For example, the cardiac sympathetic nerves arise in the lateral horns of thoracic spinal cord segments T1 through T4(T5). Therefore, the visceral sensory fibers that travel in reverse from the heart follow the cardiac sympathetic fibers and synapse in spinal cord segments T1 through T4(T5). This distribution of visceral sensory fibers that run with the cardiac sympathetic nerves accounts for specific patterns of pain that arise from the heart.

The convergence theory of referred pain indicates that visceral pain fibers in the spinal cord converge on the same second-order neurons that receive input from the somatic sensory neurons. The information is then conveyed to suprasegmental levels, where the CNS interprets the pain as arising from the somatic region (Fig. 2-9).

TABLE 2-3. Comparisons Between the Sympathetic and Parasympathetic Nervous Systems

Feature	Sympathetic Nervous System	Parasympathetic Nervous System
Location of preganglionic cell bodies	Lateral horns T1–L2 (thoracolumbar outflow)	Brainstem and sacral spinal cord S2–S4 (craniosacral outflow)
Location of ganglia	Sympathetic trunk and collateral ganglia	In organs of the gastrointestinal tract, pelvic organs, or close to other organs
Length of fibers	Short preganglionic fibers, long postganglionic fibers with exception of the named splanchnic nerves	Long preganglionic fibers, short postganglionic fibers
Ratio of preganglionic fibers to post ganglionic fibers	Approximately 1 to 33	Approximately 1 to 2–5
Postganglionic transmitter	Norepinephrine (except sweat glands, which use acetylcholine)	Acetylcholine

TABLE 2-4. Classification of Fiber Types That Supply Trunk and Limbs

Classification	Function	Structure Innervated	Embryologic Origin
General somatic afferent (GSA)	Pain, touch, temperature, proprioception (deep sensation)	Skin, skeletal muscle, parietal serous membranes	Ectoderm, somites, somatic lateral mesoderm
General somatic efferent (GSE)	Motor innervation to voluntary muscles	Skeletal muscle of the trunk and limbs	Somites
General visceral afferent (GVA)	Visceral afferents for silent information from receptors for blood pressure, serum chemistry, as well as referred pain	Organs such as cardiovascular, respiratory, gastrointestinal and urogenital systems	Visceral lateral mesoderm, intermediate mesoderm, endoderm
General visceral efferent (GVE)	Autonomic innervation	Organs such as cardiovascular, respiratory, gastrointestinal and urogenital systems	Visceral lateral mesoderm, intermediate mesoderm

●●● CLASSIFICATION OF NEURONAL FIBERS

The fibers of the above neurons are classified according to the structures they supply and the embryologic origin of these structures. The somatic motor and sensory fibers arise from cell bodies in the spinal cord or dorsal root ganglia. Thus, they are widely distributed and their fibers are classified as general somatic sensory (afferent) or motor (efferent) fibers. The autonomic nervous system supplies all of the viscera, so these fibers are also classified as general visceral motor (efferent) fibers, while the sensory fibers from the organs that run with the autonomic nerves are classified as general visceral afferent fibers (Table 2-4).

●●● DEVELOPMENT OF THE SPINAL CORD AND PERIPHERAL NERVOUS SYSTEM

The CNS develops from the neural tube, whereas the peripheral nervous system develops from parts of the neural tube and neural crest cells (Fig. 2-10).

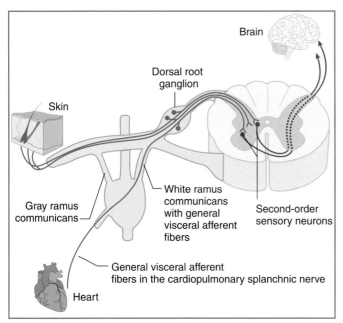

Figure 2-9. Convergence theory of referred pain points out that both somatic sensory fibers and visceral sensory fibers have the cell bodies in the same dorsal root ganglion and synapse on the same second-order neurons in the spinal cord.

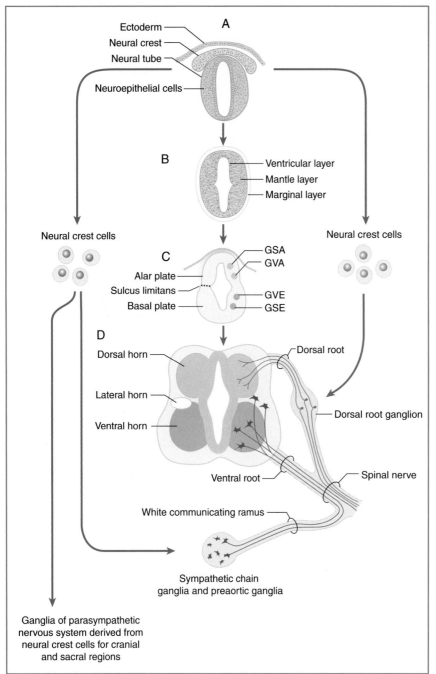

Figure 2-10. Development of spinal cord and peripheral nervous system.

The neuroepithelial cells surrounding the neural canal go through three waves of proliferation and differentiation (see Fig. 2-10). Initially, they differentiate into neuroblasts that will become the neurons of the CNS. This layer is called the ventricular layer. These newly formed neuroblasts then migrate peripherally to form a new concentric layer called the mantle layer (see Fig. 2-10B). The neuroblasts in the mantle layer further differentiate into primitive neurons. This layer will ultimately become the gray matter of the spinal cord (see Figs. 2-10B to 2-10D). The processes (axons and dendrites) of the primitive neurons in the mantle layer then extend peripherally to form the outermost layer called the marginal zone. As the oligodendrocytes myelinate the axons, this layer will become the white matter (see Figs. 2-10B and 2-10 D).

In the second wave of differentiation, the neuroepithelial cells in the ventricular layer proliferate and differentiate into glioblasts that will ultimately become oligodendrocytes and astrocytes, the glial or supporting cells of the CNS.

In the third wave, the neuroepithelial cells form the ependymal cells that line the lumen of the neural tube.

Cells from the adjacent mesoderm form the covering layers, called *meninges*, that surround the CNS. These layers, starting from the white matter, are called the pia mater, arachnoid mater, and dura mater, respectively. During development, the neural tube's central lumen narrows owing to the extensive development of the mantle and marginal zones and is now referred to as the *central canal*. The canal is lined by ependymal cells (which originate from the neural tube's original neuroepithelium) and is located in the center of the transverse portion of gray matter. (The central canal is normally patent throughout life although its terminal ventricle enlargement within the conus medullaris typically regresses in middle age.)

As differentiation continues, the tube enlarges in an asymmetric manner. When viewed in the transverse plane, the mantle (developing gray matter) layer's ventral and dorsal components (plates) have enlarged and the region between them remains relatively narrow (see Figs. 2-10C and 2-10D). The paired, enlarged dorsal portions of the developing gray matter become the alar plates, while the paired ventral portions are called *basal plates*. The narrow groove between the dorsal and ventral plates is the sulcus limitans (see Figs. 2-10C and 2-10D). The ventral and dorsal horns are concerned with the derivatives of the somites.

The alar plates contain developing sensory fibers and second-order neurons in the future dorsal horn (see Fig. 2-10D). The basal plates are the future ventral horns (see Figs. 2-10C and 2-10D). They are found anterior to the sulcus limitans and are the sites of developing neurons whose axons migrate out of the spinal cord to innervate the muscles developing from the adjacent somites.

The portion of the basal plate close to the sulcus limitans produces developing neurons that supply viscera (see Figs. 2-10C and 2-10D). These neurons and their fibers are part of the autonomic nervous system. This portion of the alar plate is designated as the intermediolateral horn.

Concurrent with the development of the spinal cord and somites, the neural crest cells migrate to various points including a dorsolateral position between the alar plate and the somites. Here, the neural crest cells develop into the neuronal cell bodies of the dorsal root ganglia (see Fig. 2-10), which send processes peripherally to supply sensory fibers to skin, dermis, and developing skeletal muscle and centrally to the alar plate (developing dorsal horn). The central processes penetrate the marginal layer (future white matter) to reach suprasegmental levels of the CNS, or they can synapse at this level.

The central processes of the dorsal root ganglion form the dorsal root, and the basal plate's processes form the ventral root. The two roots unite and form the spinal nerve (see Fig. 2-10). The stimulus for much of this is the development of the paraxial mesoderm, which has produced segmented pairs of somites. The somites continuously subdivide to form segmented sclerotomes, myotomes, and dermatomes. The sclerotomes form the vertebrae. The myotomes develop into skeletal muscle, while the dermatomes produce the dermis. This pattern of segmentation results in one pair of developing spinal nerves innervating a specific group of muscles, dermis, and adjacent skin. These specific regions of the body are also referred to as the myotomes and dermatomes of the adult body and are a useful tool in understanding pain or anesthesia as symptoms of injury or disease.

Neural crest cells also migrate into the visceral regions of the body to develop into autonomic ganglia and fibers (see Fig. 2-10). Some of the peripheral fibers of the developing sensory neurons in the dorsal root ganglia also accompany the neural crest cells as they migrate. These sensory fibers carry sensory impulses from viscera to the CNS.

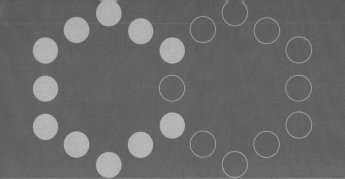

The Back

3

CONTENTS

THE BACK AND VERTEBRAL COLUMN
Vertebral Column
Curvatures of the Neonatal Vertebral Column

TYPICAL VERTEBRA
Regional Differences

DEVELOPMENT OF VERTEBRAE AND RIBS
Joints
Ligaments
Spinal Meninges

NEONATAL CHANGES IN THE SPINAL CORD
Development of the Meninges

MUSCLES OF THE BACK
Innervation
Blood Supply
Development

●●● THE BACK AND VERTEBRAL COLUMN

The back is the region between the neck and buttock, which are the prominences formed by the gluteal muscles. The major components of the back are the vertebral column, spinal cord, associated muscles, neurovascular bundles, as well as the skin and fascia located on the posterior aspect of the trunk. The back is important in support of the upper portion of the body, locomotion, and innervation of the trunk and lower limbs. It is the structural axis of the body around which the movements of the head, neck, limbs, and trunk revolve.

Vertebral Column

The central nervous system (CNS) is encased in the skull and vertebral column (or spinal column, or spine). The vertebral column is important in erect posture, locomotion, protection of the spinal cord, and weight-bearing above the pelvis.

The axial skeletal system consists of the skull, vertebral column, ribs, and sternum. The appendicular system consists of the pectoral girdle (clavicle and scapula) along with the other bones of the upper limb as well as the pelvic girdle (hip bones) and the other bones of the lower limb.

The vertebral column determines 40% of an individual's height. It consists of 32 to 34 vertebrae (depending on the number of coccygeal vertebrae), the connective tissue disks between the vertebrae, and the ligaments that hold the column together. The vertebrae are organized as follows: 7 cervical (C) vertebrae, 12 thoracic (T) vertebrae, 5 lumbar (L) vertebrae, 5 fused sacral (S) vertebrae, and 3 to 5 coccygeal vertebrae (Fig. 3-1). The coccygeal vertebrae are also referred to as *vestigial* or *caudal* vertebrae.

The vertebral column is not straight; it has four curvatures. The anterior convex cervical and lumbar curvatures are referred to as secondary curvatures, since they develop after birth. The anterior concave thoracic and sacral curvatures are referred to as primary curvatures (see Fig. 3-1).

Curvatures of the Neonatal Vertebral Column

At mid-gestation, the embryo's vertebral column is flexed so that the entire vertebral column has an anterior concave curvature. During the first 18 months of life, two secondary convex curvatures occur. A secondary anterior convex cervical curvature appears at about 3 to 4 months neonatally, when the infant begins to pick up its head. The other secondary anterior convex curvature is the lumbar curvature, which appears at about 12 to 18 months. The lumbar curvature is an adaptation of the lumbar vertebrae to support the upper body weight in the upright posture. A thoracic kyphosis is an abnormal thoracic anterior concavity, and a lordosis is an abnormal anterior convexity typically of the lumbar vertebrae.

●●● TYPICAL VERTEBRA

A typical vertebra has several named parts (Fig. 3-2). The body is the large cylindrical anterior aspect of the vertebra for weight-bearing (see Figs. 3-1 and 3-2). The posterior surface of the body has a large nutrient foramen, through which arteries and veins pass from the vertebral canal into the vertebral body. In general, the vertebral bodies increase in size from the cervical region to the lumbar region.

Extending posteriorly from the body is the vertebral or neural arch, which is composed of two pedicles and two laminae (see Fig. 3-2). The two pedicles extend from the body,

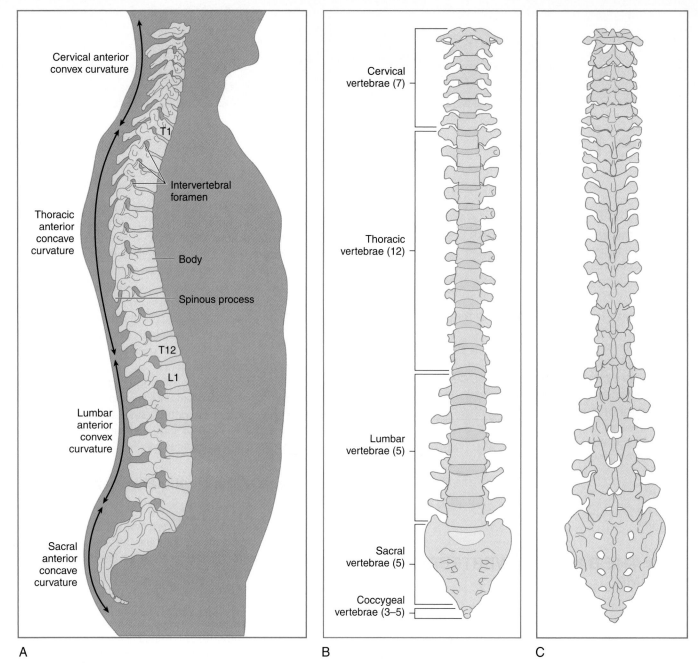

Figure 3-1. Curvatures of the vertebral column. An adult vertebral column. **A,** Lateral view. **B,** Anterior view. **C,** Posterior view.

while the two laminae extend from the pedicles. The body and the vertebral arch form a vertebral foramen (see Fig. 3-2). When the vertebrae are stacked on each other, the vertebral foramina and the intervening intervertebral disks form the vertebral canal (see Fig. 3-1), which extends from the skull to the coccyx and contains the spinal cord, meninges, and the roots of the spinal nerves.

Each pedicle has two vertebral notches, a shallow one on its superior surface and a deeper one on its inferior surface (see Fig. 3-2). When the vertebrae and their disks articulate, the notches are aligned to form an intervertebral foramen

(Fig. 3-3). The intervertebral foramina are smallest in the cervical region and enlarged in the lumbar region. An intervertebral foramen is not an opening in a bone but rather an opening between bones (e.g., an opening between two vertebrae). Each intervertebral foramen transmits a spinal nerve and associated blood (radicular) vessels.

The two laminae form the most posterior aspect of the arch. A transverse process extends laterally (transversely) from the junction of the pedicle and lamina on each side (see Fig. 3-2). Extending posteriorly from the point where the two laminae meet is the spinous process. The length and shape of

CLINICAL MEDICINE

Scoliosis

Abnormal curvatures have associated weight-bearing and visceral pathologies. An abnormal lateral curvature of the thoracic vertebrae, which may be congenital or acquired, is called *scoliosis.* It has a 7 to 1 female predilection.

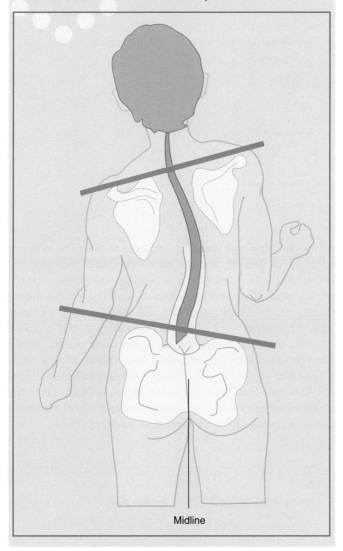

Midline

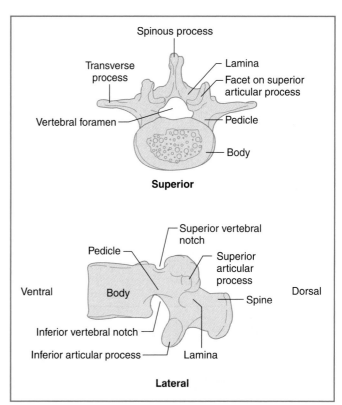

Figure 3-2. Lumbar vertebra with its various parts.

HISTOLOGY

Bone

The body is composed of a core of spongy bone surrounded by compact (dense) bone. Spongy bone is characterized by a latticework of trabeculae (beam-like structures) with interstitial spaces filled with marrow. Bone marrow consists of different types of connective tissue and stem cells that produce blood cells including erythrocytes and granulocytes. On the growing ends of the bone there is hyaline cartilage, which participates in growth or lengthening of long bones until an individual reaches about 21 years of age.

the spinous processes vary. Each vertebra has two transverse processes and one spinous process, except for the first cervical vertebra (C1), which does not have a spinous process. Back muscles attach to the transverse and spinous processes.

The two superior and two inferior articular processes extend from the vertebral arch (see Figs. 3-2 and 3-3). Each superior process has an articular facet (small face) that faces posterior or posteromedially (see Fig. 3-3). The inferior facet faces anteriorly or anterolaterally, depending on the level of the vertebrae. The superior process of one vertebra articulates with the inferior process of the adjacent vertebra, forming a plane type of synovial joint. The articulation between superior and inferior articular processes allows for a slight movement;

however, considerable movement occurs when it involves many vertebrae.

Regional Differences

Cervical Vertebrae

Each cervical vertebra has a foramen in each of its transverse processes, the foramina transversa (singular, foramen transversarium), which transmit the vertebral vessels. Each transverse foramen is formed by the fusion of the true transverse process and the adjacent costal element. (In the thorax, costal elements form the ribs.) These foramina are usually smaller in the 7 cervical vertebrae because they transmit only vertebral veins. *Only the cervical vertebrae have transverse foramina.*

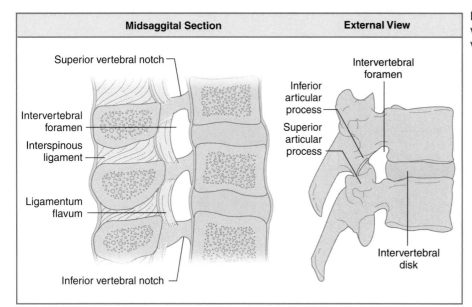

Figure 3-3. Articulation of adjacent vertebrae. Midsagittal section through the vertebral column and external view.

Midsaggital Section

Superior vertebral notch
Intervertebral foramen
Interspinous ligament
Ligamentum flavum
Inferior vertebral notch

External View

Intervertebral foramen
Inferior articular process
Superior articular process
Intervertebral disk

CLINICAL MEDICINE

Spondylolisthesis

The superior and inferior articular processes help prevent the forward movement (dislocation) of a superior vertebra on the vertebra below it. Spondylolisthesis is a forward separation of the superior articular processes, transverse processes, pedicles, and body from the remaining inferior articular processes, laminae, and spine. Spondylolisthesis can be due to trauma or disease including degeneration of the articular joints or damage to the pars interarticularis (isthmus) between the superior and the inferior articular processes. This condition is most commonly found at the level of the L5 vertebra. It results in the forward movement of L5 and the vertebral column superior to it. Potentially, the spinal roots that make up the cauda equina could be compressed as the result of a spondylolisthesis at this level.

The spinous processes enlarge until C7, which is called the vertebra prominens because its spine is usually the first spine that can be palpated (examined by touch) in the neck. The middle cervical spines from C2 to C6 are typically bifid.

Cervical transverse processes have anterior and posterior tubercles. The anterior tubercle of C6 is enlarged and called the *carotid tubercle* because the common carotid artery can be compressed against this tubercle in an emergency. The portion of the transverse process between the anterior and posterior tubercles is grooved for the passage of the spinal nerve from the intervertebral process to the adjacent tissues of the neck.

The first two cervical vertebrae are atypical. C1, the atlas, does not have a body or spinous process. It has an anterior and a posterior arch. The spinous process is replaced by a tubercle (Fig. 3-4). There are two lateral masses at the junctions

of the anterior and posterior articular arches. The superior surfaces of lateral masses articulate with the occipital condyles, the two articular processes on the inferior surface of the skull. The inferior articular surfaces of the lateral masses articulate with the axis, C2 (see Fig. 3-4). On each side, the superior surface of the posterior arch has a groove for the vertebral artery and first cervical spinal nerve. The anterior arch has a fovea facet dentis for the dens ("toothlike") process of C2. There is no disk between C1 and C2. The joint between C1 and the skull's occipital bone, the atlanto-occipital joint, allows only anteroposterior movement as in the up-and-down movement of nodding "yes."

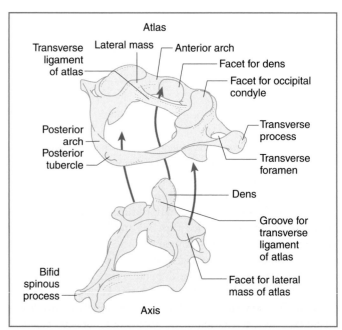

Atlas
Transverse ligament of atlas
Lateral mass
Anterior arch
Facet for dens
Facet for occipital condyle
Posterior arch
Posterior tubercle
Transverse process
Transverse foramen
Dens
Groove for transverse ligament of atlas
Bifid spinous process
Facet for lateral mass of atlas
Axis

Figure 3-4. Articulation of C1 (atlas) and C2 (axis) vertebrae.

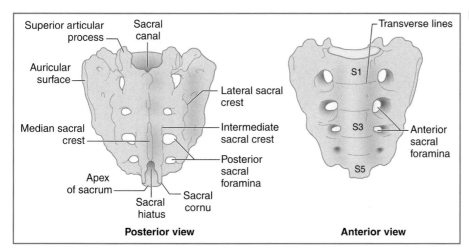

Figure 3-5. Sacrum.

The second cervical vertebra (C2 or axis) is also unusual. The superior surface of the body has the dens, which represents the body of the atlas and which separated from the atlas to fuse with the body of the axis during development. The dens articulates with the anterior arch of the atlas to form the pivot around which the atlas and skull rotate laterally from side to side as in shaking the head "no." This is the atlantoaxial joint.

Thoracic Vertebrae

The distinguishing features of the thoracic vertebrae are the articular facets for the articulation with the heads and tubercles of adjacent ribs on their bodies and on most of their transverse processes. These joints are called costovertebral and costotransverse joints, respectively. However, the transverse processes of T11 and T12 do not have articular facets (discussed in greater detail in Chapter 4).

Lumbar Vertebrae

Lumbar vertebral bodies are massive with heavier, short, quadrilateral spinous processes and thin transverse processes. They do not have costal facets or transverse foramina. The lumbar vertebral laminae are shorter than the thoracic vertebral laminae. This produces a space between the laminae of adjacent lumbar vertebrae, which is accentuated by flexion. The superior articular processes have irregular, rounded elevations called *mamillary processes* for the attachment of muscles.

Sacral Vertebrae

The five sacral vertebrae (Fig. 3-5) are fused, producing a triangular-shaped structure with a smooth anterior concave surface and a rough convex posterior surface. The bodies and transverse processes fuse to produce the lateral masses so that the intervertebral foramina are not visible. Anterior and posterior sacral foramina are for ventral and dorsal rami of sacral spinal nerves, respectively. Posteriorly, the spines of the upper four sacral vertebrae fuse to produce a median sacral crest. Articular processes fuse to produce an intermediate sacral crest. The spine and laminae of the S5 vertebra do not fuse, leaving the opening called the *sacral hiatus*. This is the site of the exit of the S5 spinal nerves and the first coccygeal nerves as well as one of the sites of injection of an anesthetic for an epidural (caudal) anesthesia.

●●● DEVELOPMENT OF VERTEBRAE AND RIBS

During development, each somite will develop into a sclerotome, myotome, and dermatome, with the arteries passing between adjacent somites. The paired sclerotomic mesenchyme rapidly proliferates anterior to the notochord to produce the vertebral body, and around the neural tube to form the vertebral arch. The rapid proliferation of the cells of the sclerotome versus the myotomes or dermatomes is referred to as differential growth.

The mesenchyme of the sclerotome surrounding the notochord initially separates into cranial and caudal halves with an intermediary cellular region between the two halves (Fig. 3-6A and 3-6B). The caudal half of one sclerotome joins the cranial half of the adjacent sclerotome to produce the centrum, which is the developing vertebral body (see Fig. 3-6C). The centrum is not equivalent to the vertebral body, since the posterolateral aspect of the body is formed by the neural arch. The mesenchyme cells between the cranial and caudal portions of the sclerotome develop into the intervertebral disk. The notochord regresses except in the region of the intervertebral disk, where it proliferates to form the nucleus pulposus. These events result in a recombination that produces vertebrae that are now located intersegmentally.

The differential growth of the sclerotome also produces the neural arch, which is composed of two laminae, two pedicles with adjacent portion of the body, and associated processes. The developing vertebrae now lie out of synchrony or in an intersegmental position to the sprouting segmentally

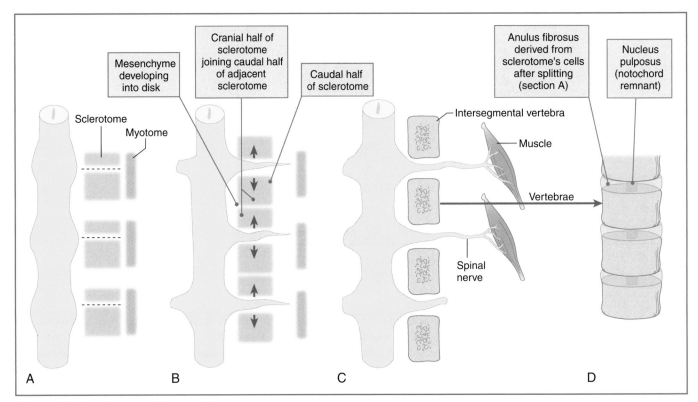

Figure 3-6. Development of the vertebrae.

arranged spinal nerves and myotomes. The nerves will lie between the developing vertebrae, while the intersegmental arteries lie ventral to the vertebrae to become intercostal and lumbar arteries.

The cranial portion of the first sclerotome fuses with the occipital somites in the development of the skull, while its caudal half forms the atlas (C1). The atlas and axis (C2) are unusual because the centrum of the atlas fuses with the centrum of the axis to become the dens of the atlas. The axis' neural arch connects to the anterior arch to complete a ring-like vertebra without a centrum (see Fig. 3-4).

The sacral vertebrae are separate from each other at birth. Fusion of the sacral vertebrae takes place in stages into adulthood.

The development of the vertebrae will proceed from the mesenchymal stage to a stage defined by the development of cartilage, which forms the vertebral body and arch. During endochondral bone formation, the cartilage is replaced with bone.

Costal elements, which are originally derived from the body wall mesenchyme, form parts of the neural (vertebral) arch and produce different vertebral structures at different levels. Typically the costal processes form most of the transverse processes. In the lumbar region, the costal elements produce most of the transverse process, while in the sacrum they contribute to the lateral mass. However, in the cervical region, the costal processes form the anterior aspect of the foramina transversa. Only in the thoracic region do the costal elements become independent and elongate to produce the ribs.

Joints

The vertebral bodies articulate with each other by means of joints characterized by intervertebral disks between adjacent bodies. The range of motion between adjacent vertebrae is limited. However, the overall effect is additive, producing a significant range of motion in the cervical, thoracic, and lumbar regions.

Intervertebral disks are part of the cartilaginous joint between the bodies of adjacent vertebrae. Each disk acts as a shock absorber. It has a central avascular (without blood supply) nucleus pulposus surrounded by fibrous tissue of the anulus fibrosus. The anulus fibrosus consists of lamellae (layers) of fibrous tissue. The innermost lamellae are formed

CLINICAL MEDICINE

Metastases Utilizing Vertebral Plexus of Veins

The vertebral plexus of veins (Batson's plexus) is a possible route of dissemination of malignant cells. Blood flow may change upon coughing, sneezing, or changes in the intra-abdominal pressure. Metastasis of malignant cells is possible from the pelvis to vertebral bodies, lung, or brain.

of fibrocartilage that surround and retain the nucleus pulposus (see Fig. 3-6D). The anulus fibrosus binds vertebral disks together to provide stability. It also permits rotation between adjacent vertebral bodies.

The nucleus pulposus, which is the remnant of the notochord, is a semigelatinous mass containing hyaluronic acid and 70% to 80% water. It is noncompressible but can be deformed or distorted between the bodies of adjacent vertebrae, thereby acting as an equalizer of stresses. This feature allows the disk to absorb compression forces and allows one vertebra to move, or rotate, on another. The axis of movement between adjacent vertebrae runs through the nuclei pulposus. There are no disks between the atlas and the occipital bone or between the atlas and axis.

Joints between adjacent articular processes of vertebral arches (zygapophyseal joints) are classified as synovial joints, since they have a synovial membrane and fluid. These joints are also classified as gliding joints and are innervated by dorsal rami of spinal nerves.

Ligaments

The bodies and disks are held together by a series of ligaments. Interspinous and supraspinous ligaments attach the spines. In the cervical region, the supraspinous ligaments are expanded and thickened to form the ligamentum nuchae, which extends from the occipital bone to the C7 vertebra. It serves as an attachment site for the cervical musculature.

Each ligamentum flavum is one of two paired ligaments found between the anterior surface of the lamina above and the posterior surface of the lamina below, making it a series of discontinuous ligaments that connects vertebrae vertically. These ligaments form part of the posterior wall of the vertebral canal. The elastic connective tissue gives these ligaments a yellow color (hence their name). The ligamenta flava are prominent in the lumbar region because the laminae are narrower than the respective bodies and do not overlap here. Flexion further separates the laminae (e.g., during lumbar puncture).

The anterior longitudinal ligament is broad and is attached to both disks and bodies from the occipital bone to the sacrum. This ligament prevents hyperextension of the vertebral column.

The posterior longitudinal ligament is narrower and attaches to the upper and lower aspect of the body. However, the posterior longitudinal ligament expands as it passes over and attaches to the disks. It prevents hyperflexion.

Spinal Meninges

The meninges (Fig. 3-7) are three membranes that surround the CNS. The spinal and cranial meninges are continuous at the foramen magnum; however, they have specific differences. The three spinal meninges are the dura, arachnoid, and pia mater.

The outermost layer, the dura mater (see Fig. 3-7), is a thick membrane. It is dense connective tissue composed of fibrous collagen and some elastic connective tissue. *It extends from*

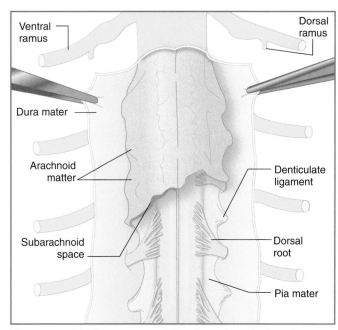

Figure 3-7. Meninges surrounding thoracic spinal cord.

the foramen magnum to the S2 vertebra. Fibrous slips attach the dura mater to the foramen magnum and the posterior aspects of the C2 and C3 vertebral bodies and to the posterior longitudinal ligament especially at caudal vertebral levels. Below the level of the S2 vertebra, the dura surrounds the filum terminale to end at the posterior aspect of the coccyx, where it blends with its periosteum.

The spinal dura also has a tubular prolongation around the spinal roots and spinal nerve, which becomes continuous with the epineurium (outermost connective tissue covering of the nerve) at or slightly beyond the intervertebral foramen.

The epidural space is located between the dura and periosteum of the vertebral canal. It contains fat, loose connective tissue and the internal vertebral venous plexus. The vertebral venous plexus consists of both external and internal vertebral plexuses that communicate with each other. They do not have valves, and they communicate with basivertebral veins that drain vertebral bodies centrally.

The subdural space is a potential or artificial space produced by the separation of the arachnoid from the dura as the result of trauma or a pathologic event. The subdural space does not communicate with the subarachnoid space.

The arachnoid mater (see Figs. 3-7 and 3-8) extends from the foramen magnum to the S2 vertebra. It is a delicate, avascular, loose, irregular type of connective tissue membrane.

The subarachnoid space is located between the arachnoid and pia mater. It contains numerous delicate connective tissue trabeculae and cerebrospinal fluid (CSF). Wider intervals of this subarachnoid space are called cisterns. The lumbar cistern is located between the end of the spinal cord with its attached pia at the level of L1–L2 and the distal end of the arachnoid and dura at the level of S2.

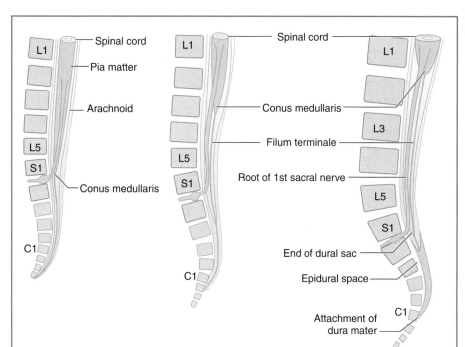

Figure 3-8. Differential growth of vertebral column versus spinal cord.

CSF supports, buffers, and nurtures the CNS. The weight of the brain is approximately 1500 grams, although its apparent weight in CSF is reduced to approximately 50 grams.

The pia mater is a loose connective tissue membrane. It is intimately associated with the spinal cord and passes into its sulci. The pia sends extensions along nerve roots, which blend with the covering of the nerve. The spinal pia contains a plexus of minute blood vessels held together by loose connective tissue, but it is less vascular than cerebral pia. Large arteries are found in the subarachnoid space. However, these arteries are not directly bathed by cerebrospinal fluid, since they are separated from the CSF by a layer of pia, sometimes only one cell thick, that covers them.

The pia has one pair of denticulate ligaments with 21 processes (see Fig. 3-7) that extend from the lateral aspect of the spinal cord and attach to the arachnoid and to the dura. They lie on the lateral side of the spinal cord between adjacent spinal nerve roots with the apex of the triangle attached to the dura. The ventral roots are ventral to the denticulate ligaments and dorsal roots are dorsal to the denticulate ligaments.

Inferiorly, the pia continues beyond the end of the spinal cord, which is called the conus medullaris. Here, it forms a thin band called the filum terminale internum (Figs. 3-8 and 3-9). The filum terminale internum is joined at the level of the S2 vertebra by the arachnoid and dura. Together, they form the filum terminale externum, which extends through the sacral hiatus to end on the periosteum of the posterior surface of the first coccygeal vertebra, where it is often referred to as the coccygeal ligament.

●●● NEONATAL CHANGES IN THE SPINAL CORD

There is an ascent of spinal cord in the vertebral column, which is most pronounced in the lumbar, sacral, and coccygeal spinal cord levels. Early in development, the spinal cord fills the vertebral canal and the spinal nerves leave through intervertebral canals closely associated with the origin of the spinal nerve roots. However, owing to differential growth of the vertebral column versus the spinal cord, the spinal cord ascends.

At birth the conus medullaris is located at the L3 vertebra level. By the age of 6 months, however, the conus medullaris has ascended approximately to the level of the L1 and L2 disk space. This difference in length explains the long lower lumbar, sacral, and coccygeal nerve roots that form the cauda equina. The ascent of the spinal cord also accounts for the presence of the filament-like extension of the pia as the filum terminale internum.

NEUROSCIENCE

Cerebrospinal Fluid

CSF is a clear, slightly alkaline fluid with few cells that is secreted by the choroid plexus of the brain. It flows from the fourth ventricle into the subarachnoid space. The CSF returns to the venous system by means of arachnoid granulations into the dural venous sinuses of the neurocranium, and possibly by venous plexuses of the vertebral, posterior intercostal, and lumbar veins.

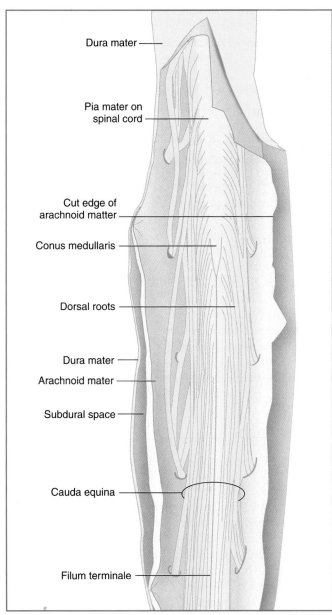

Figure 3-9. Cauda equina, filum terminale, and meninges.

Labels on figure:
- Dura mater
- Pia mater on spinal cord
- Cut edge of arachnoid matter
- Conus medullaris
- Dorsal roots
- Dura mater
- Arachnoid mater
- Subdural space
- Cauda equina
- Filum terminale

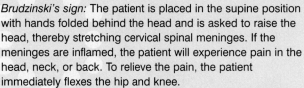

CLINICAL MEDICINE

Signs of Meningitis

Brudzinski's sign: The patient is placed in the supine position with hands folded behind the head and is asked to raise the head, thereby stretching cervical spinal meninges. If the meninges are inflamed, the patient will experience pain in the head, neck, or back. To relieve the pain, the patient immediately flexes the hip and knee.

Kernig's sign: The patient is placed in the supine position with the hands folded behind the head and is asked to elevate one of the lower extended limbs. Upon hip flexion, the patient cannot fully extend the knee because of pain. The test is considered positive if this maneuver elicits pain in the neck, head, or back that is relieved by hip and knee flexion.

Lumbar puncture (spinal tap) is performed in cases of meningitis to determine the cell count, to culture bacteria, and to perform chemical analysis of the CSF. The lumbar cistern of the subarachnoid space is an enlargement of the subarachnoid space. It does not contain the spinal cord but does contain the cauda equina or roots of lumbar, sacral, and coccygeal nerves. The patient is placed in the lateral decubitus position (in bed and flexed on the side) to increase the size of the spaces between adjacent lumbar laminae. The spine of the L4 vertebra is located by finding the imaginary line that passes through the highest point of the iliac crest (the intercristal line). *The adult spinal cord ends as the conus medullaris at the bodies of the L1 and L2 vertebrae.* The subarachnoid space can be entered between the spines of L3 and L4 or L4 and L5. In a newborn child, a lower position is required, because the spinal cord may extend to the level of L2 and L3. In the midline, the needle passes through skin, superficial fascia, deep fascia, supra- and interspinous ligaments, possibly fused margins of ligamenta flava, epidural space, dura, subdural space, and arachnoid before reaching the subarachnoid space.

●●● MUSCLES OF THE BACK

The back muscles fall into two categories—superficial and deep layers—based not only on location but also on function and innervation. These muscle groups consist of incompletely separated components that have specific names depicting length and region (e.g., longissimus thoracis).

The superficial group of back muscles is organized into several layers (Fig. 3-10), which are associated with the upper limb or ribs.

Layer 1 consists of the trapezius and latissimus dorsi.

Layer 2 consists of the levator scapulae and rhomboid major and minor muscles.

Layer 3 consists of the serratus posterior superior and serratus posterior inferior, which may be associated with respiration.

Development of the Meninges

The meninges develop from the mesenchyme surrounding the neural tube. The external layer develops into the dura mater. The internal layer, or leptomeninges, develops into the arachnoid and pia mater. The subarachnoid space develops between the arachnoid and pia upon secretion of CSF.

Meningitis

Meningitis is an inflammation of the meninges produced by viral, bacterial, fungal, or parasitic microorganisms. The infection usually extends through the subarachnoid space.

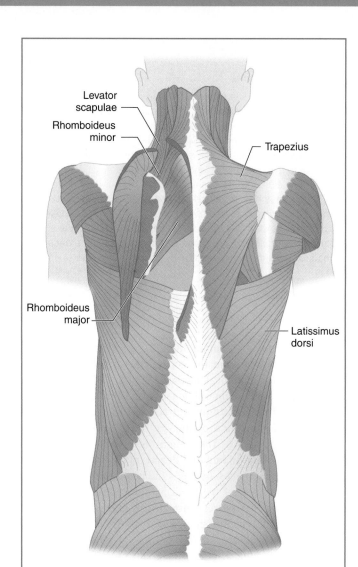

Levator
scapulae

Rhomboideus
minor

Trapezius

Rhomboideus
major

Latissimus
dorsi

Figure 3-10. Superficial back muscles.

The deep muscles are the true or intrinsic muscles of the back, which are arranged in longitudinal layers that typically extend over multiple vertebral levels. They are divided into spinotransverse and transversospinales muscles (Table 3-1).

The spinotransverse muscles consist of the erector spinae and splenius muscles. The erector spinae muscle is a group of muscles that stretches from the sacrum and adjacent structures and ascends to insert into the ribs. This muscle is found along both sides of the vertebral column and is subdivided into three columns medial to lateral: spinalis, longissimus, and iliocostalis (see Table 3-1). The splenius muscles are splenius capitis and cervicalis.

The transversospinal muscles originate on the transverse processes and run to a superior vertebra. They are, superficial to deep, the semispinalis, multifidus, and rotatores.

Innervation

The superficial muscle layers are innervated by ventral rami of the spinal nerves except for the trapezius, which is innervated by cranial nerve XI. The deep muscle layers are innervated by segmental dorsal rami. These divisions are rooted in the development of the trunk skeletal muscle.

Blood Supply

Segmental arteries arising from the aorta supply the back of the trunk. These include the 11 pairs of intercostal, 1 pair of subcostal, and 4 to 5 pairs of lumbar arteries. In the neck, the vertebral and to a lesser extent the branches of the occipital and costocervical trunk supply the muscles. Most of these arteries also send radicular arteries through the intervertebral foramina to anastomose with the one anterior and two posterior spinal arteries that run the length of the spinal cord.

Development

Each myotome divides into a ventrally located hypomere and a dorsally located epimere. The hypomere develops into the hypaxial muscles of the lateral and ventral trunk wall and limbs, while the epimere develops into the true back muscles. The developing spinal nerves migrating to specific muscles or muscle bundles follow a similar pattern by dividing into ventral and dorsal rami. The dorsal ramus of the spinal nerve migrates to and innervates the epimere-derived muscles while the ventral ramus migrates to and innervates the hypomere-derived muscles. The ventral rami pass between the three layers of the thoracic epimeric-derived muscles to reach the more ventral muscle group. These layers are actually columns of muscles that extend into the lateral abdominal wall as the external oblique, internal oblique, and transverse abdominal muscles.

The somitic myoblasts also migrate into the developing limb to develop into the limb musculature, but they do not form the limb skeleton or the trunk wall connective tissue and tendons. These structures are derived from the somatic lateral plate mesoderm.

TABLE 3-1. Intrinsic Muscles of the Back

Muscle	Origin	Insertion	Action	Innervation and Development
Spinotransverse group: superficial layer of the intrinsic muscles of the neck that arise from spines and ligamentum nuchae; these muscle fibers run superolaterally				
Splenius capitis	Inferior portion of ligamentum nuchae and spinous processes of C7, T1–T3(4)	Mastoid process and adjacent superior nuchal line	Extends neck and rotates head to ipsilateral side	Dorsal rami Epimere
Splenius cervicalis	Thoracic spinous processes of T3–T6	Upper cervical transverse processes	Lateral flexion and rotation to ipsilateral (same) side	Dorsal rami Epimere
Erector spinae muscle is subdivided into iliocostalis, longissimus, and spinalis components, which can be further subdivided into lumbar, thoracic, and cervical components				
Iliocostalis	(a) Common origin from sacrum, lumbar vertebrae, iliac crests (b) Lower ribs (c) Upper ribs	(a) Ribs (b) Upper ribs (c) Cervical transverse processes	Extends vertebral column	Dorsal rami Epimere
Longissimus	Mostly from lumbar and thoracic transverse processes, also from sacrum, lumbar vertebrae, iliac crests	Thoracic and cervical transverse processes as well as mastoid process	Extends vertebral column	
Spinalis	Lumbar spinous processes	Thoracic spinous	Extends vertebral column	Dorsal rami Epimere
Transversospinal group: deep to erector spinae; arise from transverse processes and insert into higher vertebrae				
Semispinalis	Transverse processes of thoracic and cervical vertebrae	Spinous processes of cervical and thoracic vertebrae	Extensor of thoracic, cervical, and head vertebral column; rotates vertebral column to contralateral side	Dorsal rami, cervical and thoracic nerves
Thoracis	T5–T7	Spinous processes C7, T1–T5	Extensor of vertebral column; rotates vertebral column to contralateral side	Dorsal rami Epimere
Cervicalis	Transverse processes T2–T5	Spinous processes of C2–C5	Extensor of cervical vertebral column; rotates vertebral column to contralateral side	Dorsal rami, cervical and thoracic nerves Epimere
Capitis	Transverse processes of T1–T5 and articular processes C4–C7	Occipital bone between superior and inferior nuchal lines	Extends head	Dorsal rami, cervical nerves Epimere
Multifidus	Sacrum, sacroiliac ligament, mamillary processes of the lumbar vertebrae, transverse processes of thoracic vertebrae, and articular processes of C4–C7	Spinous processes of vertebrae above origin	Rotates vertebral column to contralateral side	Dorsal rami Epimere
Rotatores	Best developed in thorax from transverse process	Base of spine of vertebrae above origin	Rotate vertebral column to contralateral side; possibly function as muscles of proprioception	Dorsal rami Epimere

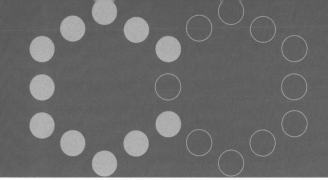

The Thorax

4

CONTENTS

THORACIC WALL
Rib Cage
Superior Thoracic Aperture
Inferior Thoracic Aperture
Musculature of the Thoracic Wall
Neurovascular Structures of the Thoracic Wall

DIAPHRAGM
Function
Innervation
Blood Supply
Embryology

SURFACE ANATOMY OF THE THORAX
Reference Lines of the Thoracic Cavity

THORACIC CAVITY
Development of the Thoracic Cavity
Pleural Cavity
Lungs

MEDIASTINUM
Anterior Mediastinum
Middle Mediastinum
Pericardium

HEART
Surfaces of the Heart
Sulci on the Surface of the Heart
Coronary Arteries
Venous Drainage of the Heart
Interior of the Heart
Innervation of the Heart
Cardiac Referred Pain
Conduction System of the Heart
Lymphatics in the Heart
Auscultation of Heart Sounds
Development of the Heart

SUPERIOR MEDIASTINUM
Thymus
Veins of the Superior Mediastinum
Arteries of the Superior Mediastinum
Trachea
Esophagus
Azygos Vein
Vagus Nerve

POSTERIOR MEDIASTINUM
Bifurcation of the Trachea
Esophagus
Descending Thoracic Aorta

Azygos System of Veins
Thoracic Duct
Sympathetic Trunk
Thoracic Lymph Nodes

The thorax is the area of the body located between the neck and the diaphragm. It contains the heart and lungs with their associated serous cavities, the lower respiratory system, the esophagus, and the neurovascular structures that run between the neck, upper extremities, and abdomen.

●●● THORACIC WALL

Deep to skin and superficial fascia of the thoracic wall lies the musculoskeletal system wrapped by the outer investing layer of deep fascia. While this layer of deep fascia is not very distinguishable from the muscular fascia, the superficial layer of muscle that covers the thoracic wall is very prominent. Several large muscles on the ventral thoracic wall arise from the ribs and insert into the humerus and scapula, which are components of the appendicular (limb) skeleton. These muscles include the pectoralis major and minor and the serratus anterior and will be considered with the upper limb.

Rib Cage

The rib cage (Fig. 4-1) comprises
- Twelve thoracic vertebrae and intervertebral disks
- Twelve pairs of costae (ribs) and their cartilages
- Sternum
- Superior thoracic aperture
- Inferior thoracic aperture
- Intercostal spaces

The thorax is not equated with the rib cage. The rib cage is a substantially larger structure than the thorax, protecting the organs of the thorax and those of the upper abdomen as well. Abdominal organs that are protected by the rib cage are the liver on the right and the stomach and spleen on the left, as well as the upper poles of the kidneys.

The thorax is conical in shape. It is widest at the level of the fourth to fifth costal cartilage, which corresponds to approximately the T6–T7 vertebral levels. However, the superior

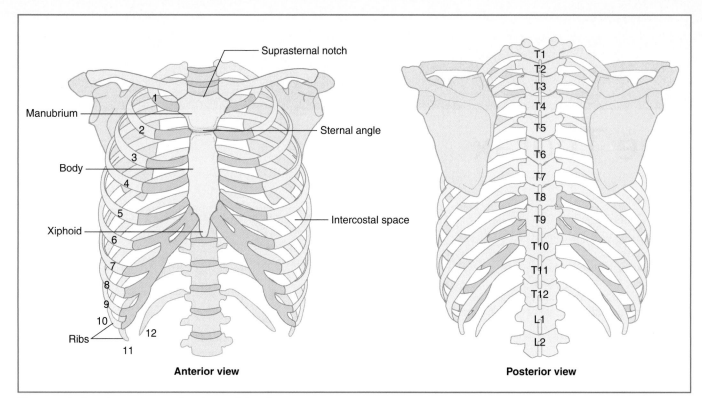

Figure 4-1. Anterior and posterior views of the rib cage.

aspect of the thorax is narrowest at the level of the T2–T3 vertebrae because of the anterior curvature of the thoracic vertebral column.

Ribs

There are 12 pairs of ribs (see Fig. 4-1). Ribs are thin, narrow, curved, and elongated bones. They articulate with the vertebral column posteriorly. The shaft of the rib initially runs posterior and laterally from the vertebral column and then runs anteriorly and medially toward the sternum. The anterior terminal end is always located inferiorly in position when compared with the posterior end of the rib. The vertical distance between the two ends of the same rib is approximately the length of two thoracic vertebrae.

Parts of the Rib

The head has a superior and an inferior facet separated by a crest (Fig. 4-2). It articulates with facets on the bodies of two adjacent vertebrae, the same numbered vertebra as the rib and the vertebra above.

The neck is the narrow portion connecting the head to the shaft. It is just anterior to the adjacent transverse process.

The tubercle of the rib is located on its external surface at the junction of the neck and body (shaft). The tubercle is a bony projection that has an articular facet for articulation with the transverse process of the same numbered vertebra.

The shaft is the longest part. It is long and flat and has an angle where the rib changes direction from posterolateral to anterolateral. The angle of the rib is in the same plane as the

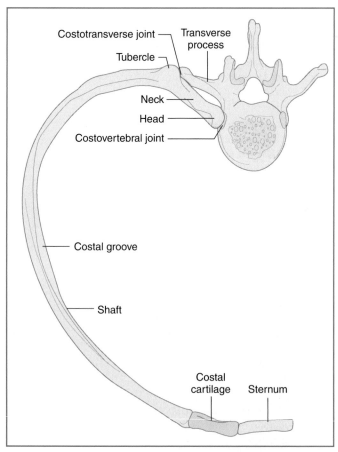

Figure 4-2. Articulation of a typical rib with a vertebra.

same numbered spinous process. In the supine position, a person is lying on the vertebral spines and the angles of the ribs.

The superior border of the shaft is typically rounded. The inferior border has a costal groove, which contains the intercostal neurovascular bundle. The components of the intercostal neurovascular bundle have a characteristic orientation from superior to inferior: vein, artery, and nerve (VAN).

The shaft continues curving anteromedially and inferiorly so that the anterior terminal end is inferior in position to the head of the rib. The costal cartilage connects the end of the rib to the sternum. Costal cartilages 1–3 run in the same general plane as the anterior terminal ends of those ribs. However, the ventral portions of costal cartilages 4–10 are angled superiorly in direction. This angle increases from ribs 4 to 10.

Classification of Different Ribs

The costal cartilages of ribs 1–7 articulate directly with the sternum. These ribs are referred to as *true ribs* (see Fig. 4-1).

The costal cartilages of ribs 8–12 do not articulate directly with the sternum. These ribs are known as *false ribs* (see Fig. 4-1). The costal cartilages of ribs 8, 9, and typically 10 articulate with the costal cartilage above. Thus, the cartilage of the eighth rib articulates with the cartilage of rib 7 rather than directly with the sternum. The junction of these cartilages forms the costal margin. Both costal margins together form the costal arch.

The costal cartilages of ribs 11 and 12 are not attached anteriorly; these are the *floating ribs*. Often, the tenth costal cartilage does not articulate with the ninth costal cartilage. If the tenth rib does not participate in the formation of the costal margin, it is considered to be a floating rib. This is the reason that counting ribs from the costal margin is unreliable.

The costal cartilages are avascular and therefore regenerate slowly. Aggressive intervention is necessary to prevent infection that is capable of spreading down both costal margins.

Unique Features of Various Ribs

The first rib is the shortest and strongest and articulates with only one vertebra—T1. The superior surface of the first rib has a prominent tubercle, called the scalene tubercle, for the attachment of the anterior scalene muscle. There are two grooves, one on each side of the scalene tubercle, for the subclavian artery and vein. The subclavian artery and inferior trunk of the brachial plexus run in the posterolateral groove, while the subclavian vein runs in the anteromedial groove. Therefore, the anterior scalene muscle separates the subclavian vein from the subclavian artery. Ribs 1–7 progress in length. The first is the shortest, and the seventh is the longest. Ribs 8–12 decrease in length, and the twelfth rib is longer than the first rib.

Ribs 11 and 12 do not have tubercles and therefore do not articulate with the vertebral transverse processes.

Articulations of the Ribs

Most ribs articulate with the vertebral column in two places: (1) at the costovertebral joint, where the head of the rib

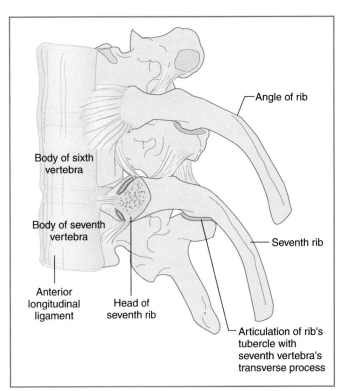

Figure 4-3. Anterior and lateral views of the sternum.

articulates with the vertebral bodies, and (2) at the costotransverse joint between the rib's tubercle and the vertebra's transverse process (see Fig. 4-2).

The superior articular facet of the typical head of the rib articulates with the body of the vertebra above while the inferior articular facet of the head of the rib articulates with the vertebral body having the same number as the rib. For ribs 2–10, the facets on adjacent vertebral bodies along with the intervertebral disk form a complete socket for the articulation with the head of the rib (see Figs. 4-2 and 4-3).

The tubercle of a typical rib articulates with the transverse process of the same number vertebra (for ribs 1–10). These so-called costotransverse joints of ribs 1–10 are encapsulated. Three adjacent ligaments run from different points on the rib's neck to the adjacent transverse process or the transverse process above (see Fig. 4-3).

Sternum

The sternum (Fig. 4-4) is defined as a flat bone that has three parts: manubrium, body, and xiphoid process.

Manubrium

The manubrium (Latin, "handle") is the quadrilateral, superior part of the sternum. The manubrium corresponds to the T3–T4 vertebral levels. It is the widest and thickest part and has the following features:
- A concave superior border has a deep midline notch called the *jugular* (Latin, "neck") or *suprasternal notch*, which can be easily palpated (felt or touched).

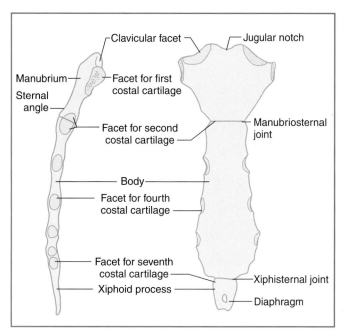

Figure 4-4. Anterior and lateral views of the sternum.

- There are two clavicular notches for articulation with the clavicles. The clavicular notches are lateral to the jugular notch. The joints between the clavicles and manubrium are the sternoclavicular joints and are important anatomic landmarks.

The manubrium's lateral edge has 1½ costal facets or notches for the articulations with the first costal cartilage and the superior half of the second costal cartilage. The first costal cartilage is located posterior to the sternoclavicular joint, making it difficult to accurately palpate.

Corpus Sterni (Body of Sternum)

The body of the sternum is twice the length of the manubrium (10–14 cm). The manubrium slopes anteroinferiorly, whereas the body is almost vertical in position. Therefore, articulation of the manubrium and body of sternum produces a definite easily palpated morphologic protrusion or ridge on the sternum's external surface called the *sternal angle (of Louis)*. The sternal angle always coincides with the articulation of the second costal cartilage with the sternum. This constant relationship allows for the accurate identification of the second costal cartilages and ribs, thereby allowing one to locate with great certainty the remaining ribs and intercostal spaces that serve as landmarks for underlying structures. The first rib is typically not useful when counting ribs because its articulation with the manubrium may be obscured by the sternoclavicular articulation.

The body of the sternum has four complete costal notches on each side along with two hemifacets. The hemifacet on the manubrium joins the hemifacet on the body to produce the complete facet or notch for the second costal cartilage, while the hemifacet on the xiphoid process joins the hemifacet on the body for the articulation with the seventh

costal cartilage. The body of the sternum corresponds to T5–T9.

Xiphoid Process

The xiphoid process is a small, elongated cartilaginous process that may be pointed or bifid. The xiphoid process is cartilaginous in young individuals and ossifies with age. It articulates with the seventh costal cartilage, but this joint is harder to palpate than the sternal angle. The xiphisternal articulation corresponds approximately to the level of T9.

The sternum is not a common site for fractures. When a fracture does occur, posterior displacement is rare because of the support from the endothoracic fascia found on the internal surface of the sternum.

Superior Thoracic Aperture

The superior thoracic aperture is formed by
- The first pair of ribs and their cartilages
- The superior surface of the manubrium
- The T1 vertebra

The jugular notch projects posteriorly to the level of the disk space between T2 and T3. Thus, the posterior aspect of the superior thoracic aperture, which is found at the level of T1, is higher and slopes to a lower anterior level. This opening is for the passage of structures between the neck and the thorax (e.g., neurovascular bundles, esophagus, trachea). The superior portion of the lung is called the apex of the lung, and its pleural covering is referred to as the cupola. These structures also pass through the superior aperture. The apex of the lung and its cupola are found approximately 3–4 cm above the medial third of the clavicle.

Inferior Thoracic Aperture

The inferior aperture is formed by
- The xiphoid process with xiphisternal articulation
- The margins of the costal cartilages 7–10
- The tips of ribs 11 and 12
- The T12 vertebra

The diaphragm closes the inferior thoracic aperture.

Musculature of the Thoracic Wall

The space between adjacent ribs is called the intercostal space. There are 11 intercostal spaces on each side of the rib cage. The intercostal spaces are wider anteriorly than posteriorly. The upper intercostal spaces are also wider than the lower intercostal spaces. This is especially true of the third and fourth intercostal spaces.

There are three layers of intercostal muscles, which fill in the intercostal spaces, protect against pressure changes, and participate in forced respiration (Figs. 4-5 and 4-6).

External Intercostal Muscle

This muscle forms the most external layer (see Figs. 4-5 and 4-6). The external intercostal muscle runs from the inferior

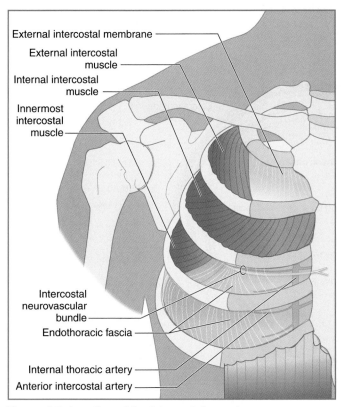

External intercostal membrane

External intercostal muscle

Internal intercostal muscle

Innermost intercostal muscle

Intercostal neurovascular bundle

Endothoracic fascia

Internal thoracic artery

Anterior intercostal artery

Figure 4-5. Location of the intercostal muscles.

border of one rib to the superior border of the next lower rib. These fibers are directed anteriorly and inferiorly. The external intercostal muscles begin near the vertebral column at the tubercle of the rib and fill the intercostal space up to the costochondral junction (i.e., the point where the bony portion of the rib ends). Here, the external intercostal membrane replaces the muscle fibers. The muscle fibers, therefore, do not reach the sternum. The external intercostal muscles are muscles of inspiration because they elevate the ribs.

Internal Intercostal Muscles

The internal intercostal muscles form the layer just deep to the external intercostal muscles. These muscle fibers run posteriorly and inferiorly, at right angles to the muscle fibers of the external intercostal muscles (see Figs. 4-5 and 4-6). The internal intercostal muscle runs from the sternum to the angle of the rib. The internal intercostal membrane fills in the remaining space (see Fig. 4-6).

The portion of the internal intercostal muscle between adjacent bony ribs depresses the rib and is a muscle of forced expiration. However, the portion of these muscles between adjacent cartilages (intercondylar portion) elevates the rib and is a muscle of inspiration.

Innermost Intercostal Muscle

The innermost intercostal muscle is the deepest muscle in the intercostal space and extends approximately from the anterior axillary line to the angle of the rib. The innermost intercostal muscle's fibers run in the same direction as the internal intercostal muscle. These muscles are best demonstrated by the presence of the intercostal neurovascular bundle (see Fig. 4-6), which separates the internal intercostal muscle from the innermost intercostal muscles.

There are two other muscles that occupy the innermost position of the thoracic wall in the anterior aspect of the rib cage and the posterior aspect of the rib cage. They are the transversus thoracis muscle and the subcostal muscles, respectively.

The transversus thoracis muscle arises from the sternum (xiphoid process and body) and runs superiorly and laterally to insert into the internal surfaces of the costal cartilages of ribs 2–6. This is a muscle of expiration.

The subcostal muscles are found in the posterior thoracic wall near the angle of the rib. They pass over one or two intercostal spaces to insert into the rib's superior border. They are considered to be similar in direction to the innermost intercostal muscles and therefore have a similar function.

Breast

The breasts, or mammary glands, are modified sweat glands located in the superficial fascia of the thoracic wall. The base of each breast is circular with its medial side at the lateral border of the sternum and its lateral border at the axilla. The superior and inferior borders are approximately at the second and sixth rib. The deep surface of the breast is concave and adjacent to the pectoralis major, serratus anterior, and external oblique muscles. However, the breasts are separated from the deep fascia covering these muscles by a layer of loose connective tissue known as the retromammary space. This allows for movement of the breasts on the chest wall.

The mammary gland has 15 to 20 lobes that are each drained by a single lactiferous duct that leads to the nipple. The breasts are not developed in males or prepubescent females. The lobes are delineated by connective tissue septae called *suspensory ligaments (of Cooper) of the breast*. The glandular tissue of the lobes is surrounded by varying amounts of adipose tissue that gives the breast its shape. Both the glandular tissue and the adipose tissue are under hormonal control. During pregnancy the increase in glandular tissue is due to estrogen and progesterone. The adipose tissue is sensitive to levels of estrogen.

The breasts are highly vascularized with branches from the internal thoracic artery and vein, thoracoacromial artery and vein, and lateral thoracic arteries and veins. The lymphatic drainage of the breast follows the venous drainage. It is important to note that because of the tear-drop shape of the breast, 75% of the breast is lateral to the nipple so 75% of the lymph drains to the anterior axillary (pectoral) nodes.

Four percent of women have malignant tumors of the breast. Scirrhous (hard) tumors of the breast often place traction on the suspensory ligaments (of Cooper), which causes dimpling of the skin of the breast. This cancer can metastasize (spread) to other areas through the lymphatic system. The breast's lymphatics drain primarily into the anterior axillary (pectoral) lymph nodes. However, cells from

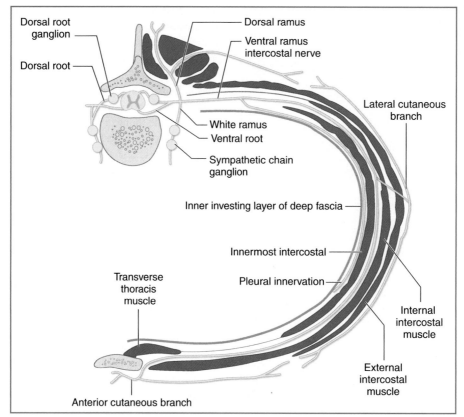

A

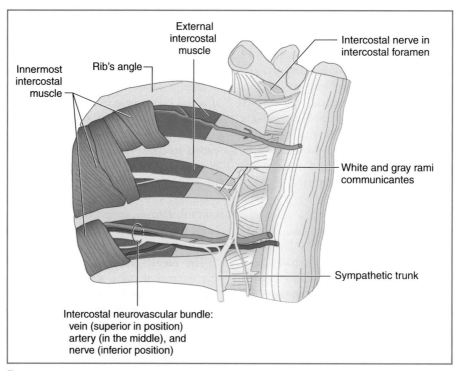

B

Figure 4-6. A, Intercostal neurovascular bundles. **B,** Intercostal muscles and the intercostal neurovascular bundle.

a tumor in the medial part of the breast would drain toward the internal thoracic nodes (parasternal nodes).

Neurovascular Structures of the Thoracic Wall

The intercostal nerves are the ventral rami of the first 11 thoracic spinal nerves. The ventral ramus of the 12th thoracic spinal nerve is called the subcostal nerve. The intercostal nerves exit from the vertebral canal through the intervertebral foramen, enter the intercostal spaces, and run between the innermost and internal intercostal muscles (see Fig. 4-6).

The T1 nerve has a large superior division that helps form the inferior trunk of the brachial plexus and a smaller inferior division that is the first intercostal nerve. The first intercostal nerve does not provide cutaneous branches in the thorax wall.

Arterial Supply
Posterior Blood Supply

Intercostal spaces 3–11 have posterior intercostal arteries that are branches of the descending thoracic aorta. The artery below the twelfth rib is the subcostal artery. These arteries run in the plane of the subfascia or extraserous fascia. They run between the pleura and the inner investing layer of deep (endothoracic) fascia, penetrating the endothoracic fascia to reach the costal groove.

The supreme (highest) intercostal artery arises from the costocervical trunk of the subclavian artery and descends across the first two ribs. The supreme intercostal artery supplies the upper two posterior intercostal spaces with posterior intercostal arteries. The sympathetic trunk is on the supreme intercostal artery's medial side and the first thoracic nerve is on its lateral side.

Anterior Blood Supply

The internal thoracic artery is also a branch of the subclavian artery. It gives rise to the anterior intercostal arteries, which supply intercostal spaces 1–6 (see Fig. 4-5). The anterior intercostal arteries in intercostal spaces 4–6 run on the external surface of the transversus thoracis muscle.

The internal thoracic artery ends at the sixth intercostal space by branching into the superior epigastric artery and the musculophrenic artery. The superior epigastric artery is always the medial branch, and the musculophrenic artery is always the lateral branch.

For intercostal spaces 7–9, the anterior intercostal arteries arise from the musculophrenic artery. The lower two intercostal spaces do not have anterior intercostal arteries. They receive blood only from the last two posterior intercostal arteries.

There are nine pairs of posterior intercostal arteries that are branches of the descending aorta.

Venous Drainage

The venous drainage follows the arterial supply with anterior and posterior intercostal veins. The anterior intercostal veins drain into the musculophrenic and internal thoracic veins. The internal thoracic veins in turn drain into the brachiocephalic veins.

The posterior intercostal veins drain into the azygos system of veins. There are many variations in the azygos system of veins (see posterior mediastinum section). The first posterior intercostal vein on both sides often, but not always, drains into the brachiocephalic vein and is referred to as the highest or supreme intercostal vein. The next two to three posterior intercostal veins are different. The second, third, and fourth posterior intercostal veins unite to form the superior intercostal vein. The left superior intercostal vein drains into the left brachiocephalic vein, while the right superior intercostal vein drains directly into the azygos vein. The azygos vein drains into the posterior aspect of the superior vena cava.

Lymphatics

The lymphatics of the intercostal spaces drain anteriorly to the parasternal nodes associated with the internal thoracic artery that in turn drain into bronchomediastinal nodes (lymphatic vessels arising from the union of the efferent lymphatics from the tracheal [paratracheal] and superior mediastinal nodes). The lymphatics associated with the posterior intercostal arteries drain into the thoracic duct, right main lymphatic duct, and diaphragmatic nodes. The diaphragmatic nodes lie on the thoracic surface of the diaphragm and receive afferents from the lower intercostal spaces, pericardium, and liver. These nodes drain into the parasternal nodes.

●●● DIAPHRAGM

The diaphragm is a skeletal muscle that partitions the thorax and abdomen by closing the inferior thoracic aperture. It arises from the periphery on the body wall and inserts into the central tendon. It is important but not essential for respiration. The origins of the thoracic diaphragm form an oblique peripheral ring as this skeletal muscle arises from the body wall.

Function

Contraction of its skeletal muscle results in the diaphragm moving inferiorly. This increases the vertical volume of the thoracic cavity during inspiration. Elevation of the ribs increases the volume of the ribs in two planes.
- Elevation of ribs 7–10 produces a bucket-handle-like action that increases the transverse (side-to-side) plane of the rib cage.
- Elevation of ribs 2–6 produces an elevation of the sternum that increases the pump-handle (anterior to posterior) volume of the rib cage. This is due to the oblique slope of the rib from posterior to anterior.

Innervation

The phrenic nerves supply the general somatic efferent (motor, or GSE) fibers to the diaphragm. The neuronal cell bodies of these GSE fibers are located in C3–C5 spinal cord segments. The general somatic afferent (sensory, or GSA) fibers to most of the diaphragm arise from cell bodies located in the dorsal root ganglia of C3–C5 spinal cord segments. This reflects the diaphragm's embryologic origin from mesoderm that migrates from the rostral portion of the embryo during craniocaudal folding. Even though the right crus crosses the midline, the left phrenic nerve supplies the portion of the right crus to the left of the midline.

The sensory innervation of the diaphragm is dual in nature, with thoracic spinal nerves 6–10 supplying the lateral and posterior peripheral aspects of the diaphragm, and the phrenic nerves supplying the sensory fibers to the central portion of the diaphragm. Therefore, pain stimulated by irritation of the central aspects of the diaphragm is referred to dermatomes C3, C4, and C5 (shoulder tip pain). However, pain from the peripheral aspects of the diaphragm is referred to the lateral and posterior aspects of thoracic dermatomes 6–10.

The postganglionic sympathetic fibers to the diaphragm arise from cell bodies located in the superior and middle cervical sympathetic ganglia. These postganglionic sympathetic fibers reach the ventral rami of C3–C5 spinal nerves by means of gray rami communicantes.

CLINICAL MEDICINE

Neural Paralysis of the Diaphragm

Neural paralysis of the diaphragm results in a paradoxical movement. Loss of one phrenic nerve results in the elevation of the diaphragm on the affected side upon inspiration. Instead of descending upon inspiration, the denervated portion of the diaphragm is elevated by the increased abdominal pressure.

Blood Supply

The superior surface of the diaphragm is supplied by the following: the pericardiacophrenic artery (a branch of the internal thoracic artery, which accompanies the phrenic nerve), the musculophrenic artery (a branch of the internal thoracic artery), and the paired superior phrenic arteries from the descending thoracic aorta. Each of these three sources has minor branches to the inferior surface of the diaphragm as well.

However, the major source of blood to the inferior surface of the diaphragm is the paired inferior phrenic arteries, which are the first paired branches off the abdominal aorta.

Embryology

The diaphragm develops from the following four embryologic entities (Fig. 4-7): septum transversum, pleuroperitoneal membranes, dorsal mesentery of the esophagus, and body wall mesoderm. The septum transversum originally lies cranial to the buccopharyngeal membrane but moves to its definitive location in the thoracic region during longitudinal folding of the embryo. This accounts for the innervation to the central part of the diaphragm by the phrenic nerves (C3, C4, and C5). The pleuroperitoneal membranes grow toward the septum transversum from the posterolateral aspect of the intraembryonic coelom and fuse with septum transversum and dorsal mesentery of the esophagus. This partitions the pleural cavity from the peritoneal cavity. Body wall mesoderm then forms the periphery of the diaphragm. The most common congenital malformation of the diaphragm is a congenital diaphragmatic hernia that results from a failure of the pleuroperitoneal membranes to completely fuse with the septum transversum, usually on the left side. This allows abdominal viscera to herniate into the thorax and can cause

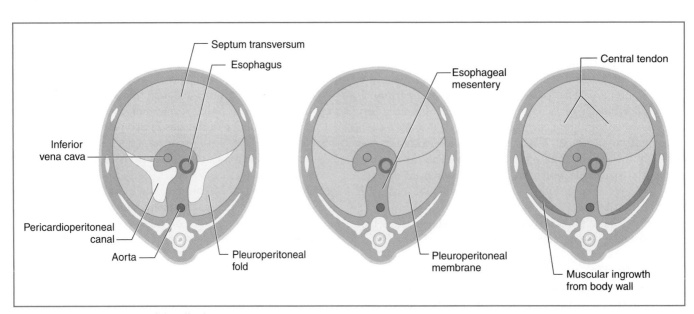

Figure 4-7. Development of the diaphragm.

pulmonary hypoplasia, which is the diminished development of the lung.

●●● SURFACE ANATOMY OF THE THORAX

Reference Lines of the Thoracic Cavity

There are vertical lines that are used as reference points (Fig. 4-8) for locating deeper structures in the thorax and for performing pleural punctures and insertion of chest tubes.

The midsternal line passes through the middle of the sternum. In cardiac surgery, an incision is most often made along this line. The rib cage can then be opened similarly to opening a book.

The midclavicular line runs perpendicular to the clavicle at its midpoint (see Fig. 4-8). The mammary gland is located at the level of ribs 4–6 in the midclavicular line. In men, the nipple is located approximately at the fourth intercostal space. This relationship is variable in women.

The axillary lines are three lines that can be traced vertically downward from the axilla (the armpit; see Fig. 4-8). The anterior axillary line (see Fig. 4-8) is a vertical line passing inferiorly from the anterior axillary fold, which is formed by the skin, fascia, and lateral margin of the pectoralis major muscle moving to its humoral insertion. The midaxillary line (see Fig. 4-8) is a vertical line passing inferiorly from the midway point that intersects the anterior and posterior axillary folds or lines. The posterior axillary line (see Fig. 4-8) is a vertical line passing inferiorly from the posterior axillary fold, which is formed by the skin, fascia, and margin of the latissimus dorsi muscle and teres major muscle.

The parasternal line is a vertical line equidistant from the sternal and midclavicular lines. It passes through the costal cartilages. The internal thoracic artery passes along this line. Lymphatic nodes that follow the internal mammary chain are the parasternal nodes.

The scapular line, in the anatomic position, extends vertically through the inferior angle of the scapula and the seventh rib (the rib number will change when the arm is abducted).

●●● THORACIC CAVITY

The thoracic cavity is found internal to the endothoracic fascia, which is the boundary that separates the thoracic wall from the thoracic cavity. It extends from the superior thoracic aperture to the diaphragm and from the sternum to the T12 vertebra and the ribs. The thoracic cavity contains the following serous sacs: two pleural sacs that surround the lungs and the pericardial sac that surrounds the heart. The thoracic cavity also contains the lower respiratory system, cardiovascular system, esophagus, and posterior neurovascular structures.

Development of the Thoracic Cavity

During the fourth week of development, the splitting of the lateral plate mesoderm and the embryonic folding create the intraembryonic coelom that will ultimately subdivide into four serous cavities—two pleural cavities associated with two lungs, one pericardial cavity associated with the heart, and the peritoneal cavity associated with the gastrointestinal system. Partitioning of the intraembryonic coelom begins when the septum transversum moves from a cranial position (cranial to buccopharyngeal membrane) to a more caudal and ventral position as a result of longitudinal folding of the embryo. This partially divides the intraembryonic coelom into an early pericardial cavity and a peritoneal cavity. These two cavities remain connected through openings posteriorly called pericardioperitoneal canals. The primitive pericardial

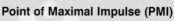

CLINICAL MEDICINE

Point of Maximal Impulse (PMI)

The apical beat is also called point of maximal impulse, which is due to the hardening of the apex of the heart during contraction. The apex of a normal heart and the PMI are located approximately at the left fifth intercostal space in the midclavicular line. The PMI may move inferolaterally in the patient with cardiomegaly.

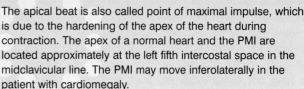

Midclavicular line

Anterior axillary line

Midaxillary line

Posterior axillary line

Figure 4-8. Reference surface lines.

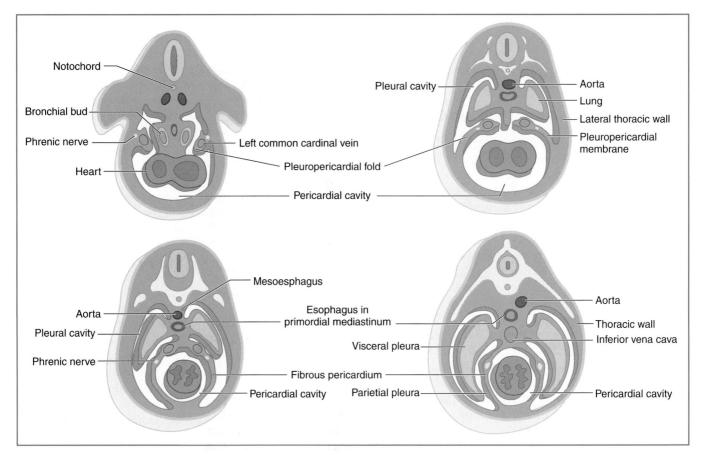

Figure 4-9. Partitioning of the primitive pericardial cavity.

cavity further subdivides as pleuropericardial folds grow toward each other from the sides of the region. When they meet and fuse with each other, three cavities are formed—left and right pleural cavities and a definitive pericardial cavity (Fig. 4-9). Later, additional folds called pleuroperitoneal folds close off the pericardioperitoneal canals that will contribute to formation of diaphragm (see Fig. 4-8) and create definitive peritoneal cavity. The mesothelial linings of these cavities are composed of simple squamous epithelium that produces serous fluid. Thus, these membranes are called serous membranes and their associated cavities are called serous cavities.

Pleural Cavity

Features and Nomenclature

The nomenclature of the pleural cavities is based on its embryologic development. The lungs develop as outgrowths of the cranial foregut. As each lung bud enlarges and grows laterally, it becomes surrounded by the medial side of the developing pleural sac (Fig. 4-10). This part of the pleural sac now associated with the developing lung is known as the *visceral pleura*, since it is developing with the lung. The parts of the pleural sac that are not in contact with the lung but rather with the body wall are known as the *parietal pleura*.

It is important to note that during development, the space between the two membranes—the pleural cavity—becomes a double-walled structure so that the two layers face each other. It is a closed continuous cavity, whose layers are separated by only a few milliliters of serous fluid. The points at which the parietal and visceral serous membranes are continuous are referred to as the sites of reflection. In the pleural cavity, this occurs at the hilum of the lung.

Nomenclature Describing the Parietal Pleura

Nomenclature of the parietal pleura is derived from its relationship to adjacent structures.

The costal pleura is the pleura found in relation to the ribs. The diaphragmatic pleura is associated with the diaphragm. The mediastinal pleura faces the mediastinum. Below the root of the lung, the mediastinal parietal pleura extends inferiorly as a two-layered fold of pleura called the *pulmonary ligament*. The pulmonary ligament is continuous with the site of reflection at the hilum of the lung. It extends in an inferoposterior direction toward the esophagus and diaphragm. The pulmonary ligament only contains a few lymph nodes.

The cupola is the cervical pleura or the parietal pleura over the apex of the lung. The apex of the lung and pleura rise approximately 3 cm above the clavicle at the first rib's anterior aspect. The cupola is reinforced by fascia derived from the scalene muscles of the neck called the suprapleural

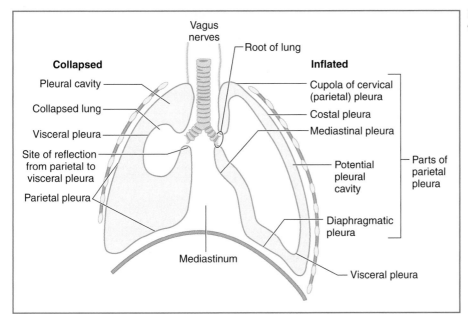

Figure 4-10. Relationship between visceral and parietal pleurae.

membrane (Sibson's fascia). This fascia is attached anteriorly to the first rib and posteriorly to the transverse process of the C7 vertebra.

Recesses of the Pleural Cavity

The parietal and visceral pleurae do not have the same contours. The visceral pleura stays in intimate contact with the lung and therefore takes the shape of the lung. It dips into the fissures of the lung that separate the lung into lobes.

The parietal pleura takes the shape of the body wall, which extends farther inferiorly than do the lungs. Thus, there are parts of the cavity where visceral pleura *is not* directly opposite parietal pleura. Even during forced inspiration, the lung does not completely fill the pleural cavity. Therefore, there are regions of the cavity where parietal pleura abuts parietal pleura with no intervening visceral pleura. These regions are called the *recesses of the pleural cavity.*

The costodiaphragmatic recess is found where the parietal pleura passes from the ribs onto the diaphragm. Inferiorly, both the lung and attached visceral pleura extend to the sixth rib in the midclavicular line, the eighth rib in the midaxillary line, and the tenth rib in the scapular line (Figs. 4-11 and 4-12). However, the parietal pleura reflects from the chest wall onto the diaphragm at the eighth rib in the midclavicular line, the tenth rib in the midaxillary line, and the twelfth rib in the scapular line. The potential space between these points is the costodiaphragmatic recess. This potential space represents a low point in the pleural cavity. It is larger posterolaterally than anteromedially owing to the contours of the diaphragm. Clinically, blood, pus, or serous fluid can collect in this recess of the pleural cavity. In the patient, this material can safely be removed by inserting a chest tube through the appropriate intercostal space.

The costomediastinal recess is located in the anterior plane behind the sternum and is smaller than the costodiaphragmatic recess. Here, the costal pleura reflects to become continuous with the mediastinal pleura. The costomediastinal recess is better developed on the left because of the presence of the heart and bare area of the pericardium.

Neurovascular Supply of the Pleura
Parietal Pleura

Since the parietal pleura develops from somatic mesoderm, the innervation of the parietal pleura follows the innervation of the adjacent body wall. The costal parietal pleura receives GSA sensory fibers from the intercostal nerves and pain is localized to the chest wall.

The central diaphragmatic and mediastinal parietal pleura is associated with the diaphragm and is innervated by the phrenic nerve. Therefore, irritation of the central portion of the diaphragmatic pleura is referred to (perceived to come from) the shoulder tip and neck, which are regions supplied by the same cervical spinal nerves that form the phrenic nerve (C3, 4, and 5).

The peripheral diaphragmatic parietal pleura receives GSA fibers from adjacent the intercostal nerves. Therefore, irritation of the peripheral portion of the diaphragmatic

CLINICAL MEDICINE

Thoracentesis

To obtain a sample of fluid from the pleural cavity for analysis, a needle is inserted through the thoracic wall at the level of the seventh or eighth intercostal space (over the top of the rib to avoid the intercostal nerve). The appropriate intercostal space can be confirmed by percussion, a diagnostic procedure to determine the density of a body cavity by the sound produced by tapping the surface with the finger. To determine the effect of diaphragm movements on the position of organs, percussion is done accompanied by deep inspiration and then forced expiration.

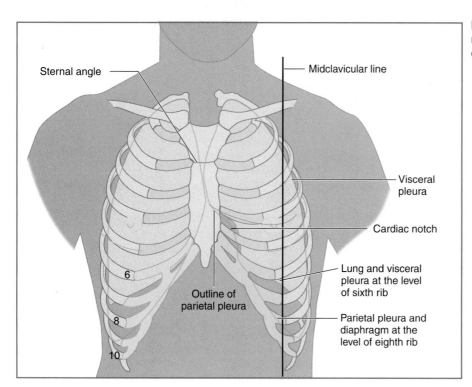

Figure 4-11. Anterior view of the pleural membranes in relationship to the rib cage.

Labels: Sternal angle — Midclavicular line — Visceral pleura — Cardiac notch — Lung and visceral pleura at the level of sixth rib — Outline of parietal pleura — Parietal pleura and diaphragm at the level of eighth rib — 6 — 8 — 10

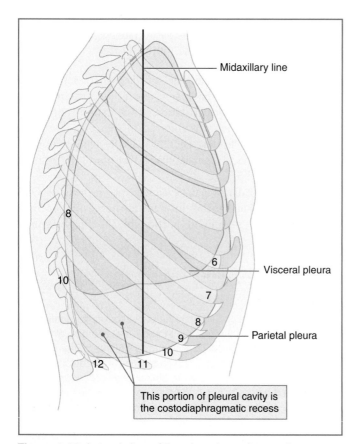

Figure 4-12. Lateral view of the pleural membranes in relationship to the rib cage.

Labels: Midaxillary line — Visceral pleura — Parietal pleura — 8 — 10 — 6 — 7 — 8 — 9 — 10 — 12 — 11 — This portion of pleural cavity is the costodiaphragmatic recess

pleura is referred to (perceived to come from) the lower thoracic and lumbar regions and can mimic pain owing to abdominal processes.

The blood supply of the parietal pleura includes branches of the intercostal, pericardiacophrenic, and superior phrenic arteries.

Visceral Pleura

The visceral pleura develops from splanchnic (visceral) mesoderm. Therefore, it is innervated by general visceral afferent (GVA) fibers for stretch. Otherwise it is believed that the visceral pleura is insensitive to pain.

Respiration

Pleural pressure is the fluid pressure found normally in the pleural cavity. This pressure is generated in part by the outward pull on the parietal pleura (because of its adherence to the thoracic wall and diaphragm) and the inward pull (retractile force) on the visceral pleura owing to its association to the lung. The inward pull of the lung and bronchi, etc. is due to the elastic connective tissue content of these structures. The retractile force of the lung tissue, transmitted by the pleural membranes along with the continual suction of pleural fluid into the lymphatics, creates a negative pleural pressure, which will increase during normal inspiration.

During inspiration, the superior-inferior, anteroposterior, and transverse dimensions of the thorax increase owing to the action of the diaphragm, the external intercostal muscles, and the portion of the internal intercostal muscles between the costal cartilages. During forced inspiration, other muscles such as the sternocleidomastoid, pectoral, and scalene muscles aid in the expansion of the thoracic wall.

Expiration is normally a passive process relying on diaphragmatic relaxation and the lung's elastic recoil. However, during *forced expiration* the internal intercostal (the portion between the shafts of the ribs) and abdominal muscles contract to aid in exhalation.

Lungs

External Features

Each lung presents three surfaces (costal, mediastinal, and diaphragmatic) as well as an apex, base, and hilum; the root is the collection of structures entering and leaving the hilum, so it is not part of the lung. It is part of the middle mediastinum. The hilum is the "indentation in an organ where the neurovascular bundle enters and leaves an organ," while the root of the lung is "all the structures entering or leaving the lung at the hilum."

The right lung is larger and weighs more than the left. The right lung has two fissures (oblique and horizontal) that divide the lung into superior, middle, and inferior lobes. The right oblique fissure begins posteriorly at the level of the body of the T3 vertebra, crosses the angle of the fifth rib, and ends anteriorly at the sixth rib's costochondral junction. The oblique

PATHOLOGY

Pleural Cavity

Air (pneumothorax), blood (hemothorax), or pus (pyothorax or empyema) may invade the pleural cavity. These conditions may involve only one side, since the two pleural cavities are independent.

If air enters the pleural cavity upon inspiration, it can produce a positive air pressure in the pleural cavity, which normally has a *negative* pressure. This leads to retraction and collapse of the lung. The positive air pressure in the damaged pleural cavity can displace the organs in the mediastinum (midline septal region of the thorax) to the opposite (contralateral) side, compromising the functioning lung. To remove air, the needle is placed into the highest point of the chest (since air rises upward). This is the second intercostal space in the midclavicular line. Since the lung is collapsed, there is less danger of puncturing the lung.

fissure can be approximated by the medial border of the scapula when the arm is partially abducted (e.g., the patient places the hand behind the head). The horizontal fissure begins posteriorly at the level of the head of the fifth rib. It extends from the sixth rib to end at the fourth costal cartilage. Impressions made by other organs include the trachea, esophagus, superior vena cava, right brachiocephalic vein, azygos vein, heart, and inferior vena cava (Fig. 4-13).

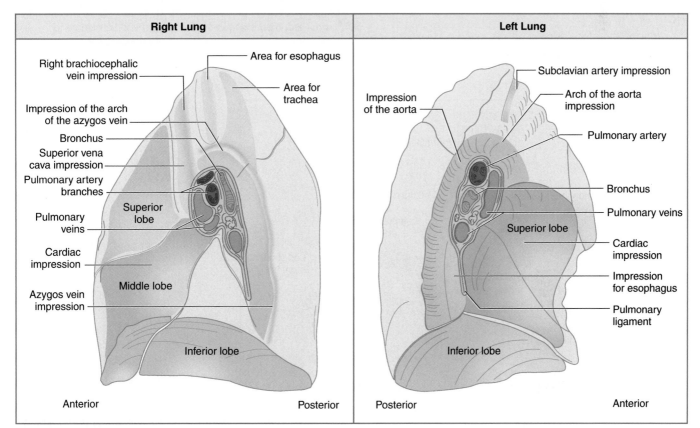

Figure 4-13. Impressions on the mediastinal surface of the lungs.

The left lung is similar to the right except that it has only one fissure and therefore only two lobes, superior and inferior, and is smaller in volume. The left lung's anterior medial border is notched (cardiac notch) and is located in intercostal spaces 4–5 on the left parasternal line.

The left oblique fissure is found posteriorly at the level of the angle of the fifth rib, continues across the fourth rib's lower border in midaxillary line, and ends anteriorly at the sixth rib's costochondral junction.

The tongue-like extension of the superior left lobe is called the "lingula," and it is homologous (similar in structure and embryologic origin) to the right middle lobe. Impressions made by other organs include the aorta, trachea, left subclavian artery (on superomedial aspect of the apex), left brachiocephalic vein, heart, and esophagus. The heart makes a deeper impression on the left lung than on the right (see Fig. 4-13).

In determining the lobe in which an abnormality is found by means of a radiograph, it is necessary to have both the lateral projection as well as the frontal (anteroposterior) view, since the apex of the lower lobe is posterior to the base of the upper lobe.

Anterior auscultation will primarily be of the upper lobe. Posterior auscultation will primarily be of the lower lobe (owing to the orientation of the oblique fissure). Pneumonia affects mostly the lower lobes; therefore, the physician listens to the lower lobe in the posterior thorax. Tuberculosis lesions usually affect the upper lobes, so the physician should listen to the anterior aspect of the patient's thorax.

Root of the Lung

The root of the lung contains all the neurovascular structures leaving and entering the hilum of the lung. They include the bronchi, pulmonary arteries, bronchial arteries, pulmonary veins, autonomic nerves, and lymphatics.

Internal Features of the Lung
Bronchi

The trachea divides into two main, or principal, bronchi at the level of the sternal angle, or the intervertebral disk between the fourth and fifth thoracic vertebrae. The tracheal bifurcation is marked internally by the carina (an inverted cartilage that resembles the keel of a boat).

Each main bronchus subdivides into secondary (lobar) bronchi that supply the lobes of the lungs. Therefore, there are two lobar bronchi for the left lung and three lobar bronchi for the right lung. These lobar bronchi then give rise to segmental bronchi (10 segmental bronchi on the right and 8 or 9 on the left). The first right secondary bronchus arises above its corresponding pulmonary artery and is referred to as the eparterial bronchus (Fig. 4-14 and Table 4-1). All others arise below the corresponding artery and are hyparterial

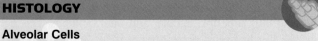

HISTOLOGY

Alveolar Cells

The alveoli in the lung are lined by type I and type II pneumocytes. Type I pneumocytes are highly attenuated cells that cover about 95% of the lining of the alveoli and are not capable of cell division. Type II pneumocytes are cuboidal cells that synthesize and secrete surfactant, a surface-active agent important for the proper functioning of the lung. When the lung is injured, type II pneumocytes undergo cell division and proliferation to restore both types of pneumocytes.

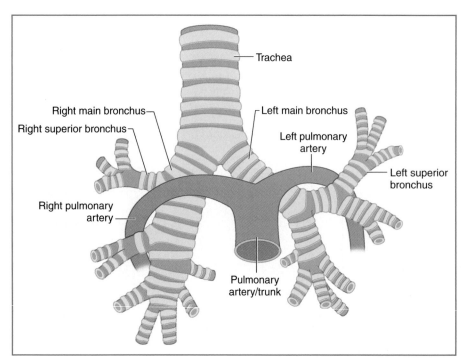

Figure 4-14. Relationships of bronchi to the pulmonary arteries.

TABLE 4-1. Comparisons of Characteristics and Relationships Between Right and Left Bronchi

Feature	Right Bronchus	Left Bronchus
Orientation	Nearly vertical	Nearly horizontal
Length	Shorter (3 cm)	Longer (5 cm)
Width	Wider (12–16 mm)	Narrower (10–14 mm)
Predisposition to aspirated items	Foreign bodies often found within	Foreign bodies not usually found within
Impressions it makes	None	Makes an impression on the esophagus
Relationships at the root	Azygos vein arches over the root to anastomose with the posterior surface of the superior vena cava	Arch of the aorta curves over the left root to become the descending aorta
Anterior relationships	Small portion of superior vena cava, right atrium and right phrenic nerve, anterior pulmonary plexus, and pulmonary artery are anterior	Left phrenic nerve and left anterior pulmonary plexus are anterior; pulmonary artery is anterosuperior
Posterior relationships	Right vagus nerve and posterior pulmonary plexus are posterior	Left vagus nerve, posterior pulmonary plexus, and descending aorta are posterior

bronchi. When the diameter of a segmental bronchus has decreased by branching to about 1 mm, it is called a bronchiole. The terminal bronchioles further divide into respiratory bronchioles and finally into alveoli. Gas exchange occurs in the specialized structures called alveoli.

Bronchopulmonary Segments

Bronchopulmonary segments are pyramidal areas of the lung supplied by one segmental bronchus. These zones are radiologic units as well as surgical units that may be resected. They are supplied by segmental bronchi and arteries and are separated from each other by connective tissue septa that contain the pulmonary veins. The septa with the veins define the surgical line of resection.

Blood Supply to the Lung

The lungs have a dual blood supply: nutritive and pulmonic. The bronchial arteries are the nutritive blood supply to the larger components of the bronchial tree. The left lung receives two bronchial arteries from the aorta while the right lung receives one bronchial artery from either the third intercostal artery or one of the left bronchial arteries. The bronchial arteries supply blood only to the level of the terminal bronchioles.

There is one bronchial vein per lung. The right bronchial vein empties into the azygos vein, and the left bronchial vein empties into the posterior intercostal vein or the hemiazygos veins.

There is one pulmonary artery to each lung. They lie in a plane ventral to the bronchus. The pulmonary arteries arise from the bifurcation of the pulmonary trunk. Branches of the pulmonary artery follow the airways.

Each lung has two pulmonary veins that bring oxygenated blood into the left atrium of the heart. One is located anteriorly and the other inferiorly at the hilum of the lung. They do not have valves.

Innervation

The lungs are supplied by the pulmonary plexuses that are located both anteriorly and posteriorly in the root of the lung. A plexus is a redistribution of nerve fibers. These plexuses contain preganglionic parasympathetic fibers from the vagus nerves that synapse on postganglionic parasympathetic neuronal cell bodies in the small ganglia located within these plexuses. Postganglionic parasympathetic fibers that arise from these neuronal cell bodies supply the smooth muscle and glands of the bronchial tree.

The anterior and posterior pulmonary plexuses also contain postganglionic sympathetic fibers that intermingle with the parasympathetic fibers. These postganglionic sympathetic

CLINICAL MEDICINE

Diseases of the Lung

Pulmonary atelectasis is the partial or total collapse of the lung. In cases of partial atelectasis, the collapse may involve patches of pulmonary alveoli, a bronchopulmonary segment, or a pulmonary lobe. Atelectasis occurs because of two conditions: (1) obstruction of airway passages causing the collection of fluid or air in the pleural cavity and (2) compression on the lung from the outside.

Emphysema is a condition in which there is permanent enlargement of the air spaces distal to the bronchioles. It is usually associated with destruction of the alveolar walls.

Pulmonary edema is abnormal accumulation of fluid in the lungs. The serous fluid from capillaries may infiltrate the pulmonary tissues or invade the alveoli.

Pulmonary embolism is the obstruction of the pulmonary trunk or one of its tributaries by a clot from the heart or from the superior or inferior vena cava and its tributaries. An embolus is a plug composed of a circulating thrombus or mass of bacteria that can obstruct a vessel. Bubbles of air and drops of fat may provoke pulmonary embolism as well.

Hypoxia, or *anoxia*, is a reduction of oxygen in body tissues below physiologic levels. This condition is frequently caused by respiratory abnormalities.

Bronchiectasis is the chronic dilatation of one or more bronchi, resulting in cough, fevers, and sputum production. Identification is made by radiologic examination of the bronchial tree (bronchography).

fibers arise from their neuronal cell bodies in the thoracic sympathetic chain ganglia T2–T5. The preganglionic sympathetic fibers that synapse on the postganglionic neuronal cell bodies arise from the lateral horn cells of spinal cord segments T2–T4 or T5. The pulmonary plexuses are continuous with the cardiac plexus.

General visceral afferent fibers for stretch reflexes follow the vagus nerves. The parasympathetic fibers produce bronchoconstriction, vasodilation, and secretion by the bronchial glands. The sympathetic fibers produce bronchodilation and vasoconstriction. Inhalers used by patients with asthma deliver adrenergic drugs, which are bronchodilators.

Lymphatics

Lymph drains from the lung into the pulmonary nodes, then to the bronchopulmonary nodes at the hilum of the lung. It continues into the tracheobronchial nodes, which are superior and inferior to the carina, and empties into the tracheal (paratracheal) nodes. These nodes join with the anterior mediastinal nodes to form the bronchomediastinal trunk that will empty into the thoracic duct on the left and right lymphatic duct.

Development of the Lung

The development of the lung begins in the fourth week of gestation as an endodermal diverticulum that grows out of the ventral wall of the foregut. The diverticulum grows in length, and as it does, the esophagotracheal septum forms, which separates the diverticulum from the foregut (Fig. 4-15). At the distal end of the diverticulum, two endodermal lung buds begin to grow laterally into the surrounding mesoderm. By the end of the fifth week, these lung buds have formed the left and right main bronchi. The right bronchus then forms three secondary bronchi and the left bronchus forms two secondary bronchi, presaging the three lobes of the right lung and the two lobes of the left lung, respectively. The straight portion of the diverticulum that is cranial to the lung buds will become the trachea. The lining of all the structures that form from the diverticulum is endodermally derived, whereas the surrounding mesoderm induces the branching patterns of the growing respiratory system and forms the cartilage, the smooth muscle associated with the airways, the connective tissue, the visceral pleura, and the vasculature.

The lung then goes through four phases of development. The first phase is called the *pseudoglandular phase* (5–17 weeks of gestation) and is characterized by further branching of the secondary bronchi to form smaller airways called bronchioles. Infants born prematurely during this phase are not viable.

The second phase is called the *canalicular phase* (13–25 weeks) and involves the formation of the terminal bronchioles and lung vasculature. Infants born during this phase may survive.

The third phase is called the *terminal phase* (24–36 weeks) in which the epithelium of the airways becomes attenuated and the type II pneumocytes develop and mature. Type II pneumocytes synthesize and secrete surfactant, a compound

CLINICAL MEDICINE

Respiratory Distress Syndrome

Infants born prematurely in the early part of the terminal phase usually suffer from respiratory distress syndrome (RDS) because the type II pneumocytes have not yet produced surfactant, a mixture of phospholipids and proteins, to allow the airways to inflate upon exhalation. Infants born during this period must be given surfactant, placed in an oxygen incubator, and given corticosteroids, which accelerate the development of the terminal portions of the respiratory system.

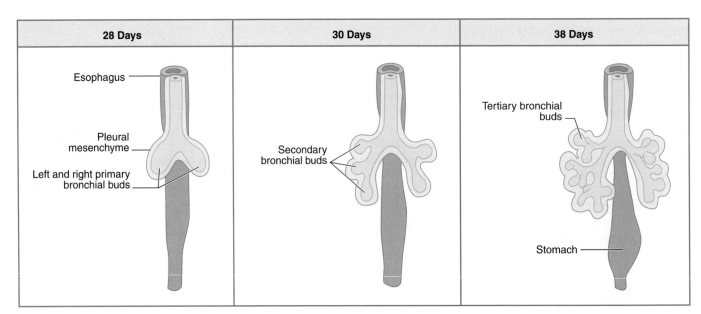

Figure 4-15. Development of the lungs.

that lowers the surface tension of the airways. Infants born during the latter part of this period have a better outcome.

The *alveolar phase* is the last phase (36 weeks to 8 years of age), when terminal sacs become alveolar ducts and mature alveoli. There are 20 to 80 million alveoli formed before birth, and an additional 220 million are formed by the age of 8 years.

●●● MEDIASTINUM

The mediastinum is the midline visceral space or cavity of the thorax. It is bounded laterally by the mediastinal parietal pleura, posteriorly by the 12 thoracic vertebrae, and anteriorly by the sternum. The mediastinum's superior boundary is the superior thoracic aperture, and its inferior boundary is the thoracic diaphragm. It contains all the structures of the thoracic cavity except the pleural sacs and the lungs.

The mediastinum is divided into four parts by the presence of the pericardial sac (Fig. 4-16). The anteroposterior (horizontal) plane that passes through the superior margin of the pericardium separates the mediastinum into superior and inferior divisions. Note that this plane also passes through the sternal angle (of Louis) anteriorly. If an imaginary line were passed transversely from the sternal angle to the vertebral column, it would pass through the intervertebral disk between the T4 and T5 vertebrae. If a similar line were drawn starting at the xiphisternal articulation, it would typically pass through T9 (see Fig. 4-16).

The four subdivisions of the mediastinum are as follows:
1. The superior mediastinum is found above the superior border of the pericardium.
2. The anterior mediastinum is the region between the anterior pericardial surface and the body of the sternum.
3. The middle mediastinum includes everything within the pericardium (heart and parts of the great vessels), the roots of the lungs, plus the phrenic nerves.

4. The posterior mediastinum is the region behind the pericardium (i.e., between the pericardium and the T5 to T12 vertebrae). Owing to the dome shape of the lateral and posterior portions of the diaphragm, the superior-inferior dimensions of the posterior mediastinum are greater than those of the anterior mediastinum.

Surgically, the mediastinum may be reached by a midline (median) sternotomy (incision through the sternum).

Anterior Mediastinum

The structures found within this region include the sternopericardial ligaments, several lymph nodes, and in some cases, the tail of the thymus.

Middle Mediastinum

The middle mediastinum contains the pericardium and its contents, along with the phrenic nerve that runs in the fibrous parietal pericardium. The middle mediastinum lies at the level of T5–T8 (see Fig. 4-16) and the body of the sternum and costal cartilages 2–6. The middle mediastinum is located between the posterior mediastinum and the anterior mediastinum.

Pericardium

The pericardium is the serous membrane that surrounds the heart and parts of the great vessels, including the two venae cavae, the pulmonary veins, the pulmonary trunk, and the aorta. Like other serous membranes, the pericardium has a parietal layer, which is derived from somatic mesoderm and is associated with the body wall. The visceral serous pericardium is derived from visceral mesoderm and is intimately adherent to the heart (Fig. 4-17). This visceral layer is usually called the *epicardium.*

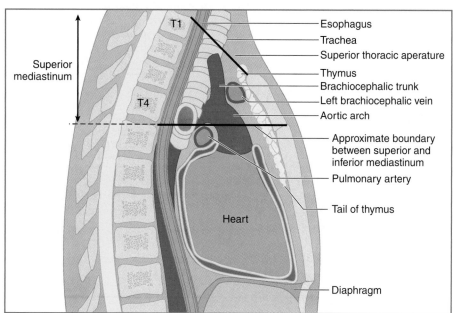

Superior mediastinum

T1

T4

Esophagus
Trachea
Superior thoracic aperature
Thymus
Brachiocephalic trunk
Left brachiocephalic vein
Aortic arch
Approximate boundary between superior and inferior mediastinum
Pulmonary artery
Tail of thymus

Heart

Diaphragm

Figure 4-16. Midsagittal section through the mediastinum.

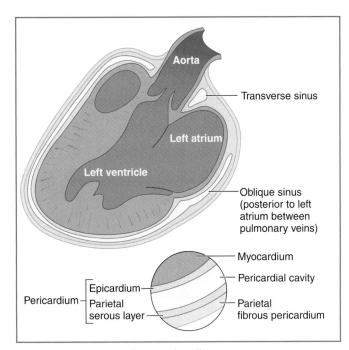

Figure 4-17. Layers of the pericardium.

The potential space between the parietal and visceral layers of pericardium is called the *pericardial cavity*, which contains small amounts of serous fluid. The parietal pericardium has an additional specialization reinforcing it externally called the *fibrous pericardium*. The fibrous pericardium is derived from the embryologic pleuropericardial folds that contain body wall mesenchyme which is added to the somatic mesoderm, forming the parietal serous pericardium. The fibrous layer cannot be separated from the parietal serous pericardium. The union of the serous and fibrous layers gives the pericardial sac its distinctive toughness (see Fig. 4-17). The pericardial sac is adherent to the central tendon of the diaphragm. This arrangement anchors the pericardial sac to the diaphragm. However, the pericardium is not so adherent to the muscular portion of the diaphragm

and to the adjacent posterior mediastinal structures. The pericardial sac is attached to the body of the sternum by means of two variable sternopericardial ligaments.

The pleural membranes partially encircle the anterior surface of the pericardium except for an anterior segment lying between the pericardium and sternum. This portion of the pericardium is referred to as the *bare area of the pericardium*. It is one of the potential sites used to enter the pericardial cavity without damaging the pleura, thereby avoiding a pneumothorax. The bare area of the pericardium can be entered by inserting a needle into the left fifth intercostal space aided by imaging.

Pericardial Sinuses

The visceral pericardium is continuous with the parietal serous pericardium at two sites of reflection, one at the venous end and one at the arterial end. These sites of reflection are called the *pericardial sinuses*. The embryonic heart (Fig. 4-18) starts out as a tube with a venous end and an arterial end hanging within the developing pericardial cavity by the mesocardium. As the heart tube undergoes looping so that the arterial end (pulmonary artery and aorta) comes to lie anterior to the venous end (venae cavae and pulmonary veins), these reflections are found just posterior to the heart, and the mesocardium degenerates, allowing passage between the arterial and venous channels. The transverse pericardial sinus is the reflection associated with the arterial end. It can be located by passing a finger around the left side of the pulmonary artery, then behind the pulmonary artery and the aorta, and finally around the right side of the aorta. Thus, the transverse sinus of the pericardial cavity is posterior to the pulmonary trunk and ascending aorta (anterior boundary), anterior to the superior vena cava, and superior to the left atrium. Since it is part of the pericardial cavity, it communicates with the rest of the pericardial cavity on both the right and left sides.

The site of reflection associated with the venous end of the heart (see Fig. 4-18) forms the boundary of the oblique pericardial sinus of the pericardial cavity. Once the

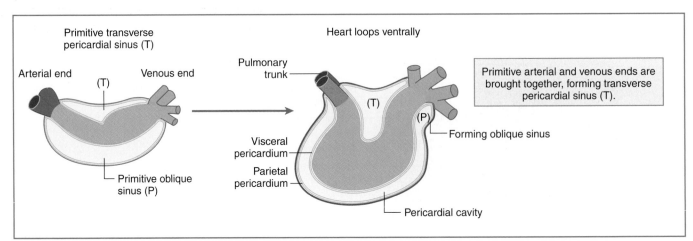

Figure 4-18. Formation of sinuses of the pericardial cavity.

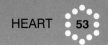

pericardial sac has been opened, the oblique pericardial sinus can be found by pulling the apex of the heart anteriorly, and exploring the pericardial cavity behind the heart. The oblique pericardial sinus is bounded by the pericardium on the left atrium, inferior vena cava, pulmonary veins, and the pericardium that overlies the posterior mediastinum.

Arterial Supply to the Pericardium

Branches of bronchial, esophageal, and superior phrenic arteries along with the pericardiacophrenic arteries supply the parietal pericardium.

The coronary arteries supply the epicardium.

Innervation of the Pericardium

The pericardial sac receives sensory, or GSA, fibers and postganglionic sympathetic fibers from the phrenic nerves. Irritation of the pericardial sac is very painful owing to its somatic innervation and is often felt in the neck, shoulder tip, and over the angle of the mandible. These are regions innervated by cervical spinal nerves derived mostly from the C3 to C5 ventral roots. Thus, these cutaneous cervical spinal nerves share a common origin with the phrenic nerve, with the fourth cervical spinal nerve being the most important. Postganglionic sympathetic (vasomotor) fibers reach these cervical ventral rami and contribute to the phrenic nerve by means of gray rami communicantes from the superior and middle cervical ganglia.

The epicardium does not receive any somatic sensory fibers.

●●● HEART

The heart is the muscular pump of the circulatory system and is found within the pericardial sac. The heart lies in the middle mediastinum oriented anteriorly, inferiorly, and laterally. Like most thoracic organs, the heart is higher in a cadaver than in a living person. In general, the heart is not completely located in the midline but lies under the sternum

and to the left. However, a small part of the heart projects to the right of the sternum onto the right costal cartilages.

The heart consists of four chambers: the right and left atria and the right and left ventricles. Veins carry blood to the heart while arteries carry blood away from the heart. Blood from the body (systemic circulation) and heart enters the right atrium by means of the superior and inferior vena cava, the anterior cardiac veins, and the coronary sinus. Blood flows from the right atrium to the right ventricle through the right atrioventricular (tricuspid) valve. Upon contraction of the right ventricle, blood passes through the pulmonic semilunar valve into the pulmonary trunk and the right and left pulmonary arteries to the lungs. Blood is returned to the left atrium from the lungs (pulmonic circulation) by means of the four pulmonary veins. Blood flows from the left atrium into the left ventricle through the left atrioventricular (mitral) valve and from the left ventricle into the aorta by means of the aortic semilunar valve. Thus, the systemic circulation consists of the entire circulatory system except for the pulmonary vessels going to and from the lungs.

Surfaces of the Heart

The anterior surface lies just posterior to the sternum, right and left costal cartilages, and left ribs. This surface is also called the *sternocostal surface* (Figs. 4-19 and 4-20) and is formed predominately by the right ventricle, partly by the right atrium, by the left ventricle, and sometimes by a small portion of the left auricle.

The diaphragmatic (inferior) surface (Fig. 4-21) sits over the central tendon of the diaphragm and is formed primarily by the left ventricle and some of the right ventricle. The coronary sulcus separates the diaphragmatic surface from the base of the heart. The diaphragmatic surface extends approximately from the left fifth intercostal space in the midclavicular line to the right sixth costal cartilage.

The right border (see Fig. 4-20) is formed by the right atrium. This border is posterior to the right costal cartilages, just to the right of the sternum. The right border extends from the sixth right costal cartilage to the superior surface of the third right costal cartilage, where it is continuous with the superior vena cava.

The left border is formed primarily by the left ventricle and a small portion of the left auricle. This margin of the heart extends from the fifth intercostal space in the midclavicular line to approximately the second left intercostal space about a centimeter to the left of the sternum.

The base of the heart (see Fig. 4-21) is formed mostly by the left atrium with a small contribution from the right atrium and is the site of the entrance of the great veins of the heart. The atria are located posterior to their respective ventricles. This is the most static part of the heart. The base of the heart projects posteriorly onto vertebrae T5(T6)–T8(T9). The base also forms the heart's superior border since it faces superiorly, posteriorly, and to the left.

The apex of the heart is the tip of the left ventricle and is normally located at the level of the fifth intercostal space or

---

CLINICAL MEDICINE

Cardiac Tamponade

The pericardial sac is inelastic because of the presence of the fibrous layer of pericardium. Intrapericardial effusion is a rapid effusion of greater than 150 mL that can provoke cardiac tamponade (a compression of the heart). The patient may go into shock or die. This condition is frequently seen in cardiac trauma with intrapericardial hemorrhage (hemopericardium).

Pericardial tap (pericardiocentesis) is indicated to diagnose or remove either exudate or transudate in the pericardial cavity. This procedure requires a puncture of the thoracic wall upward on the left side of the xiphisternal junction or in the left fifth intercostal space, so as not to endanger the pleural membrane.

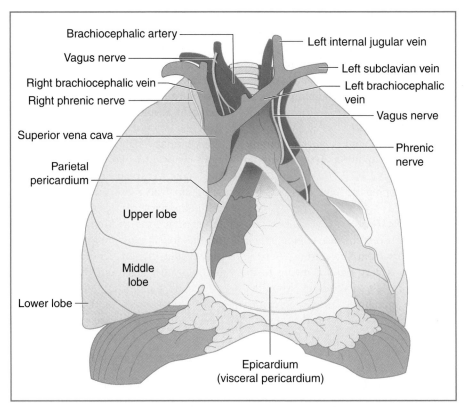

Figure 4-19. Anterior view of the mediastinum.

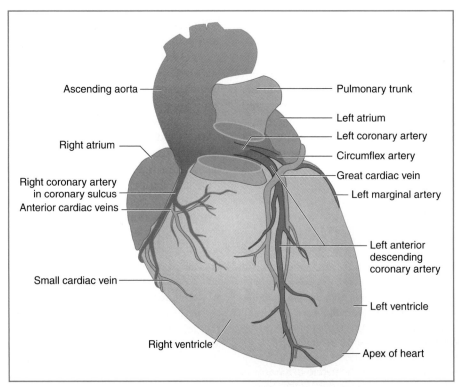

Figure 4-20. Anterior (sternocostal) surface of the heart.

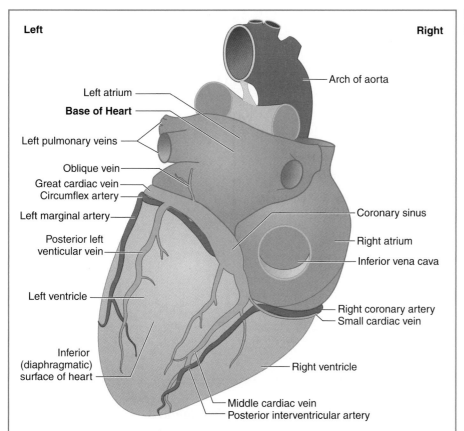

Figure 4-21. Posterior (base) and inferior (diaphragmatic) surfaces of the heart.

Labels in figure:
Left
Right
Arch of aorta
Left atrium
Base of Heart
Left pulmonary veins
Oblique vein
Great cardiac vein
Circumflex artery
Left marginal artery
Posterior left ventricular vein
Coronary sinus
Right atrium
Inferior vena cava
Left ventricle
Right coronary artery
Small cardiac vein
Inferior (diaphragmatic) surface of heart
Right ventricle
Middle cardiac vein
Posterior interventricular artery

even the sixth costal cartilage along the left midclavicular line. The apex is oriented to the left and anteroinferiorly. It is separated from the chest wall by the intervening portion of the left lung and adjacent pleura.

Sulci on the Surface of the Heart

There are two sulci, or grooves, on the surface of the heart that correspond to the division of the heart into four underlying chambers. They are occupied by the coronary vessels, which supply the heart. The sulci are initially difficult to find because they are filled with varying amounts of epicardial fat.

The coronary sulcus (atrioventricular groove; see Fig. 4-20) surrounds the heart, separating the atria from the ventricles. Anteriorly, the pulmonary trunk interrupts the coronary sulcus.

The interventricular sulcus (see Figs. 4-20 and 4-21) represents a groove on the surface of the heart that corresponds to the septum which separates the two ventricles. Anterior and posterior interventricular sulci are found on the anterior and diaphragmatic surfaces of the heart, respectively.

Coronary Arteries

The coronary arteries arise from aortic sinuses (of Valsalva), which are dilatations of the aorta above the cusps of the aortic valve. The arteries are analogous to the vasa vasorum (vessels that supply the walls of the large vessels).

Right Coronary Artery and Its Branches

The right coronary artery (RCA; see Fig. 4-20) arises from the aorta and initially runs *between the pulmonary trunk and right auricle*. The right coronary artery passes inferiorly and to the right in the coronary sulcus between the right atrium and ventricle.

Its first branch, the first atrial artery, encircles the right auricle and the superior vena cava to supply the atrium and sinoatrial (SA) node as the artery to the SA node (nodal artery).

As it travels toward the right and inferior margins of the heart, the RCA has many smaller branches that supply either the right atrium or the right ventricle. At the right margin of the heart, the RCA gives rise to the right (acute) marginal artery on the right ventricular border.

The RCA then continues in the coronary sulcus between the posterior and inferior surfaces of the heart, where it often passes beyond the crux of the heart to help supply the left ventricle and atrium.

The major branch of the RCA descends in the posterior interventricular sulcus as the posterior interventricular artery (see Fig. 4-21).

A small branch to the atrioventricular (AV) node arises at the point of intersection of the coronary sulcus and the posterior interventricular sulcus. This latter landmark is referred to as the crux of the heart (Fig. 4-22).

The RCA often has posterior left ventricular branches. The RCA also anastomoses with the circumflex branch of the left coronary artery on the posterior surface of the heart,

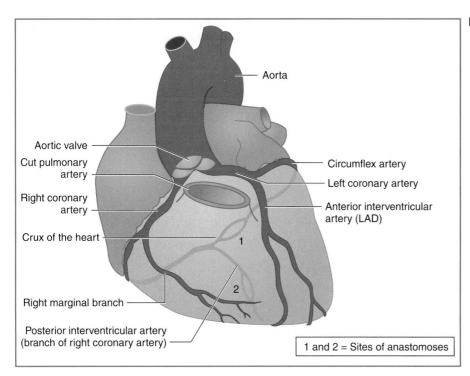

Figure 4-22. Coronary arteries.

Aorta

Aortic valve

Cut pulmonary artery

Right coronary artery

Crux of the heart

Right marginal branch

Posterior interventricular artery (branch of right coronary artery)

Circumflex artery

Left coronary artery

Anterior interventricular artery (LAD)

1

2

1 and 2 = Sites of anastomoses

but this anastomosis is insufficient to supply the heart tissue. The posterior interventricular artery anastomoses with the anterior interventricular artery approximately at the apex of the heart.

Thus, the RCA typically supplies most of the right atrium, right ventricle, SA and AV nodes, posterior third of the interventricular septum, and some of the diaphragmatic portion of the left ventricle.

Left Coronary Artery and Its Branches

The left coronary artery (LCA; see Fig. 4-20) arises from the aorta and passes behind the pulmonary artery and in front of the root of the left auricle. The left coronary artery is also called the left main coronary artery. Much shorter than the RCA, the left coronary artery divides almost immediately into the anterior interventricular artery (left anterior descending artery, or LAD) and the circumflex artery at the left margin of the pulmonary artery.

The anterior interventricular artery has several important diagonal branches to the left ventricle as well as septal branches to the anterior two thirds of the interventricular septum supplying most of the AV bundle and its branches.

The circumflex artery travels in the coronary sulcus to the left (obtuse) margin of the heart, where it gives off the left marginal artery.

The circumflex artery continues in the coronary sulcus, where it may anastomose with the RCA. The circumflex artery usually has several posterior left ventricular branches to the diaphragmatic surface of the left ventricle.

Thus, the left coronary artery typically supplies the left ventricle, the anterior two thirds of the interventricular septum, the adjacent portion of the right ventricle, and the left atrium.

Coronary Artery Dominance

In most cases, the right coronary artery is dominant, since it sends branches to the right and left ventricles and interventricular septum. In 20% of the reported cases, the left coronary artery is dominant. In this event, its circumflex branch crosses the crux of the heart and supplies branches to the right ventricle's diaphragmatic surface, posterior interventricular septum, and adjacent posterior left ventricular wall.

Venous Drainage of the Heart

The cardiac veins (see Figs. 4-20 and 4-21) accompany the coronary arteries in the sulci.

The coronary sinus (see Fig. 4-21) is a short venous swelling, or trunk, on the posterior portion of the coronary sulcus that receives most of the cardiac veins and empties into the right atrium. The coronary sinus is a vein that begins at the point where the oblique vein (of Marshall) of the left atrium joins the great cardiac vein. The oblique vein is an embryologic remnant of the left common cardinal vein that forms the distal end of the coronary sinus. However, the oblique vein is often difficult to find. Therefore, the origin of the coronary sinus can be approximated at the junction of the posterior vein of the left ventricle and the great cardiac vein.

The great cardiac vein (see Figs. 4-20 and 4-21) begins on the anterior surface of the heart in the anterior interventricular sulcus next to the anterior interventricular artery. After ascending in the sulcus, it runs with the circumflex artery to drain into the coronary sinus on the posterior aspect of the heart.

The middle cardiac vein (see Fig. 4-20) lies on the diaphragmatic surface of the heart in the posterior interventricular sulcus with the posterior interventricular (descending) artery. It ascends to drain into the coronary sinus.

The small cardiac vein (see Fig. 4-21) begins as the right marginal vein next to the right marginal artery and travels with the RCA in the coronary sulcus to reach the coronary sinus.

The anterior cardiac veins drain the anterior surface of the right ventricle and empty directly into the right atrium.

The smallest cardiac veins (thebesian veins, or venae cordis minimae) are found in the walls of *all* four chambers, but they are most numerous in the atria. These veins empty directly into the chamber with which they are associated, *not* into the coronary sinus.

Interior of the Heart

Right Atrium and Its Features

The right atrium (see Fig. 4-20) is located posterior to the sternum and the third to sixth right costal cartilages. As such, it forms part of the sternocostal surface and right margin of the heart. However, a portion of the right atrium is found posterior to the right ventricle.

The right atrium can be divided into two parts: a larger smooth-walled posterior part called the *sinus venarum (sinus of the venae cavae)*, which is derived from the incorporation of the right horn of the sinus venosus and an anterior part composed of the atrium proper; and the auricle, which is a blind (ear-like) sac derived from the primitive atrium. The border between these two parts is marked on the inside by a ridge called the *crista terminalis*. The crista terminalis extends from the anterior surface of the superior vena cava to the partial valve of the inferior vena cava. The small pectinate muscles that characterize the inside surface of the auricle extend from the crista terminalis into the auricle.

The superior vena cava, inferior vena cava, and coronary sinus all enter the right atrium in the sinus venarum. The orifice of the superior vena cava does not have a valve. However, the orifice of the inferior vena cava usually has a rudimentary fenestrated valve. This valve does not have a function in adults, but it may function to direct blood flow through the inferior vena cava to the foramen ovale in the fetus. The orifice of the coronary sinus has a valve that helps prevent blood from back-flowing when the atrium is filling.

The crista terminalis corresponds to the sulcus terminalis on the external surface of the heart. Note that the sinoatrial node is in the atrial wall, approximately where the sulcus terminalis (or crista terminalis) bisects the superior vena cava. The SA node consists of cardiac muscle that is specialized for conduction.

The interatrial septum is thin-walled. As seen from the right atrium (Fig. 4-23), it forms the atrial wall that lies posterior and to the left. The following landmarks characterize it. The fossa ovalis (see Fig. 4-23) is a depression on the middle of the septum with a ridge called the limbus of the fossa ovalis located laterally, superiorly, and medially. In fetal life, this fossa was the foramen ovale, a communication

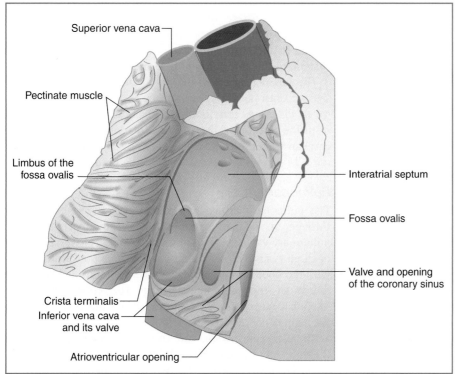

Figure 4-23. Internal features of the right atrium.

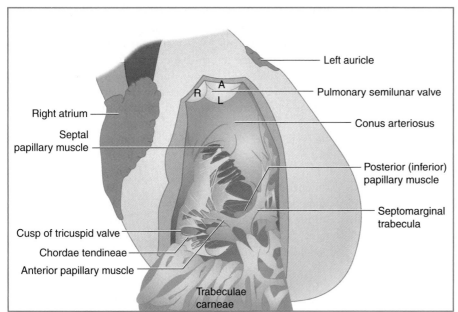

Figure 4-24. Internal features of the right ventricle.

Left auricle

Pulmonary semilunar valve

Conus arteriosus

Posterior (inferior) papillary muscle

Septomarginal trabecula

Right atrium

Septal papillary muscle

Cusp of tricuspid valve

Chordae tendineae

Anterior papillary muscle

Trabeculae carneae

between the two atria. An overlapping flap valve persists in 20% of the population with no concurrent pathology.

The AV node is part of the conduction system of the heart. It is found within the interatrial wall above the orifice of the coronary sinus and between the fossa ovalis and AV orifice.

The atrioventricular orifice is the site of communication between the atrium and the ventricle. On the right side, this opening is guarded by the tricuspid valve—a valve with three cusps. A cusp is formed mostly from dense connective tissue that is attached to a fibrous ring called the *annulus fibrosus*. There are four rings, annuli fibrosi, that surround each of the four valves of the heart and form the fibrous skeletal system of the heart. The annuli fibrosi compose the heart's fibrous connective tissue skeletal system for the attachment of the valves' cusps. For the tricuspid valve, the anterior cusp is the largest, the posterior cusp is the smallest, and the septal cusp is intermediate in size. Blood flows freely from the atrium into the ventricle during ventricular diastole. However, the tricuspid valve prevents regurgitation of blood from the ventricle into the atrium during ventricular systole.

Right Ventricle and Its Internal Features

The right ventricle (Fig. 4-24) receives blood from the right atrium and is responsible for sending it on to the lungs for reoxygenation. It has a thick muscular wall that is thrown into irregular ridges of cardiac muscle called *trabeculae carneae*. In addition, there are muscular projections with a nipple-like appearance called *papillary muscles*. Three papillary muscles are continuous with the rest of the cardiac muscle. From them, chordae tendineae extend to the ventricular surface and margin of the cusps. The *chordae tendineae* prevent the valve from being everted into the right atrium during ventricular contraction (systole); therefore, they prevent valve prolapse. The chordae tendineae are attached to the

ventricular surface and margins of the cusps and thereby strengthen the cusp.

The large anterior papillary muscle arises from the anterior wall and is attached by chordae tendineae to the anterior and posterior cusps. The posterior (also referred to as inferior) papillary muscle is intermediate in size. It arises from the inferior wall and is attached to the posterior and septal cusps. The small septal papillary muscle or muscles arise from the upper septum and are attached to the anterior and septal cusps.

The *septomarginal* or *moderator band* is composed of trabeculae carneae that extend from the septum to the anterior papillary muscle. It carries a portion of the right branch of the atrioventricular bundle, part of the conducting system, to the anterior papillary muscle.

The superior aspect of the right ventricle is smooth-walled, since it does not have any trabeculae carneae. This region is called the *conus arteriosus* or *infundibulum* and is separated from the portion of the ventricle marked by the trabeculae carneae by a muscular ridge known as the *supraventricular crest*. The conus arteriosus leads to the pulmonary trunk.

Pulmonary Artery

The pulmonary artery, or trunk, leaves the right ventricle through an opening guarded by a semilunar valve, the pulmonary valve (see Figs. 4-24 and 4-25). This valve consists of three cusps. The semilunar cusps have a pocket-like shape with the open end of the pocket facing superiorly toward the lumen of the pulmonary artery. The convexity of the semilunar cusp faces the ventricle, while the concavity faces the lumen of the artery. As the blood is forced out during ventricular contraction, the cusps are forced peripherally, thereby opening the valve. When the contraction is over, blood flows back toward the ventricle, filling the cusps, which

Open Position	Closed Position

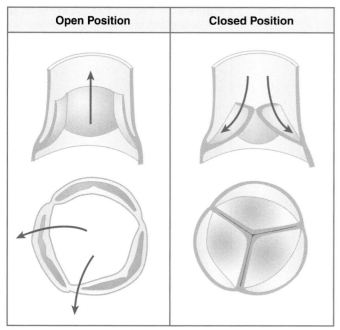

Figure 4-25. Position of cusps of aortic or pulmonic semilunar valve during opening and closing.

in turn closes the valve until the next contraction. The cusps are situated in an anterior, right (and posterior), and left (and posterior) configuration.

Left Atrium and Its Features

The left atrium is slightly larger than the right atrium and has openings without valves for four pulmonary veins, which bring oxygenated blood from the lungs.

The atrium proper is smooth-walled and is derived from the incorporation of the pulmonary veins during development. There is also a very small, ear-like, blind sac (*auricle*) derived from the primitive atrium, which is rough-walled owing to the presence of pectinate muscles. Note that there is *no* crista terminalis in the left atrium. Also note that the auricle on the left side is much smaller than on the right side.

There is no fossa ovalis on the left side of the interatrial septum. However, the thinner, crescent-shaped portion of the interatrial septum that corresponds to the fossa ovalis is often referred to as the valve of the foramen ovale.

The left atrioventricular orifice is an opening between the left atrium and ventricle, which is guarded by the bicuspid (mitral) valve. The anterior leaflet of this valve is sail-like and larger than the posterior leaflet or cusp.

Left Ventricle and Its Internal Features

The left ventricle (Fig. 4-26) has a thick muscular wall, which is much thicker than the right ventricular wall. The thickness of the ventricular wall is approximately proportional to the work that it performs. The left ventricle produces approximately 120 mm Hg of pressure, compared with 20 mm Hg of pressure produced by the right ventricle. The left ventricular wall is rough owing to the presence of trabeculae carneae that are surprisingly finer and more numerous than in the right ventricle.

The mitral valve has only two papillary muscles, anterior and posterior, and only two cusps, which are anterior and posterior. The anterior interventricular artery supplies the anterior papillary muscle. The posterior interventricular artery supplies the posterior papillary muscle.

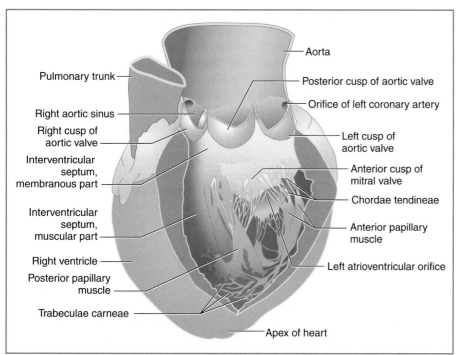

Figure 4-26. Morphology of the right and left ventricles.

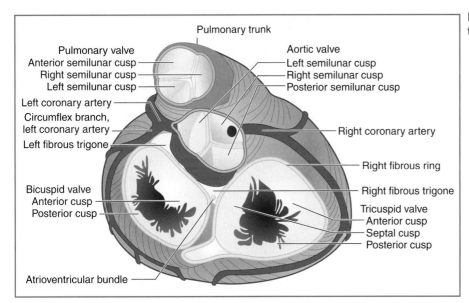

Figure 4-27. Section through the heart at the level of the atrioventricular junction.

The anterosuperior aspect of the left ventricle is smooth-walled without trabeculae carneae. This is similar to part of the right ventricle. This smooth-walled region is referred to as the *aortic vestibule* and is the outflow tract from the left ventricle to the aorta. The walls of the aortic vestibule are formed by part of the interventricular septum and are fibrous in nature.

The interventricular septum consists of two parts: a membranous portion and a muscular portion.

The membranous interventricular septum is superior, thin-walled, and separates the right and left ventricles. The annulus fibrosus for the mitral valve inserts at a slightly different level on the membranous septum than the annulus of the tricuspid valve, leaving this small portion of the membranous septum, the atrioventricular portion, separating the right atrium from the left ventricle.

The membranous interventricular septum is a common site of a developmental anomaly called an interventricular defect. When a defect occurs, the greater pressure of the left side shunts blood to the right side of the heart.

The remainder of the interventricular septum is thick-walled and is continuous with the cardiac muscle of the ventricles. The muscular portion of the septum separates the two ventricles only.

The aorta is separated from the left ventricle by the aortic valve (Fig. 4-27). Like the pulmonic valve, this consists of three pocket-like leaflets or semilunar cusps, called right, left, and posterior (noncoronary). Dilatations or bulges of the aortic wall above the cusps are called aortic *sinuses* (*of Valsalva*). The coronary arteries take origin from two of these sinuses.

Note that the anterior cusp of the mitral valve virtually touches the aortic valve (see Fig. 4-27). The anterior cusp of the mitral valve separates the blood passing through the mitral valve from the blood leaving the heart by means of the aortic valve. Thus, the large anterior cusp helps direct the flow of blood both into and out of the left ventricle. In the right ventricle, the pulmonic valve and the tricuspid valve are separated by the conus arteriosus.

Innervation of the Heart

The heart can beat outside the body without autonomic innervation (vagus and sympathetic nerves). These nerves, which form the cardiac plexuses, only serve to speed up (*sympathetic*) or slow down (*vagus*) the heart rate.

The cardiac plexus contains postganglionic sympathetic fibers, pre- and postganglionic parasympathetic fibers, and, of course, the ganglia that contain the postganglionic parasympathetic neuronal cell bodies. This plexus has superficial and deep divisions. The superficial cardiac plexus is located just inferior to the arch of the aorta and receives postganglionic sympathetic fibers from cervical and upper thoracic sympathetic ganglia as well as branches of the vagus nerves that are preganglionic fibers. The deep cardiac plexus is located at the bifurcation of the trachea and also receives the sympathetic cardiac branches and the cardiac branches of the vagus. By definition, all postganglionic sympathetic fibers pass through the cardiac plexus without a synapse. However, the small cardiac ganglia that are found in the cardiac plexuses or close to the heart receive preganglionic parasympathetic vagal fibers that synapse on postganglionic neuronal cell bodies in these ganglia. Postganglionic parasympathetic fibers and sympathetic fibers run to the SA node and the AV node.

Cardiac Referred Pain

The cardiac general visceral sensory pain fibers follow the sympathetics back to the spinal cord and have their cell bodies located in thoracic dorsal root ganglia 1–4(5). It is not a coincidence that these are the same spinal cord levels that gave rise to the preganglionic sympathetic fibers. As a general

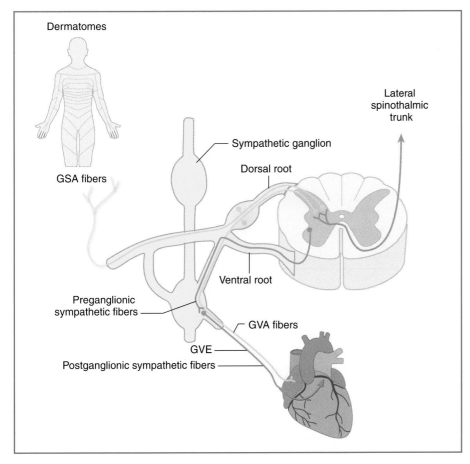

Figure 4-28. Cardiac referred pain.

rule, in the thorax and abdomen, GVA pain fibers follow sympathetic fibers back to the same spinal cord segments that gave rise to the preganglionic sympathetic fibers (Fig. 4-28). The central nervous system (CNS) perceives pain from the heart as coming from the somatic portion of the body supplied by the thoracic spinal cord segments 1–4(5).

Angina pectoris, severe chest pain produced by ischemic heart muscle that results in deprivation of oxygen, is carried by general visceral sensory fibers that follow the sympathetic fibers. Angina pectoris is *usually* perceived as substernal pain and left-sided pain that radiates down the medial side of the arm and forearm, sometimes into the medial hand and little finger. The dermatomes of this region of the body wall and upper limb have their neuronal cell bodies in the same dorsal root ganglia (T1–T5) and synapse in the same second order neurons in the spinal cord segments (T1–T5) as the general visceral sensory fibers from the heart. The CNS does not clearly discern whether the pain is coming from the body wall or from the viscera, but it perceives the pain as coming from somewhere on the body wall. Such visceral referred pain, while intense and even crippling, often does not seem to have the specificity of location on the body wall as somatic pain does.

GVA fibers from the vagus nerve carry impulses from interoceptive receptors (baroreceptors and chemoreceptors) for blood pressure and blood oxygen and carbon dioxide pressures. Baroreceptors are found in the venae cavae, pulmonary veins, arch of the aorta, aorta, and carotid arteries to sense changes in blood pressure. Chemoreceptors are associated with the ascending aorta, pulmonary trunk, and carotid arteries.

Conduction System of the Heart

The sinoatrial node initiates the heartbeat (Fig. 4-29). It is found in the myocardium close to the epicardium and is about 3 mm wide and 8 mm long. The SA node is described as a specialized type of cardiac tissue that can spontaneously depolarize. Although it cannot be grossly seen, it can be located approximately at the point where the sulcus terminalis bisects the superior vena cava. The impulses travel to the AV node by means of tracts that can be demonstrated physiologically; however, they do not appear to correspond to any established morphologic tracts in the atrial wall.

HISTOLOGY

Purkinje Fibers

Purkinje fibers are modified cardiac muscle cells that are specialized for conduction. They are much larger than regular cardiac muscle cells and contain more glycogen. They are located in the subendocardial layer of the endocardium.

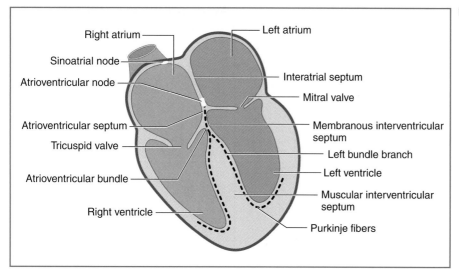

Figure 4-29. Cardiac conducting system.

CLINICAL MEDICINE

Bundle Block

A myocardial infarct (an area of necrosis or damage resulting from sudden insufficiency of the blood supply) can damage the AV bundle. The resultant scar tissue can partially replace the AV bundle. Improper impulse conduction may result in a lack of coordination between atrial and ventricular contractions and is known as heart block (impairment of the normal conduction between the atria and ventricles). In a complete AV bundle block, no impulses can reach the ventricles. Therefore, the atria and ventricles beat independently. In such cases, a cardiac pacemaker could be implanted to normalize the heart rate.

The AV node (see Fig. 4-29) is situated in the interatrial septum just above the opening of the coronary sinus and between the fossa ovalis and the atrioventricular orifice. The AV node sends impulses along the AV bundle (bundle of His), which is about 2 mm thick and represents the only muscular connection between the atria and the ventricles. The AV bundle runs for a centimeter before it penetrates the fibrous skeletal system of the heart, which is attached to the membranous septum.

The AV bundle divides into left and right branches, or crura, that have an inverted Y arrangement. Each bundle branch runs down the interventricular septum just beneath the endocardium (subendocardial layer). The left and right branches end as terminal ramifications or Purkinje fibers (a term often used for lower vertebrates) in the myocardium. On the right side, a specialized band of trabeculae carneae called the moderator (septomarginal) band carries its own Purkinje fibers to reach the anterior papillary muscle.

Lymphatics in the Heart

The cardiac lymphatic plexus empties into the right and left cardiac lymphatic trunks. These trunks drain into the tracheobronchial chain on the left and the superior mediastinal nodes on the right.

Auscultation of Heart Sounds

Listening to sounds arising within an organ (auscultation) is usually done with a stethoscope. Listening to the valve sounds, which are projected onto the chest wall, helps diagnose diseased valves. An echocardiogram is usually prescribed to determine or confirm the severity of disease.

The physician listens over an intercostal space, not over a rib. Since all the valves are found posterior to, or close to, the sternum, a particular valve sound can be heard best in the area where the sound of the blood passing through the valve is projected onto the chest wall. However in that area, sounds from other parts of the heart may also be heard to a lesser degree (Fig. 4-30).

- The pulmonary valve sound projects to and is heard at the level of the second intercostal space on the left.
- The aortic valve sound can best be heard in the second intercostal space just to the right of the sternum.
- The mitral valve sound can best be heard in the left fifth intercostal space in the midclavicular line.
- The tricuspid valve sound is the most difficult to hear, since it projects behind the sternum. It can be heard in either the fifth intercostal space slightly to the left of the sternum or the fifth intercostal space just to the right of the sternum.

Development of the Heart

Two things must be considered in understanding the development of the heart. First, blood must be able to flow continuously through the developing heart. Second, the fetal circulation is very different from the postnatal circulation. In utero the heart is concerned only with pumping blood to the placenta and the systemic systems, since the lungs are not yet mature. So the developing four-chamber heart

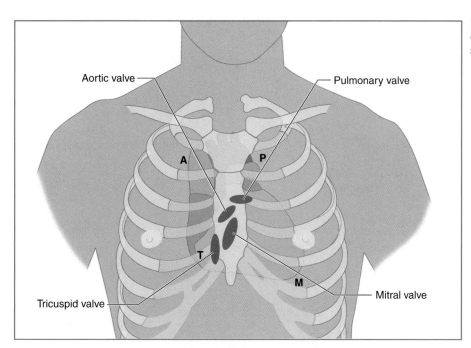

Figure 4-30. Location of heart valves and classical areas for auscultation of heart sounds.

essentially functions as one chamber by utilizing two shunts—an interatrial shunt and the ductus arteriosus from the pulmonary trunk to the arch of the aorta. The blood that enters the heart is then distributed to both atria through the interatrial shunt, and the blood leaving from both ventricles gets mixed together as the ductus arteriosus meets the descending aorta. The resistance in the pulmonary system is high because the lungs are not functioning, and the systemic blood pressure is low because of the inclusion of the low-pressure placenta. Thus, prenatally the pressure on the right side of the heart is higher than on the left side. Within hours after birth, the two shunts close down and the right side of the heart begins pumping into the pulmonic circulation and left side empties into the systemic system. Thus, the pressure on the left side of the heart is now higher than on the right side of the heart.

The heart begins development in the third week from splanchnic mesoderm as a pair of endocardial tubes that fuse in the midline during the lateral folding of the embryo. The heart tube has six regions. Listed from caudal to cranial, in the direction of blood flow, they are sinus venosus, primitive atrium, primitive ventricle, bulbus cordis, truncus arteriosus, and truncoaortic sac (Fig. 4-31).

The heart tube undergoes a rightward bend and rotation called cardiac looping (see Fig. 4-31). The sinus venosus and primitive atrium move cranially and posteriorly to where they will ultimately form the definitive right and left atria, respectively. The primitive ventricle and the bulbus cordis, which will become the left and right ventricles, respectively, assume a caudal position. The truncus arteriosus will be divided into the aortic and pulmonary arteries (Table 4-2).

During weeks 4 and 5, partitioning of the heart must take place. Partitioning of the single atrium (Fig. 4-32) into the left and right atria involves the formation of the septum primum, a crescent-shaped flap that grows down from the posterosuperior wall to meet the endocardial cushions. Just

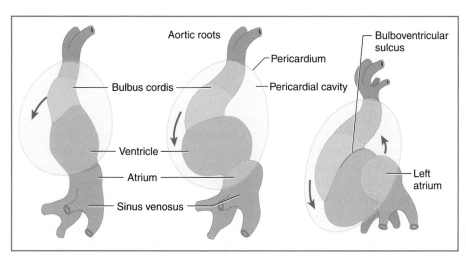

Figure 4-31. Early cardiac development—cardiac looping.

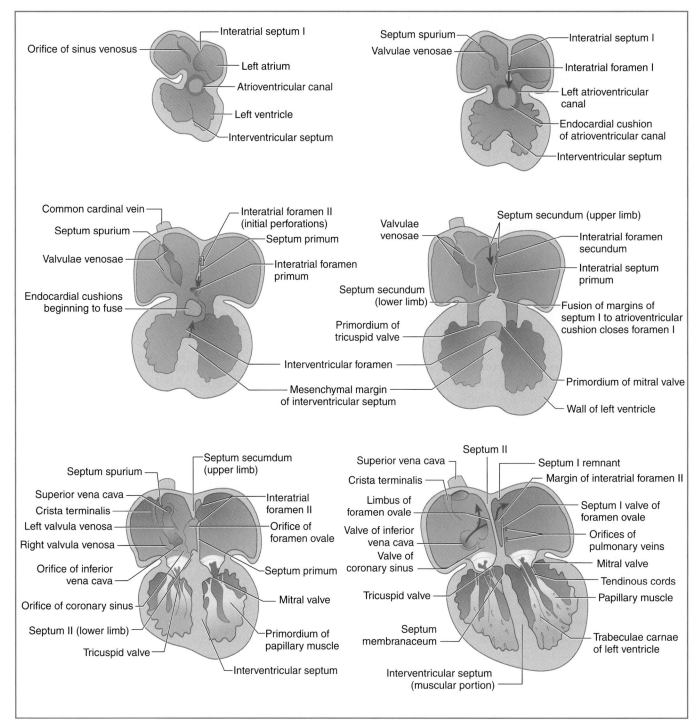

Figure 4-32. Stages in the partitioning of the atria and ventricles.

before the septum primum fuses with the endocardial cushions, an opening forms in the septum primum, the ostium secundum, to preserve the communication between the two developing atria. A second flap grows down on the right side of the septum primum, the septum secundum. It, however, does not fuse with the endocardial cushions. This leaves two openings—the ostium secundum and the foramen ovale—through which the oxygenated blood from the placenta can move from the right atrium to the left atrium

during fetal life. After birth, the now higher pressure on the left side of the heart forces the septum primum against the septum secundum, thus closing the foramen ovale and separating the two atria. This physiologic closure occurs within a few hours after birth and becomes an anatomic closure within a few months. A defect in the interatrial septum that allows blood from the left atrium to pass to the right atrium can lead to pulmonary hypertension because of the extra blood entering the pulmonic system (Fig. 4-33).

TABLE 4-2. Correlations of Primitive and Definitive Heart Areas

Primitive Area of the Heart	Definitive Area of the Heart
Sinus venosus	Right atrium
Primitive atrium	Left atrium
Primitive ventricle	Left ventricle
Bulbus cordis	Right ventricle
Truncus arteriosus	Aorta and pulmonary trunk

Concurrently with the interatrial partitioning, the partitioning of the ventricles begins with an outgrowth of the muscular wall of the primitive ventricle called the *muscular interventricular septum*. However, it cannot become complete at this time because the blood is still entering the left ventricle and leaving the heart through the right ventricle. The partitioning of the ventricles will be completed by the eighth week when the endocardial cushions and the truncoconal ridges fuse with the muscular interventricular septum (see Fig. 4-32). The most common heart defect is a ventricular septal defect, which results from the failure of this fusion to take place (see Fig. 4-33).

The final step in the development of the heart is the partitioning of the conus cordis and truncus arteriosus during weeks 7 and 8, when the growing truncoconal ridges spiral around and fuse to each other, converting the single outflow tract into the aorta and pulmonary trunks (Fig. 4-34).

Three potential defects are associated with this process (Fig. 4-35). If the truncoconal ridges do not spiral, then the aorta will arise from the right ventricle and the pulmonary trunk will lead from the left ventricle. This is called *transposition of the great vessels* and must be accompanied by either a ventricular septal defect or a patent ductus arteriosus for the infant to survive. Alternatively, if the separation of the outflow tract is not complete, the defect is called *persistent truncus arteriosus*. This allows partially oxygenated blood to go to both the lungs and the systemic circulation. The third defect arises when the outflow tract is not partitioned equally. This is typical of *tetralogy of Fallot* and combines four defects: pulmonary stenosis, ventricular septal defect, overriding aorta, and right ventricular hypertrophy. For the infant to survive, there must also be a patent ductus arteriosus.

●●● SUPERIOR MEDIASTINUM

The superior mediastinum lies above the pericardium, which can be visualized externally by the level of the sternal angle. The boundaries of the superior mediastinum (see Fig. 4-16) are the manubrium, Tl–T4 vertebrae, parietal pleura above the root of the lung, and medial portion of the superior thoracic aperture. The superior mediastinum is organized around the arch of the aorta.

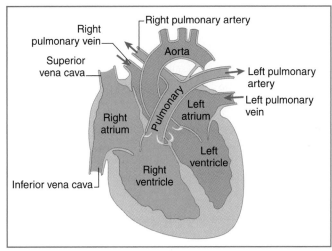

A

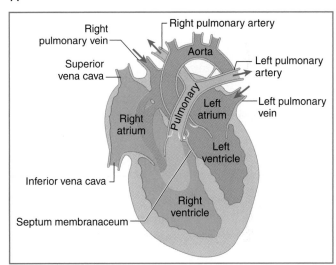

B

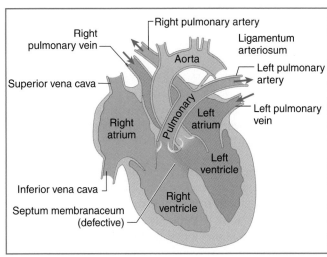

C

Figure 4-33. Heart defects related to partitioning of the four chambers. **A,** Normal heart. **B,** Interatrial defect. **C,** Interventricular defect.

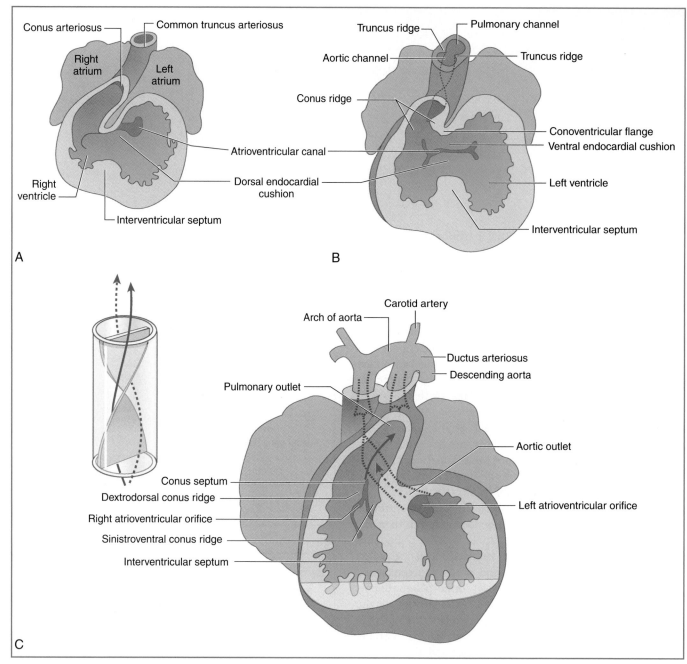

Figure 4-34. Conversion of single outflow tract into the aorta and pulmonary trunk. **A,** Single outflow tract. **B,** Growth of truncoconal ridges. **C,** Aorta and pulmonary trunk formed.

The ascending aorta starts within the pericardial sac, therefore within the middle mediastinum. However, the arch of the aorta lies above the pericardium in the superior mediastinum. The descending aorta is within the posterior mediastinum.

The major structures found in the superior mediastinum are described below, as found from anterior to posterior.

Thymus

The thymus is a bilobed gland found just posterior to the manubrium and the strap muscles that arise from the manubrium. The thymus extends inferiorly into the anterior mediastinum and superiorly into the neck, just anterior to the trachea. This primary lymph gland distributes early generations of T lymphocytes to other lymphoid organs. Its relative weight is greatest in the neonate, but its total weight is greatest at puberty. After puberty, the thymus atrophies, and it is usually observed in old age as bilobed glandular tissue that is embedded in the fascia and fat of the mediastinum.

Blood Supply

The internal thoracic and inferior thyroid arteries supply the thymus. Venous drainage of the thymus is into the left brachiocephalic, inferior thyroid, and internal thoracic veins. Lymphatic drainage of the thymus is into the adjacent lymph nodes including the tracheobronchial and superior

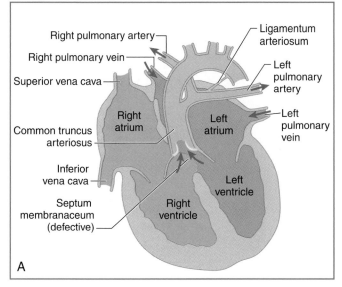
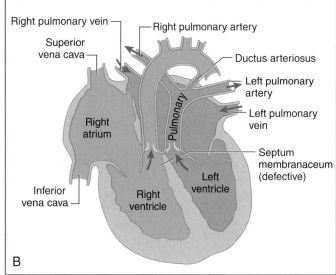
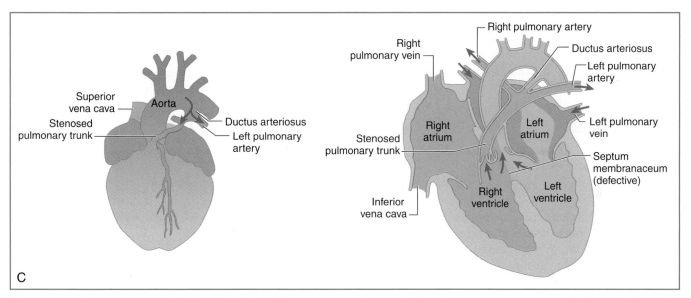

Figure 4-35. Defects associated with partitioning of the truncus arteriosus. **A,** Persistent truncus arteriosus. **B,** Transposition of the great vessels. **C,** Tetralogy of Fallot.

mediastinal nodes. Note that the thymus has no afferent lymphatics, which protects it from foreign antigens when it is producing progeny T cells.

Innervation

The innervation of the thymus consists of postganglionic sympathetic fibers from cervical and upper thoracic sympathetic ganglia. The parasympathetic fibers, if any, would be preganglionic parasympathetic fibers from the vagus.

Veins of the Superior Mediastinum

Each brachiocephalic vein drains blood from the head, neck, and upper extremity regions and is formed posterior to the sternoclavicular joint by the union of the subclavian vein and the internal jugular vein (Fig. 4-36). The left brachiocephalic vein crosses anteriorly to the aortic arch and the origin of its three branches, joining the right brachiocephalic vein to form the superior vena cava. Therefore, the left brachiocephalic vein is much longer than the right brachiocephalic vein and only the left brachiocephalic vein is found in the midsagittal plane. The left brachiocephalic vein drains the left inferior thyroid, vertebral, superior intercostal, and sometimes both left and right internal thoracic veins. The right brachiocephalic vein crosses the right pleura and lung to drain the right vertebral and inferior thyroid veins and, often, the right internal thoracic vein as well.

The superior vena cava is formed on the right side of the mediastinum posterior to the first right costal cartilage or the first intercostal space. The arch of the azygos vein passes over

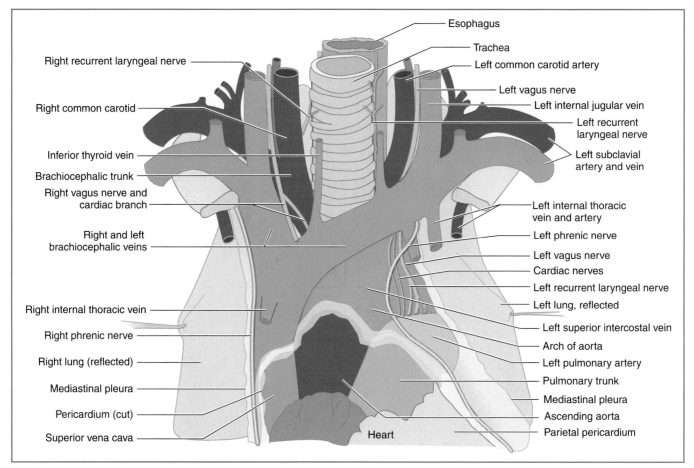

Figure 4-36. Superior mediastinum.

the root of the right lung and empties into the posterior wall of the superior vena cava. The azygos vein drains the posterior wall of the thorax, as well as a portion of the abdomen. The superior vena cava passes posteriorly to the right costal cartilages to enter the right atrium.

Arteries of the Superior Mediastinum

The arch of the aorta begins and ends at the level of the intervertebral disk between T4 and T5, which corresponds to the sternal angle. In the superior mediastinum, the aorta arches to the left and posteriorly over the root of the left lung and then continues inferiorly as the descending aorta. Three large arteries arise from the arch of the aorta.

The brachiocephalic (innominate) artery is the first and largest branch. This artery starts in the same plane as the second right costal cartilage and gives rise to the right common carotid and the right subclavian arteries just posterior to the sternoclavicular articulation.

The left common carotid artery ascends directly from the arch.

The left subclavian artery ascends from the aortic arch as it passes posteriorly and to the left. The left subclavian artery now passes posteriorly to the left sternoclavicular articulation, over the first rib and posterior to the anterior scalene muscle.

This artery makes an impression on the medial anterior aspect of the apex of the left lung.

Development of Vessels in the Superior Mediastinum

The cranial end of the truncus arteriosus is the aortic sac. After the truncus arteriosus has divided into the ventral aorta and the pulmonary trunk, the aortic sac forms right and left horns and gives rise to six symmetric aortic arches (Fig. 4-37). The left horn gives rise to the proximal portion of the arch of the aorta, and the right horn forms the brachiocephalic trunk. The arches end laterally in the right and left dorsal aortae. The arches do not form simultaneously but rather in a cranial-to-caudal fashion. The fifth arch actually never fully forms and then regresses. As development proceeds, the symmetry is gradually lost. The first two arches give rise to vessels in the head. The common carotid artery and first part of the internal carotid artery are formed from the third aortic arch on each side. The external carotid artery forms as a branch of the third aortic arch, while the cranial ends of the two dorsal aortae form the distal ends of the internal carotid arteries. The left and right fourth aortic arches do not form symmetric vessels. The left side forms the portion of the arch of the aorta between the left common carotid artery and the

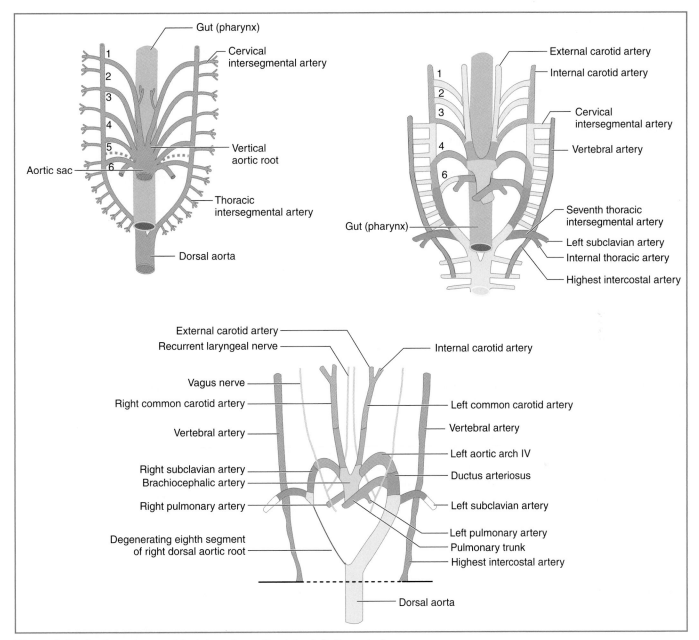

Figure 4-37. Aortic arches and their transformation into definitive arteries.

left subclavian artery. On the right side, the fourth arch forms the beginning of the right common carotid artery (Table 4-3).

Trachea

The trachea is found posterior to the V-like interval formed by the brachiocephalic trunk and left common carotid arteries as they arise from the arch of the aorta. The trachea passes posteriorly and to the right of the aortic arch.

Morphology

The trachea (wind pipe) is made of C-shaped cartilages with the open end of the cartilages facing posteriorly. The trachea deviates slightly to the right owing to the arch of the aorta. This results in a longer and more horizontal left bronchus.

The right vagus, the brachiocephalic artery, and mediastinal pleura are to the right of the trachea. Here, the trachea makes a slight impression on the right lung above the hilum. The left recurrent branch of the left vagus nerve, arch of the aorta, and left common carotid and subclavian arteries lie to the left of the trachea, while the left brachiocephalic vein lies anterior to the trachea.

Blood Supply and Innervation

The inferior thyroid and bronchial arteries give off branches that supply the trachea. The vagus nerves and the left recurrent laryngeal nerve supply preganglionic parasympathetic fibers, which synapse in small ganglia close to the trachea. Postganglionic sympathetic fibers reach the trachea from the cervical and upper thoracic ganglia.

TABLE 4-3. Derivatives of the Aortic Arches

Aortic Arch	Artery Formed	
First arch	Maxillary artery	
Second arch	Lingual and stapedial arteries	
Third arch	Common carotid artery (proximally) and internal carotid artery (distally)	
Fourth arch	Part of aortic arch on left side	Proximal part of right subclavian on the right side
Fifth arch	Never fully forms	—
Sixth arch	Left side—proximal part of left pulmonary artery and ductus arteriosus	Right side—proximal part of right pulmonary artery

Esophagus

The esophagus extends from the pharynx in the neck to the stomach in the abdomen. As it enters the thorax through the superior thoracic aperture, the esophagus lies posterior to the trachea. In the superior mediastinum, the arch of the aorta moves the esophagus to the right of the midline. Here, it makes an impression on the right lung above the hilum. The esophagus has a slight relationship with the left lung above the aortic arch. The esophagus appears as a collapsed muscular tube.

Innervation

The neurovascular supply of the upper esophagus is somewhat different from the esophagus in the posterior mediastinum and abdomen. The entire esophagus is innervated by the vagus nerves. However, the upper half of the esophagus receives somatic innervation due to the voluntary nature of swallowing mediated by special visceral efferent fibers from the vagus nerves and their recurrent branches, whereas the lower half of the esophagus receives vagal preganglionic parasympathetic fibers. The sympathetic innervation to the cervical and upper thoracic esophagus is from the cervical sympathetic trunk.

Blood Supply

The blood supply to the upper portion of the esophagus is from the descending branches of the inferior thyroid arteries and veins, which anastomose with the vessels of the lower half of the esophagus.

Azygos Vein

The azygos vein (Fig. 4-38) drains most of the posterior thoracic wall (intercostal spaces) and part of the posterior abdominal wall. It arises from the right ascending lumbar and subcostal veins and empties into the posterior surface of the superior vena cava by arching over the root of the right lung. Only the arch of the azygos vein and its entry into the superior vena cava are prominent structures in the superior mediastinum. The rest of the azygos system of veins is described with the posterior mediastinum, below.

Vagus Nerve

The vagus nerve is cranial nerve X. It carries preganglionic parasympathetic fibers to the thorax and abdomen. It also carries general visceral sensory (GVA) fibers from the thoracic and upper abdominal viscera. The vagus nerve and the left recurrent laryngeal nerve also carry special visceral efferent (SVE) fibers, which are discussed with the head and neck in Chapter 10.

Right Vagus

In the superior mediastinum, the right vagus nerve enters the thorax between the right brachiocephalic vein and artery and runs along the right lateral surface of the trachea, posterior to the root of the lung, onto the posterior surface of the esophagus (see Fig. 4-38). The right recurrent laryngeal branch of the right vagus is not in the thorax. The nerve recurs around the right subclavian artery in the root of the neck.

Left Vagus

The left vagus nerve enters the thorax with the left common carotid artery, crosses the arch of the aorta, and passes posteriorly to the root of the lung on the anterior surface of the esophagus (see Fig. 4-38). At the arch of the aorta, the left vagus has a large branch, the left recurrent laryngeal nerve, which passes posteriorly to the arch of the aorta and the ligamentum arteriosum. The ligamentum arteriosum is the fibrous remnant of the fetal ductus arteriosus, which is a bypass from the pulmonary artery to the arch of the aorta. The left recurrent laryngeal nerve runs in the tracheoesophageal groove to reach the larynx.

●●● POSTERIOR MEDIASTINUM

The posterior mediastinum is located anterior to the lower thoracic vertebrae (T5–T12) and posterior to the pericardium. It is bounded laterally by the mediastinal parietal pleura, superiorly by an imaginary plane that passes through the sternal angle and vertebral disk between T4 and T5, and inferiorly by the thoracic diaphragm. It is continuous with the superior mediastinum and contains the esophagus (with associated vagal fibers), descending thoracic aorta, thoracic duct, azygos system of veins, and bifurcation of the trachea in the living.

Bifurcation of the Trachea

The trachea ends by bifurcating and forming the right and left main bronchi. The bifurcation occurs approximately at the level of T5 at the carina, which is a single cartilage with the open end of the "C" facing superiorly instead of posteriorly. The trachea moves dynamically during respiration because

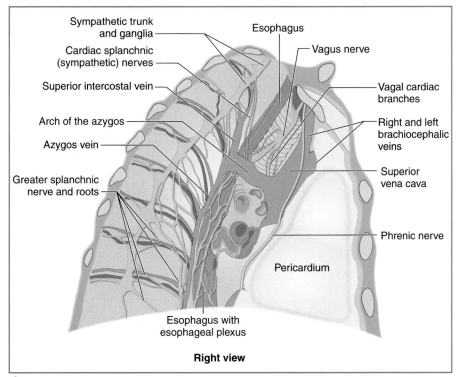

Sympathetic trunk
and ganglia

Cardiac splanchnic
(sympathetic) nerves

Superior intercostal vein

Arch of the azygos

Azygos vein

Greater splanchnic
nerve and roots

Esophagus

Vagus nerve

Vagal cardiac
branches

Right and left
brachiocephalic
veins

Superior
vena cava

Phrenic nerve

Pericardium

Esophagus with
esophageal plexus

Right view

A

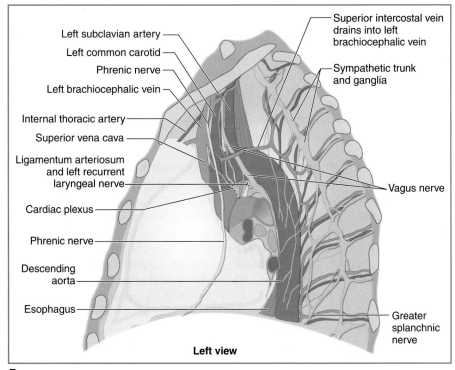

Left subclavian artery

Left common carotid

Phrenic nerve

Left brachiocephalic vein

Internal thoracic artery

Superior vena cava

Ligamentum arteriosum
and left recurrent
laryngeal nerve

Cardiac plexus

Phrenic nerve

Descending
aorta

Esophagus

Superior intercostal vein
drains into left
brachiocephalic vein

Sympathetic trunk
and ganglia

Vagus nerve

Greater
splanchnic
nerve

Left view

B

Figure 4-38. Lateral view of the right (**A**) and left (**B**) sides of the mediastinum.

of its elastic connective tissue. During this movement, it can descend to the level of T6 or even T7.

Esophagus

In the posterior mediastinum, the esophagus makes an impression on both lungs. After making an impression on the right lung, the esophagus moves back to the left, making an impression just anterior to the impression produced by the descending aorta (see Fig. 4-38B). The esophagus passes through the esophageal hiatus in the right crus of the diaphragm approximately at the level of the 10th thoracic vertebra.

In the thorax, several structures make impressions on the esophagus. In the superior mediastinum, the aortic arch

TABLE 4-4. Relationships of the Esophagus in the Posterior Mediastinum

Structures Found Anterior to the Esophagus	Structures Found Posterior to the Esophagus
Trachea	Descending thoracic aorta
Left bronchus	Thoracic vertebral bodies
Left atrium	Right posterior intercostal arteries
Anterior esophageal plexus	Azygos vein
	Posterior esophageal plexus
	Thoracic duct (to vertebral level T5)

TABLE 4-5. Blood Supply and Innervation to the Esophagus by Region

Region	Arterial Supply	Venous Drainage	Innervation
Cervical region	Inferior thyroid artery	Inferior thyroid vein	Vagus (via recurrent laryngeal nerves), sympathetics from cervical sympathetic trunk
Thoracic region	Bronchial arteries and descending aorta branches	Azygos and hemiazygos veins	Vagus, sympathetics from cervical sympathetic trunk
Lower thoracic and abdominal region	Descending aorta and branches of left gastric artery	Left gastric vein	Vagus, sympathetics from greater splanchnic nerve

CLINICAL MEDICINE

Transesophageal Echocardiogram

The relationship of the left atrium to the esophagus can be used to detect an enlarged left atrium. An enlarged left atrium may impinge on the esophagus, making an additional impression that can be observed by endoscopy or radiography. During a transesophageal echocardiogram (TEE), the transducer is placed in the esophagus to obtain better images of the heart, especially the left atrium and mitral valve. During valve replacement, TEE gives the surgeon real-time feedback regarding the competency of the repaired valve.

pushes the esophagus to the right of the midline and makes an impression on the left side of the esophagus.

In the posterior mediastinum, the left bronchus makes a distinct impression on the esophagus as it crosses the esophagus anteriorly at the level of the fifth thoracic vertebrae. The esophagus then curves posterior to the pericardium and left atrium.

The esophagus lies on the left side of the midline as it courses inferiorly toward the esophageal hiatus. Thus, the esophagus follows a path that runs from the left side of the body, over to the right side, and back again to the left side, making impressions on both lungs (Table 4-4).

Blood Supply to the Esophagus

Since the esophagus travels through three regions of the body—cervical, thoracic, and abdominal—its blood supply comes from vessels originating in all three regions (Table 4-5). In terms of venous drainage, two venous plexuses drain the esophagus. The longitudinal submucosal esophageal plexus lies between the esophageal mucosa (inner lining of the esophagus) and the connective tissue of the esophagus. It drains superiorly and inferiorly but has numerous branches that drain to the external esophageal plexus. The external esophageal plexus is located on the outer surface of the

esophagus and drains to vessels in the three regions through which the esophagus travels (see Table 4-5). The left gastric (coronary) vein drains the most inferior portion of the esophagus. The left gastric vein is a tributary of the portal venous system. A potential collateral venous circulation exists between the portal system and the azygos system that drains into the superior vena. This material will become important in studying the abdomen.

Innervation to the Esophagus

In the posterior mediastinum, the esophageal plexus innervates the esophagus. This plexus consists of preganglionic parasympathetic and GVA fibers from the vagus nerves and postganglionic sympathetic and GVA fibers for pain that run with the sympathetics. The preganglionic parasympathetic vagal fibers synapse in ganglia found in the wall of the esophagus. The very short postganglionic parasympathetic fibers supply the smooth muscle and glands of the esophagus.

The sympathetic innervation to the lower esophagus is best understood after reading the section on splanchnic nerves, below. The sympathetic preganglionic cell bodies responsible for this portion of the esophagus are located in the lateral horns of spinal cord segments T5 and T6. These cell bodies give rise to fibers that join the greater splanchnic nerve to synapse in ganglia closer to the esophagus. The postganglionic sympathetic fibers join the esophageal plexus. Owing to the origin of the preganglionic fibers at spinal cord level T5 and T6, pain from the esophagus would be referred to thoracic dermatomes 5 and 6. Acid reflux disease is often the cause of substernal pain in dermatomes 5 and 6. It can be mistaken for angina pectoris and vice versa.

Descending Thoracic Aorta

The descending thoracic aorta passes through the aortic hiatus behind the diaphragm at the T12 vertebral level. It gives rise to both parietal and visceral branches while in the thorax. The descending thoracic aorta starts just to the left of the intervertebral disk between the fourth and fifth thoracic vertebrae. As it descends, it passes back toward the midline. In the inferior portion of the posterior mediastinum, it is found posterior to the esophagus, and anterior to thoracic vertebrae T11, T12 before it passes behind the diaphragm.

Branches of the Descending Aorta

Nine pairs of posterior intercostal arteries supply the lower intercostal spaces and one pair of subcostal arteries supplies the upper posterior abdominal wall below the 12th rib. The first two posterior intercostal arteries are branches of the highest intercostal artery, which in turn is a branch of the subclavian artery's costocervical trunk.

Two left bronchial arteries supply the left lung. The right bronchial artery arises from the third right posterior intercostal artery.

Three to six esophageal arteries supply the lower esophagus.

The superior phrenic arteries arise just superior to the diaphragm to supply the superior surface of the diaphragm.

Mediastinal branches supply the connective tissue and lymph nodes of the mediastinum.

Azygos System of Veins

The azygos system of veins is highly variable. It drains blood from the posterior aspect of the thoracic and abdominal wall (Fig. 4-39). Note that the azygos vein lies slightly to the right side of the midline and therefore drains the right side of the posterior body wall while the hemi-azygos and accessory hemiazygos veins lie significantly on the left side of the midline and drain the left side.

Azygos Vein

The roots of the azygos vein are the right subcostal vein, inferior vena cava, and the right ascending lumbar vein, which is formed by the lumbar veins in the posterior abdominal wall (see Fig. 4-34). The azygos passes through the right crus of the diaphragm or the aortic hiatus to the right of the aorta. It ascends on the bodies of the thoracic vertebrae to the level of T4. The azygos vein also drains the posterior intercostal veins from intercostal spaces 5 to 11. The arch of the azygos vein passes over the root of the right lung. Here, it drains into the posterior surface of the superior vena cava at the level of the second costal cartilage.

The right posterior intercostal veins from spaces 2, 3, and 4 form a common trunk, the superior intercostal vein, which drains into the azygos vein.

Hemiazygos Vein

The roots of the hemiazygos are the left ascending lumbar vein and the left subcostal vein. It also frequently communicates with the left renal vein (see Fig. 4-34). The root from the left renal vein is variable and may drain into either the azygos or the hemiazygos. The hemiazygos vein passes directly through the thoracic diaphragm's left crus.

The hemiazygos vein usually drains the left posterior intercostal veins from intercostal spaces 9, 10, and 11. Traveling superiorly to the level of T8(T9), the hemiazygos vein crosses the midline to join the azygos vein. It passes posteriorly to the aorta, esophagus, and the thoracic duct.

Accessory Hemiazygos Vein

The accessory hemiazygos vein drains the left intercostal veins from intercostal spaces 5–8 and then crosses the midline to join the azygos vein at about T7 or joins the hemiazygos vein (see Fig. 4-34).

The second, third, and fourth posterior intercostal veins make up the left superior intercostal vein, which drains into the left brachiocephalic vein by crossing the arch of the aorta between the phrenic and vagus nerves.

The first intercostal spaces on the left and right side are drained by their respective supreme (highest) intercostal veins, which may drain into the adjacent brachiocephalic veins.

Remember that there is significant variation in the azygos system of veins.

Thoracic Duct

The thoracic duct is the largest lymphatic vessel in the body and serves as the connection between the lymphatic system and the venous system. It is responsible for draining all of the body except the right upper quadrant, which is done by the right lymphatic duct. The right and left lumbar lymphatic trunks collect lymph from the lower limbs and the pelvic region. They join the intestinal trunk, which drains lymph from the abdominal viscera, to form the cisterna chyli. The cisterna chyli is a lymphatic dilatation usually found posterior to and to the right of the aorta at approximately L1 or L2. The thoracic duct ascends through the aortic hiatus to the right of the aorta.

After passing through the aortic hiatus, the thoracic duct ascends through the posterior mediastinum on the anterior surfaces of the vertebral bodies. Here, it lies between the aorta and the azygos vein, posterior to the esophagus.

At the level of the sternal angle, the duct moves to the left of the midline and to the left side of the esophagus. Essentially, the duct passes between the veins and the arteries. In the superior aspect of the trunk, the thoracic duct receives lymph from the posterior intercostal and left superior mediastinal nodes.

The thoracic duct passes posteriorly to the left brachiocephalic, left internal jugular, and the left subclavian veins. However, it passes anteriorly to the left vertebral and subclavian arteries. The thoracic duct empties into either the left internal jugular vein or left subclavian vein or

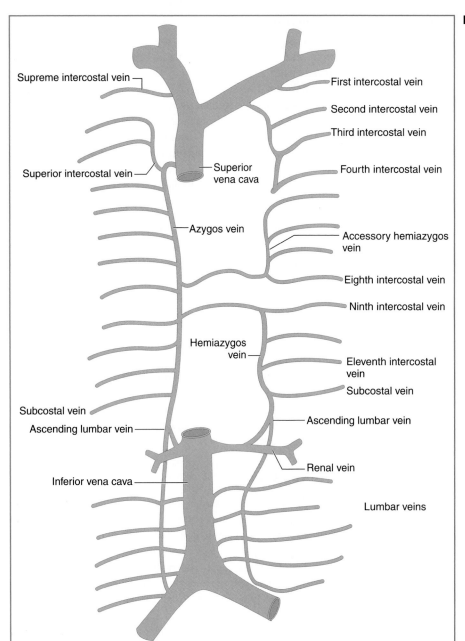

Figure 4-39. Azygos system of veins.

Supreme intercostal vein

First intercostal vein

Second intercostal vein

Third intercostal vein

Superior intercostal vein

Superior vena cava

Fourth intercostal vein

Azygos vein

Accessory hemiazygos vein

Eighth intercostal vein

Ninth intercostal vein

Hemiazygos vein

Eleventh intercostal vein

Subcostal vein

Subcostal vein

Ascending lumbar vein

Ascending lumbar vein

Renal vein

Inferior vena cava

Lumbar veins

into the confluence where they meet to form the left brachiocephalic vein.

Sympathetic Trunk

The sympathetic trunk is not in the posterior mediastinum. It is found posterior to the parietal pleura. However, the splanchnic nerves pass into the posterior mediastinum.

Sympathetic nerves originate from their cell bodies located in the lateral horns of spinal segments Tl to L2. They travel from the spinal cord with the ventral roots of the spinal nerves and leave the mixed nerves' ventral rami as white rami communicantes. The fibers in the white rami can synapse in the ganglia of the sympathetic chain. Some of the postganglionic fibers rejoin the spinal nerves as gray rami communicantes

to innervate the "visceral" structures in the body wall, such as the smooth muscle of blood vessels, the erector pili muscles, and the sweat glands. Sympathetic chain ganglia T1 to L1 are located in the thorax.

Splanchnic Nerves

There are four pairs of splanchnic nerves, which are composed of preganglionic fibers and which leave the lateral horns from levels T5 to L2. These fibers pass through the sympathetic chain ganglia without synapsing to supply structures in the abdomen and pelvis. They are called the greater, lesser, least, and lumbar splanchnic nerves.

The roots of the greater splanchnic nerves arise from sympathetic ganglia T5 to T9, with fibers arising from neuronal cell bodies located in spinal cord segments

T5–T9. The roots form a greater splanchnic nerve on each side that passes through the crus of the diaphragm to synapse in the celiac and superior mesenteric ganglia.

The lesser splanchnic nerves arise from neuronal cell bodies located in spinal cord segments T10–T11. These preganglionic sympathetic fibers synapse primarily in the aorticorenal ganglia.

The least splanchnic nerves arise from neuronal cell bodies located in spinal cord segment T12 and synapse in the renal plexus on renal sanglia.

The lumbar splanchnic nerves arise from neuronal cell bodies located in lumbar spinal cord segments 1 and 2 and synapse in the inferior mesenteric ganglia. These splanchnic nerves are discussed with the abdomen and pelvis in Chapters 5 to 7.

Thoracic Lymph Nodes

The lymphatics of the skin and superficial fascia of the thorax drain into the axillary lymph nodes.

Preaortic nodes are located just anterior to the aorta, and they drain the esophagus. Lymph nodes found lateral to the aorta are called para-aortic lymph nodes and drain the posterior intercostal spaces. Lymph from the anterior intercostal spaces and the anterior mediastinum drain into parasternal lymph nodes. Parasternal lymph node samples can be obtained for examination through left intercostal spaces 1–3.

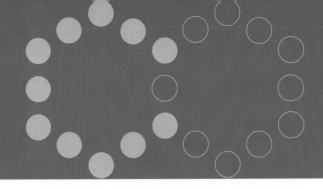

The Abdomen

5

CONTENTS

ANTERIOR ABDOMINAL WALL
Regional Divisions of the Abdominal Wall

LAYERS OF THE ANTERIOR ABDOMINAL WALL
Skin
Abdominal Muscles
Bony Components of the Anterior Abdominal Wall

MUSCLES OF THE ANTERIOR ABDOMINAL WALL
Inner Investing Layer of Deep Fascia (Endoabdominal Fascia)
Subserous (Extraserous) Fascia
Rectus Sheath
Formation of the Rectus Sheath
Ligaments
Innervation of the Anterior Abdominal Wall

VASCULATURE OF THE ANTERIOR ABDOMINAL WALL
Arterial Supply
Venous Drainage

INGUINAL REGION AND INGUINAL CANAL
Boundaries of the Inguinal Canal in the Anatomic Position
Openings of the Inguinal Canal
Contents of the Inguinal Canal
Layers of the Scrotum and Spermatic Cord
Development of the Inguinal Canal

PERITONEUM
Embryology of the Peritoneum
Anatomy of the Peritoneum

ABDOMINAL VISCERA
Esophagus
Stomach
Sensory Innervation (Abdominal Pain)

DEVELOPMENT OF THE STOMACH AND OTHER FOREGUT ORGANS
Arterial Supply to the Foregut and the Midgut

DEVELOPMENT OF THE CAUDAL FOREGUT
Development of the Liver
Rotation of the Stomach and Formation of the Lesser Sac
Formation of the Peritoneal Ligaments from the Dorsal Mesogastrium

DEVELOPMENT OF THE PANCREAS

DUODENUM
The Four Parts of the Duodenum
Blood Supply to the Duodenum
Innervation of the Duodenum

JEJUNUM AND ILEUM
Blood Supply to the Jejunum and Ileum
Innervation of the Jejunum and Ileum

LARGE INTESTINE, OR COLON
Cecum
Appendix
Ascending Colon
Transverse Colon
Descending and Sigmoid Colon
Blood Supply to the Colon
Venous Drainage of the Colon
Lymphatics of the Colon
Innervation of the Colon

LIVER
Anatomy of the Liver
Relationships of the Liver
Peritoneal Ligaments of the Liver

GALLBLADDER
Anatomy of the Gallbladder
Blood Supply to the Gallbladder
Innervation of the Gallbladder

SPLEEN
Anatomy of the Spleen
Blood Supply to the Spleen
Innervation of the Spleen

PANCREAS
Anatomy of the Pancreas
Blood Supply to the Pancreas
Innervation of the Pancreas

EXTRAHEPATIC BILIARY DUCTS

DEVELOPMENT OF THE MIDGUT
Physiologic Herniation
Physiologic Reduction
Fixation
Congenital Abnormalities of the Midgut

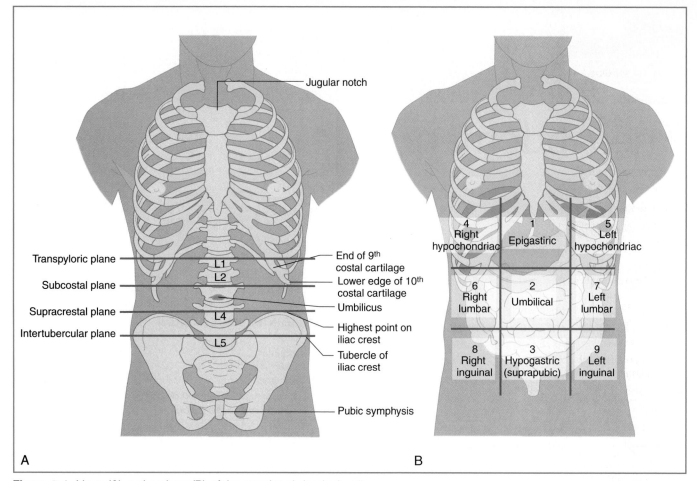

Labels in figure A (left to right):
- Jugular notch
- Transpyloric plane
- Subcostal plane
- Supracrestal plane
- Intertubercular plane
- L1
- L2
- L4
- L5
- End of 9th costal cartilage
- Lower edge of 10th costal cartilage
- Umbilicus
- Highest point on iliac crest
- Tubercle of iliac crest
- Pubic symphysis

A

Labels in figure B (nine regions):
- 4 Right hypochondriac
- 1 Epigastiric
- 5 Left hypochondriac
- 6 Right lumbar
- 2 Umbilical
- 7 Left lumbar
- 8 Right inguinal
- 3 Hypogastric (suprapubic)
- 9 Left inguinal

B

Figure 5-1. Lines (**A**) and regions (**B**) of the anterior abdominal wall.

●●● ANTERIOR ABDOMINAL WALL

Regional Divisions of the Abdominal Wall

The anterior abdominal wall can be subdivided into quadrants or into nine regions for either anatomic or clinical descriptive purposes. Several lines or planes (Fig. 5-1) are used to subdivide the anterior abdominal wall into regions. A line is a mark or streak, while a plane is two-dimensional. A line often denotes the presence of a two-dimensional plane and often has the same name.

The abdominal wall can be subdivided into four quadrants by a horizontal and a vertical line through the umbilicus. This division produces four quadrants: right upper, left upper, right lower, and left lower (Table 5-1).

The abdominal wall can also be divided into nine regions by using four lines: two horizontal lines and two sagittal (vertical) lines (see Fig. 5-1A). The two sagittal lines are the mid-inguinal lines. These lines are found halfway between the anterior superior iliac spine and the pubic tubercle. The two horizontal lines are the transpyloric plane and the intertubercular line.

The transpyloric plane (see Fig. 5-1A) passes through the first lumbar vertebra posteriorly (L1) and usually the ninth costal cartilage anteriorly. The transpyloric line is usually described as being half the distance between the jugular notch and the pubis or approximately half the distance between the xiphoid process and the umbilicus. The transpyloric plane passes through the pylorus of the stomach (sometimes), gallbladder, duodenojejunal juncture, neck and body of the pancreas, and the hila of both kidneys. (A hilum is the part of an organ that receives its neurovascular bundle.) The transpyloric line is *not* the subcostal line that connects the inferior margins of 10th costal cartilages.

The subcostal plane passes through the third lumbar vertebra. Many clinicians use the subcostal plane at the level of the 10th costal cartilage instead of the transpyloric plane as the superior horizontal line.

The intertubercular (transtubercular) line passes through the tubercles of the iliac crest approximately at the level of the fifth lumbar vertebra.

These lines produce nine regions (see Fig. 5-1B). The epigastric region is located above the transpyloric line between the mid-inguinal lines. The right and left hypochondriac regions are found lateral to the mid-inguinal lines at the same level as the epigastric region. The umbilical region is located between the transpyloric, or subcostal, line and the intertubercular line and between the mid-inguinal lines. Lateral to the mid-inguinal lines on each side of the umbilical region are the lumbar or lateral regions. The hypogastric (suprapubic) region is below the transtubercular line and between the mid-

TABLE 5-1. Organs Associated with the Four Abdominal Quadrants

Right Upper Quadrant	Left Upper Quadrant
Liver (right lobe), gallbladder	Liver (left lobe)
Pylorus of stomach	Stomach (body and fundus)
Duodenum	Jejunum and proximal ileum
Right kidney (upper pole)	Left kidney (upper pole) and suprarenal gland
Head of pancreas	Spleen
Right suprarenal gland	Body and tail of pancreas
Ascending colon	Splenic (left colic) flexure
Hepatic (right colic) flexure	Adjacent transverse and descending colon
Transverse colon	
Right Upper Quadrant	**Left Upper Quadrant**
Right kidney (lower pole)	Left kidney (lower pole)
Right ureter	Left ureter
Small intestine	Small intestine
Cecum and beginning ascending colon	Inferior descending colon
Right spermatic cord	Sigmoid colon
Appendix	Left spermatic cord
Right ovary, uterine tube	Left ovary, uterine tube
Abdominal portion of right ureter	Abdominal portion of left ureter
Enlarged uterus	Enlarged uterus
Extended urinary bladder	Extended urinary bladder-

inguinal lines, while the inguinal regions are located lateral to the mid-inguinal lines.

●●● LAYERS OF THE ANTERIOR ABDOMINAL WALL

Skin

The major landmark is the umbilicus, a depressed scar marking the site of the umbilical cord in the fetus. In a normal recumbent individual of average weight, the umbilicus is found at the level of the disk space between the third and fourth lumbar vertebrae. The umbilicus usually lies just above the level of the supracrestal line (connecting the top of the iliac crests), which is also at the level of the fourth lumbar vertebra. Upon standing, and in children and overweight individuals, the umbilicus will be lower.

Internally, the following structures are connected to the umbilicus. All three structures run in the plane of the extraperitoneal fascia.

- The ligamentum teres (round ligament) of the liver is the remnant of the umbilical vein. It runs superiorly from the umbilicus to the liver.

- The median umbilical ligament is the remnant of the fetal urachus, which stretches from the vertex of the bladder to the umbilicus.
- The medial umbilical ligaments represent the obliterated umbilical arteries.

Superficial Fascia

The superficial fascia of the abdominal wall is continuous with the corresponding layer in the thorax, and both have two components. In the abdominal wall these layers are

- An outer fatty layer (Camper's fascia) that is continuous into the thigh.
- An inner membranous layer (Scarpa's fascia) that is continuous into the scrotum and thigh. In the thigh, it fuses with the deep fascia about 2 cm below the inguinal ligament. This arrangement produces the *fold* in the inguinal region that denotes the separation of the trunk and thigh.

Deep Fascia

Deep fascia includes inner and outer investing layers as well as layers that invest the muscles of the abdominal wall (muscular fascia). The outer investing layer is quite thin. The inner investing layer of the abdominal wall deep fascia is well formed and is clinically important because it forms much of the posterior wall of the inguinal canal.

Abdominal Muscles

The muscle layer includes four paired muscles arranged such that the three lateral muscles are in three layers that will have aponeurotic insertions that form a sheath around the fourth, medially placed muscle (Fig. 5-2). An aponeurosis is a thin but very strong connective-tissue, ribbon-like or dense tendinous insertion.

Bony Components of the Anterior Abdominal Wall

Parts of the rib cage serve as the superior bony attachments of the abdominal muscles, while parts of the pelvis are the inferior bony attachments of these muscles. Only the lumbar vertebrae are found below the ribs and above the iliac crests of the pelvis, indicating the flexible nature of this portion of the anterior abdominal wall.

Inferiorly, the abdominal musculature is attached to parts of the hip bones. The pelvis consists of the sacrum, the coccyx, and two hip bones. Each hip bone consists of three bones: the ilium, pubis, and ischium. Only parts of the ilium and pubis contribute to the bony attachment of the muscles of the anterior abdominal wall.

The superior aspect of the pelvis consists of the iliac crests (Fig. 5-3). Each iliac crest has an anterior superior iliac spine projecting from its anterior surface.

The two pubic bones articulate in the midline by means of the pubic symphysis (see Fig. 5-3). The superior and inferior pubic rami are two branches of bone that extend laterally

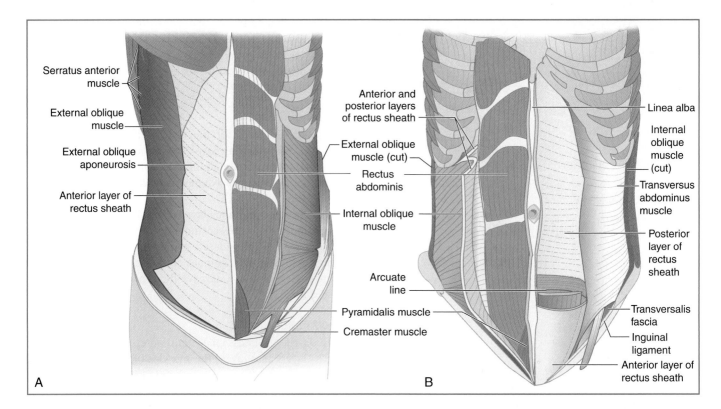

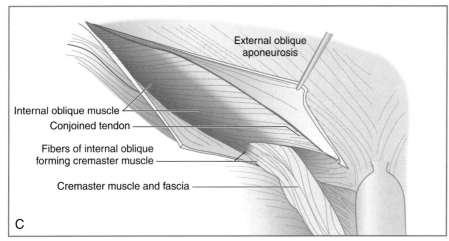

Figure 5-2. Muscles of the anterior abdominal wall.

from the body. The superior pubic ramus extends toward the ilium. The superior pubic ramus has a sharp line on the posterior margin of its superior surface. This line is referred to as the pecten of the pubis or the pectineal line. On the anterosuperior surface of the pubis is the pubic crest, which extends laterally and somewhat anteriorly to be continuous with the pubic tubercle (see Fig. 5-3). The pubic tubercle projects laterally from the pubis and is palpable.

●●● MUSCLES OF THE ANTERIOR ABDOMINAL WALL

The external oblique muscle (see Fig. 5-2) is the thickest of the three lateral muscles. Its anatomic origin is from the external surface of the lower seven or eight ribs, where it is often continuous with the adjacent external intercostal muscles. The muscle fibers run obliquely downward to insert on the anterior half of the outer lip of the iliac crest. Between the ribs and iliac crest, the origin of the external oblique has a free margin that faces the latissimus dorsi muscle. However, most of the muscle fibers that run toward the midline end as an aponeurosis that inserts into the linea alba. The caudal portion of this aponeurosis stretches between the pubic tubercle and iliac crest's anterior superior iliac spine as the inguinal ligament. The inguinal ligament is an important thickening of the aponeurosis of the external oblique.

The external abdominal oblique muscle compresses the abdomen in *forced expiration*. One side, acting alone, will bend the vertebral column laterally. Both sides working together will flex the trunk. It is innervated by spinal nerves T6–T12.

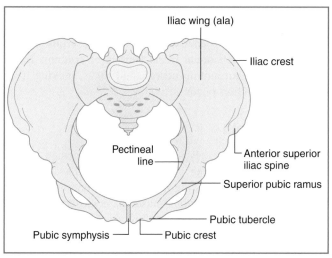

Figure 5-3. Superior view of the pelvis.

Thoracic spinal nerves T6–T11 are often referred to as thoracoabdominal nerves, while T12 is called the subcostal nerve.

The internal oblique muscle (see Figs. 5-2 and 5-4) arises from approximately the lateral two thirds of the inguinal ligament, anterior two thirds of the middle lip of the iliac crest, and lower portion of the lumbar fascia (the posterior layer of the thoracolumbar fascia). Since it is attached posteriorly to the thoracolumbar fascia, the internal oblique does not have a posterior free margin.

The fibers of the internal oblique muscle pass superiorly toward the midline. These fibers insert into the cartilages of the last three or four ribs along the costal margin. This insertion appears to be almost continuous with the lowest three internal intercostal muscles on the external surfaces of the ribs, making the separation of the internal oblique from the rib and costal cartilage difficult. Most of the insertion is in the form of an aponeurosis that inserts into the rectus sheath, the linea alba, and into the pubic crest and pectineal line (with the transversus abdominis) as the conjoined (conjoint) tendon (falx inguinalis).

The muscle compresses the abdomen in forced expiration and acts like the external oblique muscle to flex the vertebral column. Both muscles, working together, help flex the trunk. The internal oblique is innervated by spinal nerves T7–T12 and L1.

The transversus abdominis muscle (see Figs. 5-2 and 5-4) is the thinnest of the three lateral muscles. The transversus abdominis muscle arises from the lateral third of the inguinal ligament, anterior three fourths of the inner lip of the iliac crest, thoracolumbar fascia, and inner surfaces of the cartilages of the last six ribs. This latter origin is almost continuous with the origins of the diaphragm, being separated from the diaphragm by only a thin raphe. It inserts into the rectus sheath and as a part of the conjoined tendon. It is innervated by spinal nerves T7–T12 and L1.

The rectus abdominis muscle (see Figs. 5-2 and 5-4) is a long, flat muscle that arises from the pubis crest and the ligaments covering the pubic symphysis. The rectus abdominis inserts into the xiphoid process and costal cartilages of ribs 5 to 7 as well as the ventral surfaces of the ribs themselves. The rectus muscles help flex the trunk and are innervated by the ventral rami of the lower 6 or 7 thoracic nerves.

The two rectus abdominis muscles (see Fig. 5-4) are separated at the midline by the linea alba, and each muscle is enclosed in an aponeurotic sheath. The rectus abdominis muscle is adherent to the anterior layer of the rectus sheath but can be easily separated from the posterior layer. The muscle flexes the trunk and is innervated by spinal nerves T7–T12.

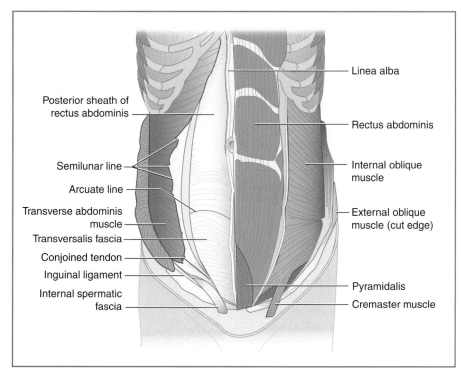

Figure 5-4. Anterior abdominal wall muscles with posterior lamina of the rectus sheath.

The pyramidalis muscle (see Fig. 5-4) is a small triangular muscle that arises from the pubic crest to insert into the linea alba. This muscle lies anterior to the rectus abdominis within the rectus sheath. The pyramidalis muscle tenses the linea alba and is innervated by the subcostal nerve.

Inner Investing Layer of Deep Fascia (Endoabdominal Fascia)

The investing layer of the deep fascia (endoabdominal fascia; see Fig. 5-2) is a continuous layer found deep to the skeletal muscles. It covers the entire abdominal surface of the posterior and anterior abdominal walls and the diaphragm, including the crura, and contributes to the arcuate or lumbocostal arches (the fascial origins of the diaphragm). It is continuous with the endopelvic fascia at the brim of the pelvis. It separates the body wall from the abdominal cavity.

The endoabdominal fascia usually contains no fat except in obese people and appears as a gray, felt-like membrane. The endoabdominal fascia on the anterior wall is also called the *transversalis fascia*. Part of the transversalis fascia forms much of the posterior wall of the inguinal canal, which makes it a clinically important structure during inguinal hernia repair.

Subserous (Extraserous) Fascia

The subserous (extraserous) fascia is the external fascial backing of a serous membrane. Thus, the extraserous fascia is found between the inner investing layer of fascia and the parietal peritoneum. The peritoneum is the serous membrane of the abdominopelvic cavity. Hence, the extraserous fascia is also called extraperitoneal fascia. This layer contains blood vessels, organs, autonomic nerves, and ducts, making it an important dissection plane.

Rectus Sheath

The rectus sheath (see Figs. 5-2 and 5-4) is formed by the aponeuroses of the three lateral muscles of the abdominal wall plus the inner investing layer of deep (endoabdominal) fascia. Each rectus abdominis muscle is enclosed separately in its own connective tissue envelope (rectus sheath), which holds this muscle in its anatomic position. This arrangement prevents the muscle from bulging forward (bow stringing) while flexing the trunk. The subserous fascia and peritoneum lie deep to the sheath and are not considered part of the sheath.

Formation of the Rectus Sheath

At the lateral border of the rectus abdominis (linea semilunaris), the aponeuroses of the three lateral muscles form two layers: the anterior and posterior laminae (layers) of the rectus sheath (Fig. 5-5). The anterior and posterior layers of the rectus sheath are formed differently at different points in the anterior abdominal wall. *The major difference occurs*

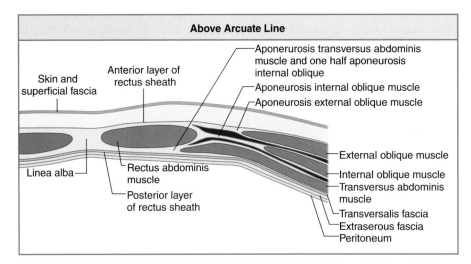

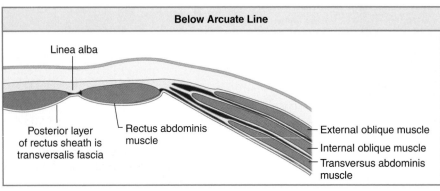

Figure 5-5. Cross-section of the anterior abdominal wall above and below the arcuate line.

approximately halfway between the pubis and umbilicus at a point designated the arcuate line.

The aponeurosis of the external oblique always contributes to the anterior lamina (layer) of the rectus sheath. Above the arcuate line, the aponeurosis of the internal oblique splits into anterior and posterior lamellae, which enclose the rectus abdominis, whereas the aponeurosis of the transversus abdominis muscle contributes only to the posterior lamina (see Figs. 5-4 and 5-5).

Below the arcuate line, *all three aponeurotic layers* of the lateral muscles contribute only to the anterior rectus sheath lamella (see Figs. 5-2 and 5-4). The posterior lamella of the rectus sheath is formed solely by the transversalis fascia (see Figs. 5-4 and 5-5).

Thus, the arcuate (semicircular) line represents the point at which the aponeuroses of the internal abdominal oblique and transversus abdominis muscles join the aponeurosis of the external oblique (see Fig. 5-5). Accordingly, all three layers of lateral muscles now contribute only to the anterior lamella of the rectus sheath. The arcuate line can be quite distinct and appear as an abrupt curved line, or it can be quite diffuse (see Fig. 5-4).

The extraserous (subserous) fascia separates the posterior lamina of the rectus sheath from the peritoneum. This arrangement permits the inferior epigastric vessels to arise from the external iliac vessels and to run in the plane of the extraserous fascia, where they mark the lateral boundary of the inguinal triangle. The inferior epigastric vessels then *penetrate* the transversalis fascia below the arcuate line to enter the rectus sheath posterior to the rectus abdominis muscle. The inferior epigastric vessels then run on the posterior surface of the rectus abdominis and anastomose with the superior epigastric vessels.

The linea alba (see Figs. 5-4 and 5-5) is the midline connective tissue band (raphe) running from the xiphoid process to the pubis. It represents the union or common insertion of the aponeuroses of the right and left lateral muscles after they have formed the layers of the right and left rectus sheaths. The linea alba is up to 2 cm wide above the umbilicus, making it quite easily recognized. However, it is difficult to define below the umbilicus.

Ligaments

The inguinal ligament (Fig. 5-6) is the thickened lower border of the aponeurosis of the external oblique muscle, which extends from the anterior superior iliac spine to the pubic tubercle (Table 5-2). It is attached to the fascia lata (thickening of the outer investing fascia of the thigh). The aponeurosis of the external oblique is folded posteriorly (inward) to form a shelf at a right angle to the external oblique aponeurosis. This is especially true at its medial end, where these fibers have an almost horizontal configuration. This shelf or fold is the part of the inguinal ligament that supports the spermatic cord in the male or the round ligament in the female at the medial end. The lacunar ligament (see Fig. 5-6) is the curved medial end of the pubic insertion of the inguinal ligament. It is

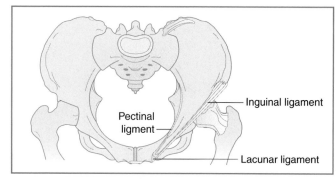

Figure 5-6. Inguinal, lacunar, and pectineal ligaments.

TABLE 5-2. Alternative Names for Structures of the Inguinal Region	
Structure	**Eponyms**
Fatty layer superficial fascia	Camper's fascia
Membranous layer superficial fascia	Scarpa's fascia
Inguinal ligament	Poupart's ligament
Lacunar ligament	Gimbernat's ligament
Conjoint ligament	Falx inguinalis, Henle's ligament
Interfoveolar ligament	Hesselbach's ligament
Pectineal ligament	Cooper's ligament

formed by an expansion of the inguinal ligament in a posterior direction from the pubic tubercle and crest to the pectin of the pubis (pectineal line). This free edge also forms the medial border of the femoral ring, the abdominal opening of the femoral canal. Laterally, the femoral neurovascular bundle and the iliopsoas muscle pass posteriorly to (deep to) the inguinal ligament to enter the thigh. The femoral artery can be palpated at the mid-inguinal line.

The pectineal ligament (see Fig. 5-6) appears as a continuation of the lacunar ligament along the pectinate line of the superior ramus of the pubis. The pectineal ligament is posterior to the femoral artery and vein, which are continuous with the external iliac artery and vein. It is firmly attached to the bone and diminishes as it approaches the iliopectineal (iliopubic) eminence.

The conjoined (conjoint) tendon or falx inguinalis is the lower terminal portion of the aponeuroses of the internal oblique and transversus abdominis muscles as they come together to insert into the pubic crest and pectineal line. This insertion is immediately deep (posterior) to the superficial inguinal ring and strengthens this potentially weak spot.

Innervation of the Anterior Abdominal Wall

The ventral rami of thoracic spinal nerves 6 to 12 plus the iliohypogastric (L1) and ilioinguinal (L1) nerves of the lumbar plexus supply the abdominal wall. The 6th to 11th thoracic

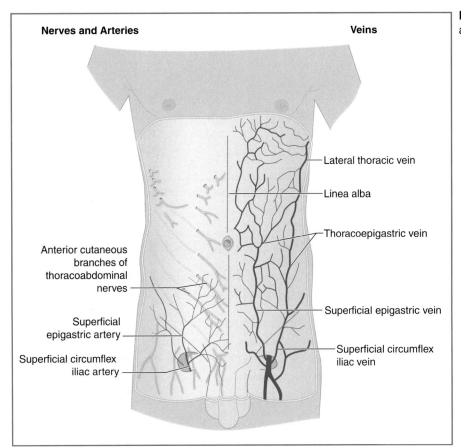

Nerves and Arteries

Lateral thoracic vein

Linea alba

Thoracoepigastric vein

Anterior cutaneous
branches of
thoracoabdominal
nerves

Superficial
epigastric artery

Superficial circumflex
iliac artery

Veins

Superficial epigastric vein

Superficial circumflex
iliac vein

A

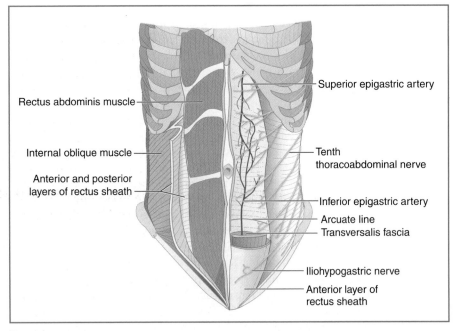

Rectus abdominis muscle

Internal oblique muscle

Anterior and posterior
layers of rectus sheath

Superior epigastric artery

Tenth
thoracoabdominal nerve

Inferior epigastric artery

Arcuate line

Transversalis fascia

Iliohypogastric nerve

Anterior layer of
rectus sheath

B

Figure 5-7. Superficial (**A**) and deep (**B**) abdominal neurovascular structures.

spinal nerves start as intercostal nerves and are referred to as thoracoabdominal nerves (Fig. 5-7), since they supply both thoracic and abdominal walls. The 12th thoracic spinal nerve passes inferiorly to the 12th rib and is referred to as the subcostal nerve. This innervation is both general somatic motor and sensory to the muscles and general somatic sensory to the skin and parietal peritoneum. These nerves also carry postganglionic sympathetic fibers.

The thoracoabdominal nerves pass between the internal oblique and transversus abdominis muscles, penetrate the rectus sheath, and supply the three lateral muscles as well as the rectus abdominis muscle (see Fig. 5-7). The thoracoabdominal nerves have anterior cutaneous branches that penetrate the rectus sheath and supply the overlying skin. As a reference point, the periumbilical region surrounding the umbilicus is innervated by the 10th thoracic spinal nerve. These nerves have muscular branches to the external and internal oblique muscles and the transversus abdominis muscle as well as lateral cutaneous branches that supply the lateral cutaneous regions of the abdominal wall.

The iliohypogastric nerve innervates the skin around the pubis and the lateral buttock. The ilioinguinal nerve escapes through the superficial inguinal ring to innervate the skin over the pubis, anterior scrotum or labia majora, and medial thigh.

The diaphragmatic parietal peritoneum receives sensory fibers from the phrenic nerve. The parietal peritoneum is highly sensitive to pain because it is derived from the somatic mesoderm of the lateral plate. The motor innervation to the abdominal wall is arranged segmentally. Each somite is invaded by a single spinal nerve that innervates all the muscles derived from that somite. This is of great importance during surgery of the abdominal wall, since cutting more than two nerves could result in a large area of muscle paralysis and evagination (protrusion of the abdominal viscera).

●●● VASCULATURE OF THE ANTERIOR ABDOMINAL WALL

Arterial Supply

The superior portion of the anterior abdominal wall (see Fig. 5-7) is normally supplied by the following arteries: the superior epigastric and musculophrenic arteries, which are the terminal branches of the internal thoracic artery, the posterior intercostal and subcostal arteries from the aorta, and the lateral thoracic artery, a branch of the axillary artery (see Fig. 5-7).

The inferior portion of the anterior abdominal wall is normally supplied by the inferior epigastric and deep circumflex iliac arteries, which are branches of the external iliac artery, and the superficial epigastric and superficial circumflex iliac branches of the femoral artery. The latter two arteries run in the superficial fascia and anastomose with the lateral thoracic artery. The inferior epigastric runs between the posterior lamella of the rectus sheath and the rectus abdominis muscle to anastomose with the superior epigastric artery. The deep circumflex iliac artery runs between the internal oblique and transversus abdominis muscles, and it will anastomose with the descending branch of the musculophrenic artery.

Venous Drainage

Venous drainage of the abdominal wall has two venous paths, superficial and deep (see Fig. 5-6). These different venous drainage pathways can form collateral circulations circumventing the inferior vena cava or hepatoportal venous pathway.

The deep venous drainage path consists of the superior epigastric vein and the descending branches of the musculophrenic veins superiorly and the inferior epigastric and deep circumflex iliac veins inferiorly.

The superficial veins (see Fig. 5-7) include the superficial circumflex iliac, superficial epigastric veins inferiorly and mostly lateral thoracic or axillary, but also the intercostal veins superiorly. The superficial epigastric veins normally drain into the greater saphenous branch of the femoral vein, while the lateral thoracic vein normally drains into the axillary vein. The superficial veins anastomose to form the thoracoepigastric veins, which can open up to form a collateral venous drainage when there is increased portal pressure or obstruction of the inferior vena cava.

●●● INGUINAL REGION AND INGUINAL CANAL

The inguinal region of the anterior abdominal wall is not the same as the inguinal canal. The inguinal region is lateral to the suprapubic region and only includes the inguinal canal's deep ring.

The inguinal canal is a 4- to 5-cm passageway through the anterior abdominal wall with all the layers of the wall taking part in the formation of the canal. It is formed by the aponeuroses and muscle fibers of the three lateral muscles and the transversalis fascia. Its openings allow posterior abdominal wall structures to communicate with the scrotum in males or the labium majus in females. The canal enables the spermatic cord in men and the round ligament in women to leave the abdominal cavity. The canal extends from approximately the mid-inguinal line to the pubic tubercle

Boundaries of the Inguinal Canal in the Anatomic Position

The anterior wall (Fig. 5-8) is formed by the aponeurosis of the external oblique throughout the length of the canal. A small portion of the lateral aspect of the anterior wall is formed by the internal oblique's origin from the inguinal ligament. Thus, the internal oblique forms a small portion of the anterior wall only in the region of the deep inguinal ring (see Fig. 5-8). Skin and superficial fascia cover the anterior wall.

The inferior inguinal wall (see Figs. 5-6, 5-8, and 5-9) consists of the inguinal ligament throughout the length of the canal and the lacunar ligament at the medial end.

The superior wall (see Fig. 5-8) is formed by the arching fibers of the internal oblique and transversus abdominis muscles. This is a dynamic (moving) wall owing to the contraction of these muscles. The superior wall starts, in part, anterior and superior to the deep ring. It then passes superiorly and finally passes posteriorly to the spermatic cord, where it inserts as the conjoined tendon. Contraction of the canal's muscles and an increase in intra-abdominal pressure lengthens and narrows the canal. The superior wall descends, the posterior wall pressess against the anterior

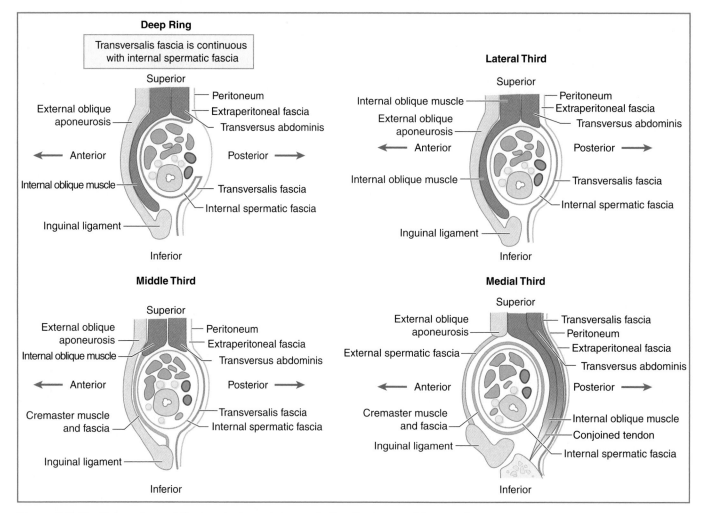

Figure 5-8. Sagittal sections of the inguinal canal demonstrating the layers of the canal.

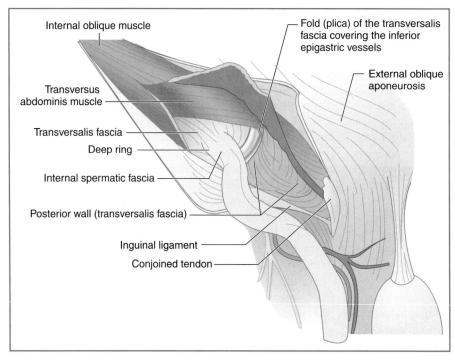

Figure 5-9. Posterior wall of the inguinal canal.

wall, and the internal oblique fibers overlying the deep ring cell contracts producing a protective effect.

The transversalis fascia (the inner investing layer of deep fascia) is the major component of the posterior wall (see Figs. 5-8 and 5-9). Medially, the conjoined tendon reinforces the posterior wall (see Fig. 5-8). The inferior epigastric vessels are located just medial to the deep ring, making this a key relationship. However, these vessels are in the plane of the subserous (extraperitoneal) fascia, which is deep to the transversalis fascia.

The posterior wall is also referred to as the inguinal or Hesselbach's triangle. The boundaries of the inguinal triangle consist of the inferior epigastric artery (laterally), inguinal ligament (inferiorly), and the lateral margin of the rectus sheath (medially).

The peritoneum and subserous (extraserous or extraperitoneal) fascia are found deep to the posterior inguinal wall.

Openings of the Inguinal Canal

The lateral or internal end of the canal is the deep (internal) inguinal ring, while the medial or external end of the canal is the superficial (external) inguinal ring.

The deep inguinal ring is the point where the transversalis fascia is extended out over the spermatic cord as a tubular fascial investment called the internal spermatic fascia (see Figs. 5-8 and 5-9). This is not an interruption or defect of the transversalis fascia, but is an out-pocketing, or evagination, of the fascia that looks like a dimple from the internal view. When viewed from the peritoneal cavity, the deep ring is always found just lateral to the lateral umbilical fold of peritoneum covering the inferior epigastric vessels, and it can be projected anteriorly to the midpoint of the inguinal region. When viewed from the inguinal canal, the deep ring is always found just lateral to the fold of the transversalis fascia covering the inferior epigastric vessels (see Fig. 5-8). The deep inguinal ring has a U slit–like shape when viewed internally with the open end of the U facing superolaterally almost in a vertical plane.

The superficial inguinal ring (see Fig. 5-8) is an opening in the inferomedial border of the external oblique aponeurosis. The superficial ring is triangular in shape, with the base being the pubic crest and apex facing superolaterally. It is just superior and lateral to the pubic tubercle and, in males, allows the spermatic cord to pass from the inguinal canal into the scrotum. The lateral (inferior) crus is stronger than the medial crus and is composed of aponeurotic fibers that are continuous with the inguinal ligament, and it attaches to the pubic tubercle with the inguinal ligament. The medial (superior) crus is formed by the aponeurotic fibers that insert into the pubic crest and symphysis. There are intercrural fibers running between the two crura, which prevent the crura from separating. The opening is covered with the outer investing layer of deep fascia (external oblique fascia, which is prolonged over the spermatic cord as the external spermatic fascia). The reflected inguinal ligament consists of fibers that arise from the lateral crus. The reflected inguinal ligament

passes posteriorly to the medial crus and anterior to the conjoint tendon to attach to the contralateral reflected inguinal ligament at the linea alba. The superficial ring is only one third to one half as large in women as in men because of the size of the round ligament versus the spermatic cord.

Contents of the Inguinal Canal

In females, the round ligament of the uterus and the ilioinguinal nerve (L1) are found in the inguinal canal. The ilioinguinal nerve provides general somatic sensory fibers to the anterior aspect of the labia majora, pubis, and medial thigh. This nerve does *not* enter the canal through the deep ring. It pierces the internal oblique near the anterior superior iliac spine to run obliquely downward and anteriorly between external and internal oblique muscles to enter the inguinal canal, where it lies anterolateral to the round ligament. However, in both sexes, the ilioinguinal nerve passes through the superficial ring.

In males, the spermatic cord and the ilioinguinal nerve are located in the inguinal canal. The ilioinguinal nerve enters the inguinal canal as described above. Thus, the nerve is on, but not in, the spermatic cord. The ilioinguinal nerve provides general somatic afferent (GSA) and postganglionic sympathetic fibers to the anterior scrotal wall, pubis, and medial thigh.

The spermatic cord is the neurovascular bundle of the testis and consists of the following structures:

- Ductus (vas) deferens
- Artery of the ductus deferens (a branch of the internal iliac artery)
- Testicular artery (a branch of the abdominal aorta)
- Pampiniform (vine-like) plexus of veins (which will drain into the testicular vein, which on the right drains into the inferior vena cava and on the left into the left renal vein)
- Cremasteric artery (a branch of the inferior epigastric artery)
- The genital branch of the genitofemoral nerve (L1–L2), providing motor innervation to the cremaster muscle and sensory innervation to the anterior scrotal wall
- Postganglionic sympathetics with general visceral afferents and probably parasympathetic fibers
- Lymphatics

The lymphatic drainage from the scrotum is to the inguinal lymph nodes, drainage from the ductus deferens is to the external iliac nodes, and drainage from the testis is to the lumbar lymph nodes.

Layers of the Scrotum and Spermatic Cord

In the scrotum, the outer fatty layer of superficial fascia (Camper's fascia) loses its fat and is replaced by a smooth muscle layer. This smooth muscle layer fuses with the inner membranous layer of superficial fascia (Scarpa's fascia) to form the *dartos tunic* (dark brown layer). Sympathetic nerves innervate the dartos tunic (Table 5-3).

TABLE 5-3. Comparison Between the Layers of the Anterior Abdominal Wall and the Scrotum Plus the Spermatic Cord

Anterior Abdominal Wall	Corresponding Layers of Scrotum and Spermatic Cord
Skin	Skin
Superficial fascia	Dartos tunic (smooth muscle [musculus dartos] plus membranous superficial fascia)
Outer investing layer of deep fascia on external oblique aponeurosis	External spermatic fascia
Internal oblique muscle and fascia	Cremaster muscle and fascia
Transversalis fascia	Internal spermatic fascia
Subserous fascia (also called extraperitoneal fascia)	Areolar fascia (both layers are found in the spermatic cord)
Peritoneum	Tunica vaginalis (sac partially surrounding testis that develops from processus vaginalis)

There is no external spermatic fascia within the inguinal canal. It is added to the cord at the superficial inguinal ring. In addition, there is no contribution of the transversus abdominis muscle to the layers surrounding the spermatic cord and of the scrotum.

The cremaster muscle (see Figs. 5-4 and 5-8) consists of loops of skeletal muscle, which arise from the internal oblique to run onto the spermatic cord down to the testis and up to the pubic tubercle (see Table 5-3). Fibers are best observed anterior to the spermatic cord as it passes posteriorly to the internal oblique muscle. The genital branch of the genitofemoral nerve (spinal cord segments L1–L2) innervates the cremaster muscle.

The cremaster reflex is a somatic reflex. Stroking the anteromedial aspect of the thigh of a male, which is innervated by the femoral branch of the genitofemoral nerve, will produce an elevation of the testis. The femoral branch of the genitofemoral nerve is the general somatic sensory arm of this reflex, while the genital branch of the same genitofemoral nerve is the general somatic motor arm. The fibers of the genitofemoral nerve arise from the L1 and L2 spinal cord segments. Therefore, this reflex is used to test the status of the L1 and L2 spinal cord segments.

The transversalis fascia is extended into the inguinal canal at the deep ring as the internal spermatic fascia (see Figs. 5-8 and 5-9 and Table 5-3).

The tunica vaginalis is the peritoneal covering of the testis. The visceral layer of the tunica vaginalis covers most of the testis except the posterior surface.

Development of the Inguinal Canal

The undifferentiated gonad along with a connective mass begins to develop in the posterior abdominal wall in the plane of the extraperitoneal fascia at the level of the 10th thoracic vertebra. The connective tissue mass forms a cord identified as the genitoinguinal ligament, which extends from the gonad to the developing labioscrotal swellings (Fig. 5-10A). The latter structures will develop into the labia majora in females or the scrotum in males. Both the genitoinguinal ligament and gonad lie external to the peritoneum. The abdominal wall forms with the genitoinguinal ligament maintaining its attachment to the labioscrotal swelling, thus the genitoinguinal ligament maps out the path of the future inguinal canal. In the male, the distal end of the genitoinguinal ligament is called the gubernaculum while in the female it is called the round ligament.

CLINICAL MEDICINE

Inguinal Hernia

A hernia is a protrusion of an organ from its normal anatomic position usually into or through the body wall. An inguinal hernia carries with it the normal anatomic coverings that exist between the body cavity and its new position. These coverings form a sac. Ten percent of males suffer from an inguinal hernia during their lifetime.

An indirect hernia is a congenital hernia in which the processus vaginalis of the peritoneum is not completely obliterated and still extends through the deep inguinal ring into the inguinal canal. The processus vaginalis is an embryologic outgrowth of the peritoneal cavity that moves along a preformed path. As it moves into the labioscrotal swellings, the processus vaginalis carries the layers of the wall with it to form the inguinal canal. In an indirect hernia, the neck of the herniating sac is at the site of the origin of the processus vaginalis, which is the deep inguinal ring. The key relationship is that the deep ring is lateral to the plane of the inferior epigastric vessels. Since the herniating sac passes through the deep ring, it is within the spermatic cord covered by all the layers of the spermatic cord in the inguinal canal, and thus, the spermatic cord appears fat.

In a direct hernia, the neck of the herniating sac is always found medial to the inferior epigastric vessels in Hesselbach's triangle, which is the posterior wall of the canal. A direct inguinal hernia usually occurs along the weakest portion of the canal, along the lower margin of the internal oblique muscle. The herniating organ and its visceral peritoneum pushes the parietal peritoneum and extraperitoneal fascia posterior to the wall and the transversalis fascia anteriorly, forcing the posterior wall ahead of it into the inguinal canal and often through the superficial inguinal ring. It should be clear that a direct inguinal hernia never passes through the deep ring.

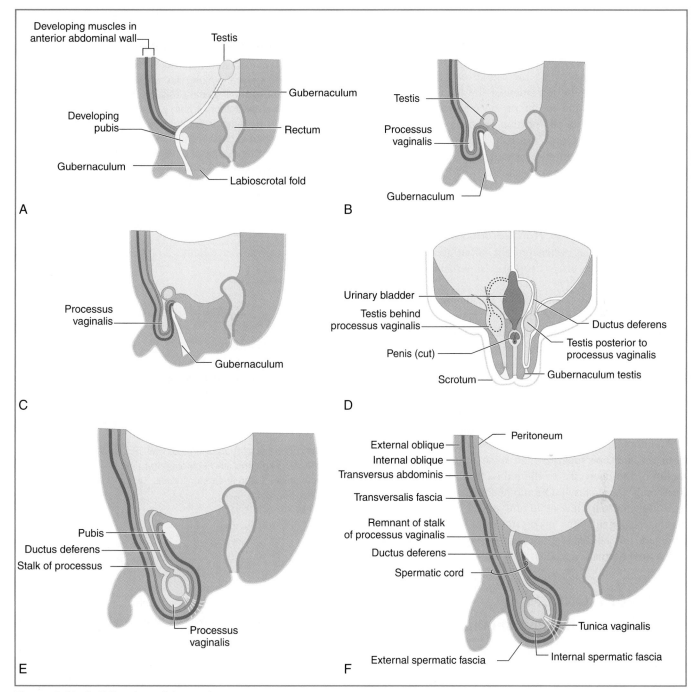

Figure 5-10. A–F, Descent of the testis.

Descent of the Testis

The descent of the testis has two stages: an intra-abdominal descent and an inguinal descent into the scrotum. The testis descends from the posterior abdominal wall to the position of the deep ring by week 26 (see Fig. 5-10B). It has been suggested that this phase of descent may be due to enlargement of the fetal pelvis, elongation of the embryo's trunk, or thickening of the gubernaculum, which is the distal, surviving portion of the genitoinguinal ligament in the male. At about the seventh month, an outpocketing of the peritoneal cavity, the processus vaginalis, passes through the abdominal wall, forming the inguinal canal (see Figs. 5-10B and 5-10C). Thus,

all layers of the lateral abdominal wall form some component of the canal and, excepting the transversus abdominis muscle, form the layers of the spermatic cord (see Figs. 5-10D and 5-10E and Table 5-3).

In the male, the testis descends posterior to the processus vaginalis but *not* in it, since the processus is part of the peritoneal cavity. The testis has migrated into the scrotum and is surrounded by the three layers of the spermatic cord. The processus vaginalis is normally obliterated from the superior pole of the testis to the deep ring (see Fig. 5-10F). This last, important step separates the inguinal canal and scrotum from the abdominal peritoneal cavity.

Descent of the Ovary

The ovary descends to the level of the developing pelvic brim. The cranial end of the genitoinguinal ligament in the female becomes the connective tissue of the suspensory ligament of the ovary while the caudal end is divided into two components by the formation of the uterus. The portion between the ovary and the uterus becomes the ligament of the ovary proper, and the portion between the uterus and labium majus is the round ligament. The processus vaginalis pushes through the anterior abdominal wall, forming the inguinal canal. The processus vaginalis is obliterated, and the female inguinal canal contains the round ligament of the uterus and the ilioinguinal nerve.

Specializations of the Transversalis Fascia

These specializations, when present, often allow for identification of structures either deep to or superficial to the transversalis fascia.

The interfoveolar ligament is a thickening of the transversalis fascia from the level of the transversus abdominis muscle to the inguinal ligament and on to the superior pubic ramus. It is found at the *medial boundary of the deep inguinal ring*. The interfoveolar ligament marks the presence of the inferior epigastric vessels, which are found deep to it in the plane of the extraperitoneal fascia. This ligament can be used to identify the inferior epigastric artery, which is not visible, since it lies in the plane of the extraperitoneal fascia.

The iliopubic tract is a thickening of the transversalis fascia from the anterior superior iliac spine or possibly from the region of the deep ring to the pubis. It marks the transition from transversalis fascia to femoral sheath. It is only evident from the internal view as it runs posteriorly (deep) to the inguinal ligament. This makes the iliopubic tract a useful landmark for the inguinal ligament during laparoscopy repair of inguinal hernia (Fig. 5-11).

CLINICAL MEDICINE

Cryptorchidism (Undescended Testis)

Cryptorchidism means hidden testis. The undescended testis can be found anywhere along the normal path of descent—inside the abdomen, inguinal canal, or upper scrotum. If the testis does not enter the scrotum within the first year, the individual has a greater incidence of sterility because spermatogenesis is dependent on a lower body temperature. In addition, cryptorchidism is a risk factor for testicular cancer and is associated with an increased incidence of indirect inguinal hernia. The pathophysiology is uncertain, but hormonal factors appear to play a role. Hormones such as human chorionic gonadotropin and gonadotropin-releasing hormone are used in the treatment with varying degrees of success.

CLINICAL MEDICINE

Sliding Inguinal Hernia

In a sliding hernia, the peritoneum of an organ, usually the sigmoid colon or cecum, forms one of the walls of the sac. When the surgeon attempts to separate the organ from the sac, the surgeon must be careful not to damage (perforate) the organ or the blood supply to that portion or segment of the organ.

Other hernias of the abdominal wall include femoral, umbilical, epigastric, and spigelian hernias. A spigelian hernia passes through the linea semilunaris, typically below the arcuate line.

●●● PERITONEUM

Embryology of the Peritoneum

The abdominal cavity is lined by a continuous serous membrane called the *peritoneum*, which consists of a thin layer of connective tissue lined by mesothelial cells (Fig. 5-12). Like other serous membranes, the peritoneum has two components: a *visceral peritoneum*, which is in intimate contact with the viscera and forms all of the peritoneal ligaments and mesenteries, and the *parietal peritoneum* in contact with the body wall. The embryonic lateral plate mesoderm splits into visceral (splanchnic) and somatic (parietal) mesoderm. The visceral peritoneum is derived from the visceral mesoderm, while the parietal (somatic) peritoneum is derived from the somatic mesoderm.

Anatomy of the Peritoneum

The peritoneal cavity is the potential space between the two layers of peritoneum—parietal and visceral—containing small amounts of serous fluid. *No* organs are within the peritoneal cavity. The peritoneal cavity is closed in males and open in females by means of the uterine tubes. The peritoneal cavity has two major subdivisions: the greater sac and the lesser sac. The greater sac consists of the entire cavity excluding the lesser sac. This subdivision for the most part is found posterior to the stomach and its attached peritoneal ligaments. These ligaments are the lesser omentum (Latin, "apron"), which consists of hepatoduodenal and hepatogastric ligaments, the greater omentum, and the peritoneum on the posterior abdominal wall (see Figs. 5-12 and 5-13).

Lesser Sac

The lesser sac (omental bursa) has an upper recess found anterior to the caudate lobe of the liver and a lower recess between the layers of the greater omentum (see Figs. 5-12 and 5-14). The boundaries of the lesser sac are the lesser omentum; the visceral peritoneum over the stomach; the greater omentum; the parietal peritoneum over the posterior

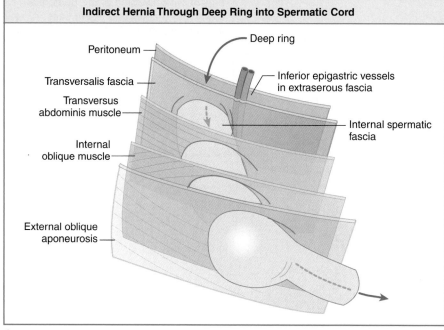

Indirect Hernia Through Deep Ring into Spermatic Cord

Peritoneum

Transversalis fascia

Transversus abdominis muscle

Internal oblique muscle

External oblique aponeurosis

Deep ring

Inferior epigastric vessels in extraserous fascia

Internal spermatic fascia

A

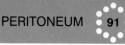

Figure 5-11. Path of indirect (**A**) and direct (**B**) hernia.

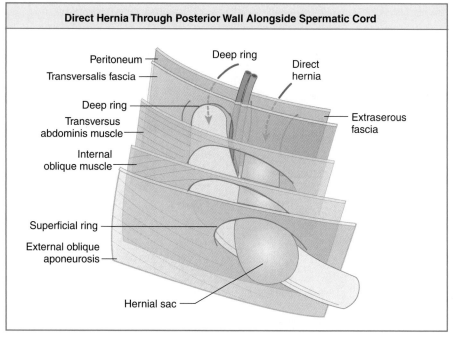

Direct Hernia Through Posterior Wall Alongside Spermatic Cord

Peritoneum

Transversalis fascia

Deep ring

Transversus abdominis muscle

Internal oblique muscle

Superficial ring

External oblique aponeurosis

Hernial sac

Deep ring

Direct hernia

Extraserous fascia

B

abdominal wall and diaphragm; the posterior leaf of the coronary ligament; on the left, the splenorenal and gastrosplenic ligaments; and on the right, the omental (epiploic) foramen (of Winslow).

The omental (epiploic) foramen (epiploon is Greek for omentum) is the site of communication between the lesser sac and the remainder of the peritoneal cavity or the greater sac (see Figs. 5-12 and 5-14). Its boundaries are anteriorly, the hepatoduodenal ligament; posteriorly, the peritoneum over the inferior vena cava and right crus of the diaphragm; superiorly, the peritoneum over the caudate lobe of the liver; and inferiorly, the peritoneum over the duodenum and the reflection of the hepatoduodenal ligament.

Peritoneal reflections are the points at which the parietal and visceral peritoneal layers are continuous. At these points, the peritoneum extends from the body wall to the organ it will surround. The peritoneum extending from the body wall as peritoneal ligaments or mesenteries to the intraperitoneal

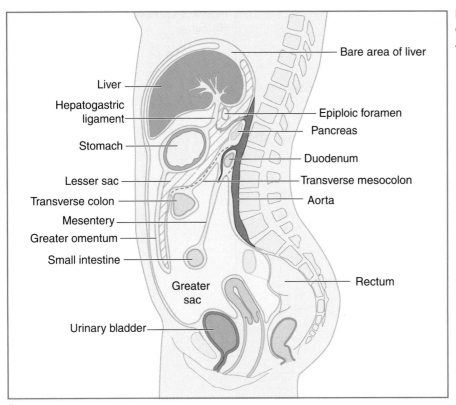

A

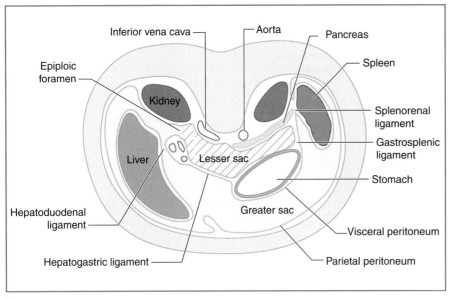

B

Figure 5-12. Division of the peritoneal cavity into greater and lesser sacs. **A,** Sagittal section. **B,** Cross-section.

organs is visceral peritoneum (see Figs. 5-12 and 5-13). Peritoneal ligaments are double layers of visceral peritoneum that stretch from the abdominal wall to an organ or from organ to organ. Many of these ligaments contain neurovascular bundles from the body wall to the intraperitoneal organs. Mesentery is a double layer of peritoneum that is attached to the abdominal wall and contains an organ and its neurovascular bundle. The mesentery (see Fig. 5-12) is similar to a peritoneal ligament but "slings" the intestine from the posterior abdominal walls. As such it is longer than the peritoneal

ligaments. An example is the "mesentery" (see Figs. 5-12A and 5-13) that suspends the jejunum and ileum from the posterior wall and contains intestinal branches of the superior mesenteric artery and vein as well as autonomic nerves and lymphatics that run with the superior mesenteric vessels. Examples of peritoneal ligaments are the splenorenal and gastrocolic ligaments (see Fig. 5-14). However, some ligaments do not contain neurovascular bundles.

Intraperitoneal organs are those organs which are surrounded and suspended by peritoneum. The peritoneal

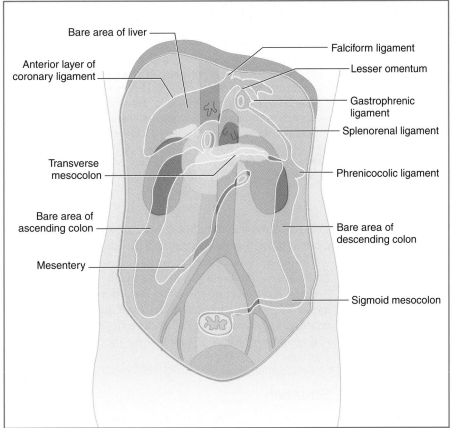

Figure 5-13. Retroperitoneal structures and posterior peritoneal sites of reflection.

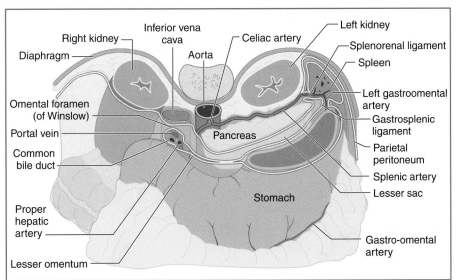

Figure 5-14. Lesser sac and stomach.

ligaments are also derived from the visceral mesoderm and are therefore classified as visceral peritoneum.

Retroperitoneal organs are those organs which may have peritoneum on one or more sides but are not suspended by peritoneum. These retroperitoneal organs are usually embedded in subserous (extraperitoneal) fascia in the body wall. Retroperitoneal organs may develop in a retroperitoneal position, or they may initially develop as intraperitoneal organs that become retroperitoneal by a process called fixation. These

latter organs are often referred to as secondarily retroperitoneal organs (Table 5-4).

●●● ABDOMINAL VISCERA

The abdominal cavity consists of all the structures found internal to the inner investing layer of deep fascia (endoabdominal fascia). This layer is also named according to the muscle that it is related to. Thus, the transversalis fascia is the

TABLE 5-4. Intraperitoneal and Retroperitoneal Organs

Intraperitoneal Organs	Retroperitoneal Organs
Stomach	Second and third portions of the duodenum
Liver and gallbladder	
Spleen	Pancreas (except the tail)
First and fourth parts of duodenum	Ascending colon
	Hepatic flexure
Jejunum and ileum	Splenic flexure
Cecum and appendix	Descending colon
Transverse colon	Rectum
Sigmoid colon	Kidneys and suprarenal glands

CLINICAL MEDICINE

Gastroesophageal Reflux Disease (GERD)

The function of the lower esophageal sphincter (LES) is to keep the acidic gastric contents out of the esophagus. The esophagus serves as a pump, the LES as a valve, and the stomach as a reservoir. In general, the intra-abdominal pressure is lower than the intraesophageal pressure. The etiology of gastroesophageal reflux disease (GERD) can involve any component of this system, including poor esophageal peristalsis, decreased LES pressure, and delayed gastric emptying.

inner investing layer of deep fascia internal to the transversus abdominalis muscle, the quadratus lumborum fascia is internal to the quadratus lumborum muscle, and the iliacus fascia is internal to the iliacus muscle. These fasciae are parts of a continuous fascial structure.

Esophagus

The portion of the esophagus found in the abdomen is about 1 cm of its total length. It enters the abdomen through the esophageal hiatus in the right crus of the diaphragm at vertebral level T10, to the left of the midline. The esophagus notches the superior visceral surface of the liver.

The esophagus empties into the stomach's cardiac region (Fig. 5-15). The lower esophageal (gastroesophageal) sphincter (LES) is composed of esophageal circular smooth muscle, which extends for 2 to 5 cm above the gastroesophageal junction. This sphincter is usually closed, but as the peristaltic wave approaches, the sphincter relaxes under the influence of the vagus nerves to allow the esophageal content to enter the

stomach. Subsequently, the sphincter closes, preventing regurgitation of the gastric content into the esophagus.

The lower esophagus receives preganglionic parasympathetic fibers from the vagus nerves, which synapse in its wall. Preganglionic sympathetic fibers arise from spinal cord segments T5 and T6, which for the most part synapse in the celiac ganglia or small ganglia close to the esophagus. The abdominal esophagus is supplied by the left gastric artery and vein.

Stomach

The stomach (see Fig. 5-15) is a mobile, dilated, J-shaped organ. Its main function is digestion, breaking food down into a semiliquid mass called *chyme*. The stomach has three layers of smooth muscle making up part of its wall: an innermost oblique, middle circular, and outermost longitudinal.

The stomach has two curvatures and two surfaces (see Fig. 5-15). It has a greater and a lesser curvature and anterior and posterior surfaces. The lesser curvature of the stomach lies to the right of the esophagus. It faces superiorly and to the right. The greater curvature is about four times larger than the lesser curvature and faces inferiorly and to the left. It is also

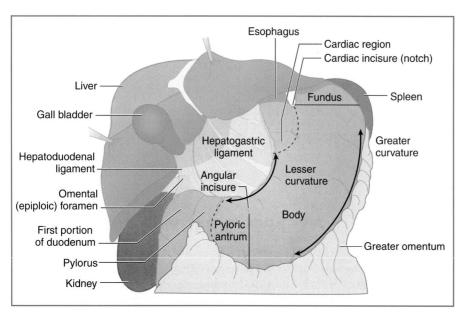

Figure 5-15. Stomach and the lesser omentum (hepatogastric and hepatoduodenal ligaments).

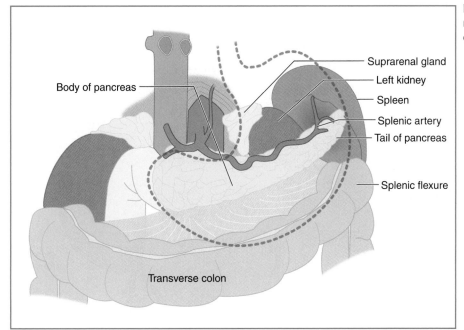

Figure 5-16. The outline of the stomach is represented with a dashed line to demonstrate the "bed of the stomach."

continuous with the fundus. The outer longitudinal smooth muscle layer is best developed at the curvatures. The stomach's cardiac incisure (notch) separates the esophagus from the stomach's fundus to the left.

In general, viscera with mesenteries are mobile. Most of the stomach is mobile owing to the presence of peritoneal ligaments (e.g., the lesser omentum, and the greater omentum; see Figs. 5-12 and 5-15). The embryonic *dorsal mesogastrium* produces most of the stomach's peritoneal ligaments: consisting of the greater omentum, the gastrosplenic, splenorenal, gastrophrenic, and gastrocolic ligaments. The embryonic *ventral mesogastrium* produces the lesser omentum, which consists of the hepatogastric and hepatoduodenal ligaments. In general, the stomach is located deep to the rib cage and costal margin on the left, but it may extend inferiorly for a varying length.

The stomach is fixed at the junction of the esophagus and stomach and again at the junction of the pylorus and duodenum. The esophageal junction is located at the level of the seventh costal cartilage to the left of T10–T11. The pyloric junction is to the right of the midline in the transpyloric plane (level of first lumbar vertebra).

The parts of the stomach (see Fig. 5-15) include the cardiac region, which is associated with the gastroesophageal junction; fundus; body; pyloric antrum; and pylorus.

The cardiac region is located at the gastroesophageal junction or where the esophagus joins the stomach. This region is separated from the pericardium of the heart by the diaphragm.

The fundus (blind end of a sac) is the upper distended region of the stomach, close to the left dome of the diaphragm. It is found to the left of the gastroesophageal (cardiac) region and is usually filled with gas or air. The fundus and cardiac portions meet at the cardiac notch (incisure). On the left, the fundus is continuous with the greater curvature. The spleen,

diaphragm, and gastrosplenic and gastrophrenic ligaments are posterior to it. The splenorenal ligament contains the splenic vessels, tail of the pancreas, lymph nodes, and sympathetic nerves. The gastrosplenic ligament, which is continuous with the splenorenal ligament, contains the left gastroepiploic vessels, short gastric vessels, and the sympathetic fibers and lymphatics that supply the fundus.

The body (see Fig. 5-15) is the major portion of the stomach. On the lesser curvature, it extends from the cardiac notch to the angular notch. On the greater curvature, it extends from the fundus to the pylorus.

The pyloric (Greek, "gatekeeper") region is the most distal constricted region of the stomach and is located at the junction of the stomach and duodenum. It begins at the angular notch and consists of the pyloric antrum just distal to the body; the pyloric canal, or the narrowing of the pyloric antrum; and the pyloric sphincter, which is a thickening of the inner circular layer of smooth muscle around the orifice or pylorus. The gastroduodenal vessels and the bile duct (common bile duct) are posterior to the pylorus.

Relationships

Structures found *anterior* to the stomach are the liver, greater peritoneal sac, left costal margin, and anterior abdominal wall (see Figs. 5-12 and 5-15). The lateral segment of the left lobe of the liver is anterior to the superior aspect of the stomach's body and lesser curvature. The pylorus makes an impression on the quadrate lobe, just to the left of the gallbladder.

The structures that are located *posterior* to the stomach (Fig. 5-16) are referred to as the "bed of the stomach." These structures include the

- Left suprarenal gland
- Superior pole of the left kidney
- Gastric surface of the spleen

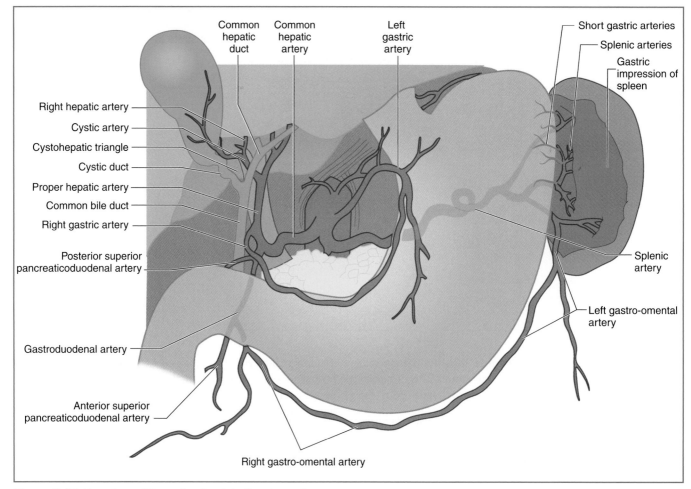

Figure 5-17. Branches of the celiac trunk to the stomach.

CLINICAL MEDICINE

Gastrotomy

A gastrostomy tube is used to feed a patient who can no longer swallow as a result of a disease such as cancer of the throat, Parkinson's disease, or stroke. The direct relationship between the anterior abdominal wall and the anterior surface of the stomach allows for the placement of a gastrostomy tube by means of an incision in the anterior wall and another in the anterior surface of the stomach.

- Body and tail of the pancreas
- Splenic artery just superior to the pancreas
- Transverse colon (which is often tucked posterior to the lateral aspect of the greater curvature)

Blood Supply to the Stomach

The blood supply to the stomach consists of celiac artery branches: the left and right gastric arteries to the lesser curvature, the four to six short gastric arteries to the fundus, and the left and right gastro-omental (gastroepiploic) arteries to the greater curvature (Figs. 5-17 and 5-18). The celiac artery is a branch of the aorta that immediately gives rise to the left gastric artery, common hepatic artery, and splenic artery.

The left gastric artery is a relatively large vessel. It runs along the posterior abdominal wall to reach the reflection of the lesser omentum at the lesser curvature. Here, it anastomoses with the much smaller *right gastric artery*. The right gastric artery is variable in its origin. It can be a small branch of the proper hepatic, or common hepatic, artery. It passes through the lesser omentum to anastomose with the left gastric artery.

The right gastro-omental artery is one of the terminal branches of the gastroduodenal artery. The latter artery is a branch of the common hepatic artery. The right gastro-omental artery runs in the gastrocolic (ligament) portion of the greater omentum. The short gastric arteries are branches of the splenic artery (see Fig. 5-17) and reach the fundus by passing through the gastrosplenic ligament. The left gastro-omental artery (see Fig. 5-17) is also a branch of the splenic artery. It also reaches the greater curvature by running in the gastrosplenic ligament to reach the gastrocolic portion of the greater omentum on the left. A careful examination of these arteries reveals that there is a complete collateral circulation around the stomach and that every major branch of the celiac trunk participates (see Figs. 5-17 and 5-18).

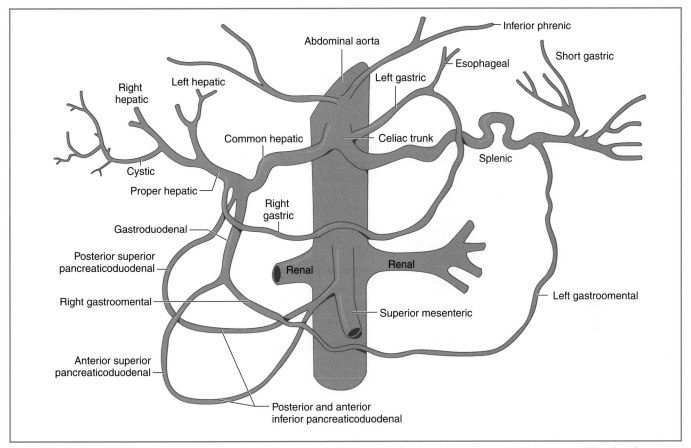

Figure 5-18. Branches of the celiac trunk have pancreaticoduodenal branches that anastomose with pancreatoduodenal branches of the superior mesenteric artery.

Since the arteries follow the curvatures, the anterior and posterior surfaces of the stomach do not receive as good a blood supply as do the curvatures. Thus, the midpoints of either the anterior or posterior surfaces are the best points to incise and enter the stomach in order to minimize bleeding.

The stomach's venous drainage is by veins that follow the arterial supply. These veins drain into the portal vein, which is formed by the splenic vein joining the superior mesenteric vein posterior to the neck of the pancreas. The left gastric vein, also called the coronary vein, drains much of the lesser curvature and the lower portion of the esophagus. The short gastrics and the left gastro-omental veins drain into the splenic vein, while the right gastro-omental vein usually drains into the superior mesenteric vein.

Innervation of the Stomach

The innervation of the stomach includes parasympathetic and sympathetic nerves. The parasympathetic supply is from the *vagus* nerves, which (Fig. 5-19) form the anterior and posterior esophageal plexuses in the thorax. These plexuses in turn form the *anterior and posterior vagal trunks* just before they enter the abdominal cavity. Here, they continue on the anterior and posterior surfaces of the esophagus and then onto the anterior and posterior surfaces of the stomach, about 1 or 2 cm from the lesser curvature.

The anterior vagal trunk follows the lesser curvature to reach the pylorus. However, this nerve has a hepatic branch that reaches the liver and gallbladder by passing through the lesser omentum.

The posterior vagal trunk divides high on the cardiac region. This nerve has a celiac branch that reaches the celiac plexus by running with the left gastric artery. The posterior vagus nerve does *not* synapse in the celiac plexus but continues along the aorta to the root of the superior mesenteric artery to reach the superior mesenteric plexus. The posterior vagus nerve then continues along the superior mesenteric artery and its branches to synapse in the wall of the organs derived from the midgut.

The stomach's preganglionic sympathetic innervation arises from neuronal cell bodies in the lateral horn of spinal cord segments T6–T9. These neuronal cell bodies give rise to fibers that pass through the established pathway to thoracic sympathetic chain ganglia T6–T9. These preganglionic fibers do *not* synapse in these sympathetic ganglia but pass through them to give rise to the root of the *greater splanchnic nerve* (see Fig. 2-7), which passes through the crura of the diaphragm (see Fig. 5-19). The greater splanchnic nerve synapses in the celiac ganglia, which are located tightly around the origin of the celiac trunk. Sympathetic fibers from the celiac plexus supply the stomach. Postganglionic sympathetic fibers from the

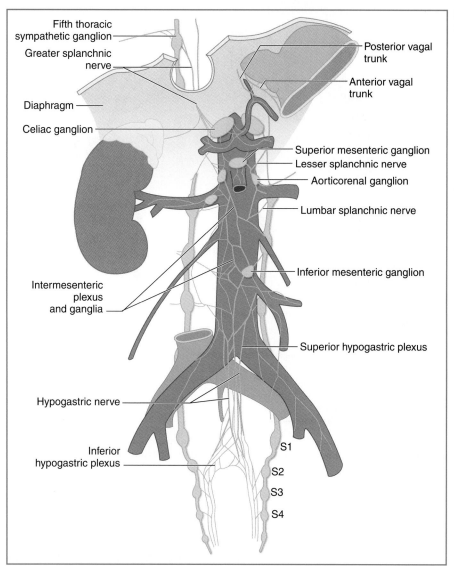

Figure 5-19. Abdominal sympathetic nerves, ganglia, and plexuses.

Fifth thoracic sympathetic ganglion

Greater splanchnic nerve

Diaphragm

Celiac ganglion

Intermesenteric plexus and ganglia

Hypogastric nerve

Inferior hypogastric plexus

Posterior vagal trunk

Anterior vagal trunk

Superior mesenteric ganglion

Lesser splanchnic nerve

Aorticorenal ganglion

Lumbar splanchnic nerve

Inferior mesenteric ganglion

Superior hypogastric plexus

S1

S2

S3

S4

Sensory Innervation (Abdominal Pain)

General visceral afferent fibers for pain from stomach and other parts of the abdominal gut follow the sympathetic fibers that innervate the specific organ. For example, pain fibers from the stomach follow the postganglionic fibers from the celiac ganglion and then the greater splanchnic nerves back to the T5 to T9 nerves. *For all organs* supplied by the greater splanchnic nerves, pain (GVA) fibers enter the thoracic spinal nerves 5–9, have their neuronal cell bodies in the dorsal root ganglia T5–T9, and synapse in spinal cord segments T5–T9. The GSA fibers from thoracic dermatomes T5–T9 share the same dorsal root ganglia that receive general visceral sensory fibers from the stomach. The *key point* is that both the general somatic sensory fibers from the abdominal wall and the general visceral sensory fibers from the stomach

celiac ganglia follow the arteries to reach the stomach and other organs supplied by the celiac plexus (i.e., organs derived from the caudal foregut).

converge on and synapse with the same second-order sensory neuronal cell bodies in the spinal cord. The patient perceives the referred pain in the somatic region that coincides with dermatomes T5–T9, which in the case of the stomach would be the epigastric and left hypochondriac region. However,

CLINICAL MEDICINE

Abdominal Pain

Many factors are involved in interpreting abdominal pain. Acute pain is often produced by rupture of an organ and may involve the body wall (somatic pain). Pain that has a gradual onset and is poorly localized is often produced by distention of the organ's lumen, ischemia (decreased blood supply), or a gradual increase of inflammation. It is imperative that the examiner take a careful history first and examine the patient carefully to interpret the pain properly. Pain can begin as referred pain and spread or shift to another region if the parietal peritoneum becomes inflamed.

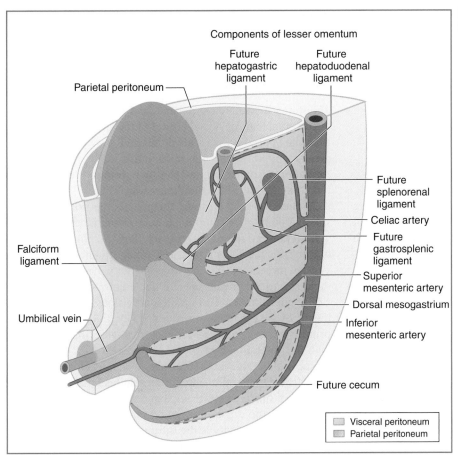

Figure 5-20. Arterial supply of caudal foregut, midgut, and hindgut.

different organs can receive sympathetic fibers from different spinal cord levels, such as the spleen T6–T8.

●●● DEVELOPMENT OF THE STOMACH AND OTHER FOREGUT ORGANS

Arterial Supply to the Foregut and the Midgut

The parts of the future abdominopelvic gut are the caudal end of the foregut, the midgut, and parts of the hindgut. Each segment of the gut, starting with the caudal foregut, midgut, and hindgut, is supplied by a single major artery (Fig. 5-20). These arteries supply the organs that develop from that part of the gut.

The celiac artery supplies the caudal foregut, which gives rise to the esophagus, stomach, duodenum up to the duodenal papilla, pancreas, biliary ducts, gallbladder, and liver.

The superior mesenteric artery supplies midgut organs. The midgut organs include the remainder of the duodenum, ileum, cecum, ascending colon, and proximal half to two thirds of the transverse colon.

The inferior mesenteric artery supplies the hindgut organs, which consists of the remainder of the transverse colon, descending colon, sigmoid colon, rectum, and anal canal to the pectinate line.

Transitional regions are supplied by two of the above arteries. Anatomically, the foregut is continuous with the midgut just distal to the duodenal papilla (the common opening for both the common bile duct and pancreatic duct into the duodenum). The midgut is continuous with the hindgut approximately where the proximal half to two thirds of the transverse colon meets the remaining distal portion of the transverse colon. The hindgut is continuous with the somatic portion of the anal canal at the pectinate line.

These transitional points represent regions of collateral circulation that can be identified by knowledge of the development of the gut. The foregut-midgut collateral circulation occurs just distal to the duodenal papilla, where the superior pancreaticoduodenal arteries, which arise from the celiac trunk branches, anastomose with the inferior pancreaticoduodenal arteries, which arise from the superior mesenteric artery (see Figs. 5-18 and 5-20). The midgut-hindgut collateral circulation occurs across the transverse colon. Here, the middle colic branch of the superior mesenteric artery anastomoses with the left colic branch of the inferior mesenteric artery to form the marginal artery (of Drummond). The visceral-somatic collateral circulation takes place across the pectinate line of the anal canal, where the superior rectal branch of the inferior mesenteric artery anastomoses with the inferior rectal artery of the pudendal artery. The superior rectal artery also anastomoses with the middle rectal branch of the internal iliac artery.

●●● DEVELOPMENT OF THE CAUDAL FOREGUT

Development of the Liver

The gut begins as a simple tube suspended from the posterior wall by the primitive *dorsal mesentery* (see Fig. 5-20). Initially, a swelling of the caudal foregut develops into the future stomach. At the same time, a cord of endoderm and adjacent visceral mesoderm starts just distal to the developing stomach and grows into the septum transversum as the liver bud, which develops into the biliary ducts, gallbladder, and liver. The ventral pancreatic bud is an outgrowth of the gut that originates very close to the origin of the liver bud, while just proximal to the origin of the liver bud another outgrowth occurs that is the dorsal pancreatic bud.

The liver begins developing in the septum transversum. It quickly outgrows the septum transversum, extending caudally into the peritoneal cavity. However, it retains an association with the developing diaphragm that becomes the bare area of the liver in the adult. Here, the liver comes into contact with the fascia of the inferior surface of the diaphragm. As the liver outgrows the diaphragm, it grows into the ventral mesentery. There is no mesentery ventral to the developing gut below the level of the foregut; i.e., the midgut and hindgut do not have a ventral mesentery. The liver now occupies the ventral mesentery that lies between the fetus's ventral wall and the stomach. The mesentery posterior to the gut is the dorsal mesentery. The dorsal mesentery of the stomach is referred to as the dorsal mesogastrium.

All of the peritoneal ligaments associated with the liver and the lesser curvature of the stomach are derived from the ventral mesentery. The falciform (sickle-shaped) ligament is the portion of the ventral mesentery between the ventral wall and the liver, since it is sickle-shaped. The lesser omentum stretches between the liver and the stomach and first portion of the duodenum. It can also be separated into the hepatogastric ligament, which stretches between the liver and the lesser curvature, and the hepatoduodenal ligament, which stretches between the liver and the duodenum. The coronary ligament of the liver is the peritoneal reflection from the diaphragm to the liver that is found at the margins of the liver's bare area. Peritoneal ligaments typically have two contiguous layers. However, the coronary ligament is unusual in that the bare area separates its two layers of peritoneum from each other so that the coronary ligament's superior and inferior layers have separate sites of reflection. However, the two layers do come together in the typical manner in the formation of the right and left triangular ligaments, the falciform ligament, and the lesser omentum.

Unlike the liver, the spleen is not an outgrowth of the foregut. It develops coincidentally with the gut in the dorsal mesogastrium but independently of the gut. However, its splenic artery is a branch from the celiac trunk.

Rotation of the Stomach and Formation of the Lesser Sac

The stomach primordium enlarges and broadens in the anteroposterior plane. The dorsal border of the stomach grows faster than the ventral border. This differential growth produces the greater curvature and lesser curvature of the stomach. The formation of the lesser sac can be accounted for by several phenomena that occur simultaneously.

At the level of the caudal foregut, the peritoneal cavity is subdivided into a right and left component by the dorsal and ventral mesenteries of the stomach (Figs. 5-21 and 5-22). That is not true for the midgut and hindgut, since they lack a ventral mesentery. The peritoneal cavity becomes partially divided into the greater sac and the lesser sac, which is posterior to the stomach. These two subdivisions communicate by means of the omental foramen (see Figs. 5-12 and 5-13). The primitive dorsal mesogastrium is relatively thick compared with the ventral mesogastrium. Active excavation of the dorsal mesogastrium and rotation results in the development of the lesser sac. On its right side, little vacuoles form and coalesce to make a single cavity that expands transversely and superiorly within the dorsal mesogastrium and to the right of the esophagus. This cavity is the future lesser sac. The developing diaphragm and the liver cut off the uppermost part of the developing lesser sac.

Rotation of the Stomach

Rotation of the stomach with a concurrent rearrangement of its mesenteries is the second step in this process. The liver, stomach, spleen, aorta, and visceral peritoneum forming the ligaments are initially found in the midline (see Figs. 5-20 and 5-21). The stomach undergoes a 90-degree clockwise rotation to the right through its longitudinal axis (see Figs. 5-21 and 5-22). This results in the liver, ventral mesentery, and lesser curvature of the stomach moving to the right. As the right side of the stomach becomes its dorsal surface, the right vagus is now located on the posterior aspect of the lesser curvature of the stomach and attached esophagus. The stomach's greater curvature, spleen, and dorsal mesentery (the future greater omentum) will move to the left. As rotation results in the stomach's left side becoming its ventral surface, the left vagus is now located on the anterior surface of the lesser curvature and the attached esophagus.

Owing to the differential growth of the greater curvature and 90-degree rotation, the axis of the stomach shifts from a longitudinal (sagittal) plane to a coronal plane (see Figs. 5-21 and 5-22). The second rotation takes place in the coronal plane. The distal end of the foregut, which is the pylorus and proximal duodenum, rotates from its caudal position to a position superior and to the right. This rotation brings the pylorus and adjacent duodenum into close proximity to the liver. In the adult, these organs make impressions on the liver's visceral surface. This narrowing of space between

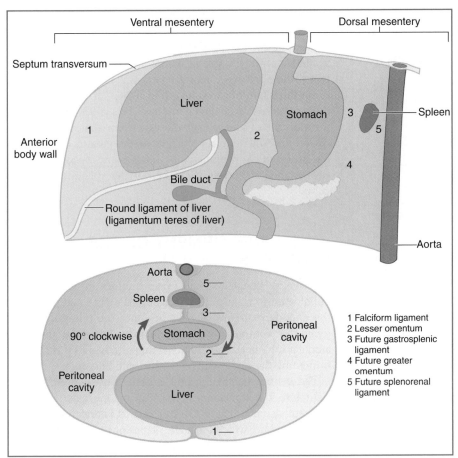

Figure 5-21. Before the 90-degree clockwise rotation of the stomach.

1 Falciform ligament
2 Lesser omentum
3 Future gastrosplenic ligament
4 Future greater omentum
5 Future splenorenal ligament

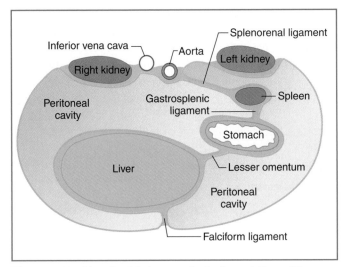

Figure 5-22. After the 90-degree clockwise rotation of the stomach.

the pylorus and liver contributes to the formation of the omental foramen.

Formation of the Lesser Sac

The lesser sac (omental bursa) (Figs. 5-23 and 5-24) has an upper recess found anterior to the caudate lobe of the liver and a lower recess between the layers of the greater omentum.

The peritoneum is reflected over the duodenum to contribute to the hepatoduodenal ligament. This point is the right gastropancreatic fold, and this is where the hepatic portal vein, proper hepatic artery, and bile duct enter the hepatoduodenal ligament. It is important to remember that the peritoneal cavity is considered one unit that is subdivided into the greater and lesser sacs.

Formation of the Peritoneal Ligaments from the Dorsal Mesogastrium

The differential growth of the dorsal border of the stomach is accompanied by a simultaneous growth of the dorsal mesogastrium. The presence of the spleen is used to separate the continuous dorsal mesogastrium into the splenorenal and gastrosplenic ligaments (see Figs. 5-21, 5-23, and 5-24). Upon extensive growth, the inferior portion of the dorsal mesogastrium becomes the greater omentum. However, since they are all subdivisions of the dorsal mesogastrium, they are continuous with each other. This allows the splenic artery to run from the posterior wall through one ligament (the splenorenal ligament) to reach the spleen and then continue through a continuous ligament (the gastrosplenic ligament) to reach the fundus, or through the anterior layers of the greater omentum to reach the right side of the greater curvature of the stomach.

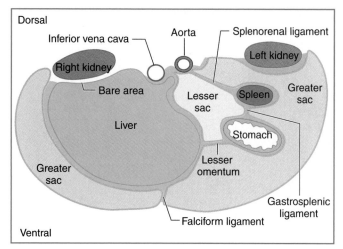

Figure 5-23. Development of greater and lesser sacs of the peritoneal cavity.

The greater omentum (see Fig. 5-12) attaches the greater curvature of the stomach to the posterior abdominal wall. As the stomach's greater curvature develops, the adjacent greater omentum also grows to accommodate this differential growth and coronal rotation. Consequently, the greater omentum folds upon itself, producing a four-layered peritoneal structure that consists of two anterior and two posterior layers (see Fig. 5-12). The inferior recess of the lesser sac is found between the anterior and posterior layers of the greater omentum (see Fig. 5-12). After birth, these four layers are usually fused inferiorly, forming a variably fat-filled omental apron. The anterior two layers contain the gastro-omental arteries and veins, which are found close to the greater curvature of the stomach. In addition, following the concurrent midgut rotation, the transverse mesocolon will fuse with the greater omentum's two posterior layers (see Fig. 5-12).

The splenorenal ligament was originally in the midline of the embryo (see Fig. 5-21). It migrates anterior to the left kidney during the 90-degree rotation of the stomach. This ligament carries the splenic artery and vein to the spleen. The tail of the developing pancreas extends into this ligament to reach the hilum of the spleen (Fig. 5-24).

The gastrosplenic ligament (see Figs. 5-23 and 5-24) is the portion of the dorsal mesogastrium that connects the spleen and the superior portion of the greater curvature of the stomach. It contains the short gastric vessels and left gastro-omental vessels (branches of the splenic artery and vein).

●●● DEVELOPMENT OF THE PANCREAS

The ventral pancreatic bud arises in close proximity to the initial site of origin of the liver bud. The proximal portion of the endodermal cord of cells becomes the bile duct, which joins the ventral pancreatic duct to form the duodenal ampulla (of Vater). The duodenal ampulla typically is the duct formed by the main pancreatic duct and bile duct.

The ventral pancreatic bud is carried dorsally and to the right into the dorsal mesogastrium by the rotation of the adjacent stomach (Fig. 5-25). It is carried inferior to the dorsal pancreatic bud, which forms the superior portion of the head, neck, body, and tail of the pancreas. The ventral pancreas, which forms the inferior portion of the head and the uncinate process, has a separate duct. The ducts of the ventral and dorsal pancreas join. The ventral pancreatic duct becomes the main passageway for secretion for both the inferior pancreatic head and its body and tail derived from the dorsal pancreatic bud. Often an accessory pancreatic duct remains as a remnant of the proximal portion of the dorsal pancreatic duct (see

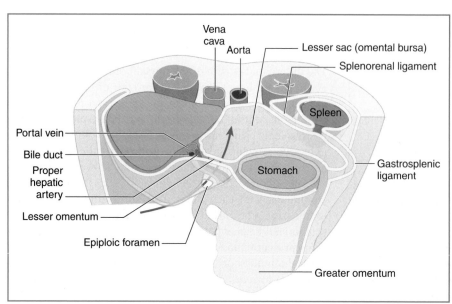

Figure 5-24. Lesser sac (omental bursa) of the peritoneal cavity.

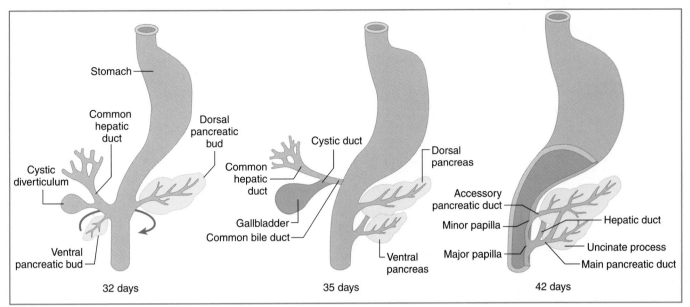

Figure 5-25. Development of the pancreas.

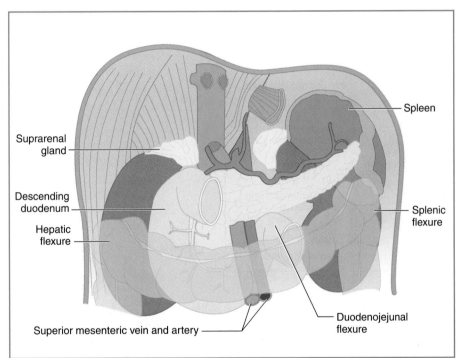

Figure 5-26. Anterior relationships of the duodenum.

Fig. 5-25). It will always enter the duodenum proximal to the duodenal papilla. This papilla is the nipple-like elevation that marks the entrance of the duodenal ampulla.

●●● DUODENUM

The duodenum (Figs. 5-26 and 5-27) is the C-shaped first section of the small intestine, which is mostly retroperitoneal. It is approximately 12 inches long. Its wall has only two layers of smooth muscle—an inner circular and an outer longitudinal. The primary functions of the duodenum are the digestion of chyme and the absorption of the breakdown products.

The Four Parts of the Duodenum

The superior segment has a proximal part and a distal part. The proximal part of this segment, into which the pylorus protrudes, is an *intraperitoneal* structure. The superior duodenal segment runs superiorly to the right and posteriorly at approximately vertebral level L1. Here, it makes an impression on the visceral (posteroinferior) surface of the liver just to the right of the neck of the gallbladder (see Figs. 5-19 and 5-28).

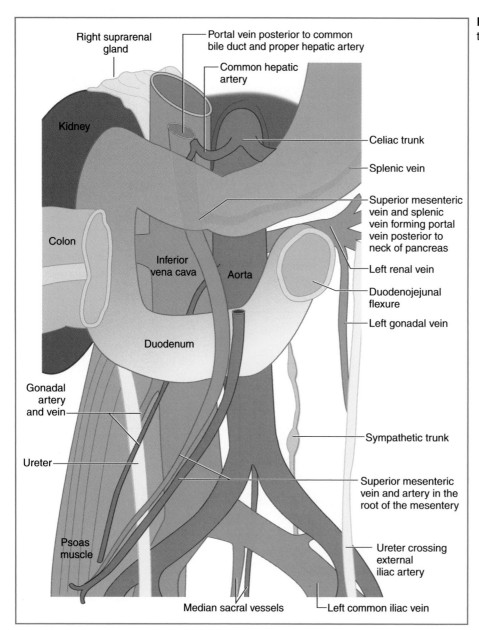

Figure 5-27. Posterior relationships of the duodenum.

Right suprarenal gland

Portal vein posterior to common bile duct and proper hepatic artery

Common hepatic artery

Kidney

Celiac trunk

Splenic vein

Superior mesenteric vein and splenic vein forming portal vein posterior to neck of pancreas

Colon

Inferior vena cava

Aorta

Left renal vein

Duodenojejunal flexure

Left gonadal vein

Duodenum

Gonadal artery and vein

Ureter

Sympathetic trunk

Superior mesenteric vein and artery in the root of the mesentery

Psoas muscle

Ureter crossing external iliac artery

Median sacral vessels

Left common iliac vein

The first part of the superior segment is found in the hepatoduodenal ligament and is freely mobile (see Fig. 5-12). This portion of the duodenum is the inferior boundary of the omental foramen (of Winslow). The bile duct, gastroduodenal artery, and portal vein are found posterior to the superior segment of the duodenum (see Fig. 5-24).

The descending segment begins at the superior duodenal flexure and is retroperitoneal. The bile duct and the main pancreatic duct join to form the hepatopancreatic ampulla (of Vater) within the major duodenal papilla (see Fig. 5-28). An ampulla is a dilated portion of a duct or canal. The major duodenal papilla (of Vater) is located on the posteromedial aspect of the longitudinal folds, or plica, of the duodenum. A minor duodenal papilla for the accessory pancreatic duct may be present just superior to the major duodenal papilla.

The fundus and body of the gallbladder are often found on the lateral side of the upper portion of the descending segment. A diseased gallbladder or duodenum may produce adhesion and subsequently a fistula here. The descending segment of the duodenum passes anteriorly to the right renal hilum and sinus, renal vessels, and ureter (renal pelvis) to the level of the inferior pole of the right kidney (see Fig. 5-27). Thus, it is in contact with the medial side of the right kidney as it descends from the level of the first lumbar vertebra to the inferior margin of the third lumbar vertebra. The descending duodenum is crossed by the transverse mesocolon, which lies anterior to this segment (see Fig. 5-26). The head of the pancreas is found in intimate contact with the medial aspect of the descending duodenal segment.

The horizontal (transverse) segment, which begins at the inferior duodenal flexure, is also retroperitoneal. It lies anterior to the right psoas major muscle, inferior vena cava, aorta, right ureter, gonadal vessels, and the third lumbar vertebra (see Fig. 5-27). The superior mesenteric vein and artery and

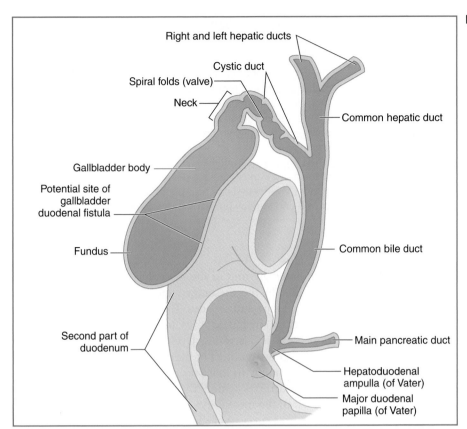

Figure 5-28. Major duodenal papilla.

Labels in figure:
- Right and left hepatic ducts
- Cystic duct
- Spiral folds (valve)
- Neck
- Common hepatic duct
- Gallbladder body
- Potential site of gallbladder duodenal fistula
- Fundus
- Common bile duct
- Second part of duodenum
- Main pancreatic duct
- Hepatoduodenal ampulla (of Vater)
- Major duodenal papilla (of Vater)

the root of the mesentery are anterior to the horizontal segment.

The ascending segment is still retroperitoneal. It ascends and turns anteriorly at the level of the second lumbar vertebra about 2 cm to the left of the midline. The duodenojejunal flexure is supported by the suspensory ligament of the duodenum (of Treitz), which passes from the right crus of the diaphragm in front of the aorta and behind the pancreas to reach the outer muscular coat of the duodenojejunal flexure. The suspensory ligament is a connective tissue ligament with striated muscle in the portion close to the crus of the diaphragm and smooth muscle close to the duodenum.

Blood Supply to the Duodenum

The first branch of the gastroduodenal artery is the supraduodenal artery, which supplies the first part of the duodenum. This artery can be used to identify the first part of the duodenum.

The duodenum's major blood supply (see Fig. 5-18) consists of the superior and inferior pancreaticoduodenal arteries. The pancreaticoduodenal arteries have both anterior and posterior branches that form arcades, which run in the groove between the head of the pancreas and the duodenum. Thus, the duodenum receives most of its blood supply from its pancreatic surface. Adjacent arteries also help supply the duodenum such as the right gastric, supraduodenal, and gastroduodenal arteries.

The superior pancreaticoduodenal arteries are branches of the gastroduodenal artery. The anterosuperior pancreaticoduodenal artery is a terminal branch of the gastroduodenal artery, while the posterosuperior pancreaticoduodenal artery arises higher from the gastroduodenal artery and runs to the right to wind around the bile duct to reach the posterior surface of the pancreas (see Fig. 5-18). The inferior pancreaticoduodenal artery is the first branch of the superior mesenteric artery. This artery divides into anterior and posterior branches that *anastomose* with the branches of the anterior and posterosuperior pancreaticoduodenal arteries, respectively. Thus, these anastomoses occur between branches of the celiac trunk and the superior mesenteric artery. They represent the only anastomosis between vessels that supply embryonic foregut and midgut derivatives. The venous drainage is provided by means of tributaries of the portal vein.

Innervation of the Duodenum

The parasympathetic innervation to the duodenum is the vagal trunks. The duodenum receives postganglionic sympathetic fibers from the celiac ganglia and plexus as well as the superior mesenteric ganglia. Preganglionic sympathetic fibers to this plexus are from both the greater and lesser splanchnic nerves. The fibers of the greater splanchnic nerve for the duodenum arise from spinal cord segments (levels) T7–T9. The lesser splanchnic nerve fibers for the duodenum arise

CLINICAL MEDICINE

Ligament of Treitz

The ligament of Treitz is used to locate the duodenojejunal flexure. It is also the *clinical* dividing line between the upper and lower gastrointestinal tracts. Most gastrointestinal hemorrhage is above the ligament of Treitz, coming from the esophagus, stomach, or duodenum.

HISTOLOGY

The Duodenum

The interior of the duodenum has a velvety appearance owing to the presence of thousands of villi. A villus is a finger-like projection of the mucosa into the lumen of the duodenum. The villi are composed of a loose connective tissue covered by an epithelium whose cells are specialized for digestion and absorption.

The submucosa underlies the mucosa and is a connective tissue framework. Brunner's glands are submucosal mucous glands. Their secretions help neutralize the acidity of the chyme and thereby protect the duodenal walls

from spinal cord segment (level) T10(11). The postganglionic fibers follow the branches of the arteries. Referred pain produced by duodenal peptic ulcers is perceived in the epigastric region (Table 5-5).

●●● JEJUNUM AND ILEUM

The jejunum and ileum (see Fig. 5-1) are the last two parts of the small intestine and are both *intraperitoneal* organs. Like the duodenum, they have two layers of smooth muscle in their walls. There is a gradual change from the jejunum to the ileum. Observing the proximal jejunum and terminal ileum best demonstrates their characteristic differences (Table 5-6).

Blood Supply to the Jejunum and Ileum

The blood supply to the jejunum and ileum is from the intestinal branches of the superior mesenteric artery (SMA),

which enter the root of the mesentery to reach the intestine (Fig. 5-29). In the mesentery, the intestinal arteries form a series of loops and arcades. The last arcades (see Fig. 5-29) give rise to straight arteries (*arteriae rectae*). The straight arteries are end arteries. Occlusion of these arteries could result in an infarct (area of necrosis) owing to insufficiency of the blood supply to that portion of the gut (see Fig. 5-29).

These arteries enter the mesenteric surface (surface attached to the mesentery) and then reach the antimesenteric surface (free surface) of the intestine. Transection of the small intestine followed by anastomosis of the two surfaces usually is done by means of an oblique section. This procedure retains more of the mesenteric surface than of the antimesenteric

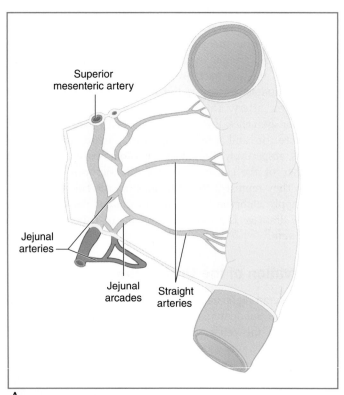

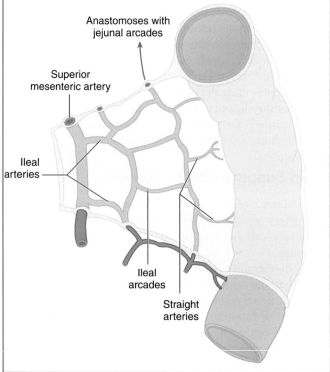

A   B

Figure 5-29. Blood supply to jejunum (**A**) and ileum (**B**).

TABLE 5-5. Sympathetic Innervation of the Abdominal Gastrointestinal Tract

Organ	Spinal Cord Level	Path of Innervation	Location of Referred Pain
Esophagus	T5–T6	Preganglionic fibers in the greater splanchnic nerves synapse on small adjacent ganglia or in the celiac ganglia Postganglionic fibers go directly to the esophagus or follow the left gastric artery	Substernal esophagitis can be confused with referred cardiac pain due to myocardial infarct of the diaphragmatic surface
Stomach	(T6)T7–T9	Preganglionic fibers in the greater splanchnic nerves synapse in the celiac ganglia Postganglionic fibers follow branches of the celiac artery to reach the stomach	Epigastric and left hypochondriac region
Duodenum (first segment only)	T7–T9	Preganglionic fibers in the greater splanchnic nerves synapse in the celiac ganglia Postganglionic fibers follow branches of the celiac artery to reach the first duodenal segment	Epigastric region
Duodenum (distal three segments)	(T9)T10–T11	Preganglionic fibers run in the lesser splanchnic nerves and synapse in the superior mesenteric ganglia Postganglionic fibers run with the arteries to reach the distal three segments of the duodenum	
Liver	T6–T9	Preganglionic fibers in the greater splanchnic nerves synapse in the celiac ganglia. Postganglionic fibers follow branches of the celiac trunk to the liver	Epigastric region and right hypochondrium Irritation of diaphragm results in pain referred to right shoulder tip
Gallbladder and bile ducts	(T6)T7–T9	Preganglionic fibers in the greater splanchnic nerves synapse in the celiac ganglia Postganglionic fibers follow branches of the celiac trunk to the gallbladder	Right hypochondrium and adjacent epigastric region
Spleen	T6–T8	Preganglionic fibers in the greater splanchnic nerves synapse in the celiac ganglia Postganglionic fibers follow the splenic artery to the spleen	Left hypochondriac region
Pancreas	T8–T9(T10)	Preganglionic fibers run in the greater splanchnic nerves (with a small contribution from the lesser splanchnic nerve) and synapse in the celiac and superior mesenteric ganglia The postganglionic sympathetic fibers follow branches of the arteries to the pancreas	Epigastric region; may overlap with upper umbilical region
Jejunum and ileum	T10–T11	Preganglionic fibers run in the lesser splanchnic nerves and synapse in the superior mesenteric and aorticorenal ganglia. Postganglionic fibers run with the branches of the artery to reach the ileum and jejunum	Umbilical region
Cecum and ascending colon	T10, T11–T12	Preganglionic fibers run in the lesser and least splanchnic nerves and synapse in the superior mesenteric and aorticorenal ganglia. Postganglionic fibers run with the inferior mesenteric artery to reach the cecum and ascending colon	Right lumbar and/or right inguinal region
Descending, and sigmoid colon	L1–L2	Preganglionic fibers run in the lumbar splanchnic nerves and synapse in the inferior mesenteric ganglia Postganglionic fibers run with the arteries to reach the descending and sigmoid colon	Left lumbar and/or left inguinal region
Colon	L1–L2	Preganglionic fibers run in the lumbar splanchnic nerves and synapse in the inferior mesenteric ganglia Postganglionic fibers run with the arteries to reach the distal colon	Suprapubic region

TABLE 5-6. Characteristics of Jejunum and Ileum

Characteristic	Jejunum	Ileum
Location	Central upper abdomen	Lower abdomen, pelvis
Diameter	Wider owing to thicker inner circular muscle	Narrower
Vascularity	More vascular, redder	Less vascular
Emptying	Rapid, vigorous peristalsis	Slower
Fat in mesentery	Little fat; many translucent windows in peritoneum	More fat, thick fat; few windows
Arcades of vessels in mesentery	Only one or two tiers; longer vasa recti	Four or five tiers; shorter vasa recti
Wall thickness	Thicker	Thinner
Lymphatics	Blind-ended lymphatic capillaries called lacteals are found in the mucosa	Lymph nodes in mesentery and in the submucosa (Peyer's patches) become more numerous in the ileum

surface, since the mesenteric surface has a better blood supply. Venous drainage is by means of the superior mesenteric vein, which is joined by the splenic vein to form the portal vein posterior to the neck of the pancreas.

The mesentery is the peritoneal structure that supports the jejunum and ileum. The root of the mesentery is the mesentery's site of reflection with the parietal peritoneum on the posterior abdominal wall. It starts just to the left of the *second lumbar vertebra* at the duodenojejunal junction and extends to the right and inferiorly to the sacroiliac joint. The root passes *anteriorly* to the following structures: the abdominal aorta, vertebral column, horizontal duodenum where this duodenal segment is crossed anteriorly by the superior mesenteric artery and vein, inferior vena cava, right ureter, and right gonadal vessels (see Fig. 5-27). The root of the mesentery contains the superior mesenteric artery and vein as well as autonomic nerves and lymphatics that supply the jejunum, ileum, cecum, appendix, ascending colon, and the proximal half of the transverse colon.

Innervation of the Jejunum and Ileum

The vagus nerves supply preganglionic parasympathetic fibers to these organs.

The lesser splanchnic nerves provide preganglionic sympathetic fibers that arise from cell bodies in the lateral horn nuclei of T10 and T11. These preganglionic fibers synapse in the superior mesenteric ganglia. Many anatomists believe that the lesser splanchnic nerves synapse in the aorticorenal ganglia. However, most physiology textbooks do not mention the aorticorenal ganglia. Although they are not synonymous, this text lists both. Postganglionic sympathetic fibers that arise from the aorticorenal ganglia and superior mesenteric ganglia follow the superior mesenteric artery and its branches to the jejunum and ileum.

GVA fibers for pain and travel back through the superior mesenteric plexus and lesser splanchnic nerves. These sensory fibers converge on the dorsal horn and second-order neurons in the spinal cord levels that give rise to the lesser splanchnic nerve, which are T10 and T11 (see Fig. 5-19). The general somatic sensory fibers from the umbilical region also have their neuronal sensory axons synapsing on second order neurons in spinal cord segments T10 and T11. Both the GVA and the GSA fibers converge on and synapse on the same second-order neurons in these spinal cord segments. Thus, pain in the umbilical region can be from the small intestine, ascending colon, or even the appendix during the early stages of appendicitis.

Other visceral sensory fibers for specific reflexes are found in the vagus nerve for thirst and various reflexes such as controlling the lower esophageal (gastroesophageal) sphincter.

●●● LARGE INTESTINE, OR COLON

The primary function of the colon is the absorption of water and salt. The divisions of the large intestine are the cecum, ascending colon, transverse colon, descending colon, and sigmoid colon (Fig. 5-30).

The diameter of the colon gradually narrows from the ascending colon to the distal sigmoid colon. The descending colon often has a diameter similar to that of the small intestine. Therefore, other criteria are used to distinguish the large intestine from the small intestine.

HISTOLOGY

The Jejunum and Ileum

The villi of the jejunum and the ileum have a layer of epithelium specialized for absorption and a rich vascular supply, which carries the absorbed amino acids and simple sugars. The center of each villus is occupied by a lacteal, a blind-ended lymphatic vessel. Chylomicrons enter the lacteal and from there pass through progressively larger lymph vessels to reach the cisterna chyli and the thoracic duct. Thus, fat travels to the liver by the following route: lymph vessels, cisterna chyli, thoracic duct, venous system, heart, aorta, celiac trunk, hepatic artery, and liver.

The submucosa of the ileum contains a large amount of lymphoid tissue collected into aggregates of lymphoid tissue known as Peyer's patches.

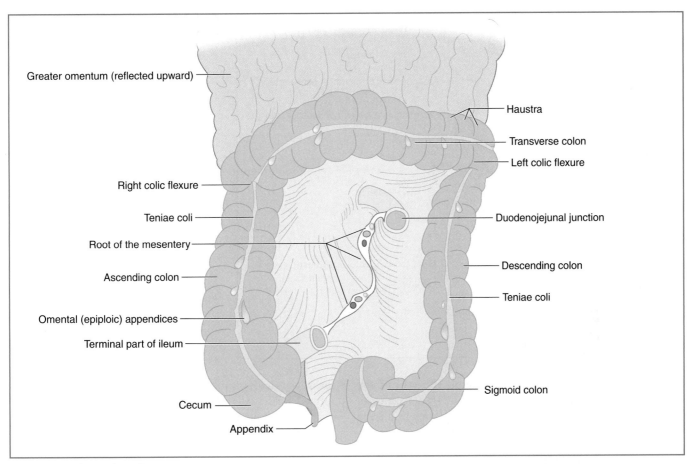

Figure 5-30. Large intestine.

In the colon (see Fig. 5-30), the longitudinal layer of smooth muscle does not completely encompass the inner circular layer but is condensed into three longitudinal bands—the *teniae coli.* The taeniae coli are shorter than the length of the colon itself. These muscular bands pull on the colon like a purse string, producing sacculations called *haustra.*

Unlike the small intestine, the colon has pockets of peritoneal fat-filled sacs hanging off the peritoneal layer. These sacs are known as omental (*epiploic*) *appendices.* They appear on the antimesenteric surface and are most numerous on transverse and sigmoid colons.

Diameter cannot be used to identify the colon versus the small intestine because of the small diameter of the descending colon. The three identifying characteristics of the colon are teniae coli, haustra, and omental appendages (see Fig. 5-30).

Cecum

The cecum is a blind pouch found in the right iliac fossa below the level of the ileocolic junction (see Figs. 5-30 and 5-31). This intraperitoneal pouch plays no role in the functioning of the colon. Due to the embryologic descent of the cecum, it typically lies in the lower right quadrant, anterior to the iliacus muscle. However, the cecum can also

be located just below the liver, subhepatically, or anywhere between these two points.

The terminal portion of the ileum penetrates the cecum at the *ileocecal junction* to produce the ileocecal valve. This valve is formed by the mucosa, submucosa, and circular muscle of the ileum as it projects into the cecum. Thus, all the layers of the ileum participate in the ileocecal valve except the outer longitudinal smooth muscle layer. The valve consists of a superior and an inferior lip (labium) that unite to produce the frenula of the valve. The frenula and labia are observed only from the lumen of the cecum. The frenula extends laterally from the two labia and indicates the separation between the base of the cecum and the ascending colon above.

Appendix

The appendix (see Fig. 5-31) is a vestigial organ not active in the functioning of the large intestine. It is a worm-like intraperitoneal process extending from the cecum usually in a posteromedial direction. Since it is derived from the developing colon, the appendix can be located by tracing the teniae coli to the base of the appendix where the teniae coli form a complete smooth muscle layer of the appendix (see Figs. 5-30 and 5-31). Although some food particles can

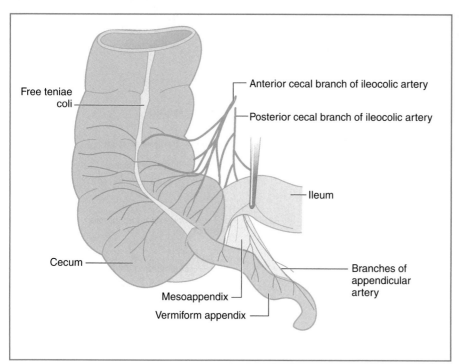

Figure 5-31. Blood supply of cecum and appendix.

enter the constricted lumen, most cannot. The wall of the appendix is full of lymphoid tissue, which in 60% of the cases of appendicitis can become enlarged and inflamed. Initially pain is felt in the umbilical (periumbilical) region. Once the parietal peritoneum is involved, pain migrates to the lower right quadrant. During the descent of the ascending colon during development, the appendix can be located in many different sites. Thus, pain due to the involvement of the parietal peritoneum from an inflamed appendix depends on the varied locations of this organ.

The appendicular artery, which is a branch of the ileocolic artery, supplies the appendix (see Fig. 5-31). The mesentery of the appendix (mesoappendix) stretches from the mesentery to the appendix and adjacent cecum by passing posteriorly to the ileum. This end artery reaches the appendix by also passing posteriorly to the ileum, through the mesoappendix.

Ascending Colon

The ascending colon is continuous with the base of the cecum at the frenulum of the ileocecal valve. It ascends on the right side of the abdominal cavity covered by peritoneum anteriorly and laterally. It is a *secondarily retroperitoneal* organ, with some aspect of its posterior surface in contact with the extraperitoneal connective tissue. The fixation of the ascending colon is variable. Almost 10% of the population has a mesentery, while others have the colon deeply embedded in the extraperitoneal fascia.

The ascending colon (see Fig. 5-30) turns to the left at the right colic (hepatic) flexure. Posterior to the ascending colon are several muscles (iliacus, quadratus lumborum, and transversus abdominis), and several branches of the lumbar plexus, (iliohypogastric, ilioinguinal, lateral femoral cutaneous) and

the lower half of the right kidney. The lumbar plexus is formed by the ventral rami of L1–L4 nerves 1–4.

The right ureter and gonadal vessels are not posterior to the ascending colon. They are medial to it. However, these retroperitoneal structures must be considered during mobilization of the ascending colon (i.e., cutting the peritoneum just lateral to the colon and moving the colon toward the midline to expose the retroperitoneal structures).

The right (hepatic) flexure is found at the ninth intercostal space approximately in the midaxillary line. The hepatic flexure is not intraperitoneal but is still a retroperitoneal structure. Superiorly, the hepatic flexure is covered by the visceral surface of the liver. At the hepatic flexure, the transverse colon is separated from the right kidney by extraperitoneal fascia.

Transverse Colon

The transverse colon is a highly mobile organ, which begins at the hepatic flexure. It becomes intraperitoneal and is suspended from the body wall by its own mesentery, the transverse mesocolon (see Figs. 5-12A and 5-30). The transverse colon crosses the abdomen approximately at the level of the second or third lumbar vertebrae, but it passes superiorly on the left side of the abdomen, typically running posteriorly to the greater curvature of the stomach. It is indirectly connected to the stomach by way of the gastrocolic ligament (part of the greater omentum) on the left side. Posterior to the transverse colon, as it runs from right to left, are the following organs: renal sinus of the right kidney, duodenum, pancreas, and lower portion of the left kidney (see Fig. 5-26). Anterior to the transverse colon, as it runs from right to left, are the right lobe of the liver and the greater curvature of the stomach.

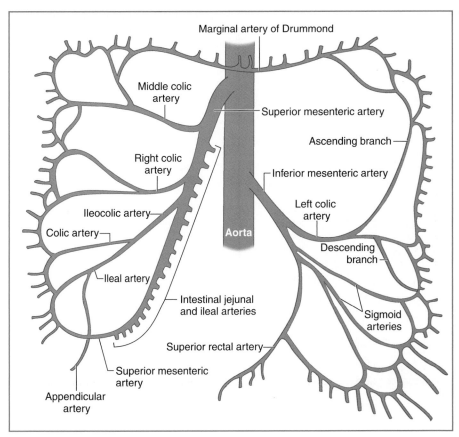

Figure 5-32. Superior and inferior mesenteric arteries. Note that the lymphatics, autonomic nerves, and veins run with the arteries to the roots of the superior and inferior mesenteric arteries. This distribution pattern is a result of midgut and hindgut development.

The transverse colon (see Figs. 5-26 and 5-30) makes a sharp inferior and posterior turn, at the left (splenic) colic flexure. Anterosuperior to the splenic flexure is the most anterior aspect of the spleen—its inferior pole. Posterior to the splenic flexure is the tail of the pancreas and renal sinus and adjacent kidney. The left colic flexure is attached to the diaphragm at the level of the 10th and 11th ribs by the phrenicocolic ligament (see Fig. 5-13).

Descending and Sigmoid Colon

The descending colon runs down the left side of the abdominal cavity retroperitoneally. The diameter of the descending colon may be less than that of the small intestine. The following structures are found posterior to the descending colon: the inferolateral aspect of the pole of the left kidney, the iliacus muscle, and several branches of the lumbar plexus (subcostal, iliohypogastric, ilioinguinal, and lateral femoral cutaneous nerves).

The sigmoid colon is the *intraperitoneal* continuation of the descending colon, which swings toward the midline. Its mesentery is the sigmoid mesocolon. The sigmoid colon can be 8 to 18 inches in length and is usually an S-shaped structure. It begins at the brim of the pelvis, continues toward, and becomes continuous with, the rectum at the level of the third sacral vertebra. The sigmoid colon in the male is found between the rectum and bladder, while in the female it is found between the uterus and the rectum. Its other relations

vary somewhat owing to the variable length of its sigmoid mesocolon. Typically, lateral to the sigmoid colon are the external iliac vessels, obturator nerve, ovary, and ductus deferens. Posterior to the sigmoid colon are the left internal iliac vessels, ureter, and sacral plexus, while superior is the ileum.

Blood Supply to the Colon

The blood supply (Figs. 5-31 and 5-32) to the colon consists of branches of either the superior mesenteric artery (SMA) or the inferior mesenteric artery (IMA) depending on the embryologic origin of the segment. The superior mesenteric artery supplies the segments of the colon that are derivatives of the embryonic midgut. Branches of the SMA to the colon are the middle colic and its right and left branches, *right colic* with its ascending and descending branches, and *ileocolic* with its colic and ileal branch. The latter branch anastomoses with the terminal portion of the superior mesenteric artery (see Figs. 5-31 and 5-32). These branches supply the cecum, appendix, ascending colon, and proximal half of the transverse colon. The middle colic artery enters the transverse mesocolon to supply the transverse colon by means of its right and left branches (see Fig. 5-32).

The inferior mesenteric artery supplies segments of the colon derived from the embryonic hindgut (see Fig. 5-32). The remaining segment of the transverse colon and the descending colon receive blood from the IMA's left colic artery. The

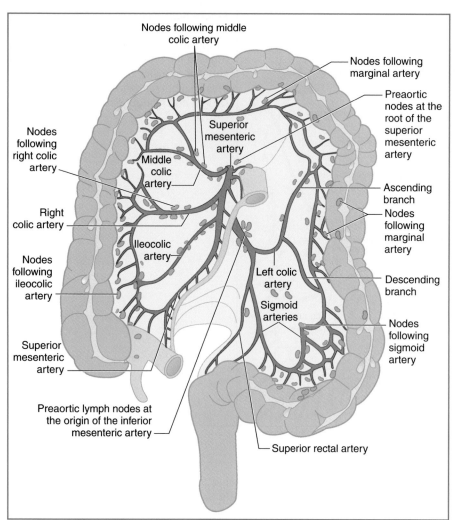

Figure 5-33. The unpaired arteries of the abdominal aorta and the accompanying lymph nodes.

Labels in figure:
Nodes following middle colic artery
Nodes following marginal artery
Preaortic nodes at the root of the superior mesenteric artery
Nodes following right colic artery
Superior mesenteric artery
Middle colic artery
Ascending branch
Nodes following marginal artery
Right colic artery
Ileocolic artery
Descending branch
Nodes following ileocolic artery
Left colic artery
Sigmoid arteries
Nodes following sigmoid artery
Superior mesenteric artery
Preaortic lymph nodes at the origin of the inferior mesenteric artery
Superior rectal artery

sigmoid colon receives blood from the sigmoid arteries, also branches of the IMA. The last sigmoid artery usually has a good anastomosis with the other sigmoid arteries.

The superior rectal artery is the continuation of the inferior mesenteric artery after it has passed over the brim of the pelvis.

Many of the arteries to the colon anastomose with each other, forming an artery that follows the mesenteric margin of the colon, the marginal artery (of Drummond) (see Fig. 5-32). This anastomosis may be incomplete, making them incompetent at certain locations where

- The ileocolic and right colic arteries anastomose.
- The left colic and middle colic arteries anastomose.
- The sigmoid arteries anastomose with the superior rectal artery.

Venous Drainage of the Colon

Venous drainage is the superior mesenteric and inferior mesenteric veins, which drain into the hepatic portal vein. The superior mesenteric vein joins the splenic vein posterior to the neck of the pancreas to form the portal vein. The inferior mesenteric vein often joins the splenic vein but can

also join either the superior mesenteric vein or the formation of the portal vein.

The inferior mesenteric vein along with the ascending branch of the left colic artery typically raises a fold of peritoneum just superolateral to the duodenojejunal junction that helps create the paraduodenal folds.

Lymphatics of the Colon

Lymphatics from the ascending and right transverse colon follow the superior mesenteric arteries (Fig. 5-33). Thus, the lymphatic drainage of the ascending colon follows the distal superior mesenteric artery and the ileocolic, right colic, and part of the middle colic arteries. These nodes drain to nodes located at the origin of the superior mesenteric artery (see Fig. 5-33). Lymphatics from the sigmoid, descending, and left transverse colon follow branches of the inferior mesenteric artery.

Innervation of the Colon

The innervation of the colon (see Fig. 5-19 and Table 5-5) is complicated by the fact that the colon is embryologically derived from both the midgut and hindgut. Thus, the vagus nerves supply preganglionic parasympathetic fibers to the colon up to approximately the middle to proximal two thirds of the transverse colon. The distal one half to one third of transverse colon, descending colon, and sigmoid colon receive preganglionic parasympathetic fibers from the pelvic splanchnic nerves. These latter fibers arise in the lateral horn of spinal cord segments S2–S4, which makes up the sacral parasympathetic outflow.

The sympathetic innervation is also dictated by the colon's development. The colon up to the middle to proximal two thirds of the transverse colon is derived from the midgut and therefore receives postganglionic sympathetic fibers from the superior mesenteric and the aorticorenal ganglia. These ganglia receive their preganglionic fibers from the lesser and least splanchnic nerves whose preganglionic cell bodies are located in the lateral horns of spinal cord segments T10–T11(T12).

The distal portions of the transverse, descending, and sigmoid colons are derived from the hindgut. They receive postganglionic sympathetic fibers from the inferior mesenteric ganglia. Preganglionic fibers are in the lumbar splanchnic nerves, which arise in the lateral horns of spinal cord segments L1–L2. These fibers synapse in the inferior mesenteric ganglia. Postganglionic fibers follow the branches of the inferior mesenteric artery.

●●● LIVER

The liver is the largest gland in the body. It is found in the right upper quadrant of the abdomen. This organ can also be described as occupying the right hypochondriac, the epigastric, and the adjacent left hypochondriac regions (see Fig. 5-1). On the right, the liver is hidden by the rib cage with just its inferior margin palpable below the costal margin. However, in the epigastric region, the liver lies below the rib cage. The liver extends superiorly under the diaphragm to the level of the right fourth intercostal space (approximate location of the nipple in the male). The superior aspect of the liver follows the diaphragm so that the superior left surface extends approximately to the left fifth intercostal space in the midclavicular line (Fig. 5-34A). The inferior margin follows the right costal margin, extending superolaterally toward the left fifth intercostal space in the midclavicular line. Indeed, a line denoting the inferior margin can be drawn from the right costal margin to the fifth left intercostal space in the midclavicular line. Remember that the inferior margin of the liver extends below the superior aspect of the right costal margin. As such, this imaginary approximate line will cross the junctions of the right eighth to ninth costal cartilages, the epigastric region, and the left seventh to eighth costal cartilages (see Fig. 5-34A). The liver is not rectangular but wedge-shaped with its thickest portion facing the right axillary lines and its narrow apex facing to the left (see Fig. 5-34B).

The fundus of the gallbladder extends below the anteroinferior margin of the liver at the point where the right ninth

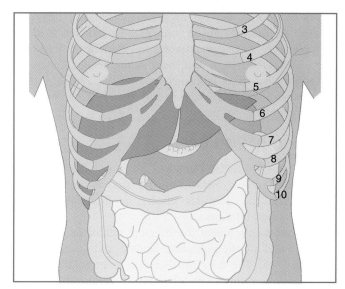

A

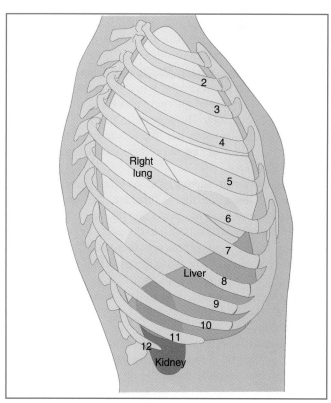

B

Figure 5-34. Surface anatomy of the liver. **A,** Anterior view of body wall. **B,** Right lateral view of surface anatomy of the liver.

costal cartilage is crossed by the lateral margin of the rectus sheath (see Fig. 5-1).

Because of the liver's close association with the rib cage, a needle biopsy of the liver is often performed by passing through the eighth to ninth intercostal spaces between the anterior and midaxillary lines (see Fig. 5-34B). The final clinical decision is made upon percussion for dullness during both inspiration and expiration. Dullness indicates that the lung is not present. Since both the thorax and abdomen share the lower portion of the rib cage, the needle will first pass through the thorax and the costodiaphragmatic recess of the pleural cavity before penetrating the diaphragm. Thus, this procedure is referred to as a transthoracic needle biopsy.

The liver has many functions including bile synthesis, toxin inactivation, storage of sugars, and synthesis of important plasma proteins.

Anatomy of the Liver

The liver has two surfaces and four anatomic lobes (Figs. 5-35 and 5-36). The two surfaces are the smooth diaphragmatic surface and the irregular visceral surface, which faces posteriorly and inferiorly.

The anatomic lobes of the liver are related to its surface structure and are the right, left, caudate, and quadrate lobes (see Fig. 5-35). The falciform ligament anatomically divides the liver into a small left lobe and a large right lobe. The posterior surface is marked by two longitudinal (sagittal) sulci (fissures), which are connected by a horizontal fissure. The right sagittal fissure is formed by two fossae (depressions). The inferior fossa, which is found closest to the anteroinferior margin, is occupied by the gallbladder. The superior fossa is the deep notch occupied by the inferior vena cava. The left sagittal fissure is produced by the continuous sulci for the ligamentum teres, located inferiorly, and the ligamentum venosum, located superiorly. The horizontal fissure is slit-like and is occupied by the porta hepatis, or doorway to the liver, which is the hilum of the liver. The sagittal fissures have a superomedial slant.

On the posterior surface, the quadrate lobe is located between the fossa for the gallbladder, the sulcus for the ligamentum teres, and the porta hepatis (see Fig. 5-36). The caudate lobe is located superior to the porta hepatis, between the sulcus for the ligamentum venosum and the fossa for the inferior vena cava (see Fig. 5-36). Because these two lobes are separated by the porta hepatis, which is surrounded by the attached lesser omentum, the caudate lobe faces the lesser peritoneal sac and the quadrate lobe faces the greater peritoneal sac.

The functional units of the liver are the hepatic segments that are supplied by independent branches of the portal vein, hepatic arteries, and bile ducts. The hepatic segments are also organized into two lobes of approximately equal size (see Fig. 5-35B). This division occurs at the main lobar fissure, which is approximately marked on the liver's posterior surface by the fossae for the inferior vena cava and gallbladder (see Fig. 5-35C). Thus, the main lobar fissure roughly corresponds to the right sagittal fissure. The quadrate lobe is part of the left physiologic lobe, while both right and left hepatic arteries supply the caudate lobe. Therefore, some authors consider the caudate lobe as part of both right and left lobes of the liver, while others consider it a special segment.

Relationships of the Liver

The following organs make impressions on the visceral surface of the liver (see Figs. 5-35C and 5-36):

- Esophagus and stomach (gastric impression) on the left lobe
- Duodenum
- Hepatic flexure and transverse colon on the right lobe
- Kidney on the right lobe
- Suprarenal (adrenal) gland with the bare area of the liver and the inferior vena cava
- Pylorus and duodenum to the left and right of the fossa of the gallbladder, respectively

Peritoneal Ligaments of the Liver

The falciform ligament attaches the liver to the anterior body wall. It contains the ligamentum teres of the liver in its inferior free margin (see Fig. 5-35A).

The coronary ligament is the peritoneum that surrounds the bare area of the liver (see Fig. 5-35C). The coronary ligament is unusual because the two layers of this ligament are separated by the bare area of the liver and each layer is given a name—the anterior layer and posterior layer of the coronary ligament. At the bare area, the liver is in direct contact with the diaphragm.

Right and left triangular ligaments are located to the right and left of the bare area. They consist of the points where the anterior and posterior layers of the coronary ligament meet. They also extend from the liver to the diaphragm. The left triangular ligament is to the left of the falciform ligament, while the right triangular ligament is actually posterior and to the right on the visceral surface of the liver (see Fig. 5-35C).

The lesser omentum (hepatogastric and hepatoduodenal ligaments) attaches the liver to the stomach and duodenum. The hepatoduodenal ligament contains the neurovascular bundle to the liver (see Fig. 5-35D).

Note that the ligaments mentioned above are peritoneal ligaments composed of two layers of visceral peritoneum. In contrast, the following two ligaments are embryonic remnants.

Ligamentum venosum is the remnant of the ductus venosus, which serves as a bypass of the liver as it runs from the portal vein at the porta hepatis to the inferior vena cava. It runs in the groove for the origin of the lesser omentum.

Ligamentum teres (see Fig. 5-35A) is the remnant of the left umbilical vein, which runs in the inferior portion of the falciform ligament between the right and left anatomic lobes to the porta hepatis. The right umbilical vein regresses in the sixth week of development. However, the left umbilical vein remains patent for some of its length and is connected to the left portal vein and ligamentum venosum.

Arterial Supply and Extrahepatic Duct

The arterial supply (Fig. 5-37) to the liver is the proper hepatic artery and its right and left hepatic branches. The cystic artery to the gallbladder is usually a branch of the right hepatic artery.

The blood supply to the liver consists of both the proper hepatic artery and the portal vein, each supplying about 50% of the O_2. The hepatic arteries supply about 25% of the total volume of blood to the liver. Typically, the right hepatic artery

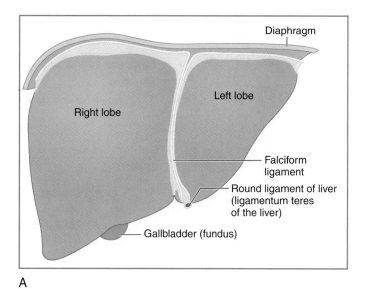

A

B

Figure 5-35. A, Diaphragmatic surface of liver with right and left anatomic lobes. **B,** Division of the liver into physiologic (functional) segments and anatomic lobes. *Continued*

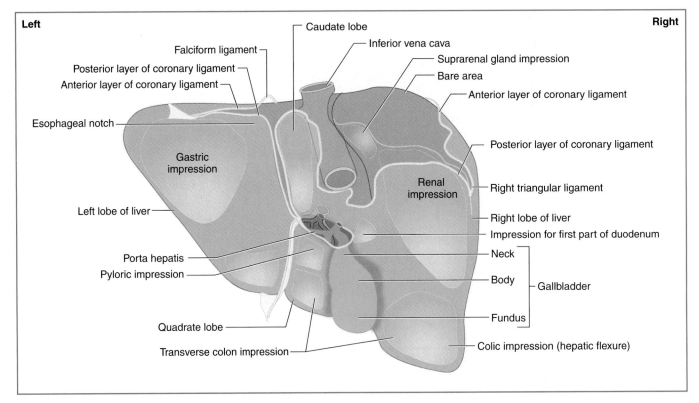

C

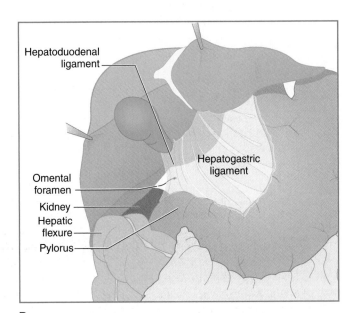

D

Figure 5-35 cont'd. C, Distribution and impression of organs on the visceral (posteroinferior) surface of the liver. **D,** Lesser omentum with hepatogastric and hepatoduodenal ligaments.

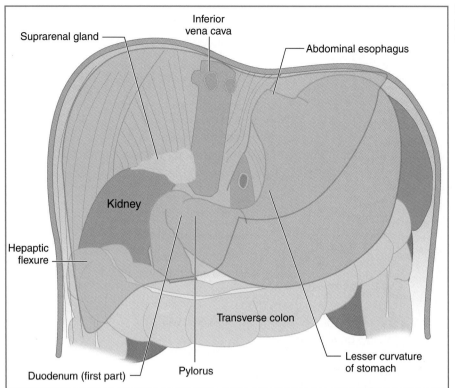

Figure 5-36. Organs that have a direct relationship with the visceral (posteroinferior) surface of the liver.

Suprarenal gland
Inferior vena cava
Abdominal esophagus
Kidney
Hepaptic flexure
Transverse colon
Lesser curvature of stomach
Duodenum (first part)
Pylorus

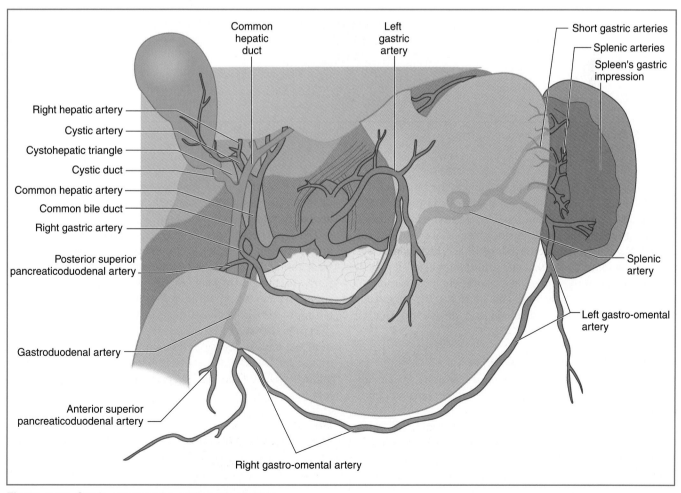

Common hepatic duct
Left gastric artery
Short gastric arteries
Splenic arteries
Spleen's gastric impression

Right hepatic artery
Cystic artery
Cystohepatic triangle
Cystic duct
Common hepatic artery
Common bile duct
Right gastric artery
Posterior superior pancreaticoduodenal artery
Gastroduodenal artery
Anterior superior pancreaticoduodenal artery
Right gastro-omental artery
Splenic artery
Left gastro-omental artery

Figure 5-37. Cystic artery and cystohepatic triangle.

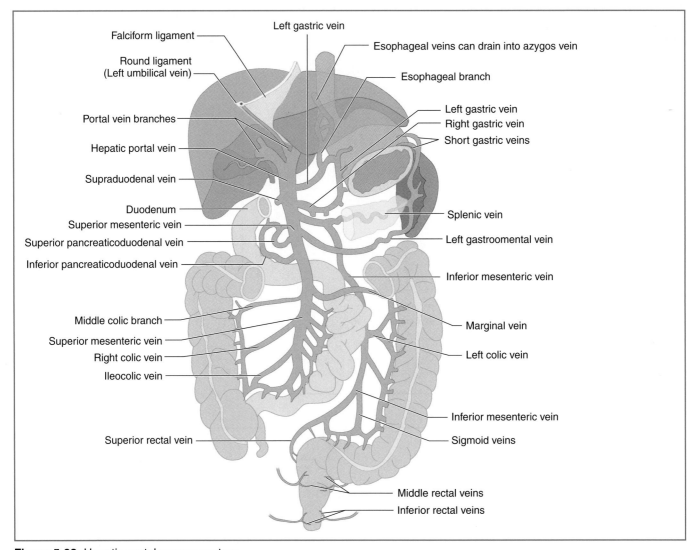

Figure 5-38. Hepatic portal venous system.

passes posteriorly to the common hepatic duct to reach the right lobe and it lies in an interval formed by the common hepatic duct, cystic duct, and the liver called the cystohepatic (Calot's) triangle. The right hepatic artery often (50% of the time) gives rise to the cystic artery to the gallbladder (see Fig. 5-37) within the cystohepatic (Calot's) triangle. This triangle is dissected early in the laparoscopic cholecystectomy to identify and protect these important structures. The left hepatic artery usually divides into lateral and medial (segmental) arteries.

Variations in the Hepatic Arteries

There are many variations in the hepatic arteries. In as many as 45% of the cases studied, the right, left, or common hepatic artery arose by some variation.

The common hepatic artery may arise from some other source than the celiac trunk, such as the superior mesenteric artery, aorta, or left gastric artery.

The left hepatic artery may arise separately from the celiac trunk or the left gastric artery. In the latter case, the left accessory gastric artery usually supplies the lateral segment or the lateral superior segment and therefore is not an accessory artery.

The right hepatic artery may arise from the celiac trunk, aorta, or even the superior mesenteric artery. When it arises from the aorta, the right hepatic artery often passes posteriorly to the portal vein. Accessory hepatic arteries often supply segments and are therefore not truly accessory arteries but rather variations of the arterial supply.

If three hepatic arteries appear in the extrahepatic dissection, the middle hepatic artery supplies the medial segment of the left lobe, while the left hepatic artery supplies the lateral segment. The right hepatic artery supplies the right lobe.

Hepatic Portal Vein

The hepatic portal vein brings blood, which contains products of digestion from the gut to the liver (Fig. 5-38). A hepatic portal system consists of a system of vessels where blood starts in a capillary bed, passes through veins to a second

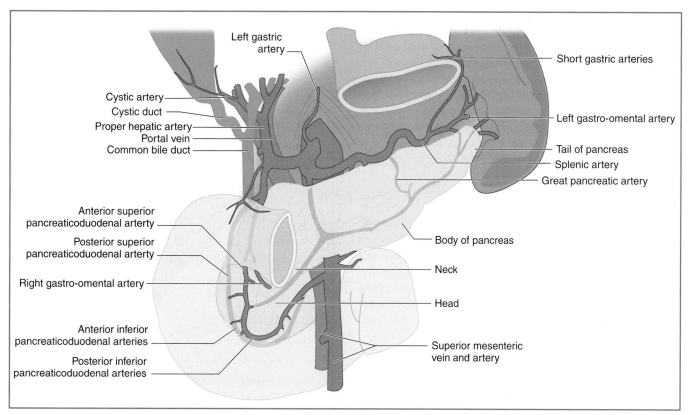

Figure 5-39. Relationship of pancreas with duodenum and left kidney.

capillary bed associated with the liver sinusoids. The hepatic portal vein provides about 75% of the liver's blood supply. It is formed posterior to the neck of the pancreas by the union of the superior mesenteric and splenic veins (see Figs. 5-27 and 5-39). The inferior mesenteric vein usually, but not always, drains into the splenic vein. Three hepatic veins drain the liver. They drain directly into the inferior vena cava, which is located in a deep notch on the liver's visceral surface by the ligament of the inferior vena cava. Thus, the three hepatic veins are very short and enter the inferior vena cava just before the inferior vena cava passes through the abdominal diaphragm. The major hepatic veins are found between the segments (intersegmental) in a similar manner to the pulmonary veins in the lungs.

Innervation of the Liver

The vagus nerve supplies preganglionic parasympathetic fibers to the porta hepatis although the function of these nerves is not certain. Postganglionic sympathetic fibers arise from the celiac ganglion and plexus. General visceral afferent fibers for pain travel with the plexus formed by the right greater splanchnic nerve and sensory fibers with the right phrenic nerve. While pain from the liver's parenchyma is felt in the right upper quadrant, inflammation of the capsule of the liver or the adjacent parietal peritoneum results in pain referred to the shoulder tip owing to the involvement of the phrenic nerve.

Lymphatics that drain the liver, gallbladder, both curvatures of the right portion of the stomach, the head of the pancreas, and adjacent duodenum drain into lumbar nodes associated with the celiac artery.

●●● GALLBLADDER

The gallbladder (see Figs. 5-28 and 5-35) stores and concentrates the bile produced by the liver. It is located under the visceral peritoneum in the right sagittal fossa lateral to the quadrate lobe of the liver, except for the surface that comes into direct contact with the liver.

Anatomy of the Gallbladder

The gallbladder has a fundus, body, and neck (see Fig. 5-28). The fundus is the enlarged blind terminal pouch that extends from the visceral surface of the liver, approximately at the level of the right ninth costal cartilage in the midclavicular line (see Fig. 5-1). The body occupies the gallbladder fossa of the liver and separates the duodenum from the quadrate lobe. Anteriorly, the body is in contact with the liver and the fundus with the body wall. Posteriorly they are in contact with the lateral side of the descending duodenum and adjacent transverse colon.

The neck has an S-shaped curve and is distinguished from the body by the entrance of the cystic artery. The mucosa of the neck is marked by ridges forming the spiral valve (of Heister) and leads to the cystic duct. The junction of right and left hepatic ducts forms the common hepatic duct. The cystic duct joins the common hepatic duct to form the common bile duct. Bile is produced in the parenchyma of the liver and secreted into the bile canaliculi. Bile then passes through the intralobular canaliculi, periportal ductules, and right and left hepatic ducts into the common hepatic duct. From here it is drawn into the cystic duct and finally the gallbladder. In the gallbladder, bile is concentrated and stored. Upon stimulation, the gallbladder contracts and bile passes through the cystic duct, the bile duct, through the hepatopancreatic ampulla (of Vater) and major duodenal papilla (of Vater) to be released into the second portion of the duodenum (see Fig. 5-28).

Blood Supply to the Gallbladder

The blood supply to the gallbladder (see Fig. 5-37) is primarily from the cystic artery and a branch (or branches) of the cystic artery that runs between the gallbladder and the substance of the liver. Venous drainage is by means of the liver and hepatic veins, which drain into the inferior vena cava. Veins from the gallbladder may also drain into tributaries of the portal vein.

Innervation of the Gallbladder

Vagal parasympathetic fibers stimulate the gallbladder to contract and release bile. Sympathetic fibers from the celiac ganglion and plexus have the opposite action.

●●● SPLEEN

The spleen is an organ of variable size and shape. It is normally found in the upper left quadrant of the abdomen and is not palpable at the costal margin. The spleen is protected by ribs 9–11 (see Fig. 5-37). The longitudinal axis of the spleen follows the axis of the 10th rib anteriorly to the midaxillary line. Its inferior pole is actually anterior and inferior while its superior pole is superior and posterior, lying to the left of the spinous process of the 10th thoracic vertebra.

Embryologically, the spleen is derived from a condensation of mesenchyme in the dorsal mesentery and is not derived from the foregut. However, it is attached to the stomach, which also develops in the dorsal mesentery.

Anatomy of the Spleen

The spleen has diaphragmatic and visceral surfaces. The diaphragmatic surface is smooth and conforms to the shape of the diaphragm. On the visceral surface is the hilum, or the site of entry of the neurovascular bundles into the spleen.

Except at the hilum, the splenic capsule is firmly attached to the adjacent peritoneum, which makes the spleen an intraperitoneal organ. The peritoneal ligament that attaches the spleen to the posterior abdominal wall is the splenorenal ligament while the gastrosplenic ligament connects the spleen with the greater curvature of the stomach (see Figs. 5-12B and 5-24). The tail of the pancreas runs in the splenorenal ligament along with the splenic vessels to reach the hilum. The branches of the splenic vessels—left gastrosplenic and short

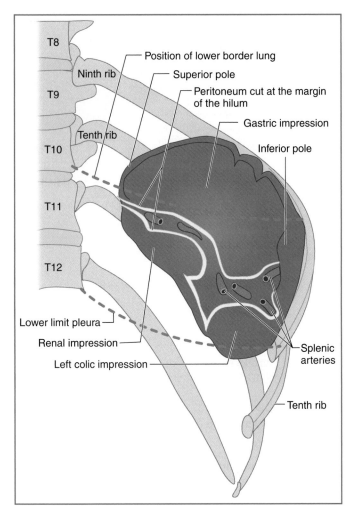

Figure 5-40. Visceral surface of the spleen.

gastric—are in the gastrosplenic ligament (see Fig. 5-14). Lymph nodes and autonomic nerves also are found in both ligaments.

The spleen lies along the 10th rib between the posterior and midaxillary lines. Thus, its posterior pole is superior in position to its anterior pole (Fig. 5-40). It has a gastric impression anterior to its hilum, a renal impression posterior to its hilum, and a colic impression for the left colic (splenic) flexure at its anterior pole. An enlarged spleen lies anterior to the midaxillary line.

The transverse colon is continuous with the descending colon just inferior to the spleen, which rests on the phrenicocolic ligament. This junction of the colon is referred to as the splenic flexure, as opposed to the hepatic flexure found in the right quadrant (see Fig. 5-26).

The spleen is suspended between the posterior abdominal wall and the stomach by the splenorenal ligament.

Blood Supply to the Spleen

The blood supply to the spleen is the splenic artery (see Figs. 5-39 and 5-40), which branches into small tributaries substance of the spleen. The superior terminal branch gives rise to the short gastric arteries. The inferior terminal branch gives rise to the left gastro-omental artery. Venous drainage is by means of the splenic vein, which joins the superior mesenteric vein posterior to the pancreatic neck to form the hepatic portal vein.

Innervation of the Spleen

Like the other organs in this region, the spleen receives parasympathetic supply from the vagus nerve and sympathetic supply from the celiac plexus. Most of the innervation of the spleen is postganglionic sympathetic fibers to blood vessels and the smooth muscle of the capsule of the spleen.

●●● PANCREAS

The pancreas is the site of synthesis of major digestive enzymes and the important hormones insulin and glucagon.

Anatomy of the Pancreas

The pancreas (see Figs. 5-39 and 5-41) is a lobulated, retroperitoneal digestive gland consisting of a head with an uncinate process, neck, body, and tail. The head lies in the C-shaped recess formed by the duodenum. Therefore, clinical problems involving the pancreas may involve the duodenum. The tail rests on the hilum of the spleen. The superior mesenteric vessels can be found just anterior to the uncinate process after they have passed posteriorly to the neck of the pancreas.

The pancreas contains a duct system for pancreatic exocrine secretions. The main pancreatic duct (of Wirsung) begins in the tail and travels the length of the gland, turning inferiorly near the neck of the pancreas. It joins the bile duct at the ampulla of Vater (see Fig. 5-28). The ducts empty together into the duodenum at the major duodenal papilla. The opening is guarded by a sphincter muscle, the sphincter of Oddi. The accessory duct (of Santorini), which continues from the pancreatic duct in the superior aspect of the pancreatic head, is eventually *superior* to the main pancreatic duct. This duct may or may not empty into the duodenum at the minor duodenal papilla (see Fig. 5-25).

Blood Supply to the Pancreas

The blood supply to the pancreas (see Fig. 5-39) includes the superior and inferior pancreaticoduodenal arteries, from the gastroduodenal and superior mesenteric arteries, respectively, to the head of the pancreas. However, pancreatic branches of the splenic artery supply the body and tail. The splenic artery runs just superior to the body of the pancreas. Venous return is through the splenic and superior mesenteric veins. The splenic vein runs posterior to the body of the pancreas. The junction of the splenic vein and superior mesenteric vein is posterior to the neck of the pancreas.

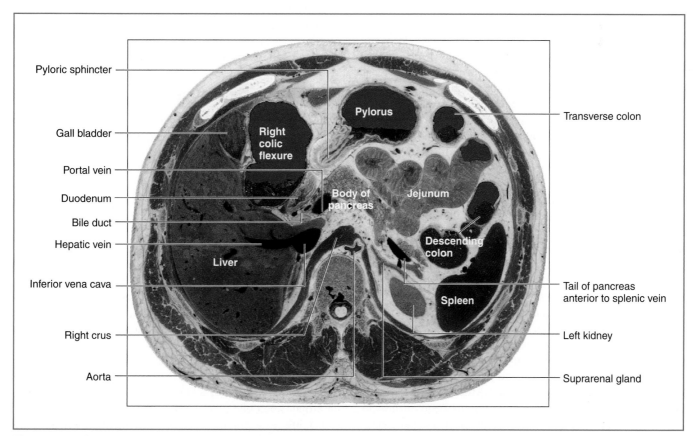

Figure 5-41. Cross-section of abdomen at T12. (Courtesy of the Visible Human Project, University of Colorado Center for Human Simulation.)

Innervation of the Pancreas

The innervation to the pancreas consists of parasympathetic fibers from the vagus and postganglionic sympathetic fibers from the celiac and superior mesenteric plexus. General visceral sensory (pain) fibers would run with the greater and a few may run with the lesser splanchnic nerves.

●●● EXTRAHEPATIC BILIARY DUCTS

The liver, gallbladder, pancreas, and duodenum are connected by a duct system, which is derived from the liver bud. The right and left hepatic ducts unite in or just inferior to the porta hepatis to form the common hepatic duct in the hepatoduodenal ligament (see Fig. 5-28).

The common hepatic duct descends in the hepatoduodenal ligament to the right of the proper hepatic artery, but anterior to the portal vein. The right hepatic artery often crosses posteriorly but sometimes anteriorly to the common hepatic duct (see Fig. 5-39).

The cystic duct connects the neck of the gallbladder to the common hepatic duct in the hepatoduodenal ligament to form the common bile duct. The bile duct is to the right of the proper hepatic artery, and both of these structures are anterior to the portal vein (see Fig. 5-39). This portion of the hepatoduodenal ligament forms the anterior boundary of the omental foramen.

The bile duct continues inferiorly to reach the posteromedial wall of the second portion of the duodenum. The bile duct has four parts.

The supraduodenal part lies in the hepatoduodenal ligament.

The retroduodenal portion is located posterior to the duodenum. Here, the bile duct is to the right of the gastroduodenal artery, which gives rise to the retroduodenal posterosuperior pancreaticoduodenal artery. This latter artery helps supply the duct and is an excellent marker for the duct. The posterosuperior pancreaticoduodenal artery initially passes anteriorly to the bile duct, then laterally to the duct, and finally posteriorly to the duct to reach the posterior surface of the pancreas.

The pancreatic portion of the bile duct passes through the posterior aspect of the pancreas to reach the posteromedial duodenal wall. The inferior vena cava is posterior to this portion of the duct.

The intramural (within the wall) portion of the bile duct passes through the duodenal wall. Here, it is joined by the main pancreatic duct to form the hepatopancreatic ampulla, or the ampulla of Vater. The ampulla empties into the duodenum by means of a single opening at the major duodenal papilla. The hepatopancreatic ampulla (of Vater) is within the duodenal papilla. However, sometimes the ducts do not anastomose. Both the bile duct and the main pancreatic duct are surrounded by smooth muscle. The circular smooth muscle is best developed around the terminal end of the bile duct. It is less well developed around the main pancreatic duct or the ampulla. The term sphincter of Oddi is often used to describe the entire sphincter system.

●●● DEVELOPMENT OF THE MIDGUT

The midgut forms most of the small intestine (except the duodenum proximal to the bile duct), cecum, appendix, ascending colon, and the proximal half of the transverse colon. The superior mesenteric artery is the blood supply to the midgut. The midgut is arranged as a loop of bowel whose axis is the superior mesenteric artery (see Figs. 5-20 and 5-42). The midgut is still attached to the yolk sac by the yolk (vitelline) stalk or duct. The midgut is suspended only by a dorsal mesentery. It has no ventral mesentery. The midgut's neurovascular bundles communicate with the body wall through the dorsal mesentery.

The superior mesenteric artery (viewed from the anterior abdominal wall) serves as the axis for the rotation of the midgut. Rotation takes place around the superior mesenteric artery, which divides the gut loop into cranial and caudal portions. When completed, the midgut is rotated 270 degrees counterclockwise. For orientation purposes, the face of a clock is applied in the coronal plane with the center of the clock at the superior mesenteric artery.

To follow the rotation, we can use the cranial and caudal limbs of the midgut loop as landmarks. The cranial limb gives rise to the duodenum distal to the duodenal papilla, the jejunum, and most of the ileum; the caudal limb differentiates into a small remaining part of the ileum, the cecum, the ascending colon, and approximately the proximal half to two thirds of the transverse colon.

There are three distinct stages in the rotation of the midgut: (1) physiologic (normal) herniation, (2) physiologic reduction of the hernia, and (3) fixation. During each step there is rotation of the intestinal tract (see Fig. 5-42).

Physiologic Herniation

A hernia is a protrusion or movement of an organ from its normal anatomic position, usually through the body wall. Herniation is due to differential growth of several organs, including the kidneys and liver. Most important is the rapid growth of the cranial limb of the midgut, which elongates faster than the caudal limb and drives the midgut loop through the umbilical opening into the umbilical cord, resulting in the midgut physiologic hernia (see Fig. 5-42A). This herniation is accompanied by a 90-degree counterclockwise rotation as viewed from the anterior surface of the fetus. The plane of rotation is through the superior mesenteric artery. The very rapid growth of the cranial limb drives it to the right of the superior mesenteric artery, and the caudal limb moves to the left of the artery (see Fig. 5-42B).

Physiologic Reduction

Physiologic reduction of a hernia is the return of an organ to its proper anatomic position. The abdominal cavity enlarges sufficiently to accommodate the midgut, which reenters the abdominal cavity in a specific manner. The proximal part of the cranial loop reenters the abdominal cavity first by passing

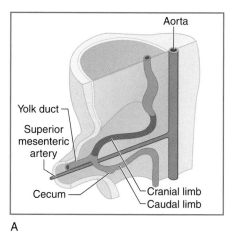

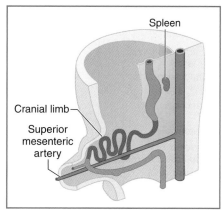

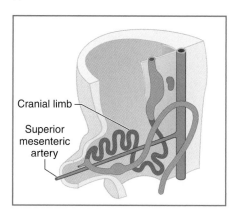

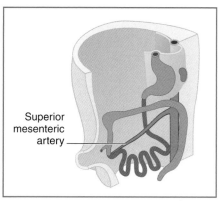

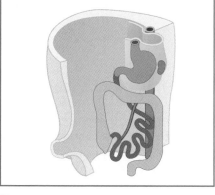

Figure 5-42. Stages of midgut rotation.

beneath the superior mesenteric artery (the axis of rotation), and it now lies to the left of both the superior mesenteric artery and midline. As reduction continues, the caudal limb enters second by passing above the superior mesenteric artery (see Figs. 5-42C and 5-42D).

Occurring first, the reduction of the cranial limb is accompanied by another 90-degree counterclockwise rotation. After passing under the axis of rotation (superior mesenteric artery), the cranial limb now is inferior to the artery. Occurring second, the reduction of the caudal limb is also accompanied by a third 90-degree counterclockwise rotation (see Figs. 5-42C and 5-42D). After passing over the axis of rotation, the caudal

limb now lies superior to the superior mesenteric artery. At the end of this stage of the midgut rotation, the proximal end of the caudal loop, which differentiates into the cecum and proximal colon, is located in the upper right quadrant of the abdomen in a subhepatic position and has undergone a total rotation of 270 degrees.

The cecum and appendix are derived from the cecal diverticulum, which appears on the antimesenteric side of the caudal midgut loop. The walls of the cecum grow unevenly with a differential growth process producing the appendix at the distal end of the diverticulum. The appendix rapidly increases in length so that it is relatively long at birth.

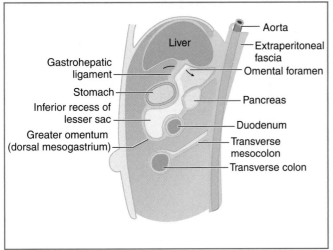

A

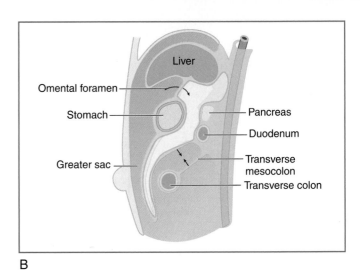

B

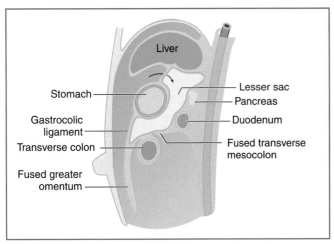

C

Figure 5-43. Lateral view of fusion of greater omentum and transverse mesocolon.

Fixation

Before fixation, all of the midgut is intraperitoneal and highly mobile. Fixation is the process by which certain mesenteries of intraperitoneal organs come into contact with the parietal peritoneum, resulting in the loss of this peritoneum. The involved organs are now firmly attached to the body walls extraperitoneal fascia. Before midgut fixation, the cecum descends from its subhepatic position to its typical position in the right lower quadrant (see Fig. 5-42D). After the descent of the cecum, the visceral peritoneum of the ascending and descending portions of the colon is now in direct contact with the parietal peritoneum of the posterior walls.

The duodenum and pancreas also become fixed at this time (Figs. 5-43A and 5-43B). The visceral and parietal peritoneal layers fuse (see Figs. 5-43B and 5-43C). The fused peritoneum is lost. These organs are now held in place by their variable relationship with the extraperitoneal fascia. However, these organs retain visceral peritoneum on the surfaces that face the peritoneal cavity. Such organs are no longer suspended by

peritoneum and are now considered secondarily retroperitoneal organs. The process of fixation stabilizes the gut to prevent a peristalsis-driven twisting (volvulus) of the gut.

During the late stages of foregut and midgut rotation (see Fig. 5-43A), rotation and the extensive growth of greater omentum contribute to the development of the lesser sac's inferior recess. The transverse colon is located just inferior to the greater curvature of the stomach, and the pancreas and duodenum are still intraperitoneal organs (see Fig. 5-43A). Fixation results in the loss of both of the visceral peritoneum on the dorsal surface of the pancreas and the duodenum as these organs become retroperitoneal organs (see Figs. 5-43B and 5-43C). The posterior layers of the greater omentum come into contact with the transverse mesocolon. The transverse mesocolon fuses with the posterior leaf of the greater omentum. The anterior and posterior layers of the omentum also fuse, leaving only a small portion of the anterior layer of the greater omentum, referred to as the gastrocolic ligament, as a potential surgical approach to the lesser sac (see Fig. 5-43C).

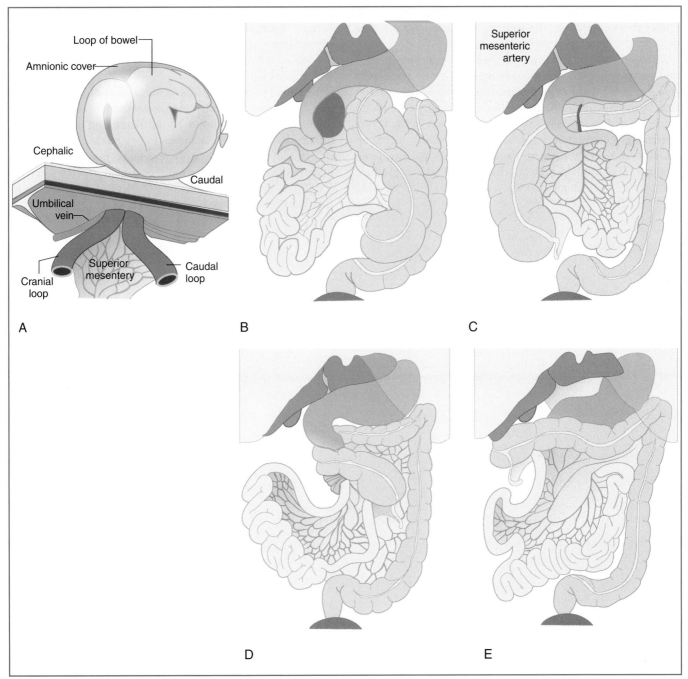

Figure 5-44. Abnormalities in midgut rotation. **A,** Omphalocele. **B,** Nonrotation. **C,** Reversed rotation. **D,** Volvulus. **E,** Subhepatic appendix.

Congenital Abnormalities of the Midgut

Many midgut abnormalities are due to malrotations or anomalies of rotation or fixation (Fig. 5-44).

Omphalocele is due to the failure of the herniated gut to return to the abdomen. It may result from a failure of the folding process to reduce the umbilicus. Omphalocele is covered by the amnion of the umbilical cord (see Fig. 5-44A).

Nonrotation occurs when the gut is reduced but there is no further rotation (loss of the last 180 degrees of rotation) (see Fig. 5-44B). The small intestine lies on the right, and the cecum

and appendix lie on the left. If everything else is normal, then the nonrotation is asymptomatic. It may become a diagnostic problem if diseases of the appendix or colon present in the left lower quadrant instead of the right lower quadrant.

Reverse Rotation

Reduction occurs in such a manner that the cranial limb is superior to the superior mesenteric artery and the caudal limb is inferior to the artery. The last 180 degrees of rotation are clockwise instead of counterclockwise. Upon fixation, the duodenum lies anterior to the superior mesenteric artery and the transverse colon posterior to the artery (see Fig 5-44C). Under these conditions, the superior mesenteric artery may obstruct the larger transverse colon.

Volvulus (twisting) occurs if fixation is incomplete. In midgut volvulus, the intestines hang from a free mesentery (see Fig. 5-44D). Upon peristalsis, the intestines can twist in such a manner to obstruct the bowel or strangle its blood supply. Poor fixation may also account for parts of the bowel becoming incarcerated beneath the mesentery, including paraduodenal hernias just to the left of the duodenojejunal flexure. A failure to completely fix the midgut can produce volvulus of the cecum or even an increased incidence of inguinal hernia.

Other anomalies associated with fixation include subhepatic cecum and retrocecal appendix. These conditions are asymptomatic and usually are important only in the event of a disease state that presents with an unusual physical position (see Fig. 5-44E).

Intestinal stenosis and atresia occur most often in the ileum and duodenum. They most commonly occur at the level of the duodenal papilla, followed by the ileum and jejunum. They are due to a failure of the lumen to recanalize either partially or completely. The failure to recanalize may be due to an interruption in the blood supply or a fetal vascular accident (produced by fetal volvulus or adhesion of the peritoneum that interferes with the blood supply).

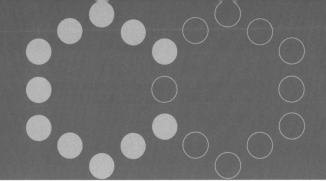

Posterior Abdominal Wall 6

CONTENTS

INTRODUCTION

MUSCLES OF THE POSTERIOR ABDOMINAL WALL

DIAPHRAGM
Openings in the Diaphragm
Fascia of the Diaphragm

KIDNEYS
Surface Anatomy of the Kidney
Fascia of the Kidney
Relationships of the Kidneys
Posteromedial Relationships of the Kidneys
Internal Anatomy of the Kidney
Arterial Supply and Venous Drainage of the Kidney
Innervation of the Kidney
Lymphatic Drainage of the Kidney
Development of the Kidneys

URETER

SUPRARENAL GLAND
Development of the Suprarenal Gland
Blood Supply and Innervation of the Suprarenal Gland

VESSELS OF THE POSTERIOR ABDOMINAL WALL
Abdominal Aorta
Inferior Vena Cava

LYMPHATICS OF THE POSTERIOR ABDOMINAL WALL

●●● INTRODUCTION

The posterior abdominal wall consists of the musculoskeletal system that supports the abdominal organs, the aorta, inferior vena cava (IVC) and its branches, as well as the innervation to the abdominal organs and body wall. The posterior abdominal wall extends from the diaphragm to the pelvic brim and the inguinal ligament. At these two points, the posterior abdominal wall is continuous with either the pelvis or the thigh (Fig. 6-1A).

The bones of the posterior wall consist of the lumbar vertebrae, the bodies of the 12th ribs, the sacral promontory and the wings (alae) of the iliac bones (see Fig. 6-1A). The lumbar vertebrae extend anteriorly as the anterior lumbar

convexity or lumbar lordoses. As such the lower abdomen is very shallow in the anteroposterior plane. The 12th ribs emerge from their articulation with the T12 vertebra, located behind the posterior origins of the diaphragm. The quadratus lumborum muscle arises from the 12th rib.

The inferior border of the posterior abdominal wall is both the inguinal ligament and the brim of the pelvis, which consists of the sacral promontory and the iliac arcuate line. The iliac arcuate line is the ridge on the inner iliac surface that marks the separation of its body and wing (see Fig. 6-1A). The iliac wing is the superior portion of the ilium that extends superiorly and laterally to end as the iliac crest. The iliac wings are the inferior aspect of the posterior abdominal wall and serve as transition zones between the abdomen and pelvis medially and the thigh laterally. In the midline, the articulation of L5 with the first sacral vertebra produces an anterior bulge called the sacral promontory (see Fig. 6-1A).

●●● MUSCLES OF THE POSTERIOR ABDOMINAL WALL

The muscles of the posterior abdominal wall include the diaphragm, quadratus lumborum, psoas major and minor, and iliacus (see Fig. 6-1). Since the psoas major and iliacus muscles insert close together on the lesser trochanter of the femur, they are often referred to as the iliopsoas muscle (see Fig. 6-1A and Table 6-1).

●●● DIAPHRAGM

The diaphragm (see Fig. 6-1B) is a skeletal muscle that partitions the thorax and abdomen by closing the inferior thoracic aperture. The origins of the diaphragm form an oblique peripheral ring as this skeletal muscle arises from the body wall and inserts into a central tendon (Table 6-2). The diaphragm is important but not essential for respiration.

The crura (a crus is any leg-like structure) arise from the lumbar vertebral bodies. The right crus is larger than the left crus and contains the entire esophageal hiatus. Half of the right crus lies to the left of the midline. The arcuate ligaments are the result of thickening of the inner investing layer of deep fascia that covers the psoas major and quadratus lumborum muscles.

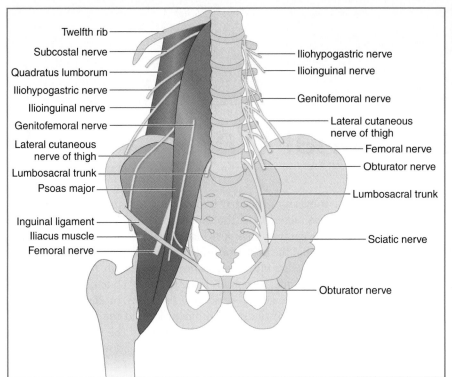

A

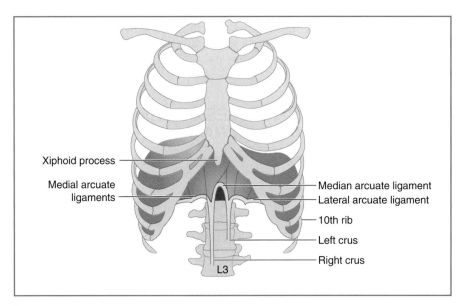

B

Figure 6-1. Muscles and nerves of the posterior abdominal wall (**A**) and diaphragm (**B**).

Labels in A:

Twelfth rib
Subcostal nerve
Quadratus lumborum
Iliohypogastric nerve
Ilioinguinal nerve
Genitofemoral nerve
Lateral cutaneous nerve of thigh
Lumbosacral trunk
Psoas major
Inguinal ligament
Iliacus muscle
Femoral nerve

Iliohypogastric nerve
Ilioinguinal nerve
Genitofemoral nerve
Lateral cutaneous nerve of thigh
Femoral nerve
Obturator nerve
Lumbosacral trunk
Sciatic nerve
Obturator nerve

Labels in B:

Xiphoid process
Medial arcuate ligaments
Median arcuate ligament
Lateral arcuate ligament
10th rib
Left crus
Right crus
L3

Openings in the Diaphragm

The dome-like curvature of the diaphragm (see Fig. 6-1B) is due to its origins, which arise from different levels of the body wall. Anteriorly the origin from the xiphoid is found at T9, and posteriorly the crura of the diaphragm arise from lumbar vertebrae. Therefore, the openings of the diaphragm that transmit structures from the thorax to the abdomen are also found at different vertebral levels.

The IVC passes through the right side of the central tendon at vertebral level T8, just lateral to the pericardium. The orifice for the IVC also transmits the right phrenic nerve.

The esophageal hiatus is in the right crus of the diaphragm at vertebral level T10. This opening also transmits the anterior

TABLE 6-1. Muscles of the Posterior Abdominal Wall

Muscle	Origin	Insertion	Action
Psoas major*	From the intervertebral disks starting from T12 to L5 vertebrae and adjacent bodies of lumbar vertebrae and from the T12 transverse processes	Inserts with iliacus into lesser trochanter	Powerful flexor of hip joint
Quadratus lumborum†	Iliac crest, iliolumbar ligament, and transverse process of L5	Twelfth rib and transverse processes of upper lumbar vertebrae	Stabilizes or depresses 12th rib during respiration, lateral bending of trunk
Iliacus‡	Anterior surface of iliac fossa	Lesser trochanter of femur	Flexor of hip joint

*Innervated by ventral rami of L1 to L3 with L1 being the most important.
†Innervated by ventral rami of L1 to L3.
‡Innervated by femoral nerve L2 to L4.

TABLE 6-2. Origins and Insertions of the Diaphragm

Origin	Insertion
Xiphoid process Costal cartilages of ribs 6–10 and tips of ribs 11 and 12 Crura: right crus arising from vertebrae L1–L3, left crus from vertebrae L1 and L2 Medial arcuate ligament (medial lumbocostal arch) stretches from the L1 vertebral body to the L1 transverse process, passing over the psoas major muscle Lateral arcuate ligament (lateral lumbocostal arch) stretches from the transverse process of L1 or L2 to the 12th rib over the quadratus lumborum muscle Median arcuate ligament connects the two crura at the level of T12 over the aorta	Central tendon or trifoliate, which has no bony attachments

and posterior vagal trunks associated with the esophagus and the abdominal blood supply to the esophagus, which consists of branches of the left gastric artery and vein.

The aortic hiatus is actually posterior to the diaphragm at vertebral level T12. It is formed by the interconnecting connective tissue fibers of the crura called the median arcuate ligament and the 12th thoracic vertebra. This passageway transmits the aorta, thoracic duct, and the azygos veins although the last also frequently penetrates the right crus instead. Often the hemiazygos vein passes posterior to the medial arcuate ligament.

The sternocostal triangle (see Fig. 6-1B) is a small opening between the sternal origin of the diaphragm (xiphoid process) and the adjacent costal cartilage. It allows the superior epigastric vessels to pass from the anterior thoracic wall into the anterior abdominal wall.

The subcostal nerve (thoracic ventral ramus 12) moves from thorax to abdomen by passing posterior to the lateral arcuate ligament (see Fig. 6-1B). The sympathetic trunk passes posterior to the medial arcuate ligament, and the splanchnic nerves pass through the crura.

The psoas major (see Fig. 6-1A and Table 6-1) passes posterolaterally in the iliac fossa, posterior to the inguinal ligament, and joins the iliacus muscle to insert on the lesser trochanter of the femur. This conical muscle is found between the laterally placed quadratus lumborum and iliacus muscles and the lumbar vertebrae and pelvic brim inlet, which are located medially. The slight groove between the psoas major and the lumbar vertebrae is occupied by the sympathetic trunk,

which can be mistaken for the adjacent paravertebral chain of lumbar lymph nodes.

The psoas minor is not always present. Although it arises from the lumbar vertebrae and the intervertebral disks, it appears to arise from the anterior fibers of the psoas major. The psoas minor passes inferiorly on the anterior surface of the psoas major to insert on the ileopubic eminence.

The psoas major overlaps the medial edge of the quadratus lumborum (see Fig. 6-1A and Table 6-1) while laterally the transversus abdominis muscle arises from the thoracolumbar (lumbodorsal) fascia.

The iliacus muscle occupies the iliac fossa found on the anterior surface of the iliac wing. All these muscles have an inner investing layer of deep fascia, extraperitoneal fascia, and parietal peritoneum covering their internal (anterior) surface.

Fascia of the Diaphragm

The muscles of the posterior abdominal wall are separated from the abdominal cavity by the inner investing layer of deep fascia, which bears the name of the adjacent muscle (e.g., iliacus fascia, diaphragmatic fascia). Anteriorly, this continuous layer of fascia is referred to as the transversalis fascia.

The inner investing layer of deep fascia also thickens to form ligaments where the diaphragm crosses the psoas major and quadratus lumborum muscles. These are the medial and lateral arcuate ligaments, which serve as important origins of the diaphragm. A similar morphology is found in the pelvis, where part of the muscles that form the pelvic diaphragm arises from the arcus tendineus (arcuate tendon), which is a

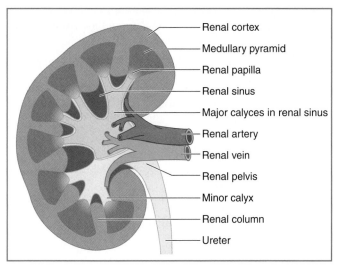

Figure 6-2. Morphology of the kidney.

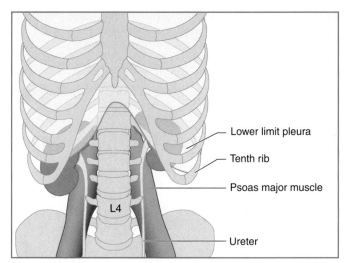

Figure 6-3. Location of the kidney (anterior view).

thickening of the inner investing layer of deep fascia of the obturator internus muscle.

The extraperitoneal (subserous) fascia is internal to the inner investing layer of deep fascia. The retroperitoneal and secondarily retroperitoneal organs occupy this layer. Internal to the extraperitoneal fascia is the peritoneum and the peritoneal cavity.

●●● KIDNEYS

The kidneys are primarily responsible for the homeostasis of fluid and electrolyte levels and the secretion of erythropoietin (stimulates production of erythrocytes), secretion of renin (involved in control of blood pressure), and regulation of calcium metabolism. The kidneys are bean-shaped organs that are longer (10 cm) than they are wide (3–4 cm). The superior and inferior ends of the kidney are referred to as the superior and inferior poles. Each kidney has an anterior/posterior surface and a medial/lateral border, but be aware that the kidney does not lie flat on the posterior abdominal wall but obliquely, so that the medial border actually faces anteromedially. The kidney has its own fibrous capsule that encloses the kidney tissue (Fig. 6-2). The capsule of the kidney is invaginated on its medial side to produce a slit-like renal hilum and an internal enlarged recess called the renal sinus. The renal artery and vein and the dilated upper end of the ureter, which is called the renal pelvis, pass through the renal sinus and hilum. The renal vein is the most anterior structure at the renal hilum, and the renal pelvis is the most posterior structure (see Fig. 6-2).

Surface Anatomy of the Kidney

The kidneys are retroperitoneal organs found below the diaphragm, along the lateral side of the psoas major muscles mostly in the upper quadrants of the abdominal cavity. The surface anatomy of the kidney in the supine position finds the superior pole of the left kidney as high as the posterior aspect of the 11th rib while the right kidney rises only to the level of the 12th rib (Fig. 6-3). This difference is due to the presence of the liver on the right. The kidneys shift inferiorly upon standing and now lie between L1 and L4. The transpyloric plane passes through the upper portion of the hilum of the right kidney and the lower portion of the hilum of the left kidney. At this point, the kidneys lie slightly medial to the plane of the ninth costal cartilage in the transpyloric plane.

The inferior pole of the right kidney can *sometimes* be palpated through the anterolateral abdominal wall just above the right iliac crest because it descends inferior to the left kidney, again owing to the presence of the liver. The superior pole is closer to the vertebral column while the inferior poles are farther apart as the kidneys lie along the lateral border of the psoas major muscle (see Figs. 6-3 and 6-4).

Fascia of the Kidney

The kidneys develop as retroperitoneal organs from the intermediate mesoderm and remain in a retroperitoneal position. The kidney and its fibrous capsule are embedded in three layers of specialized extraperitoneal (subserous) fascia. Starting at the capsule of the kidney, the pararenal fascia is the most external layer, the renal fascia is the intermediate layer, and the perirenal fascia is the most internal layer being closest to the kidney. The perirenal fascia consists of the fat and fascia that lie between the renal fascia and the kidney and serves as a soft cushion against which the kidney rests. It extends into the renal sinus, and the renal vessels and the renal pelvis are surrounded by the perirenal fascia (see Fig. 5-5B).

The kidney and its adjacent perirenal fascia are encapsulated by the renal (Gerota's) fascia. The renal fascia passes over the renal vessels medially and the suprarenal glands superiorly, where they may be separated by a septum. The anterior and posterior layers of the renal fascia fuse superiorly and are then continuous with the diaphragmatic fascia. Thus, the kidneys and suprarenal glands move with the

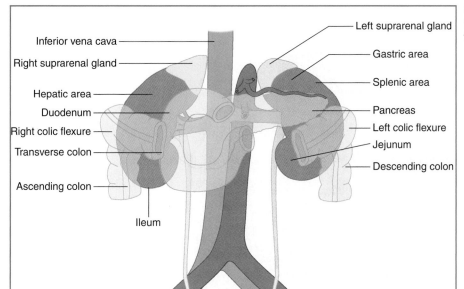

Figure 6-4. Structures that have a relationship with the anterior surfaces of the kidneys.

Inferior vena cava

Right suprarenal gland

Hepatic area

Duodenum

Right colic flexure

Transverse colon

Ascending colon

Ileum

Left suprarenal gland

Gastric area

Splenic area

Pancreas

Left colic flexure

Jejunum

Descending colon

PHYSIOLOGY

Renal Fascia

The arrangement of renal fascia and its relationship to the renal vessels dictates the course of the spread of infection. Pus or blood from a kidney is located within the renal fascia and does not find its way across the midline to the opposite kidney. However, it can track along the loose arrangement of renal fascia on the ureter and find its way into the pelvis. In addition, infection in the pelvis can track along the ureter to the kidney.

diaphragm during respiration. The renal fascia crosses the midline but in very close relationship to the renal vessels.

The thick pad of pararenal fat is usually thicker posterior to the kidney. This fascia also helps hold the kidney in place against the posterior abdominal wall.

Relationships of the Kidneys

Since the kidneys are retroperitoneal in nature, they come into relationship with both retroperitoneal and intraperitoneal organs. The kidneys are separated from the intraperitoneal organs by peritoneum as well as the extraperitoneal fascial specializations.

Right Kidney

The retroperitoneal structures found anterior or superior to the right kidney are the suprarenal gland, the second portion of the duodenum, and the right colic (hepatic) flexure (see Figs. 6-4 and 6-5).

The suprarenal gland covers the superior pole of the kidney while the descending duodenum crosses its hilum, and the right colic (hepatic) flexure is anterior to the inferolateral portion of the kidney (see Figs. 6-4 and 6-5).

The intraperitoneal structures found anterior to the right kidney are the right lobe of the liver and loops of small intestine. The liver covers the superior and lateral aspects of the right kidney. Most of the liver is covered by peritoneum. However, the posterior leaf of the coronary ligament passes from the liver anterior to the kidney, which has two important consequences.

The first consequence is part of the bare area of the liver is also anterior to the right kidney without any intervening peritoneum (see Fig. 6-5).

The second consequence is the intraperitoneal hepatorenal pouch (of Morrison) is formed by the reflection of the coronary ligament's posterior leaf from the liver onto the posterior abdominal wall anterior to the kidney. This important subhepatic peritoneal pouch is a common gathering site for disease-related entities (purulent fluids or metastatic carcinoma cells) that enter the peritoneal cavity.

The area for the small intestine (typically ileum) is inferomedial to the anterior surface of the inferior pole of the right kidney (see Figs. 6-4 and 6-5).

Left Kidney

The retroperitoneal organs associated with the left kidney are the suprarenal gland and the left colic flexure (see Figs. 6-4 and 6-5). The left suprarenal gland covers the superior pole of the left kidney. The area for the left colic (splenic) flexure covers the inferolateral aspect of the left kidney inferior to the splenic area and its inferior pole.

The intraperitoneal organs found anterior to the left kidney include the spleen, stomach, tail of pancreas, and jejunum. The spleen covers the superolateral surface of the left kidney. The body of the stomach is located anterior to the superior medial portion of the kidney just below the suprarenal gland (see Fig. 6-5). Although most of the pancreas is retroperitoneal, the tail is intraperitoneal and can be found medially over the renal hilum and directly inferior to the area for the

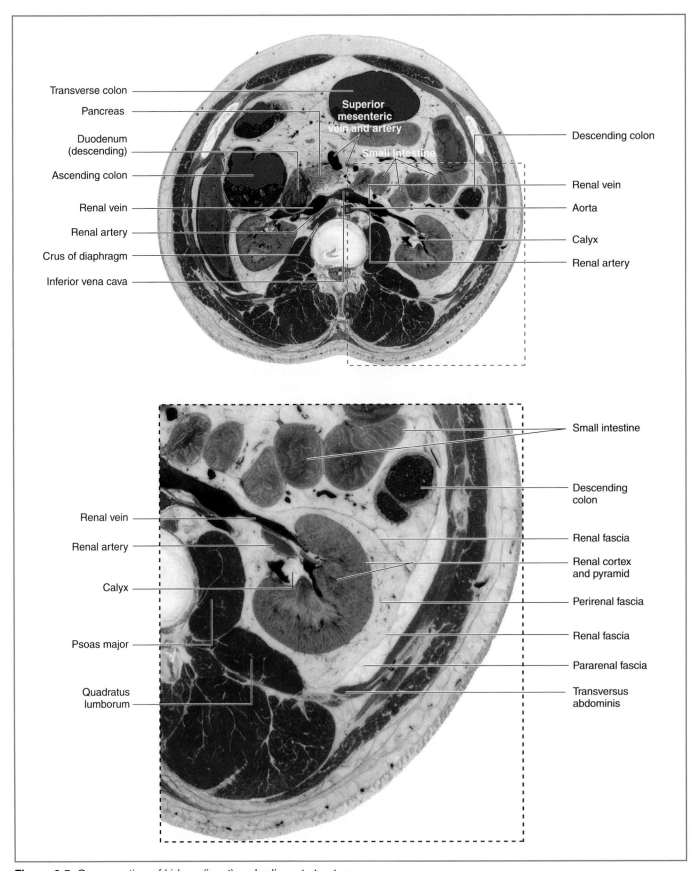

Figure 6-5. Cross-section of kidney (inset) and adjacent structures.

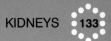

CLINICAL MEDICINE

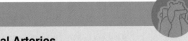

Lateral Surgical Approach to the Kidney

The costodiaphragmatic recess of the pleural cavity will be exposed if the course of the inferior surface of the 12th rib is incised during a posterolateral approach to the kidney. The pleural cavity extends to the level of the 12th rib close to the T12 vertebra. However, a transverse incision starting at the terminal end of the 12th rib would not incise the diaphragm or expose the plural cavity's costodiaphragmatic recess because the 12th rib's terminal end projects transversely to L2, which is significantly inferior to the diaphragm.

PHYSIOLOGY

Distribution of the Renal Arteries

After penetrating the parenchyma, the segmental arteries divide into the interlobar, then arcuate arteries that give off interlobular arteries. The interlobular arteries have afferent arterioles, which deliver blood to the glomerular capillary network for filtration. The efferent arterioles having glomeruli located near the capsule of the kidney join the peritubular capillary network, whereas those leaving a juxtaglomerular nephron form vasa recta, which extend into the medulla. Each of these capillary beds has different physiologic functions and venous drainage.

stomach. The left colic (splenic) flexure sits below the spleen, and a small inferomedial area for the jejunum completes the inferomedial surface of the left kidney.

Posteromedial Relationships of the Kidneys

Several muscles and associated nerves (see Fig. 6-1) are found posterior to the kidney and its fascial layers. The kidney lies anterior to the quadratus lumborum, medial and lateral arcuate ligaments, adjacent diaphragm, psoas major, and transversus abdominis muscles.

The diaphragm is posterior to the superior pole of each kidney. The psoas major muscles lie posterior to the medial border of each kidney. The quadratus lumborum muscle with the subcostal, iliohypogastric, and ilioinguinal nerves are directly posterior to the kidney (see Fig. 6-1A). The aponeurosis of the transversus abdominis is found along the posterolateral margin of the kidneys. Since the right kidney is slightly lower then the left, the 12th rib will be found posterior to the right kidney while both the 11th and 12th ribs are found posterior to the left kidney.

At the level of the costovertebral angle, which is the angle between the 12th rib and the vertebral column, the kidney is separated from the costodiaphragmatic recess (of the pleural cavity) and lung by the diaphragm. The subcostal nerve runs along the inferior surface of the 12th rib.

Internal Anatomy of the Kidney

The hilum of the kidney is the entrance/exit of the ureter's renal pelvis, renal artery and vein, lymphatics, and nerves. Like many organs, the kidney tissue has an outer cortex and an inner medulla (see Fig. 6-2).

The cortex and the medulla contain the functional unit of the kidney, the nephron, which is not visible to the unaided eye. At the macroscopic level, the cortex consists of dark red tissue and can be easily distinguished from the medulla, which consists of a dark brown tissue. The medulla is divided into 7 to 13 conical pyramids (see Fig. 6-2). The base of each pyramid delineates the medulla's outer border with the cortex or the corticomedullary junction. Dark red bands of tissues in the form of striations emanate from the base of every pyramid as medullary rays. The apex of each pyramid takes the

form of renal papillae, which project slightly into small collecting structures called minor calyces (singular, calyx). The several minor calyces unite to form a major calyx. The expanded superior end of the ureter consists of the calyces that drain into the funnel-shaped renal pelvis. Thus, two to three major calyces converge to form the renal pelvis of the ureter, which eventually narrows to become the ureter. The cortical tissue forms renal columns, which extend between the medullary pyramids (see Figs. 6-2 and 6-4). Each pyramid and associated cortical region represents a kidney lobe.

Arterial Supply and Venous Drainage of the Kidney

All of the body's blood passes through the kidneys every 5 minutes. Most of this blood is filtered in the formation of urine, but 99% of the ultrafiltrate is reabsorbed. The abdominal aorta gives rise to the renal arteries at vertebral level L2 or at the disk between L1 and L2. The right renal artery is noticeably longer than the left as it courses under the IVC (see Figs. 6-4 and 6-6). Ventral to the renal pelvis, the renal artery divides into about four or five branches to provide branches to the "renal segments."

During development renal arteries arise in the pelvis and ascend, with concurrent shifting in blood supply from the common iliac arteries to the aorta. If the transient renal arteries do not regress, they can remain as accessory renal arteries arising from the common iliac arteries and will not enter the renal hilum. Other accessory renal arteries may also arise from the aorta either above or below the main artery. Approximately 25% of the population has multiple renal arteries.

In direct contrast to the arterial supply, the venous drainage into the IVC consists of a longer left renal vein and shorter right renal vein. Each vein usually crosses anteriorly to the abdominal aorta and renal arteries.

Innervation of the Kidney

The lesser, least, and first lumbar splanchnic nerves, which arise from the lateral horn cells of T10–T12 and L1 spinal cord segments, form a synapse in the aorticorenal ganglion

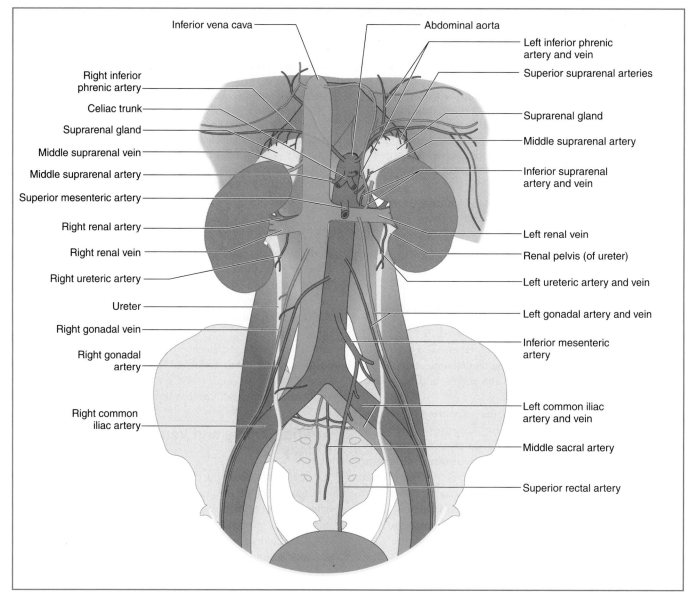

Figure 6-6. Organs and circulatory system of the abdomen.

and renal plexus associated with the renal artery. Postganglionic sympathetic fibers supply the kidney and the ureter. The sympathetic innervation to the renal arteries is important because it controls the blood flow through the kidney and therefore influences the filtration rate of the blood.

Lymphatic Drainage of the Kidney

The lymphatic drainage follows the renal vein and drains into the lumbar lymph nodes, which flow into the thoracic duct by way of the cisterna chyli.

Development of the Kidneys

The kidney and suprarenal cortex develop from intermediate mesoderm. Three sets of kidneys actually develop sequentially in the human. The first one, the pronephros, is transient and nonfunctional. The second set of kidneys, the mesonephros, functions briefly and then most of it degrades except the mesonephric duct portion that contributes to the male genital ducts. The third and permanent set of kidneys is called the metanephros and forms as an outgrowth, the ureteric bud, of the mesonephric duct. The ureteric bud forms from the distal end of the metanephric duct on each side and ultimately will form the ureter, renal pelvis, major and minor calyces, and the collecting tubules. As the bud extends into the surrounding intermediate mesoderm, it enters a region known as the metanephric blastema and begins to bifurcate. The metanephric blastema portion will form the nephrons.

Once the kidneys form in the sacral region, they ascend into their adult positions. This ascent is accompanied by a 90-degree medial rotation and several changes in blood supply.

As the kidneys ascend, they receive blood from progressively more superior vascular buds from the aorta. By the time the kidneys reach their final position, the initial kidney vessels in the sacral region have regressed. If the earlier vessels do not regress, variations in location and number of renal vessels occur.

●●● URETER

The ureter is a retroperitoneal organ that starts as the renal pelvis in the renal sinus. The renal pelvis continues as the ureter, which passes inferiorly in the extraserous fascia. The ureter lies on the psoas major muscle, which separates it from the tips of the transverse processes. The intramural portion of the ureter enters the bladder wall.

The ureter passes posterior to the gonadal vessels and anterior to the external iliac vessels over the brim of the pelvis. The abdominal ureter is supplied by the renal, gonadal, and iliac arteries and aorta. The ureters cross anterior to the genitofemoral nerve.

The right ureter is crossed by the descending duodenum, right colic vessels, ileocolic vessels, the mesentery, and the terminal ileum. The left ureter is crossed by the left colic vessels, jejunum, sigmoid colon, and its mesocolon. During mobilization of the colon and posterior abdominal wall peritoneum, the ureter may adhere to the peritoneum and may be injured.

The ureter is supplied by sympathetics whose preganglionic fibers arise in spinal cord segments T11–L1. The upper part of the ureter is supplied by spinal cord segments T11–T12, while the lower portion is supplied by L1. They also receive parasympathetic fibers from the S2–S4 spinal cord segments. In general, parasympathetic innervation increases peristalsis and sympathetics inhibit peristalsis. However, ureteric peristalsis is complicated and is not dependent on its nerves for its initiation or transmission.

●●● SUPRARENAL GLAND

The suprarenal gland is an endocrine gland found on the superomedial surface of the kidney close to the vertebral column (see Figs. 6-1 and 6-6). This retroperitoneal gland consists of an outer cortex and an inner medulla. This gland is embryologically and functionally two glands, which secrete different hormones. The cortex develops from mesoderm while the medulla develops from ectoderm. In many other organisms, these two components are found separately and the cortical component is referred to as the adrenal gland.

The cortex produces corticosteroids including mineralocorticoids, which regulate transport of sodium and water; glucocorticoids, which increase blood glucose levels; and both male and female sex hormones (testosterone and estrogen). Although the cortex secretes both sex hormones, they are secreted in small enough quantities that their effect is masked by the secretion of female or male hormones specific to the

HISTOLOGY

Glomerular Basement Membrane (GBM)

The filtration barrier in the renal glomerulus has three components: the endothelium of the glomerular capillaries, the visceral layer of Bowman's capsule consisting of podocytes, and the glomerular basement membrane. Of these three components, the GBM is the most important. The GBM has three portions: the lamina rara interna, the lamina rara externa, and the lamina densa. The lamina rara interna is adjacent to the capillary endothelium and contains a large amount of polyanions, which interfere with the passage of negatively charged proteins. The lamina rara externa is next to the podocytes and contains similarly charged components, so it is also a barrier to negatively charged proteins. Between these two layers is the lamina densa, which is composed of a meshwork of type IV collagen. Thus, the GBM by virtue of its composition provides both a physical barrier and a charge barrier for proteins. This explains why normal glomerular filtrate contains very little protein. If the concentration of protein is elevated in the urine, this is an indication that something is wrong with the GBM.

PHYSIOLOGY & PHARMACOLOGY

Renal Function

The juxtaglomerular cells are modified smooth muscle cells located in the tunica media of the afferent arteriole at the vascular pole of the glomerulus. They secrete the hormone renin in response to low blood pressure and in response to a not yet definitively identified signal from the macula densa cells. The secreted renin, in turn, converts angiotensinogen, a circulating plasma protein synthesized in the liver, into an inactive intermediate called angiotensin I. This inactive intermediate then travels to the lung, where it is converted to angiotensin II by an angiotensin-converting enzyme secreted by the endothelial cells. Angiotensin II is a vasoconstrictor and also stimulates the suprarenal cortex to secrete aldosterone, which causes the reabsorption of sodium from the distal tubules.

Individuals who are hypertensive are often treated with an angiotensin-converting enzyme (ACE) inhibitor, which blocks the conversion of angiotensin I to angiotensin II. Some individuals do not respond well to ACE inhibitors and are then treated with losartan, which is an angiotensin II receptor antagonist.

sex of the individual. However, for individuals who have a specific sex hormone–sensitive cancer (ovarian or prostate), this can sometimes lead to an adrenalectomy.

The medulla acts as a second-order sympathetic neuron that secretes epinephrine and norepinephrine into the circulatory system upon stimulation by the greater splanchnic nerve.

CLINICAL MEDICINE

Congenital Suprarenal Hyperplasia

Congenital suprarenal hyperplasia is a disorder in which excessive amounts of androgens are secreted prenatally. Typically, there is a defect in one of the enzymes involved in the synthesis of cortisol. This causes an accumulation of one of the precursors, which can be converted to testosterone in a pathway that is normally very minor. Female infants are thus exposed to unusually high levels of testosterone and are born with masculinized external genitalia.

The shapes of the right and left suprarenal glands are different, with the right gland being pyramidal and the left gland semilunar in shape (see Fig. 6-4). Both suprarenal glands are retroperitoneal and have direct relationships with the vertebral column and several midline structures. These structures consist of the diaphragmatic crura, aorta, IVC, celiac ganglia, and celiac plexus.

Anteriorly, the right suprarenal gland makes an impression on the bare area of the liver just lateral to the IVC. The gland is also found slightly posterior to the IVC as most of the gland abuts this vein posteromedially.

Anteriorly, the left suprarenal gland has a direct relationship with the body of the pancreas and the accompanying splenic vessels prior to entering the splenorenal ligament. It also forms part of the bed of the stomach, with the lesser sac found between the two organs.

Development of the Suprarenal Gland

The two parts of the suprarenal gland, the cortex and the medulla, arise from two different tissues. The cortex forms in two stages. During the 6th week, the mesothelial cells that line the posterior abdominal wall proliferate to form the fetal cortex. A second wave of proliferation of mesothelial cells surrounds the fetal cortex at 8 weeks to form the definitive cortex. However, it is not until late fetal life that the characteristic zones within the suprarenal cortex form. The suprarenal medulla develops from neural crest cells derived from adjacent sympathetic ganglia, reflecting the medulla's function as a secretor of catecholamine hormones. At birth, the suprarenal gland is 10 to 20 times larger than the adult gland relative to body weight. It will shrink in size during the first year as the fetal cortex regresses.

Blood Supply and Innervation of the Suprarenal Gland

There are three types of suprarenal arteries: superior, middle, and inferior. It is common to expect an extensive arterial supply because the suprarenal gland is an endocrine gland. However, only one large suprarenal (central) vein drains the gland (Table 6-3). The left suprarenal gland drains into the left renal vein while the right suprarenal vein drains directly into the adjacent IVC.

TABLE 6-3. Arterial Supply and Venous Drainage of the Suprarenal Glands

Vessel	Origin of Artery/Drainage of Vein
Superior suprarenal artery	Inferior phrenic with possibly 6–8 branches
Middle suprarenal artery	One or two branches from aorta
Inferior suprarenal artery	One or two branches from left renal artery
Left suprarenal vein	Drains into left renal vein
Right suprarenal vein	Difficult to find because it drains directly into the IVC posteriorly

The suprarenal gland receives its innervation from the adjacent celiac plexus and the greater splanchnic nerve. Preganglionic sympathetic fibers enter the gland to synapse directly on the medulla cells to stimulate the release of norepinephrine and epinephrine into the circulation. As is typically found in endocrine glands, the cortex receives postganglionic sympathetic fibers that are distributed with its blood vessels.

Nerves of the Posterior Abdominal Wall

Both somatic and autonomic nerves are found in the posterior abdominal wall.

The somatic nerves (Table 6-4) are found external to the inner investing layer of deep fascia. These nerves are branches of the lumbar plexus, along with the ventral ramus of the subcostal nerve, which is the ventral ramus of the T12 nerve. The subcostal nerve is found just inferior to the body of the 12th rib.

The lumbar spinal nerves emerge from the intervertebral foramina and separate into ventral and dorsal rami. The lumbar plexus arises from the ventral rami of L1–L3 with a small contribution from T12 and another from L4 (see Fig. 6-1A). This plexus is formed in the body of the psoas major muscle, where the ventral rami split into anterior and posterior divisions (see Fig. 6-1A).

The branches of the lumbar plexus emerge from the psoas major (see Table 6-4). Most of these nerves are found on the quadratus lumborum and iliacus muscles. However, the obturator nerve and the lumbosacral nerves are found on the medial side of the psoas muscle as they enter the pelvis. The branches of the lumbar plexus that emerge from the lateral side of the psoas major are the iliohypogastric (L1), ilioinguinal (L1), lateral femoral cutaneous (posterior division L2, L3), and femoral nerve (posterior division L2–L4). The genitofemoral nerve (L1, L2) emerges from the anterior surface of the psoas major, and the obturator nerve (anterior division L2–L4) emerges from the medial surface of the psoas major (see Table 6-4). The lumbosacral trunk will be considered with the sacral plexus.

The iliohypogastric and ilioinguinal nerves (see Fig. 6-1A) help supply the lateral abdominal muscles (external oblique,

TABLE 6-4. Distribution of Somatic Abdominal Nerves

Nerve	Origin	Distribution
Iliohypogastric	L1	Muscular branches to external oblique, internal oblique, transversus abdominis Cutaneous innervation to the lower hypogastric (suprapubic) region over hypogastric (suprapubic) region
Ilioinguinal	L1	Muscular branches to external oblique, internal oblique, transversus abdominis Cutaneous innervation to the superomedial thigh and the adjacent scrotum in the male or the mons pubis and labium majus in the female lower hypogastric (suprapubic) region
Genitofemoral	L1, L2	Genital branch in males supplies the cremaster muscle and helps supply the anterior scrotal wall and medial thigh; in females it helps supply the mons pubis and labium majus and medial thigh Femoral branch provides cutaneous sensation over the femoral triangle and medial thigh
Lateral femoral cutaneous	Posterior division of L2, L3	Supplies the anterolateral and posterolateral thigh to the knee
Femoral	Posterior divisions of L2–L4	Hip flexors iliacus and pectineus muscles and the knee extensor of the anterior thigh
Obturator	Anterior divisions of L2–L4	Hip adductors

internal oblique, transversus abdominis) and cutaneous innervation to the lower abdominal wall (see Table 6-4). These nerves cross the quadratus lumborum to continue to run between the transversus abdominis and internal oblique muscles (see Fig. 6-1A). The ilioinguinal nerve passes through the superficial inguinal ring but not through the deep inguinal ring. Entrapment of the iliohypogastric nerve or compression of the ilioinguinal nerve results in pain and sensory loss in the area of sensory distribution, the first lumbar dermatome.

The genitofemoral nerve penetrates the anterior surface of the psoas to run on its surface inferiorly, passing over the external iliac artery and ureter to divide into genital and femoral branches. The genital branch enters the deep inguinal ring. In males, it runs in the spermatic cord; in females, the genital branch runs on the round ligament. The femoral branch of the genitofemoral nerve passes inferior to the inguinal ligament. The femoral branch can be compressed or cut during hernia repair, resulting in pain and/or sensory loss to the skin of the femoral triangle. It can also be entrapped by resulting scar tissue.

The lateral femoral cutaneous nerve crosses the iliacus muscle in the retroperitoneal fascia as it passes towards the anterosuperior iliac spine. Here, it runs either deep to or through the inguinal ligament. The lateral femoral cutaneous nerve divides to supply the anterolateral and posterolateral thigh to the knee.

The femoral nerve (see Fig. 6-1A) is the largest branch of the lumbar plexus. It emerges from the lateral border of the psoas major. The psoas major is supplied directly by the L1, L2, and L3 ventral roots. The femoral nerve passes posterior to the inguinal ligament, lateral to the femoral artery and vein, but is excluded from the femoral sheath that encompasses the femoral vessels.

At the pelvic brim, the obturator nerve passes along the medial side of the psoas. In the pelvis, the obturator nerve passes along the lateral pelvis to the obturator foramen, where it separates into anterior and posterior divisions.

Autonomic Nerves

The greater, lesser, and least and lumbar splanchnic nerves supply the prevertebral (preaortic) ganglia and plexuses (see Fig. 5-19 and Table 5-5). The intermesenteric plexus and lumbar splanchnic nerves form the superior hypogastric plexus anterior to the bifurcation of the aorta and the L5 vertebra and medial to the two common iliac vessels. Preganglionic parasympathetic nerves that arise from the S2–S4 spinal cord levels are called the *pelvic splanchnic nerves.* Some of their branches ascend either in or close to the superior hypogastric plexus to be distributed to the abdominal portion of the hindgut by following the inferior mesenteric plexus and branches of the artery.

●●● VESSELS OF THE POSTERIOR ABDOMINAL WALL

Vessels of the posterior abdominal wall are branches of the aorta and drain into the IVC or the azygos system. These vessels lie in the extraperitoneal fascia.

Abdominal Aorta

The abdominal aorta starts in the midline at the aortic hiatus of the diaphragm, which is at the level of T12. It descends on the lumbar vertebrae moving slightly to the left and ends by bifurcating to form the two common iliac arteries at the level of the L4 vertebra (see Fig. 6-6). The abdominal aorta lies in the plane of the extraperitoneal fascia to the left of the IVC. The aorta has both somatic branches and visceral branches. The somatic branches are paired while the visceral branches can be unpaired or paired (Table 6-5; see also Chapter 5).

The inferior phrenic arteries are the first branches of the abdominal aorta (see Fig. 6-6 and Table 6-5). They arise from the anterior surface or from the celiac trunk and pass over the

TABLE 6-5. Type and Distribution of Abdominal Aorta Arteries

Artery	1—Paired/Unpaired 2—Supplies Somatic or Visceral Structure 3—Arises from Which Surface of Aorta	Structures Supplied
Inferior phrenic	1. Paired 2. Mixed 3. Anterior	Diaphragm and suprarenal gland
Middle suprarenal	1. Paired 2. Visceral 3. Lateral	Suprarenal gland
Celiac	1. Unpaired 2. Visceral 3. Anterior	Abdominal esophagus, stomach, superior and part of descending duodenum, liver, gallbladder, pancreas, spleen
Superior mesenteric	1. Unpaired 2. Visceral 3. Anterior	Inferior portion of head of pancreas, most of duodenum, jejunum, ileum, appendix, cecum, ascending colon, two thirds of transverse colon
Renal	1. Paired 2. Visceral 3. Lateral	Kidneys, part of suprarenal gland, upper portion of ureter
Ovarian	1. Paired 2. Visceral 3. Anterior	Ureter, ovary, part of uterine tube
Testicular	1. Paired 2. Visceral 3. Anterior	Ureter, epididymis, testis
Lumbar	1. Paired 2. Somatic 3. Posterior	Muscles of the posterior wall: psoas major and minor, quadratus lumborum, back muscles
Inferior mesenteric	1. Unpaired 2. Visceral 3. Anterior	Distal third of transverse colon, descending colon, sigmoid colon, rectum, anal canal up to pectinate line
Median sacral	1. Unpaired 2. Somatic 3. Posterior	Arises from posterior aspect of aorta just above its bifurcation; supplies lower lumbar vertebrae and sacrum
External iliac	Somatic branches of the common iliac	Inferior epigastric and deep circumflex iliac branches supply the anterior inferior abdominal wall

diaphragmatic crura onto the inferior surface of the diaphragm. The inferior phrenic arteries are the main supply of this muscle, and their numerous small superior suprarenal branches help supply the suprarenal gland.

The four or five pairs of lumbar arteries arise inferior to the renal arteries (see Fig. 6-6 and Table 6-5). They run between the psoas major muscle and the vertebrae to split into anterior and posterior branches. The anterior branches help supply the quadratus lumborum muscles and psoas muscles while the posterior branches supply the back.

The aorta terminates as the two common iliac arteries (see Fig. 6-6) at the level of L4. This level is approximately the same as that of the umbilicus in a thin individual. These short arteries are found medial to the psoas muscles. Each common iliac artery terminates at the lumbosacral joint, which is at the same level as the sacroiliac joint, and divides into internal and external iliac arteries. The internal iliac artery crosses the pelvic brim while the external iliac artery continues inferiorly and crosses the psoas major to pass posterior to the midpoint of the inguinal ligament (Table 6-6). Here, it becomes the femoral artery. The branches of the external iliac artery are the inferior epigastric and deep circumflex iliac arteries. Numerous important structures have a direct relationship to the external iliac arteries (see Table 6-6).

Inferior Vena Cava

The external iliac vein joins the internal iliac vein to form the common iliac vein. The right and left common iliac veins are asymmetric in that the left is longer as it joins the right common iliac vein to form the IVC to the right of the midline at the level of L5 (see Fig. 6-6). The IVC ascends anterior to

TABLE 6-6. Relationships with External Iliac Arteries

Anterior to External Iliac Arteries	Posterior to External Iliac Arteries
Ileum	Psoas major
Ureters at the level of sacroiliac joint	External iliac vein is initially posterior, but moves medial to artery so that at the inguinal ligament it is medial to the external iliac artery as it becomes the femoral vein
Ovarian artery and vein in suspensory ligament	
Testicular artery and vein	
Inguinal ligament	
Close to the inguinal ligament, testicular vessels and ductus deferens in male and round ligament (ligamentum teres) of uterus in females as these structures proceed to the deep ring	
Sigmoid colon is anterior to left external iliac artery	

TABLE 6-7. Relationships with Inferior Vena Cava (IVC)

Anterior to IVC	Posterior to IVC
Right common iliac artery	Lower lumbar vertebrae
Root of the mesentery and superior mesenteric artery and vein	Psoas major muscle
	Lumbar arteries
Horizontal (third) portion of duodenum	Right sympathetic trunk and accompanying lumbar lymph nodes
Head of pancreas	
Right gonadal artery	Right crus, but most of the crus is medial to IVC
Superior (first) part of duodenum	Right suprarenal gland is interspersed between part of IVC and diaphragm
Omental foramen (of Winslow)	
IVC lies in a groove on the visceral surface of the liver where it receives the hepatic veins	Right branches of aorta; renal and suprarenal arteries
	Ascending lumbar veins, which join with subcostal veins to form azygos and hemiazygos veins

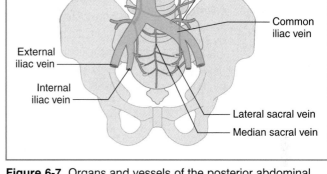

Figure 6-7. Organs and vessels of the posterior abdominal wall.

PATHOLOGY

Abdominal Aortic Aneurysm (AAA)

Abdominal aortic aneurysm is a potentially life-threatening condition. The normal aorta has an intima, media, and adventitia. The media (smooth muscle layer) is important in maintaining the aorta's structure and elasticity. Most commonly, AAA is the result of degeneration in the media. Atherosclerotic changes result in degeneration of the media followed by loss of the vessel's structural integrity and concurrent dilation of the vessel's lumen over time. This pathologic change is typically found in the abdominal aorta distal to the renal vessels.

Tributaries to the IVC include lumbar, right gonadal (left gonadal drains into left renal), renal, right suprarenal (left suprarenal drains into left renal), right inferior phrenic (left inferior phrenic drains into left renal), and most importantly the three hepatic veins (see Figs. 6-6 and 6-7 and Table 6-7).

The lumbar veins drain into the IVC and also join together to form the ascending lumbar veins (see Fig. 6-7 and Table 6-7). These veins contribute to the formation of the azygos and hemiazygos veins.

●●● LYMPHATICS OF THE POSTERIOR ABDOMINAL WALL

The lymphatics of the posterior abdominal wall, or lumbar nodes, follow the aorta and IVC. The lumbar nodes are continuous with the common iliac nodes, which receive the external and internal iliac nodes (Table 6-8). The lumbar nodes are subdivided into lateral and right lumbar nodes and

the lumbar vertebrae and to the right of the aorta starting at the level of L4. Thus, it is crossed by the right common iliac artery. The IVC ascends higher in the abdomen than the abdominal aorta, since the aorta passes through the aortic hiatus at the level of T12 while the IVC passes through its diaphragmatic hiatus at the level of T8. While still in the supracolic region of the abdomen, the aorta and IVC are separated by the right crus of the diaphragm.

TABLE 6-8. Lymphatic Drainage of the Abdominal Viscera

Structures That Drain into the Left Lateral Nodes	Structures That Drain into the Preaortic Nodes	Structures That Drain into the Right Lateral Nodes
Left common iliac	Viscera supplied by inferior mesenteric artery	Right common iliac
Left testis/ovary		Testis/ovary
Body of uterus	Viscera supplied by superior mesenteric artery	Body of uterus
Left uterine tube		Right uterine tube
Left kidney	Viscera supplied by celiac artery	Right kidney
Left suprarenal gland		Right suprarenal gland
Left posterior abdominal wall muscles		Right posterior abdominal wall muscles

preaortic nodes. The lateral nodes communicate across the midline with each other and with the preaortic nodes. The left lateral lumbar chain is related to the aorta, psoas major, and left crus while the right lateral nodes are related to the IVC, psoas major, and right crus. The preaortic nodes are somewhat variable (see Table 6-8).

The abdominal viscera as well as the posterior wall drain into the preaortic nodes.

The right and left lumbar efferent vessels on each side unite to form two lumbar lymphatic trunks. The lymphatic intestinal trunk from the superior mesenteric and celiac nodes joins the lumbar trunks to form the cisterna chyli. This lymphatic structure is the dilated beginning of the thoracic duct. It is typically found posterior and to the right of the aorta at the level of the disk between the T12 and L2 vertebrae. The thoracic duct passes into the thorax through the aortic hiatus.

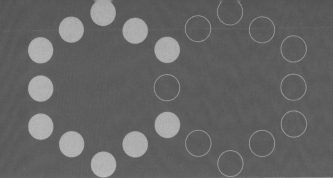

Pelvis and Perineum

7

CONTENTS

PELVIS

THE BONY PELVIS
Pubis
Ischium
Ilium
Sacrum
Coccyx

ORGANIZATION OF THE PELVIS
Greater Versus Lesser Pelvis
Ligaments Associated with the Bony Pelvis
Sex Dimorphisms
Muscles of the Pelvis
Lateral Muscles
Diaphragms

PELVIC DIAPHRAGM
Coccygeus Muscle
Levator Ani Muscle
Urogenital Hiatus

FASCIA OF THE PELVIS
Endopelvic or Inner Investing Layer of Deep Fascia
Extraperitoneal Fascia
Peritoneum and Its Pouches

NERVES IN THE PELVIS
Somatic Nerves
Autonomic Nerves

OVERVIEW OF BLOOD SUPPLY TO THE PELVIS AND GLUTEAL REGIONS
Arteries
Posterior Division of Internal Iliac Artery
Anterior Division of Internal Iliac Artery
Ovarian Artery
Veins

TERMINAL END OF THE GASTROINTESTINAL SYSTEM
Rectum
Anal Canal
Relationships of the Anal Canal and Rectum

PELVIC URINARY SYSTEM
Ureter
Urinary Bladder
Urethra

DEVELOPMENT OF URINARY BLADDER, RECTUM, AND ANAL CANAL

MALE GENITAL SYSTEM
Testis
Epididymis
Ductus Deferens
Seminal Vesicle
Prostate Gland

DEVELOPMENT OF MALE REPRODUCTIVE SYSTEM

FEMALE GENITAL SYSTEM
Ovaries
Uterine (Fallopian) Tubes (Salpinx)
Uterus
Relationships of the Uterus
Vagina
Relationships of the Vagina

DEVELOPMENT OF FEMALE REPRODUCTIVE ORGANS

PERINEUM

UROGENITAL TRIANGLE
Urogenital Diaphragm
Superficial Pouch

DEVELOPMENT OF EXTERNAL GENITALIA

ANAL TRIANGLE
Ischioanal Fossa
External Anal Sphincter Muscle

NEUROVASCULAR BUNDLES OF THE PERINEUM
Pudendal Nerve
Parasympathetic Nerves
Internal Pudendal Artery
Additional Blood Supply
Internal Pudendal Vein
Lymphatics of the Perineum

PELVIS

The pelvis is the caudal continuation of the abdominal cavity and the entire cavity can be referred to as the *abdominopelvic cavity*. The pelvis has the same basic organization and layers as the abdominal cavity.

The most striking differences between the pelvis and the abdomen are (1) the bony pelvis is inflexible, and (2) the organ systems interface with and then penetrate the somatic pelvic wall owing to the embryologic formation and subsequent rupture of the anal and urogenital subdivisions of the cloacal membrane.

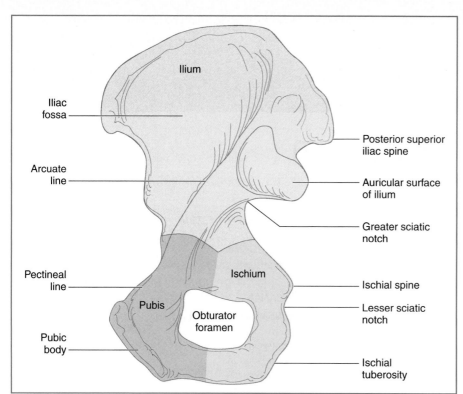

Figure 7-1. Medial view of a hemipelvis.

The pelvic region can be organized around the bony pelvis, which is rigid when compared with the anterior abdominal wall. The bony pelvis allows the body weight to be transmitted through the sacroiliac joints to the femurs during standing or to the ischial tuberosities during sitting.

The pelvic wall can be compared layer by layer to the abdominal wall. The external layers are skin and superficial fascia. The next layers consist of musculoskeletal system. The musculoskeletal system is separated from the superficial fascia by an outer investing layer of deep fascia and from the peritoneum and extraperitoneal fascia by an inner investing layer of deep fascia. The pelvic inner investing layer of deep fascia is continuous with endoabdominal (transversalis) fascia. The muscles of the pelvis are organized into an external layer of skeletal muscle and an internal layer of skeletal muscle with the bony pelvis sandwiched in between. The external layer of muscle is described with the lower limb.

●●● THE BONY PELVIS

The bony pelvis comprises the two hip bones as well as the sacrum and the coccyx. Each hip bone is composed of three fused bones: the pubis, the ilium, and the ischium (Fig. 7-1). These bones articulate at the deep socket (acetabulum) of the hip joint, found on the external pelvic surface.

The pubis is the anteromedial portion of the hip bone. The ilium is the superolateral portion, while the ischium is the inferolateral portion of the hip bone (Figs. 7-2 and 7-3). The pubic symphysis is a synchondrosis joint that separates the right and left pubic bones anteriorly. The pelvic surface of

the pubis faces superoposteriorly, while the external (perineal) surface faces inferoanteriorly in the anatomic position (see Fig. 7-1).

Pubis

As mentioned in Chapter 5, the important anterior landmarks found on the pubis are the pubic tubercle and pubic crest. The body of the pubis has two rami (branch-like extensions)—the superior and inferior pubic rami—that articulate with the ilium and with the ischium. The superior ramus is marked on its posterior superior surface by a sharp line of bone—the pectineal line or pecten—which serves as the attachment line of the pectineal (Cooper's) ligament. The point where the superior ramus articulates with the ilium is marked by an elevation of bone called the iliopectineal (iliopubic) eminence. The iliopectineal septum stretches from the inguinal ligament to the iliopectineal (iliopubic) eminence, separating this region into two small spaces, or lacunae. Lateral to the iliopectineal septum, the iliacus and psoas major muscles and femoral nerve enter the thigh in the muscular lacuna. Medial to the iliopectineal septum, the femoral artery and vein enter the thigh in the vascular lacuna. The femoral vein is the most medial of these two vessels, while the femoral nerve is lateral to the femoral artery.

The obturator groove is found on the *inferior* surface of the superior pubic ramus, in the region of the iliopubic eminence (see Fig. 7-1). The obturator neurovascular bundle occupies the obturator groove (see obturator membrane in the section on Ligaments Associated with the Bony Pelvis).

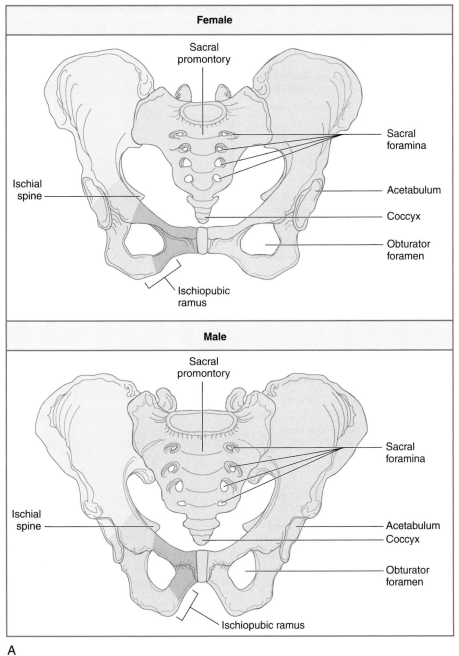

Figure 7-2. The pelvis. **A,** Anterior view, female and male.   *Continued*

A

Ischium

The ischium is the inferoposterior portion of the hip bone (see Fig. 7-1). The ischium consists of a body, spine, tuberosity, ramus, and the lesser sciatic notch. The body of the ischium participates in the formation of the acetabulum with the body of the ilium and the pubis. The inferior surface of the ischial body is enlarged as an elevated roughened bump of bone referred to as the ischial tuberosity. The ischial spine is a sharp triangular process of bone that projects posteriorly. Between the ischial spine and tuberosity is an indentation or notch known as the lesser sciatic notch. Superior to the ischial spine is the greater sciatic notch, which is a much

deeper depression. Thus, the ischial spine separates the greater and lesser sciatic notches (see Fig. 7-1). These two notches are converted into the greater and lesser sciatic foramina by the sacrospinous and sacrotuberous ligaments (see Figs. 7-2B and 7-3).

As mentioned above, the ischial ramus joins the inferior ramus of the pubis to form the ischiopubic or conjoined ramus. The obturator foramen is the large opening found in the anteroinferior aspect of the hip bone (see Fig. 7-2). It is formed by the body of the ischium, the ischiopubic ramus, and the body and the superior ramus of the pubis. Thus, no part of the ilium participates in the formation of the obturator foramen.

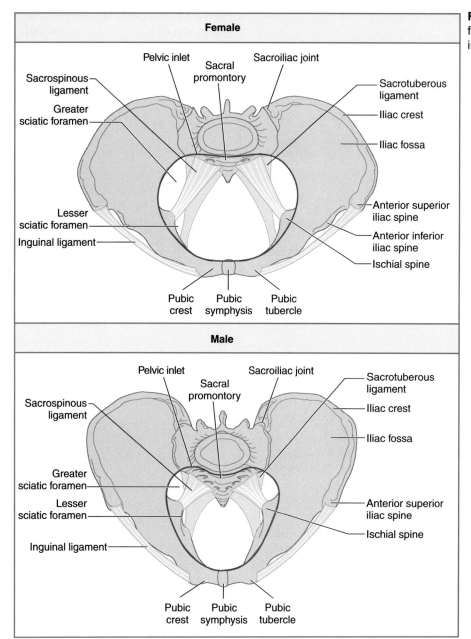

B

Ilium

The third portion of the hip bone is the ilium (see Fig. 7-1) which consists of a body at the acetabulum and a large wing (ala). Part of the body of the ilium forms the superior aspect of the acetabulum. The wing of the ilium extends superiorly and laterally and is separated from the body by the arcuate line of the pelvis. This is a curved line that is found on the medial aspect of the ilium. It extends from the pectineal line of the pubis to the sacrum. The pectineal line plus the arcuate line together are referred to as the terminal line. The anterior surface of the iliac wing is hollowed out to take the form of the ditch-like iliac fossa, which is the origin of the iliacus muscle. The superior border of the wing of the ilium is called the iliac crest. Extending posteriorly from the iliac crest is the posterior superior iliac spine, while extending anteriorly is the anterior superior iliac spine (Fig. 7-2). Recall that the iliac crest is an important attachment point for the lateral abdominal muscles (external oblique, internal oblique, and transversus abdominis muscles) and that the anterior superior iliac spine is the lateral attachment point for the inguinal ligament.

The posteromedial (sacropelvic) surface of the ilium articulates with the sacrum to form the sacroiliac joint. The iliac surface of this joint has an ear-like, roughened aspect, or "auricular" surface, which is often grooved to fit reciprocal grooves on the sacrum (see Fig. 7-1). The anterior and poste-

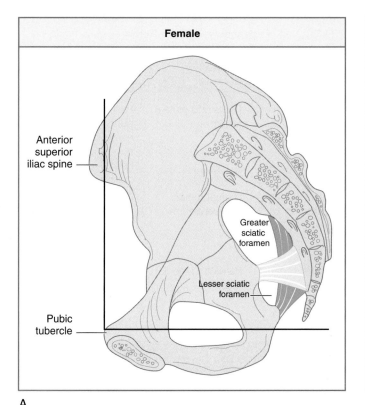

Female

Anterior superior iliac spine

Greater sciatic foramen

Lesser sciatic foramen

Pubic tubercle

A

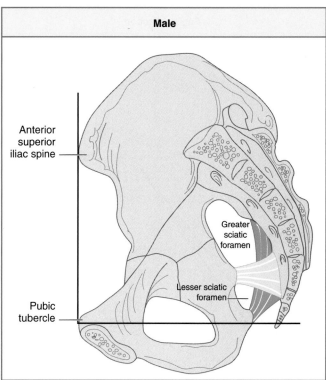

Male

Anterior superior iliac spine

Greater sciatic foramen

Lesser sciatic foramen

Pubic tubercle

B

Figure 7-3. Anatomic position of the pelvis. **A,** Female. **B,** Male.

rior sacroiliac ligaments help support this important weight-bearing joint.

Sacrum

The sacrum consists of five fused sacral vertebrae (see Fig. 7-2). The sacral vertebrae (S) begin to fuse at approximately 5 years (the costal elements first) and continue until 18 to 25 years. The disks ossify in the midline and produce transverse ridges between the bodies, which can be observed on the anterior (pelvic) concave surface. The anterior surface of S1 projects anteriorly and is called the *sacral promontory*.

The following elements fuse: costal elements, bodies, pedicle, and transverse processes forming the lateral part or mass. Owing to the fusion of the sacral vertebrae, the intervertebral foramina now lead to four pairs of anterior and posterior sacral foramina. The S5 nerves leave the sacral canal through the sacral hiatus, which is found on the posterior and inferior end of the sacral vertebral canal. The sacral hiatus is formed by the absence of the laminae and spinous process of S5. The ventral rami of the S5 nerves pass anteriorly through crescent-shaped notches just below the fourth posterior sacral foramina.

The posterior surface of the sacrum is ridged and convex. It is marked by a midline (median) sacral crest, which is formed by the fused spines and the parasagittal lateral sacral crests. The four posterior sacral foramina on each side are just medial to the lateral sacral crests. A skin dimple is usually found overlying the posterior superior iliac spine and the adjacent sacroiliac joint. A line between the two skin dimples would pass through the S2 vertebra. Just below and medial to the

adjacent lateral sacral crest is the posterior S2 foramen. This relationship may be used to find the S2 posterior sacral foramen to inject an anesthetic into the epidural space.

Coccyx

The coccyx consists of three to five coccygeal vertebrae that are arranged so that the apex is facing inferiorly with a slightly concave surface facing anteriorly. The first coccygeal vertebra has two horns (cornua) that extend superiorly from its posterior surface to articulate with the sacral cornua that are found on either side of the sacral hiatus.

●●● ORGANIZATION OF THE PELVIS
Greater Versus Lesser Pelvis

The inferior portion of the abdominopelvic cavity can be divided into the greater pelvis (false pelvis, pelvis major) and the lesser pelvis (true pelvis, pelvis minor) at the pelvic inlet. The pelvic inlet is marked by a bony line in the internal pelvic surface that consists of the terminal line (pectineal line and arcuate line) and crosses along the inferior aspect of both the lateral part and the promontory of the sacrum (see Fig. 7-2B). The area above the pelvic inlet is the greater pelvis and is part of the posterior abdominal wall while the area below the pelvic inlet is the lesser true pelvis.

The pelvic outlet (inferior aperture) is the opening marked by the inferior surface of the pubic symphysis, the ischio-pubic rami, the ischial tuberosities, and the sacrotuberous

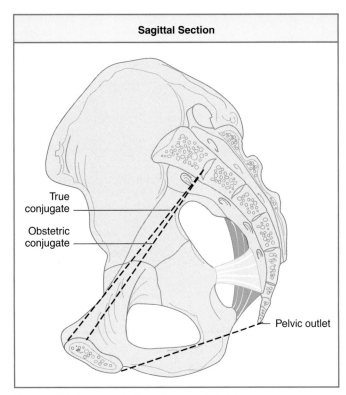

Sagittal Section

True conjugate

Obstetric conjugate

Pelvic outlet

Figure 7-4. Important diameters in obstetrics.

TABLE 7-1. Passageways in the Pelvis

Passageway	Connection Between	Structures That Pass Through
Greater sciatic foramen	Pelvis and gluteal region	Piriformis muscle, pudendal neurovascular bundle, gluteal neurovascular bundles, sciatic nerve
Lesser sciatic foramen	Gluteal region and perineum	Obturator internus, nerve to the obturator internus and pudendal neurovascular bundle
Obturator canal	Pelvis and medial thigh	Obturator neurovascular bundle

TABLE 7-2. Pelvic Sex Dimorphisms

Feature	Male	Female
Shape of pelvic cavity	Conical	Cylindric
Sacrum	Longer and narrower	Shorter and wider
Obturator foramen	Round	Triangular
Subpubic angle	50 to 60 degrees	80 to 85 degrees
Rami	Strong	Delicate
Pelvic inlet	Heart-shaped	Circular
Ischial spines	Project more medially	Do not project as medially

ligaments, which extend from the ischial tuberosities to the sacrum and the coccyx (Fig. 7-4).

Ligaments Associated with the Bony Pelvis

Several ligaments (see Figs. 7-2 and 7-3) help organize the bony pelvis. The ligaments support the sacroiliac joints and the pubic symphysis and convert notches and foramina into passageways.

The sacrospinous ligament arises from the sacrum and inserts into the ischial spine. The sacrospinous ligament is always the anterior of the two ligaments and has the coccygeus muscle attached to its anterior surface.

The sacrotuberous ligament has an extensive origin from the posterior aspect of the ilium, sacrum, and coccyx to insert into the ischial tuberosity. It serves as an origin for the gluteus maximus muscle, which is attached to its posterior surface.

The sacrospinous and sacrotuberous ligaments convert the greater and lesser sciatic notches into foramina (see Fig. 7-3).

The greater sciatic foramen is the major passageway connecting the pelvis and the gluteal region. The lesser sciatic foramen is the passageway connecting the gluteal region and the perineum (Table 7-1).

The obturator membrane is a tough ligament that fills in most of the obturator foramen and serves as part of the origin for both internal and external obturator muscles. However, the obturator groove, which is found on the superolateral aspect of the obturator foramen, is not filled in by this membrane and becomes the obturator canal.

Sex Dimorphisms

In the anatomic position, the anterior tilt of the pelvis is partially due to the lordotic curvature of the lumbar vertebrae (see Fig. 7-3). In males, the anterior superior iliac spine is in the same coronal (frontal) plane as the pubic tubercle. In addition, the superior surface of the pubic crest is in the same horizontal plane as the tip of the coccyx.

In contrast, the female pelvis is tilted forward. Thus, the coronal line through the anterior superior iliac spine falls anterior the pubic tubercle while the tip of the coccyx is above the horizontal plane of the pubic tubercle (see Fig. 7-3).

Other sex dimorphisms include the following differences. The female pelvis is shallow and cylindric. In the female, the subpubic angle is greater than in the male, with a greater pelvic outlet, everted ischial spines, and wider sciatic notches (Table 7-2; see also Fig. 7-2).

Various pelvic diameters are important in obstetrics (see Fig. 7-4). These measurements between any two specified points on the periphery of the pelvic canal are referred to as conjugate distances. The true conjugate of the pelvis inlet (conjugata vera) is the distance from the midpoint of the sacral promontory to the superior border of the pubic symphysis. Obstetric conjugate diameter (obstetric conjugate) is the shortest diameter that the infant's head must pass through. It is the distance from the midpoint of the sacral promontory to the nearest point on the posterior surface of the pubic symphysis.

Muscles of the Pelvis

The pelvic skeletal muscles are organized into two groups. The lateral or external muscles are lower limb muscles, which arise from the interior of the bony pelvis and include the obturator internus and piriformis muscles (Figs. 7-5 and 7-6

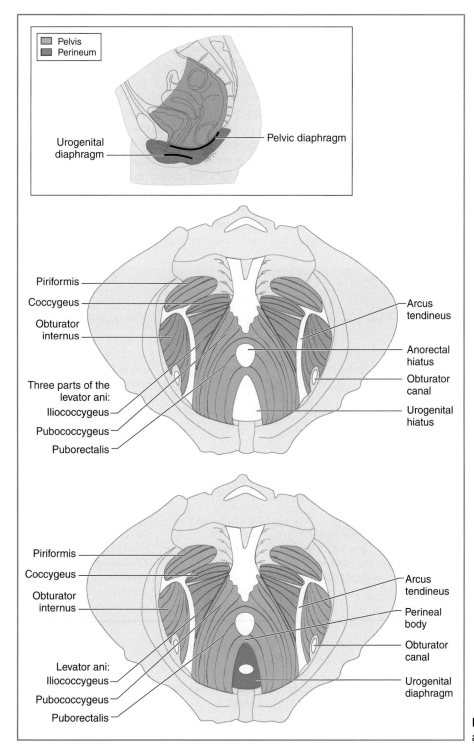

Figure 7-5. Pelvic floor with (*lower figure*) and without (*upper figure*) deep pouch.

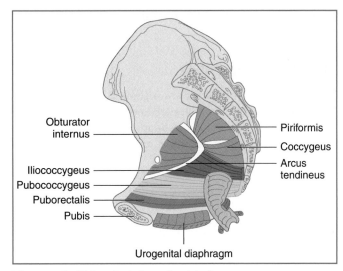

Obturator
internus

Piriformis

Coccygeus

Arcus
tendineus

Iliococcygeus
Pubococcygeus
Puborectalis
Pubis

Urogenital diaphragm

Figure 7-6. Midsagittal view of pelvic floor.

and Table 7-3). These muscles insert into the greater trochanter of the femur and are lateral rotators of the hip joint. The lateral muscles are considered here only because, as is the case with all skeletal muscles that help form a body cavity, they have the inner investing layer of deep fascia (endopelvic fascia) on their internal surface. This layer of fascia is an important building block in the pelvis.

The second group of muscles stretches from the pelvic walls to the midline in the form of the pelvic diaphragm. This diaphragm separates the pelvis from the part of the body wall referred to as the perineum (see Fig. 7-5).

Lateral Muscles

The obturator internus muscle arises from the internal surface of the obturator membrane, the ischiopubic ramus, and to a lesser extent from the superior ramus of the pubis. The muscle fibers converge on and leave the pelvis through the lesser sciatic foramen. The obturator internus muscle inserts into the greater trochanter of the femur and is the *only structure that leaves* the bony pelvis by passing through the lesser sciatic foramen.

The piriformis muscle has three origins from the anterior surface of the sacrum between the anterior sacral foramina 1–4. It also has a second head from the ilium's greater sciatic notch, which is of greater interest in the study of the lower limb. The piriformis muscle passes through the greater sciatic foramen and inserts into the greater trochanter of the femur.

Anteriorly, this muscle is covered by the sacral spinal nerves that leave the anterior sacral foramina to form the sacral plexus. In addition, many branches of the internal iliac vessels as well as the inner investing layer of deep fascia (endopelvic

TABLE 7-3. Muscles of the Pelvis

Muscle	Origin	Insertion	Function	Innervation
Lateral Muscles of Pelvis				
Obturator internus	Internal surface of obturator membrane, ischiopubic ramus, and superior ramus of pubis	Greater trochanter of femur	Rotates the hip laterally	Nerve to the obturator internus—ventral rami of L5, S1–S2
Piriformis	Anterolateral surface of the 2nd, 3rd, and 4th vertebrae, greater sciatic notch	Greater trochanter of femur	Rotates the hip laterally	Nerve to the piriformis—ventral ramus of S1–S2
Muscles That Divide Pelvis from Perineum				
Coccygeus	Ischial spine, ischium	Coccyx and sacrum	Pulls coccyx forward after defecation or parturition	Ventral ramus of S3–S4
Levator ani, iliococcygeus	Ischial spine and arcus tendineus	Coccyx and anococcygeal raphe	Supports pelvic organs	Nerve to the levator ani—ventral ramus of S3–S4—and perineal branch of pudendal nerve
Pubococcygeus	Superior ramus of pubis	Coccyx, anococcygeal raphe, and perineal body	Supports pelvic organs	
Puborectalis	Superior ramus of pubis	Contralateral puborectalis	Produces perineal flexure of rectum and ensures anal continence in conjunction with deep portion of external anal constrictor	
Urethral/ urethrovaginal sphincter	Ischiopubic ramus	Contralateral ischiopubic ramus	Protects urogenital hiatus	Perineal branch of pudendal nerve

CLINICAL MEDICINE

Prolapse of Pelvic Organs

The proper support of the pelvic organs is dependent on the integrity and tone of the pelvic diaphragm and on ligaments such as the cardinal, transverse cervical, uterosacral, and round of uterus ligaments. Multiple vaginal births, obesity, and high intra-abdominal pressure can all cause the vaginal wall, uterus, bladder, and even rectum to descend toward the vaginal vestibule. Symptoms depend on the severity of damage to the pelvic floor and which organs are involved. For example, prolapse of the vaginal wall can be asymptomatic or be associated with a sense of fullness in the vagina and a sacral backache. Prolapse of the rectum through the posterior vaginal wall or anus can cause difficulties in evacuation of feces. Treatment depends on the severity of symptoms and may include medical or surgical methods.

fascia) also cover the piriformis muscle, making it difficult to find this muscle in the pelvis.

Diaphragms

The distribution of the lateral muscles leaves a large gap in the pelvic outlet because these muscles pass laterally to leave the pelvis and to insert into the femur. Two muscle groups, the pelvic diaphragm and the urogenital diaphragm, close this gap.

The term diaphragm derives from Greek, "fence," and refers to musculomembranous structures that separate (as fences do) and are characterized by one or more openings. The pelvic diaphragm has a central urogenital hiatus, through which the urethra, vagina, and rectum pass and which is reinforced anteroinferiorly by the muscles of the urogenital diaphragm.

●●● PELVIC DIAPHRAGM

The pelvic diaphragm is composed of two pairs of muscles: the coccygeus and the levator ani (see Figs. 7-5 and 7-6 and Table 7-3). The muscles of the pelvic diaphragm pass from the lateral pelvic walls to the midline and thus close the pelvic outlet by forming *most* of the pelvic floor (see Fig. 7-5). The pelvic diaphragm is often described as a sling. However, in the living, these muscles have tone and are in a sheet-like configuration that supports the pelvic organs even during sleep. Relaxation of the pelvic diaphragm produces stretch reflexes that are responsible for the initiation of micturition.

Coccygeus Muscle

The coccygeus muscle is found on and is firmly attached to the anterior surface of the sacrospinous ligament. It arises from the spine of the ischium and inserts into the margin of the coccyx and adjacent sacrum. This muscle acts to pull the coccyx forward after posterior displacement during defecation or parturition.

Levator Ani Muscle

The levator ani muscle stretches from the walls of the pelvis toward the midline, where it meets the muscle fibers of the contralateral levator ani muscle or inserts into adjacent midline organs. The levator ani supports pelvic organs, helps retain them in their proper anatomic positions, and elevates the pelvic floor. The levator ani muscle has several parts that are named according to their origin and insertion (see Figs. 7-5 and 7-6 and Table 7-3).

The iliococcygeus muscle arises from the spine of the ischium and the arcus tendineus levator ani (tendinous arch of levator ani) and runs medially toward the midline. Here, the iliococcygeus muscle inserts into the coccyx and the anococcygeal raphe (ligament). The arcus tendineus levator ani is a condensation of the inner investing layer of deep fascia on the obturator internus muscle. It stretches from the ischial spine to the superior ramus of the pubis. Thus, the iliococcygeus arises from a fascial condensation (arcus tendineus) that lies on the internal surface of the obturator internus muscle. The anococcygeal raphe is a ligament that stretches from the anus and anal canal to the coccyx.

The pubococcygeus arises from the superior ramus of the pubis. Its fibers run posteromedially. Some of these fibers reach the coccyx and the anococcygeal raphe. Others run posteriorly and medially and insert into the perineal body (central tendon of the perineum; see Fig. 7-5), a connective tissue mass that also contains smooth muscle located between the anus and the scrotum/vagina). The medial fibers of the pubococcygeus muscle can also insert into either the false capsule of prostate as the levator prostatae muscle in males or into the vagina as the pubovaginalis muscles in females.

The puborectalis portion arises from the superior ramus of the pubis. These fibers run posteriorly around the anal canal to join with the contralateral puborectalis muscle. These muscle fibers also pass around the gastrointestinal (GI) system at the junction of the rectum and anal canal. The puborectalis muscle pulls the rectum anteriorly at this point to produce the perineal flexure of the rectum. The puborectalis muscle is inferior to the medial fibers of the pubococcygeus muscle. The puborectalis fibers blend with the deep portion of the external anal sphincter muscle. Thus, both the deep portion of the external anal sphincter and the puborectalis muscles are very important in maintaining anal continence.

Urogenital Hiatus

A reexamination of the levator ani muscle reveals a gap in this complex muscle directly posterior to the pubic symphysis. This gap in the levator ani is referred to as the urogenital (genital) hiatus. The urethra in both sexes and the vagina in females pass through this hiatus. The main function of the levator ani is to support the pelvic viscera. However, the urogenital hiatus is wide enough to require a second set of muscles to complete the floor of the pelvis. The sphincter urethrae (urethrovaginal sphincter), along with the deep transverse perineal muscles, performs this function (see Fig. 7-5). A detailed description of these muscles and their arrangement can be found in the Perineum section.

●●● FASCIA OF THE PELVIS

The fascia of the pelvis is similar to the fascia of the abdomen and is continuous at the brim of the pelvis. The inner investing layer of deep fascia in the abdomen (endoabdominal fascia) is continuous with the inner investing layer of deep fascia in the pelvis (endopelvic fascia). The subserous fascia (extraperitoneal fascia) and peritoneum are also continuous over the brim of the pelvis. Each of these layers has important specializations in the pelvis that stabilize pelvic organs. These organs are for the most part embedded in the plane of the subserous (extraperitoneal) fascia and are covered only partially by peritoneum.

Endopelvic or Inner Investing Layer of Deep Fascia

The endopelvic fascia covers the muscles on the lateral walls of the pelvis, passes onto the superior surface of the pelvic diaphragm, and extends on the sphincter urethrae and up onto the base of various pelvic organs. The endopelvic fascia separates the body wall from the body cavity. Most of the branches of the lumbosacral plexus are found external to the endopelvic fascia. Indeed, the dissector must strip away the endopelvic fascia to observe the sacral plexus anterior to the piriformis muscle. The dissector must also remove the endoabdominal fascia on the psoas major muscle in the greater pelvis to find the femoral nerve. Endopelvic fascia is usually described as having a parietal portion and visceral

portion. Note that this is an unusual circumstance because the term visceral is being used to describe a portion of somatic fascia.

The parietal aspect of the endopelvic fascia chiefly separates the internal surfaces of obturator internus muscles, the sacral plexus, and the piriformis muscles from the pelvis. The endopelvic fascia condenses between the ischial spine and the superior pubic ramus to form the arcus tendineus levator ani (tendinous arch of the levator ani), which is one of the origins of the iliococcygeus muscle (see Fig. 7-5).

The visceral aspect of endopelvic fascia also stretches from the pelvic wall to certain organs, forming supporting ligaments (Fig. 7-7). It also extends up onto these organs to form fascial layers around some organs and false capsules around others. The pubovesical ligaments in females stretch from the pubis to the neck of the bladder. The puboprostatic ligaments in males stretch from the pubis to the prostate. These ligaments, derived from visceral endopelvic fascia that may contain smooth muscle, support these organs. The false capsule of the prostate (prostatic fascia) is also derived from the endopelvic fascia. A similar but less well developed layer of endopelvic fascia forms the rectal fascia surrounding the rectum.

Extraperitoneal Fascia

The extraperitoneal (extra- or subserous) fascia is found between the endopelvic fascia and the peritoneum. This layer of fascia contains the organs, blood vessels, and autonomic nerves. In addition, the extraperitoneal fascia forms supporting ligaments, which often contain smooth muscle. These fascial ligaments along with the pelvic diaphragm and urethral

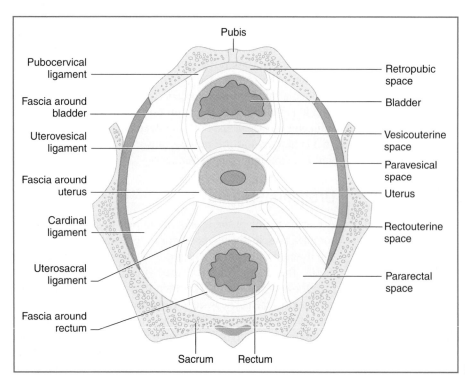

Figure 7-7. Fascia in the female pelvis.

sphincter muscle are responsible for maintaining the proper anatomic position of the pelvic organs. If these ligaments or the muscles are damaged, the organ involved can prolapse (fall through a body orifice). The uterus, and less often the bladder, can prolapse into the vaginal canal, and the rectum can prolapse through the anus.

The following ligaments are formed from extraperitoneal fascia and usually contain some smooth muscle:

- In males: (1) the rectovesical (sacrovesical) ligament and (2) the rectovesical septum (Denonvilliers' fascia)
- In females: (1) the uterosacral ligaments and (2) the transverse cervical ligaments (cardinal ligaments) of the uterus (see Fig. 7-7)

Some ligaments contain important neurovascular bundles.

Cellulitis of the extraperitoneal fascial plane and peritoneum in females occurs in pelvic inflammatory disease (PID), often a result of sexually transmitted diseases, and can be difficult to treat.

Peritoneum and Its Pouches

The peritoneum covers many structures in the pelvic cavity. However, the peritoneum only *partially* covers most of the pelvic organs, since they are retroperitoneal in position. The peritoneal cavity has pouches (pockets or recesses) produced by the peritoneum passing over an organ onto an adjacent organ. The only intraperitoneal pelvic organs are the sigmoid colon, ovaries, and uterine tubes. Loops of the ileum are found in the pelvis but have an abdominal origin. All the other organs are retroperitoneal in position and raise peritoneal folds or ligaments as the peritoneum stretches from the pelvic walls to the organs or passes from one organ to another. Examples of peritoneal ligaments are the suspensory ligaments of the ovaries, the broad ligament of the uterus, the sacrogenital folds in males and rectouterine (also called sacrogenital) folds in females, and the false (in that they are peritoneal instead of fascial) ligaments of the bladder (see Fig. 7-7).

The greater sac of the peritoneal cavity has several specializations or pouches in the pelvis as a result of the relationship of the peritoneum to the pelvic organs.

The following peritoneal pouches are found in males (Fig. 7-8). The *rectovesical pouch* is formed by the peritoneum passing from the posterior surface of the bladder onto the anterior surface of the rectum. The peritoneal coverings of the rectovesical ligaments are called the *sacrogenital folds*. These folds deepen the rectovesical pouch of the peritoneal cavity. Because the sacrogenital peritoneal folds follow the rectovesical ligaments toward the sacrum, the rectovesical pouch is also extended along the lateral sides of the rectum. However, the pouches of the peritoneal cavity that lie along the lateral aspect of the rectum are called the *pararectal pouches* of the peritoneal cavity and communicate freely with the rectovesical pouch.

In females (see Fig. 7-8), the uterus develops between the bladder and the rectum, producing a *vesicouterine pouch* and a *rectouterine pouch* (pouch of Douglas or cul-de-sac). The rectouterine pouch is the portion of the peritoneal cavity that is produced by the peritoneum passing from the posterior surface of the uterus onto the anterior surface of the rectum. The significance of this portion of the peritoneal cavity is that the ovary extends from the posterior surface of the broad ligament into the rectouterine pouch. Therefore, the ovulated ovum and any blood or other pathologic material from the ovary can enter the rectouterine pouch.

●●● NERVES IN THE PELVIS

The somatic nerves in the pelvis are the branches of the lumbosacral plexus (Fig. 7-9) while the autonomic nerves are from the pelvic splanchnic nerves, the sacral portion of the sympathetic trunk, and the superior hypogastric plexus. The somatic nerves are found in the body wall and thus are external to the inner investing layer of the deep fascia (endopelvic) fascia. In contrast, the autonomic nerves are organized into plexuses within the extraserous fascia, which is internal to the endopelvic fascia.

Somatic Nerves

The somatic nerves in the pelvic wall mainly innervate muscles associated with the lower limb and are covered in Chapter 8. However, it is important to be aware of them because tumors of pelvic viscera can invade the pelvic body wall and impinge on these neural structures and thus cause symptoms in the lower limb areas.

The lumbosacral plexus contains the ventral rami of spinal nerves L4 and L5 (from the lumbosacral trunk) and the ventral rami of spinal nerves S1–S4 (see Fig. 7-9). Most of these branches leave the pelvis through the greater sciatic foramen. They are organized somewhat by their relationship to the piriformis muscle. The superior gluteal nerve exits above the piriformis muscle while the other branches of the sacral plexus exit below the piriformis muscle. These nerves supply the muscles of the lower limb and give rise to a few branches that supply the levator ani muscles.

Autonomic Nerves

In the pelvis, the autonomic nerves are organized in multiple plexuses in the plane of the extraperitoneal (subserous) fascia (see Fig. 7-9 and Table 7-4).

Superior Hypogastric Plexus

The superior hypogastric (presacral) plexus, a continuation of the intermesenteric plexus, is located on the anterior surface of the aorta below the inferior mesenteric artery origin, and extends inferior to the bifurcation of the aorta. It contains postganglionic sympathetic fibers from the intermesenteric plexus, as well as some preganglionic sympathetic fibers and small ganglia (see Table 7-4). Visceral afferents that mediate pain from the body and fundus of the uterus are also found here traveling in conjunction with the sympathetics from T10 to T12. The postganglionic sympathetic fibers from the

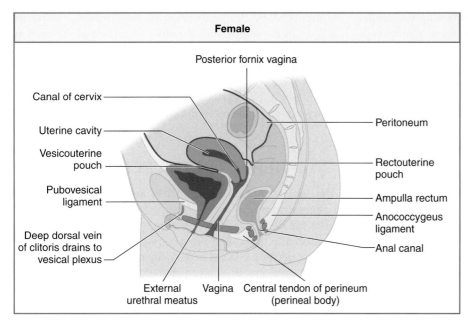

Figure 7-8. Sagittal views of female (**A**) and male (**B**) peritoneal cavities.

Female

Posterior fornix vagina

Canal of cervix

Uterine cavity

Vesicouterine pouch

Pubovesical ligament

Deep dorsal vein of clitoris drains to vesical plexus

Peritoneum

Rectouterine pouch

Ampulla rectum

Anococcygeus ligament

Anal canal

External urethral meatus   Vagina   Central tendon of perineum (perineal body)

A

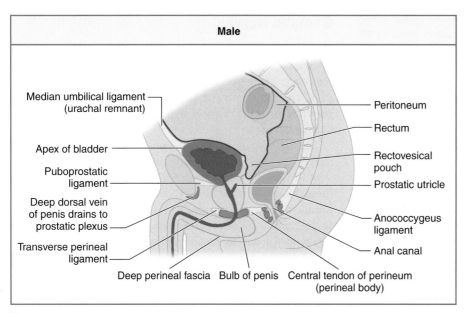

Male

Median umbilical ligament (urachal remnant)

Apex of bladder

Puboprostatic ligament

Deep dorsal vein of penis drains to prostatic plexus

Transverse perineal ligament

Peritoneum

Rectum

Rectovesical pouch

Prostatic utricle

Anococcygeus ligament

Anal canal

Deep perineal fascia   Bulb of penis   Central tendon of perineum (perineal body)

B

intermesenteric plexus and inferior mesenteric ganglia along with some preganglionic sympathetic fibers course over the sacrum and separate into right and left hypogastric nerves (see Fig. 7-9).

Hypogastric Nerves

The right and left hypogastric nerves, which are actually plexuses, originate from the superior hypogastric plexus and pass down along the right and left posterior lateral walls of the pelvis to join the inferior hypogastric plexus (see Fig. 7-9 and Table 7-4). They carry postganglionic sympathetic fibers, which are vasomotor.

Inferior Hypogastric Plexus

The inferior hypogastric plexus is actually an extended plexus (see Fig. 7-9 and Table 7-4). It has three sources: the right and left hypogastric nerves, the pelvic splanchnics, and the sacral splanchnics. The preganglionic parasympathetic cell bodies of the pelvic splanchnic nerves (nervi erigentes) are located in the lateral horn of spinal cord segments S2–S4 with S3 and S4 contributing the majority of the fibers. They leave the spinal cord and travel to the inferior hypogastric plexus, where they synapse close to their target organ if they are to supply an organ of the urogenital system or proceed directly to the hindgut organ that they supply and synapse in the wall of the organ.

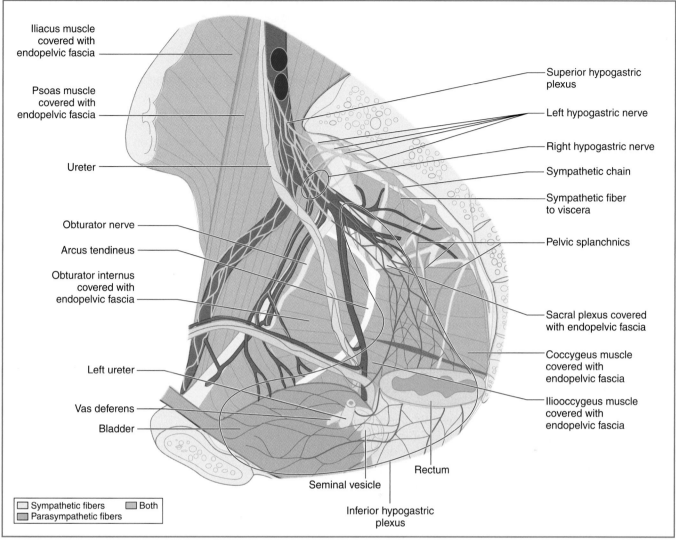

Figure 7-9. Innervation of the pelvis.

TABLE 7-4. Autonomic Plexuses of the Pelvis				
Plexus	**Location**	**Fiber Type**	**Source of Fibers**	**Synapses (If Any)**
Superior hypogastric plexus	Just inferior to the origin of the inferior mesenteric artery	Postganglionic sympathetic and a few preganglionic sympathetic Visceral afferents	Intermesenteric plexus Lumbar splanchnics from spinal cord segments L1–L3 Body and fundus of uterus	Possibly a few for preganglionic sympathetics
Hypogastric nerves	Connection between superior and inferior hypogastric plexus	Postganglionic sympathetic and possibly preganglionic parasympathetic on left side	Superior hypogastric plexus Pelvic splanchnics	None
Inferior hypogastric plexus	Against posterior lateral pelvic wall Pelvic splanchnics arising from ventral rami	Sympathetic and parasympathetic	Hypogastric nerves Sacral splanchnics Pelvic splanchnics	For some parasympathetic fibers and possibly some sympathetic fibers

The inferior hypogastric plexuses are in the extraperitoneal fascia and are named according to the organs that they innervate. In males, there are rectal, vesical, and prostatic plexuses as well as the parasympathetic supply to the erectile tissue of the penis. The last group of postganglionic parasympathetic fibers is called the *cavernous nerves*.

In females, the inferior hypogastric plexus is extended forward as the rectal, uterovaginal, and vesical plexuses. Finally, the cavernous nerves of the clitoris contain parasympathetics to the erectile tissue of the clitoris.

These autonomic pelvic plexuses, found just lateral to the organs that they innervate, are in jeopardy during pelvic surgical procedures.

Visceral Afferent Fibers

Unlike the thorax and abdomen, most of the general visceral afferent fibers from the pelvic organs are associated with the pelvic splanchnics. The general visceral sensory (GVA) fibers that accompany the pelvic splanchnics have their cell bodies located in sacral dorsal root ganglia. These sensory fibers carry visceral sensation owing to distention and contraction as well as pain from the bladder, anal canal, and lower rectum and the cervix. Pain from these organs can be referred to the portion of the body that is supplied by S2 and S3 nerves. For example, pain from the rectum can be referred to the sacrum.

However, not all organs in the pelvis have GVA fibers associated with the pelvic splanchnics. The GVA fibers from the ovary travel superiorly to the dorsal horn of spinal cord segments T10–T11, reflecting the fact that the ovary develops initially in the lower thoracic region and then descends into the pelvis during development. The ovary is supplied to a large extent by means of nerves and blood vessels traveling in the suspensory (infundibulopelvic) ligament of the ovary. Also, the GVA fibers from the body and fundus of the uterus run with the sympathetic system and, as mentioned above, are found in the superior hypogastric plexus.

●●● OVERVIEW OF BLOOD SUPPLY TO THE PELVIS AND GLUTEAL REGIONS

Arteries

The pelvis has the following arteries: median sacral artery, ovarian artery, and internal iliac artery and its branches (Table 7-5).

The median sacral artery is a branch of the aorta just above its bifurcation into the two common iliac arteries. The median sacral artery arises from the posterior surface of the aorta and passes over the promontory into the pelvis. It continues in the midline of the sacrum, sending segmental branches through the anterior sacral foramina to the contents of the sacral canal. Branches of the middle sacral artery can also anastomose with the lateral sacral arteries.

The internal iliac artery originates anteromedial to the sacroiliac joint and crosses the brim of the pelvis to enter the true pelvis. The internal iliac artery supplies the contents of

TABLE 7-5. Arteries of the Pelvis

Artery	Source	Supplies
Median sacral	Abdominal aorta	Sacral canal
Iliolumbar	Posterior division of internal iliac	Iliacus and quadratus lumborum muscles
Lateral sacral	Posterior division of internal iliac	Sacral canal
Superior gluteal	Posterior division of internal iliac	Gluteus medius, gluteus minimus, tensor fasciae latae, and gluteus maximus muscles
Inferior gluteal	Anterior division of internal iliac	Gluteus maximus and piriformis muscles
Obturator	Anterior division of internal iliac or external iliac	Adductor muscles of the thigh and obturator externus
Umbilical	Anterior division of internal iliac	Gives rise to superior vesical artery and sometimes the artery of the ductus
Inferior vesical (in males)	Anterior division of internal iliac	Base of urinary bladder; supplies seminal vesicle, prostate, lower ureter, and usually the artery of the ductus deferens
Artery of the ductus	Inferior vesical, superior vesical, or umbilical	Ductus deferens, helps supply testes, seminal vesicles, lower ureter
Vaginal	Anterior division of internal iliac	Base of bladder, vagina, vestibular bulb, lower ureter, and rectum
Uterine	Anterior division of internal iliac	Uterus, ovary, and uterine tubes
Middle rectal	Anterior division of internal iliac	Muscular wall of rectum
Internal pudendal	Anterior division of internal iliac	Perineum
Ovarian	Abdominal aorta	Ovary and uterine tubes

the pelvis and also helps supply the thigh and gluteal region. Thus, its branches are subdivided into branches that supply the body wall (parietal branches) and branches that supply organs (visceral branches). The internal iliac artery is crossed anteriorly by the ureter. In females, the ovary and uterine tube are located anterior to the artery.

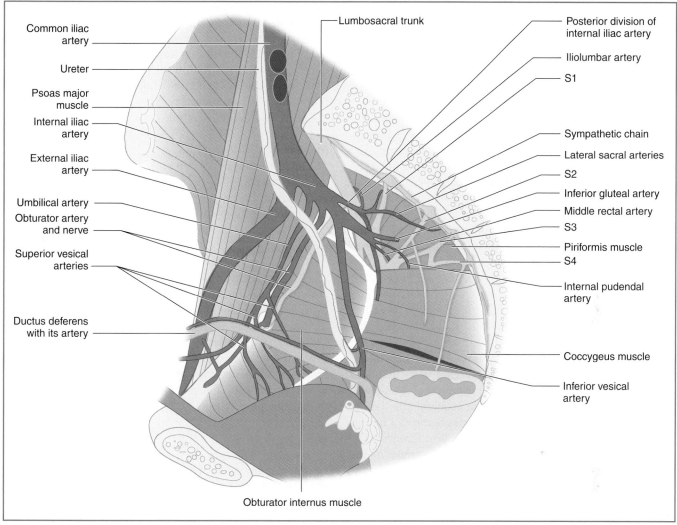

Figure 7-10. Blood supply to the pelvis: medial view of the branches of the internal iliac artery.

The internal iliac artery separates into anterior and posterior divisions (Fig. 7-10). The origin of the branches from the two divisions varies from person to person. Thus, in the pelvis, identification of an artery is best done by observing which structures the artery actually enters. Typically, the posterior division only has parietal branches while the anterior division has *both* parietal and visceral branches.

Posterior Division of Internal Iliac Artery

The posterior division (see Fig. 7-10) of the internal iliac artery has three branches: iliolumbar, lateral sacral, and superior gluteal arteries.

The first branch is the iliolumbar artery, which runs over the brim of the pelvis superiorly into the abdominal cavity. It is difficult to find because it passes posteriorly to the common iliac vein to divide into an iliac branch to the iliacus muscle and a lumbar branch. The lumbar branch ascends between the psoas muscle and the vertebral column to reach the quadratus lumborum muscle. It also sends branches through the lower

lumbar intervertebral foramina to the contents of the vertebral canal.

The lateral sacral artery runs over the lateral aspect of the sacrum to reach the anterior sacral foramina, where it sends branches into the sacral vertebral canal.

The superior gluteal artery is the largest branch of the posterior division. It passes between the lumbosacral trunk (L4 and L5) and the ventral ramus of S1 to leave the pelvis through the greater sciatic foramen above the piriformis muscle. In the gluteal region, it divides into a superficial branch that helps supply the gluteus maximus muscle and a deep division. The deep division passes between the gluteus medius and minimus muscles to supply both of these muscles and the tensor fasciae latae muscle.

Anterior Division of Internal Iliac Artery

The anterior division of the internal iliac artery has both parietal and visceral branches. There are three parietal branches (see Fig. 7-10), which typically arise from the anterior division.

The inferior gluteal artery passes through the sacral plexus usually between sacral spinal nerves S1 and S2 or between S2 and S3 to leave the pelvis through the greater sciatic foramen below the piriformis muscle. It supplies the piriformis muscle and helps supply the gluteus maximus muscle as well.

The internal pudendal artery is the last of the major branches to leave through the greater sciatic foramen. It can sometimes arise with the inferior gluteal artery. Since the internal pudendal artery is the most anterior artery to leave the pelvis through the greater sciatic foramen, it lies against the coccygeus muscle. This relationship allows identification of the internal pudendal artery with great confidence, whereas identification of the inferior gluteal artery is often a matter of elimination.

The obturator artery runs forward in the extraserous (extraperitoneal) fascia with the obturator nerve, along the lateral surface of the pelvis, to reach the obturator canal to the medial compartment of the thigh.

There are typically five visceral branches (see Fig. 7-10).

Umbilical Artery

The umbilical artery passes along the lateral surface of the pelvis up onto the abdominal wall to reach the umbilicus. In the fetus, the internal iliac artery is twice the size of the external iliac artery because of the presence of its umbilical branch, which is continuous with the umbilical cord's umbilical artery. After birth, the portion of the umbilical artery distal to the origin of the superior vesical arteries becomes a fibrous cord–like structure called the medial umbilical ligament. The superior vesical arteries supply the superior surface of the bladder. Since the umbilical artery is crossed by the ductus deferens in males, it often gives rise to the artery to the ductus.

Inferior Vesical Artery

In the male, the inferior vesical artery arises as a branch from the anterior division and runs to the base of the bladder. It also supplies the inferolateral wall of the bladder as well as the structures associated with the base and neck of the bladder. The inferior vesical artery also supplies the seminal vesicle, prostate, and lower ureter and is the usual source of the artery to the ductus deferens.

Vaginal Artery

In the female, the vaginal artery has a similar distribution to the male inferior vesical artery in that it supplies the base of the bladder and terminal portion of the ureter and helps supply the rectum. The vaginal artery reaches the vaginal wall and anastomoses with the opposite vaginal artery on the anterior and posterior surfaces of the vagina. These anastomoses produce the azygos (unpaired) arteries that run longitudinally on the anterior and posterior surfaces of the vagina. The uterine artery also has vaginal branches.

Uterine Artery

The uterine artery passes in the lateral cervical (cardinal) ligament over the ureter (in an analogous manner to the course of the ductus deferens over the ureter) to the cervix of the uterus. The cardinal ligament and the uterine artery are located in the inferior aspect of the broad ligament. The uterine artery then ascends on the lateral aspect of the body of the uterus. Here, it often has a coiled configuration, which during pregnancy and after birth, probably allows it to accommodate to changes in the size of the uterus. At the fundus of the uterus, the uterine artery gives rise to branches to both the ovary and the uterine tube.

Middle Rectal Artery

The middle rectal artery is usually the terminal branch of the anterior division of the internal iliac artery. It passes forward in the lateral ligaments (stalks) of the rectum to reach the rectum to help supply its muscular wall.

Ovarian Artery

The ovarian artery, which is a branch of the abdominal aorta, also has tubal and uterine branches. The uterine artery's ovarian and tubal branches anastomose with ovarian artery's uterine and tubal branches. This anastomosis between the ovarian and the uterine arteries across the uterine tube is very important in ectopic tubal pregnancies. The uterine tube cannot accommodate the growth of the fetus and ruptures, which in turn can damage these vessels and produce a life-threatening hemorrhage.

Veins

In general, the veins of the pelvis follow the arteries. They drain in large part to the internal iliac vein. There are, however, two clinically important venous anastomoses: the portacaval anastomoses in the rectum and anal canal region and the vesical plexus with the internal vertebral (Batson's) plexus.

●●● TERMINAL END OF THE GASTROINTESTINAL SYSTEM
Rectum

The terminal end of the GI system (Fig. 7-11) consists of the rectum, anal canal, and anus. The term rectum is derived from the Latin for "straight." However, in humans, the rectum is not straight but has two bends or flexures. It has a sacral flexure that allows it to conform to the shape of the concavity of the sacrum (see Fig. 7-11) and a perineal flexure that is produced by the anterior pull of the puborectalis portion of the levator ani. The interfacing of the puborectalis muscle with the rectum is used to delineate the anorectal line or junction. This junction also marks the terminal end of the rectum and the beginning of the anal canal. The rectum is continuous with the sigmoid colon above and to the left.

The rectum (see Fig. 7-11) begins at approximately the third sacral vertebra, which is slightly lower in the pelvis than one would expect. Another landmark to identify the junction of the sigmoid colon and the rectum is that the sigmoid colon has taeniae coli and omental appendices while the rectum

Figure 7-11. A, Rectum and anal canal. **B,** Sagittal view.

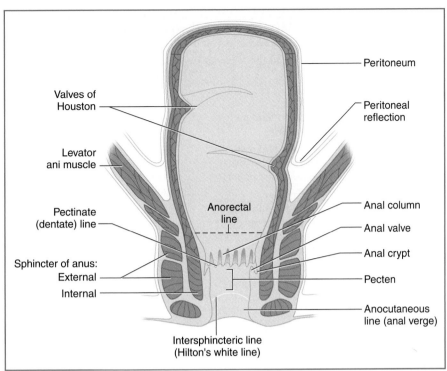

Peritoneum

Peritoneal reflection

Valves of Houston

Levator ani muscle

Pectinate (dentate) line

Anorectal line

Anal column

Anal valve

Anal crypt

Sphincter of anus:
External
Internal

Pecten

Anocutaneous line (anal verge)

Intersphincteric line (Hilton's white line)

A

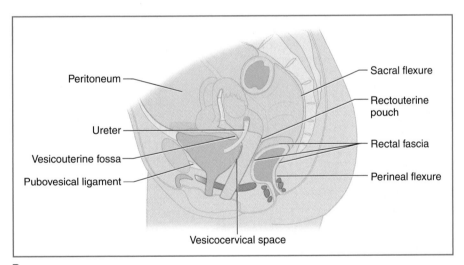

Peritoneum

Ureter

Vesicouterine fossa

Pubovesical ligament

Sacral flexure

Rectouterine pouch

Rectal fascia

Perineal flexure

Vesicocervical space

B

does not. The outer longitudinal smooth muscle layer of the rectum is organized as a complete layer, not into the longitudinal bands that produce the taeniae coli found on the sigmoid colon.

Distally, the rectum dilates into the ampulla of the rectum, which continues until the level of the pelvic diaphragm and the perineal flexure.

The lumen of the rectum is marked by the presence of three valves or folds that are the result of infolding of the circular smooth muscle layer and epithelium of the rectum. These folds are usually arranged so that there are two on the left and a middle fold on the right. These transverse rectal folds (valves of Houston) are semicircular and incomplete in nature, occupying less than half of the circumference of the lumen. This arrangement produces a step-like configuration in the lumen of the rectum.

Fascia Associated with the Rectum

The rectum is held in place posteriorly by presacral (Waldeyer's) fascia and laterally by the lateral ligaments (stalks) of the rectum, which consist of the endopelvic fascia over the middle rectal vessels. While peritoneum is found on the anterior and lateral surfaces of the upper third of the rectum, it is found only on the anterior surface of the middle third of the rectum. No peritoneum is found on the lower third of the rectum. For this reason, the rectum is classified as a retroperitoneal organ.

In females, as mentioned above, the peritoneum on the anterior surface of the rectum extends onto the posterior surface of the uterus, resulting in the formation of the rectouterine peritoneal pouch (of Douglas). Therefore, in females, the upper third of the rectum is related to the uterus through the rectouterine pouch while the lower portion is directly related to the uterus through the extraperitoneal fascia, but separated from it by the rectouterine septum.

In males, the peritoneum on the upper anterior surface of the rectum forms the posterior aspect of the rectovesical peritoneal pouch. The lower portion of the rectum is separated from the base of the bladder, prostate, and seminal vesicles by a well-developed rectovesical septum or Denonvilliers' fascia.

Anal Canal

The anal canal is continuous with the rectum. Anatomically, the anorectal junction is not well distinguished. As stated above, it is located at the intersection of the puborectalis muscle and rectum. There is a change in the epithelial layer at the anorectal junction. The rectum has simple columnar epithelium while the upper anal canal has a stratified columnar epithelium. The wall of the anal canal is continuous with the wall of the rectum and contains an inner layer of circular smooth muscle and an outer layer of longitudinal smooth muscle.

Clinically, the pectinate line is used to distinguish the upper part of the anal canal from the lower portion of the anal canal. The pectinate (dentate) line is indeed the distinguishing morphologic feature of the anal canal. This line represents the site of the anal valves, which are remnants of the fetal cloacal membrane (see Fig. 7-11 and Table 7-6).

The cloacal membrane consists of layers of ectoderm and endoderm with no intervening mesoderm. The cloacal membrane is produced in part by the ingrowth of ectoderm (proctodeum) toward the endoderm of the hindgut. Thus, the membrane has ectoderm on its external surface and endoderm on its internal surface. During normal development, the cloacal membrane is subdivided into an anal membrane and a urogenital membrane. The anal membrane ruptures, leaving the pectinate line as an approximation of the transition from the ectoderm below this line to the endoderm superior to this line. The embryology explains the many major differences that occur in the neurovascular supply to the anal canal (see Table 7-6).

Extending superiorly from the anal valves of the pectinate line are five to ten folds of submucosa and mucosa (epithelium). These folds are the anal columns (columns of Morgagni) that are formed by the five to ten internal hemorrhoidal (rectal) venous plexuses that give rise to the superior rectal veins (see Figs. 7-11 and 7-12). The recesses between the anal columns are the anal sinuses, while the folds of mucous membranes that appear to connect adjacent anal columns at their bases are the anal valves (see Fig. 7-11). About 2 cm

TABLE 7-6. Anatomic Changes at the Pectinate Line	
Inferior to the Pectinate Line	**Superior to the Pectinate Line**
Structures develop from ectoderm and parietal mesoderm	Structures develop from endoderm and visceral mesoderm
Muscles and epithelial covering are skeletal muscles and cutaneous structures	Muscles and epithelial covering are smooth muscle and columnar and cuboidal epithelium
Arteries are the inferior rectal branches of the internal pudendal artery	Arteries are branches of the inferior mesenteric artery's superior rectal artery and internal iliac artery's middle rectal artery
Venous drainage is inferior rectal vein to internal pudendal vein to internal iliac vein (systemic venous system)	Venous drainage is superior rectal vein to inferior mesenteric vein to portal system of veins
Innervation is the pudendal nerve with general somatic efferent, general somatic afferent, and postganglionic sympathetic fibers. Sensation of pain is highly localized	Autonomic innervation: postganglionic sympathetics from inferior mesenteric ganglia follow either the superior rectal artery or fibers that pass in the superior hypogastric and inferior hypogastric plexuses. Parasympathetic preganglionic fibers are part of the pelvic splanchnics. The ganglia are in the wall of the anal canal and rectum and they have very short postganglionic fibers. Sensation from this visceral region is due to distention or contraction of the gut, as is the case for the rest of the gut
Lymphatics drain to the inguinal nodes	Lymphatics drain to the lumbar nodes associated with the inferior mesenteric artery

below the pectinate line is another, but less obvious line, the intersphincteric line. The longitudinal smooth muscle layer of the anal canal becomes fibrous in nature as it terminates. This fibrous component of the longitudinal layer attaches to the submucosa of the anal canal, producing the intersphincteric line (also called white line of anal canal [or Hilton]; see Fig. 7-11). The inner circular smooth muscle terminates above the intersphincteric line by expanding to form the internal anal sphincter.

The inferior end of the anal verge (anocutaneous line), which denotes a transitional change in the epithelium, is also located approximately at the intersphincteric line. The epithelium above is stratified squamous without sweat glands or

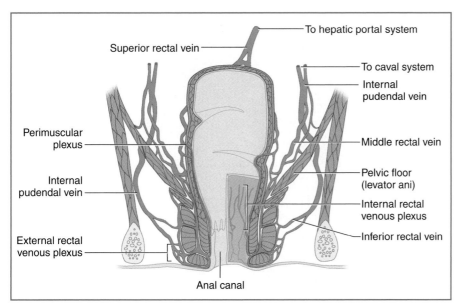

Figure 7-12. Venous drainage of rectum and anal canal.

Labels on figure:
- Superior rectal vein
- To hepatic portal system
- To caval system
- Internal pudendal vein
- Perimuscular plexus
- Middle rectal vein
- Internal pudendal vein
- Pelvic floor (levator ani)
- Internal rectal venous plexus
- External rectal venous plexus
- Inferior rectal vein
- Anal canal

hair follicles. Below the anal verge, the stratified squamous epithelium now contains hair follicles.

Finally, the *anus is the ring or circular terminal end* of the GI tract. The anus has two sphincters. The *internal anal sphincter is circular smooth muscle*. The *external anal sphincter is skeletal muscle* and has several portions described with the perineum.

Innervation

The internal anal sphincter is innervated by the autonomic nervous system, since the internal circular smooth muscle layer forms it. The parasympathetic fibers stimulate and the sympathetic fibers inhibit sphincter function. The external anal sphincter extends below the intersphincteric line and is skeletal muscle innervated by general somatic afferent and efferent fibers from the inferior rectal branches of the pudendal nerve. During digital examination, the examiner may be able to palpate the intersphincteric line found between the internal and external anal sphincters.

The result of the convergence of different embryologic planes can be readily demonstrated by the significant differences in the neurovascular supply to the specific portions of the anal canal. Since the anal canal and rectum above the pectinate line is derived from the endoderm and the visceral mesoderm as is the rest of the gut, autonomic nerves innervate the portion of the anal canal above the pectinate line. The sympathetics are from the superior and inferior hypogastric plexuses. The preganglionic parasympathetic fibers are from pelvic splanchnics in the inferior hypogastric plexus. Thus, the parasympathetic ganglia for the smooth muscle and glands of the rectum and anal canal above the pectinate line are located in the wall of the gut. Most of the general visceral sensory fibers follow the pelvic splanchnics, as illustrated by pain from the rectum being referred to the sacrum.

The innervation below the pectinate line is typical of the body wall. It consists of somatic sensory and motor fibers and postganglionic sympathetic fibers found in the inferior rectal branches of the pudendal nerve. Thus, above the pectinate line, visceral pain is carried by the autonomic fibers while below the pectinate line, the pudendal nerve carries somatic pain.

Blood Supply

The blood supply of the anal canal (see Fig. 7-12) also reflects these embryologic differences. Above the pectinate line, the arterial supply and venous drainage of the mucosa are the superior rectal artery and vein, which are branches of the inferior mesenteric artery and vein. The inferior mesenteric vein drains the internal rectal venous plexus, which is found deep to the mucosa of the anal columns, and it drains into the portal system through either the splenic or superior mesenteric veins. Below the pectinate line the arterial supply comes from the inferior rectal artery, a branch of the internal pudendal artery, and the venous drainage is to the systemic system through the inferior rectal vein. Branches of the inferior rectal vein form the external rectal venous plexus, which is found just deep to the skin. The middle rectal veins drain the muscular rectal wall into the internal iliac vessels and the internal pudendal veins.

Thus, the venous drainage below the pectinate line is to the systemic veins, while the venous drainage above the pectinate line is to the portal system of veins. This anastomosis is referred to as the portocaval anastomosis (see Fig. 7-12).

Portal hypertension, pregnancy, constipation, or any condition that applies pressure to the inferior mesenteric or superior rectal veins produces an elevation in the venous pressure found in the anal columns. Blood attempts to cross at the level of the pectinate line in the incomplete anastomotic channels between these veins and the external hemorrhoidal plexus of the inferior rectal vein. The inferior rectal vein drains into the systemic venous system by means of the internal iliac veins, and the superior rectal veins drain into the inferior mesenteric vein and the portal system. The increased venous pressure in the superior rectal vein's superior

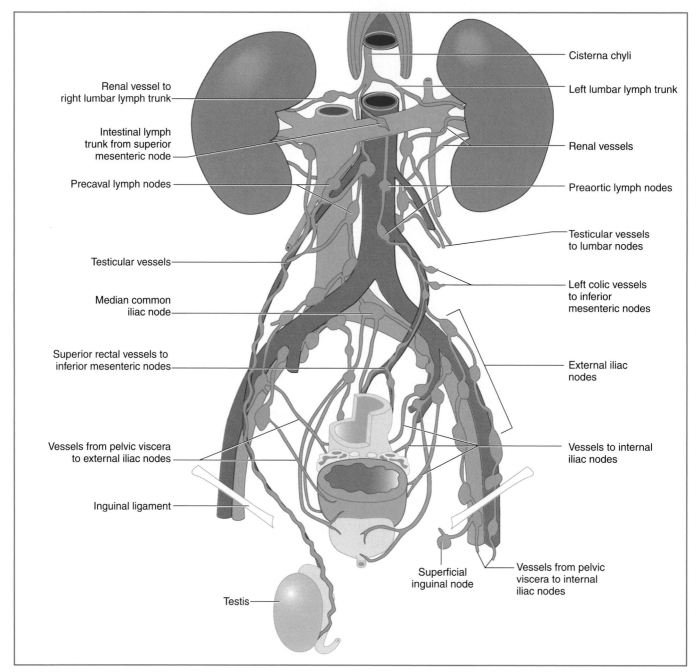

Figure 7-13. Lymphatic drainage of the male pelvis.

hemorrhoidal plexus produces an engorged or varicosed superior hemorrhoidal plexus. This condition is termed *internal hemorrhoids*.

The internal hemorrhoids can protrude into the anal lumen, and they often bleed if traumatized. Since the wall of the anal canal above the pectinate line is innervated by autonomic nerves, internal hemorrhoids are not painful but often leave the patient with the feeling of puffiness or the erroneous feeling that they are going to defecate. These are visceral sensations.

The external hemorrhoidal plexus can also become engorged and varicosed, producing *external hemorrhoids*. Since the wall of the anal canal below the pectinate line is innervated

by somatic sensory nerve fibers, external hemorrhoids are often painful. The other alternative venous anastomosis consists of the middle rectal veins from the rectal wall to the internal iliac vein. This collateral anastomosis opens and can produce rectal varicose veins.

Lymphatic Drainage

The lymphatic drainage from the GI tract usually follows the arteries. Thus, the lymphatic drainage of the rectum and anal canal above the pectinate line consists of lymphatic vessels that follow the superior rectal and inferior mesenteric arteries (Fig. 7-13). These lymphatic vessels drain into lumbar nodes associated with the aorta at the origin of the inferior mesen-

TABLE 7-7. Rectal Examination

	Male		Female	
Relationship	Normal	Pathologic	Normal	Pathologic
Anterior	Prostate	Inflammation of seminal vesicles	Cervix	Fundus of uterus if retroverted Tenderness of rectovaginal septum Pathologic content of rectouterine pouch
Posterior	Sacrum, coccyx	Enlarged sacral lymph nodes	Sacrum, coccyx	Enlarged sacral lymph nodes
Lateral	Ischial spine and conjoined ramus	Abscess in ischioanal fossa	Ischial spine and conjoined ramus	Abscess in ischioanal fossa

teric artery. Some lymphatic drainage is along nodes that follow the middle rectal artery in the lateral ligaments of the rectum to the internal iliac nodes. However, the lymphatic drainage below the pectinate line is to lymphatic vessels that follow the inferior rectal and internal pudendal arteries to the iliac nodes or to the superficial inguinal node.

Relationships of the Anal Canal and Rectum

The relationships of the anal canal and rectum are very important in clinical medicine. The high incidence of rectal and colon cancer demands examination of the rectum and anal canal. In addition, physical (digital) examination can produce significant findings about organs and anatomic regions adjacent to the anal canal or rectum (Table 7-7).

●●● PELVIC URINARY SYSTEM

Ureter

The pelvic portions of the urinary system are similar in both sexes and will be considered together. The pelvic portion of the ureter runs over the brim of the pelvis at the bifurcation of the common iliac artery and the obturator neurovascular bundle to reach the medial surface of the pelvic floor at the level of the ischial spine.

In males, the ureter passes through the rectovesical ligament under the ductus deferens and then passes slightly superiorly and laterally to the free edge of the seminal vesicle to enter the bladder (Fig. 7-14).

In females, the ureter sometimes passes posterior to the lateral pole of the ovary, since the ureter forms the posteroinferior boundary of the ovarian fossa (see female genital system). The ureter continues through the uterosacral ligament and is then inferior and posterior to the uterine artery in the transverse cervical (cardinal) ligament. It passes close to the lateral surface of the cervix and the lateral margin of

the vagina and then anteriorly to reach the bladder. Its relationships to the ovarian vessels at the brim of the pelvis and the uterine vessels in the cardinal ligament make it particularly vulnerable to injury during a hysterectomy.

Urinary Bladder

The bladder (see Fig. 7-14C) is a retroperitoneal organ found in the anterior aspect of the pelvis. It is found on the superior surface of the pubis, medial to the obturator internus muscles and the levator ani muscles and superior to the urethral sphincter muscle in the urogenital hiatus. Some of the relationships are different in the two sexes and will be described separately.

Morphology

The morphology of the bladder changes with the amount of urine that it contains (see Fig. 7-14). In the adult, the empty bladder is found completely in the pelvis. The bladder distends superiorly to accommodate the increase in urine. It extends superiorly, lifting the peritoneum with its superior surface away from the anterior abdominal wall. This relationship allows a needle to pass through the anterior abdominal wall directly into the *full* bladder without entering the peritoneal cavity to sample the bladder's content.

The empty bladder has two inferolateral surfaces: a superior surface and a posterior surface (base or fundus) (see Figs. 7-14A and 7-14B). The two inferolateral surfaces meet the superior surface behind the pubis, forming the apex of the bladder (see Fig. 7-14A). The two inferolateral surfaces also meet inferiorly with the base (fundus) to form the neck of the bladder at the superior surface of the urethral sphincter (see Fig. 7-14A). The apex of the bladder is connected to the umbilicus by means of a fibrous cord, the median umbilical ligament. This ligament is the remnant of the urachus (allantois). The neck of the bladder is held in place by several ligaments, while the superior surface can expand in the plane of the subserous fascia when the bladder is filled with urine.

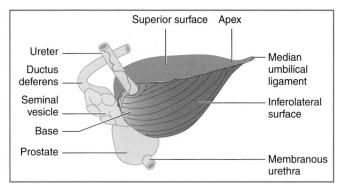

Superior surface   Apex

Ureter

Ductus deferens

Seminal vesicle

Base

Prostate

Median umbilical ligament

Inferolateral surface

Membranous urethra

A

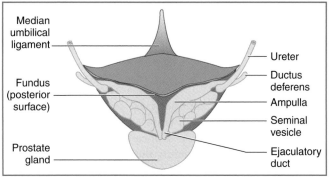

Median umbilical ligament

Fundus (posterior surface)

Prostate gland

Ureter

Ductus deferens

Ampulla

Seminal vesicle

Ejaculatory duct

B

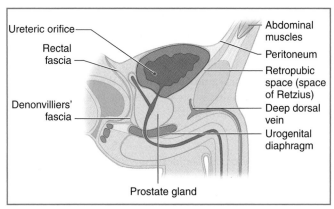

Ureteric orifice

Rectal fascia

Denonvilliers' fascia

Abdominal muscles

Peritoneum

Retropubic space (space of Retzius)

Deep dorsal vein

Urogenital diaphragm

Prostate gland

C

Figure 7-14. A, Male urinary bladder. **B,** Posterior aspect. **C,** Adjacent structures.

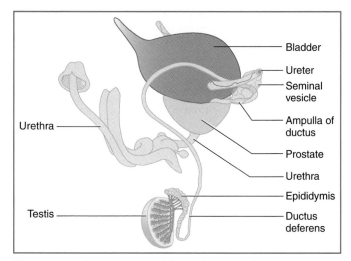

Bladder

Ureter

Seminal vesicle

Ampulla of ductus

Prostate

Urethra

Epididymis

Ductus deferens

Urethra

Testis

Figure 7-15. Components of the male urogenital system.

In females, the neck of the bladder is directly held in place by the pubovesical ligaments, while the vesicouterine ligament stretches from the bladder to the uterus and adjacent iliac vessels. In females, a much less well developed rectouterine septum exists in comparison with the male rectovesical septum.

Peritoneal Reflections

The peritoneal reflections and most of the relationships are substantially different in the two sexes. However, in both males and females there is a potential space between the bladder and the pubis in the plane of the extraperitoneal fascia. It is referred to as the retropubic space or cave of Retzius. It contains the venous plexus that connects the deep dorsal vein of the penis or clitoris to the veins of the bladder. It is a common site of pooling of urine if there is extravasation of urine due to a penetrating lesion of the bladder wall.

Peritoneum covers the superior surface of the bladder. In males, it is reflected up onto the rectum, forming the rectovesical pouch of the peritoneal cavity. In females, the peritoneum from the bladder is reflected onto the anterior surface of the uterus, forming the uterovesical (vesicouterine) pouch of the peritoneal cavity. The paravesical fossae (pouches) of the peritoneal cavity are found lateral to the bladder.

Relationships of Pelvic Structures to the Base of the Bladder

In males, the base of the bladder is anterior to the ampullae of the two ductus (vasa) deferentes and to the two seminal vesicles (see Fig. 7-14B). The ampullae of the ductus deferentes are in the midline, and the seminal vesicles are always found lateral to the ductus deferens (see Fig. 7-14B). The base of the bladder faces posteriorly and inferiorly toward the rectum. Remember that these organs can be palpated through the rectum if they are enlarged.

In females, the base of the bladder also faces posteriorly and inferiorly. However, it is loosely attached to the anterior wall of the vagina by extraperitoneal (subserous) fascia. In

Ligaments Associated with the Bladder

In males, the neck of the bladder is surrounded by the prostate gland (see Figs. 7-14 and 7-15). The puboprostatic ligaments are composed of endopelvic fascia, which stretch from the pubis to the prostate. The lateral ligaments of the bladder stretch from the lateral walls to the bladder and contain the neurovascular bundles to the bladder. The neck of the bladder with the surrounding prostate gland is connected to the rectum and iliac vessels by the rectovesical ligaments.

In addition to the rectovesical ligament, the rectovesical septum (Denonvilliers'), derived from extraperitoneal fascia, stretches from the peritoneum and passes posteriorly to the bladder and then to the floor of the male pelvis.

addition, the superior aspect of the base is separated from the supravaginal portion of the cervix by subserous fascia. The ureters pass just laterally to this aspect of the cervix and vagina to enter the superior aspect of the base.

Interior of the Bladder

The interior of the bladder is similar in both sexes. The walls of the bladder are composed of smooth muscle, the detrusor urinae, and connective tissue, and an epithelial layer lines the lumen. Most of the walls contain smooth muscle that is loosely attached to the mucous membrane. Therefore, the internal surface of the bladder that is associated with the detrusor muscle is characterized by numerous folds. The ureters enter the superior aspect of the base of the bladder and run through the wall of the bladder (intramural portion) to empty urine into the lumen of the bladder. The ureteric orifices are found near but not at the ends of the interureteric crest or fold. This fold is an elevated muscular ridge covered by mucous membrane. The interureteric crest also marks the posterosuperior boundary of the trigone of the bladder (see Fig. 7-18).

The hydrostatic pressure produced on filling the bladder flattens the intramural portion of the ureter. Urine will continue to reach the bladder by means of peristaltic waves.

The trigone (trigonum vesicae) is the triangular smooth area at the base of the bladder located between the orifices of the two ureters in the intraurethral ridge and the urethra. This part of the bladder, characterized by smooth muscle, is intimately attached to the mucous membrane of the bladder. *The trigone muscle is distinct from the detrusor urinae muscle.* There are no folds in the trigone; thus, the surface appears smooth. At the bladder's neck, this muscle forms the internal sphincter of the bladder.

The anteroinferior apex of this three-sided region of the bladder is the internal urethral orifice, which is guarded by the internal sphincter of the bladder (sphincter vesicae). Just internal to the internal urethral orifice, the trigone is sometimes elevated as the uvula of the bladder. While anatomically described as produced by the muscle of the trigone, it is not prominent except in older men with an enlargement of the median prostatic lobe. Enlargement of this lobe of the prostate can interfere with the individual's ability to void (evacuate urine), since it can obstruct the membranous urethra.

Innervation

The detrusor muscle is innervated by parasympathetic fibers from the inferior hypogastric plexus (vesical plexus), with the preganglionic parasympathetic fibers arising from the sacral spinal cord segments 2, 3, and 4. Contraction of this muscle results in voiding, while involuntary or uncontrolled contraction results in incontinence (inability to prevent the discharge of urine). The trigone muscle is thought to be innervated by sympathetic nerves and contracts during ejaculation. This contraction acts to separate the bladder from the prostatic urethra during ejaculation to prevent semen from regurgitating into the bladder. The afferent fibers follow the parasympathetic

fibers and therefore have their cell bodies located in the dorsal root ganglia of sacral spinal nerves 2, 3, and 4. These fibers carry stretch sensation from the bladder. The postganglionic sympathetic nerves reach the bladder by passing through first the superior hypogastric plexus followed by the inferior hypogastric plexus. They carry vasomotor fibers to the arteries as well as general visceral efferent fibers to the trigone smooth muscle.

Blood Supply

The arterial supply includes the superior vesical arteries from the umbilical artery to the superior surface and the inferior vesical artery to the inferior aspect and neck (see Fig. 7-10). In the male, the artery to the ductus deferens also helps supply the base. In females, the vaginal and middle rectal arteries supply branches to the base of the bladder.

In males, the prostatic venous plexus drains into the vesical venous plexus, which is found on the inferolateral surface of the bladder, and drains into the internal iliac veins. In females, the prostatic plexus is replaced by an extension of the vesical plexus, which also usually drains with the internal iliac veins. In both cases, these veins communicate with the sacral veins, which communicate with the vertebral venous plexuses (Batson's plexus). Thus, Batson's plexus can serve as a possible route of metastasis from the bladder or prostate to the thorax or the brain, since these vessels have no valves. The lymphatic drainage follows the arterial supply and is therefore via the iliac nodes (see Fig. 7-13).

Urethra

The urethra is the duct that leads from the bladder to the external environment for the discharge of urine in females and both urine and semen in males. There are also obvious sex differences.

Female Urethra

In females (Fig. 7-16A), the urethra is shorter (about 5 cm), passes through the urethrovaginal sphincter muscle and the perineal membrane, and ends as the external urethral orifice in the vestibule of the vagina. In the vestibule, the external urethral orifice is located between the clitoris and the orifice of the vagina. The urethra is fused to the anterior wall of the vagina.

Male Urethra

The male urethra (see Fig. 7-16) is longer (20 to 30 cm) and serves as a common outlet for both the urinary and genital systems. It extends from the internal urethral orifice of the bladder through the prostate, through the urethral sphincter and perineal membrane, and through the spongy portion of the penis to the external urethral orifice. The prostatic urethra passes through the prostate gland from the internal urethral orifice of the bladder to the urethral sphincter. The prostatic urethra curves forward from its origin in the neck of the bladder that is adjacent to the median lobe of the prostate gland (partly associated with the neck of the bladder). This part is

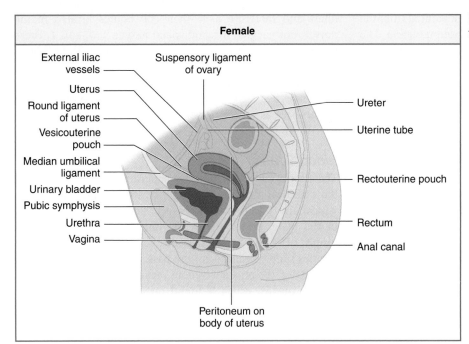

Female

External iliac vessels
Uterus
Round ligament of uterus
Vesicouterine pouch
Median umbilical ligament
Urinary bladder
Pubic symphysis
Urethra
Vagina

Suspensory ligament of ovary

Ureter
Uterine tube

Rectouterine pouch

Rectum
Anal canal

Peritoneum on body of uterus

A

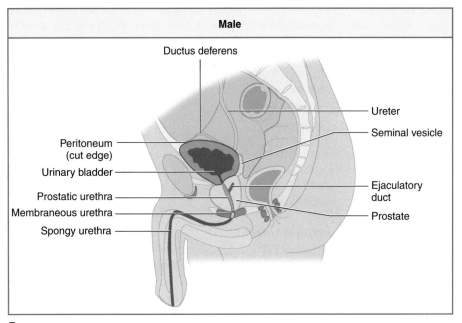

Male

Ductus deferens

Peritoneum (cut edge)
Urinary bladder
Prostatic urethra
Membraneous urethra
Spongy urethra

Ureter
Seminal vesicle

Ejaculatory duct
Prostate

B

Figure 7-16. Comparison between female (**A**) and male (**B**) urethrae.

the widest and most distensible portion of the urethra. The urethra leaves the prostate through the anterior surface of the prostate gland just above the urethral sphincter. The urethra then passes through the urethral sphincter and perineal membrane of the urogenital diaphragm about 4 cm below the pubic symphysis. This portion of the urethra is designated the *membranous urethra*. It is the least distensible portion of the urethra. Distal to the perineal membrane, the urethra continues in the spongy portion of the penis and is called the *spongy or penile urethra*. The spongy urethra will be described with the penis.

●●● DEVELOPMENT OF URINARY BLADDER, RECTUM, AND ANAL CANAL

The cloaca is the terminal portion of the hindgut that is located just internal to the cloacal membrane. It subdivides between the fourth and sixth weeks in utero into an anterior portion and a posterior portion by a down-growth of splanchnic mesoderm, called the urorectal fold, and two inferolateral folds of mesoderm form the *urorectal spetum* (Fig. 7-17). The resulting anterior portion is the primitive urogenital sinus, which will develop into the bladder, pelvic urethra, and most

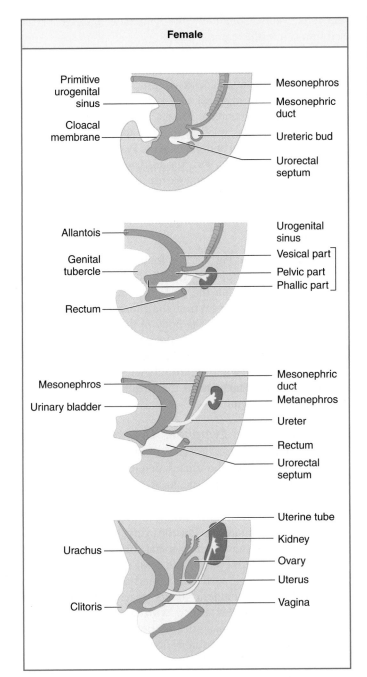

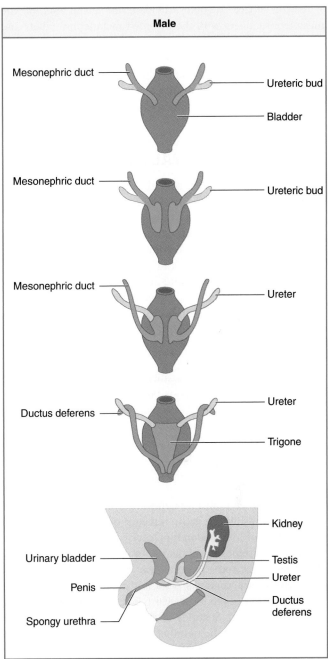

A   B

Figure 7-17. Development of urinary bladder, rectum, and anal canal in the female (**A**) and male (**B**).

inferiorly the definitive urogenital sinus. The posterior portion will develop into the rectum and anal canal. In males, the pelvic urethra will become the prostatic and membranous urethra, and in females, it will become the membranous urethra. The definitive urogenital sinus in males will become the penile urethra, and in females it will become the vestibule of the vagina. The point at which the urorectal septum reaches the cloacal membrane is the location of the future perineal body. The septum thus also subdivides the cloacal membrane

into an anal membrane and a urogenital membrane (see Fig. 7-17).

The primitive urogenital sinus is connected to the allantois, which is an outpocketing of the yolk sac that participates in the formation of the umbilical cord. It will eventually obliterate to form a ligamentous band called the urachus, which extends from the cranial portion of the bladder to the umbilicus. In the adult, the urachus becomes the median umbilical ligament.

As the cloaca becomes divided, the distal end of the mesonephric ducts with the attached metanephric ducts and ureteric buds become incorporated into the posterior wall of the developing bladder. As they do so, the two mesonephric ducts move inferiorly and medially to form the trigone of the bladder (see Fig. 7-17), and the metanephric ducts (presumptive ureters) open independently into the bladder.

●●● MALE GENITAL SYSTEM

Some parts of the male genital system are in the pelvis; however, other parts are in the perineum (see Fig. 7-16). We will consider the entire system here and return to specific parts with the study of the perineum. The specific organs in this system are the testes, epididymis, ductus (vas) deferens, seminal vesicles, prostate, and penis. All these organs are paired except the prostate and penis. The penis (more specifically, the penile urethra) is a shared outlet for both the urinary system and the genital system.

Testis

The testis (plural, testes) is an ovoid body that lies in the scrotum, which is a cutaneous pouch. Each testis is wrapped in the same fascia and muscle that wrap the spermatic cord. This fascia is derived from the body wall (see inguinal region). The spermatic cord is actually the neurovascular bundle and ductus deferens wrapped by fascia. The testis has a dense white capsule called the *tunica albuginea* that maintains its ovoid shape.

External to the tunica albuginea is a serous membrane, the tunica vaginalis, which is the remnant of an extension of the peritoneum of the abdominal cavity called the *processus vaginalis*. This serous membrane has a visceral layer, the visceral tunica vaginalis, and a parietal layer, the parietal tunica vaginalis. The tunica vaginalis does not completely enclose the posterior aspect of the testis, which is termed the *mediastinum testis*. The efferent ductules of the testis communicate with the epididymis, and the neurovascular bundle enters the testis at the mediastinum testis. Sperm is produced in the seminiferous tubules of the testis and reaches the epididymis by means of a duct system that includes the rete testis in the mediastinum and then the efferent ductules that reach the head of the epididymis (see Fig. 7-15).

Blood Supply

Blood supply to the testis is primarily the testicular artery with collateral supply from the artery of the ductus deferens and the cremasteric artery. The venous drainage is the pampiniform plexus of veins that forms the testicular vein. The right testicular vein drains into the inferior vena cava, and the left testicular vein drains into the left renal vein (see Fig. 6-6).

Lymphatic Drainage

The testicular lymphatics drain into the nodes along the aorta (left side) or inferior vena cava (IVC) (right side) just below the renal veins. Commonly the lymphatic drainage of the scrotum is into the inguinal nodes.

Innervation

Innervation to the testis consists of preganglionic sympathetic fibers that arise from spinal cord segments T10 and T11 that synapse in the aorticorenal ganglia and aortic ganglia. Thus, pain from the testes is often referred to dermatomes associated with the lateral abdominal wall. Postganglionic sympathetic fibers run mostly with the testicular artery. However, some from the inferior hypogastric plexus may reach the testis by means of the artery to the ductus deferens fibers.

Epididymis

The epididymis (see Fig. 7-15) is found on the superior and posterolateral aspect of the testis. The head of the epididymis is located superiorly on the posterior surface of the testis, where it receives the sperm from the efferent ductules. Sperm mature in the epididymis. The body of the epididymis passes inferiorly from the head down along the mediastinum testis to the tail, which continues as the ductus (vas) deferens (see Fig. 7-15). In the head, 15 to 20 efferent ductules are coiled and eventually unite to form the single duct found in the body of the epididymis.

Blood Supply and Lymphatic Drainage

The epididymis receives branches of the testicular artery as well as the artery to the ductus deferens. It has the same venous and lymphatic drainage as the testis.

Innervation

The epididymis is innervated by the sympathetic preganglionic fibers that arise from thoracic spinal cord segments T11 and T12, which pass in the lesser and least splanchnic nerves to synapse in the renal, aorticorenal, and aortic ganglia. Most postganglionic sympathetic fibers reach the ganglia by following the testicular artery, with some fibers reaching them from the superior and the inferior hypogastric plexuses by following the ductus deferens fibers.

Ductus Deferens

The ductus deferens (see Fig. 7-15) is a thick-walled muscular tube that conveys sperm from the epididymis to the ejaculatory duct. It is about 30 to 45 cm long and begins as a very coiled duct at the tail of the epididymis, located at the inferior pole of the testis. Here, it ascends medially to the epididymis, and its course straightens as it ascends. In the spermatic cord, the ductus deferens is found posteriorly, surrounded by the pampiniform plexus of veins. It is in the upper portion of the scrotum that the ductus deferens can be interrupted in a vasectomy. The ductus deferens passes through the inguinal canal and leaves the other constituents of the spermatic cord at the deep ring. After passing laterally to the inferior epigastric vessels, it bends to pass medially over the external iliac artery and vein into the pelvis.

The ductus deferens is a retroperitoneal structure once it passes into the abdominal cavity through the deep ring. Thus, it is partially covered with peritoneum. In the pelvis, it crosses the umbilical artery and its superior vesical branch. It will also cross the obturator neurovascular bundle. As the ductus deferens runs medially, it crosses anterosuperiorly to the ureter (see Fig. 7-15). Remember, the ureter hooks inferiorly to the ductus deferens. At this point, the artery of the ductus deferens gives rise to a branch to the ureter. The ductus deferens then passes along the medial surface of the seminal vesicle on the base of the bladder. This portion of the ductus is dilated and is referred to as the ampulla of the ductus deferens. The ductus deferens again becomes a narrow duct and then joins the duct of the seminal vesicle to form a common duct called the *ejaculatory duct* (Fig. 7-18).

Blood Supply

The blood supply is the artery to the ductus, which can be a branch of the umbilical, superior, or inferior vesical artery. It follows the ductus as far as the testis, which it also helps to supply.

Innervation

The innervation is the same as for the epididymis.

Seminal Vesicle

The seminal vesicle (see Figs. 7-14B and 7-15) is a coiled, elongated gland that is folded upon itself. The seminal vesicle is found lateral to the ampulla of the ductus deferens on the base of the bladder.

Each seminal vesicle is firmly attached anteriorly to the base of the bladder and is separated from the rectum by the rectovesical septum (fascia of Denonvilliers; see Fig. 7-14C). The ureter passes close to the seminal vesicle, usually just slightly above its superior pole. The vesical and prostatic veins are also present. The medial end of the seminal vesicle is just superior to the prostate gland and the ampulla of the ductus deferens. Here, the seminal vesicle narrows to form the straight duct of the seminal vesicle that joins the duct of the narrow portion of the ductus deferens to produce the ejaculatory duct. Thus, the ejaculatory duct (see Fig. 7-18) is a common outlet for both the seminal vesicle and the ductus deferens. The ejaculatory duct passes through the prostate to empty into the prostatic urethra on the colliculus, laterally and distally to the utricle. The seminal vesicle produces secretions that are necessary for the mobility of sperm, but it does not contain sperm.

Blood Supply

The seminal vesicles are supplied by branches of the artery of the ductus, the inferior vesical, and the middle rectal.

Innervation

The seminal vesicles, ductus deferens, and epididymis are innervated in a similar manner. However, the seminal vesicle also receives postganglionic parasympathetic fibers from ganglia in the inferior hypogastric plexus. These parasympathetic ganglia receive their preganglionic fibers from the pelvic splanchnics. Their function is unclear.

Prostate Gland

The prostate is an oval gland that is found (in the standing position) anteroinferiorly surrounding the neck of the bladder (see Figs. 7-14, 7-15, and 7-18). Indeed, it surrounds the neck of the bladder and the first portion of the urethra. It is a fibromuscular gland with a capsule composed of dense connective tissue with a considerable amount of smooth muscle. The prostate has a base, apex, and four surfaces: anterior, posterior, and two inferolateral surfaces. The base of the prostate is in close relationship to the neck of the bladder, separated from the bladder by only a groove, while the apex faces inferiorly and is embedded in the urethral sphincter muscle. The anterior surface faces the lower half of the pubic symphysis and the retropubic space.

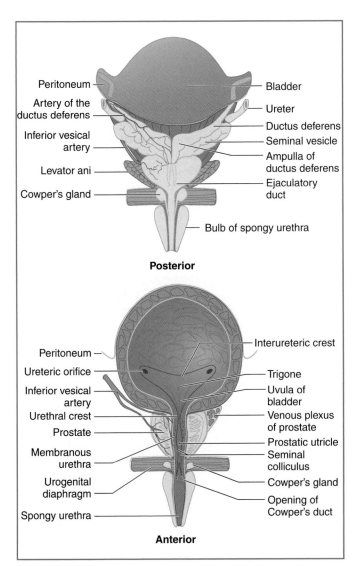

Figure 7-18. Posterior and anterior views of the prostate gland.

The posterior surface is separated from the rectum by the rectovesical septum. The seminal vesicles and ductus deferens are found just above the posterior surface on the base of the bladder. The inferolateral surfaces face the levator ani (pubococcygeus) muscles. The puboprostatic ligaments (endopelvic fascia) cross the retropubic space from the pubis to the apex of the prostate. The levator ani muscles give off slips of muscle that run below the puboprostatic ligaments to reach the posterior aspect of the apex and are called the levator prostatae muscles. The true capsule of the prostate is fibromuscular in nature. The endopelvic fascia extends up from the floor of the pelvis onto the external surface of the prostate and then up onto the bladder, producing the false capsule of the prostate gland (prostatic sheath). The false capsule is fascial in nature. Between the true and false capsules of the prostate gland is the prostatic plexus of veins, which receives the deep dorsal vein of the penis and the venous blood of the prostate and drains into the vesical plexus. This plexus usually drains into the internal iliac veins, but it also communicates with the vertebral venous plexuses via the sacral veins, which may be a route of metastasis.

The prostate gland is divided into two lateral lobes that are connected by means of a fibromuscular isthmus anterior to the urethra and a posterior lobe. Part of the posterior lobe is also referred to as the median lobe. It is found posterior to the urethra and between the right and left ejaculatory ducts. Part of the median lobe is posterior to the neck of the bladder. This lobe helps produce the uvula of the bladder. It pushes the smooth muscle of the trigone wall into the lumen of the bladder, thereby producing the bulge (uvula) of the trigone. The prostate secretes, by means of 20 to 30 prostatic ducts, directly into the prostatic urethra between the posterior wall and the colliculus seminalis (see below). The urethra enters the prostate at approximately the middle of its base. However, the urethra curves anteriorly as it passes through the prostate, emerging from its anterior surface just above the apex.

The posterior surface of the prostatic urethra has a distinctive morphology. Beginning at the internal urethral orifice and running the entire length of the posterior surface of the prostatic urethra is a fold or elevation known as the urethral crest. Approximately two thirds of the way down the length of the urethral crest is a further elevation that gives this part of the urethral crest a hill-like elevation over the rest of the urethral crest (see Fig. 7-18). This elevated portion of the urethral crest is the colliculus seminalis (seminal hillock, verumontanum). The colliculus has a pit-like depression at its eminence, which is the prostatic utricle (see Fig. 7-18). This blind pouch is often referred to as the male uterus, but actually it is homologous to the upper aspect of the vagina and serves no physiologic function. The ejaculatory ducts open onto the colliculus on either side of the prostatic utricle and are usually slightly distal to the utricle. Each ejaculatory duct is formed by the combination of the ampulla of the ductus deferens and the duct of the seminal vesicle. Thus, it carries sperm and the secretions of the epididymis, as well as secretions of the seminal vesicle.

Blood Supply

The prostatic arteries are branches of the inferior vesical artery, with some branches arising from the middle rectal artery and the artery to the ductus (Table 7-8). The prostatic venous plexus drains blood from the prostate, which then travels to the vesical plexus and into the internal iliac and sacral veins. These veins communicate with the internal vertebral plexus (of veins), known as Batson's plexus. This explains why prostate cancer often spreads to the vertebral column.

TABLE 7-8. Blood Supply and Innervation of Male Sex Organs and Ducts

Organ	Blood Supply	Venous Drainage	Lymphatics	Innervation
Testis	Testicular artery, artery of the ductus, cremasteric artery	Pampiniform plexus of veins to testicular vein	Nodes along the aorta or inferior vena cava (IVC) below renal veins	Sympathetics from T10–T11
Epididymis	Testicular artery and artery of the ductus	Pampiniform plexus of veins to testicular vein	Nodes along the aorta or IVC below renal veins	Sympathetics from T11–T12
Seminal vesicle	Artery of the ductus, inferior vesical and middle rectal arteries	Prostatic venous plexus to vesical plexus to internal iliac veins	Internal iliac nodes	Sympathetics from T11–T12 and parasympathetics
Ductus deferens	Artery of the ductus	Pampiniform plexus of veins to testicular vein	External iliac nodes	Sympathetics from T11–T12
Prostate	Branches from inferior vesical, artery of the ductus and middle rectal artery	Prostatic venous plexus to vesical plexus to sacral or internal iliac veins	Internal iliac nodes	Sympathetics from T11–L1 (also pelvic splanchnics)

CLINICAL MEDICINE

Benign Prostatic Hyperplasia (BPH)

Benign prostatic hyperplasia is a condition commonly found in older men. It is caused by an overgrowth of prostate cells that can put pressure on the prostatic urethra and thereby make it difficult to empty the bladder. BPH typically involves an enlargement of the median lobe of the prostate.

Innervation

The innervation of the prostate consists of preganglionic sympathetic fibers from spinal cord segments T11–L1 that synapse in intermesenteric and inferior mesenteric ganglia. Postganglionic fibers from these ganglia pass through the superior hypogastric plexus, and hypogastric nerves to the inferior hypogastric plexus and its prostatic plexus. These fibers cause contraction of the smooth muscle of the gland, which releases prostatic secretions into the urethra during ejaculation. The prostate also receives parasympathetic innervation that arises from S2–S4. While we are not sure exactly what they supply, it also explains why pain due to prostatitis is typically felt at the tip of the penis, which is part of the S4 dermatome.

Lymphatic Drainage

The lymphatic drainage is similar to that of the bladder (see Fig. 7-13). However, the lymphatics of the prostate begin within the false capsule of the prostate near the prostatic plexus of veins, not in the prostatic stroma. This is one explanation why metastasis from the prostate most often occurs through venous drainage.

●●●● DEVELOPMENT OF MALE REPRODUCTIVE SYSTEM

Despite the fact that the genetic sex of the embryo is determined at fertilization, all embryos look the same until about 7 weeks. The undifferentiated gonads begin to develop in the posterior abdominal wall near the T10 vertebra. There they stimulate the adjacent coelomic epithelium to proliferate and form cords of tissue called *primitive sex cords* (Fig. 7-19), which in turn cause ridges to form, called the *gonadal ridges*. As the gonadal ridges form, another pair of ducts form just lateral to the mesonephric ducts. These are called the *paramesonephric* or *müllerian ducts*.

If the embryo is genetically male, the primordial germ cells will be carrying an XY chromosomal complex. The Y chromosome contains a region called the sex-determining region (SRY) in which a gene encodes a transcription factor, testis-determining factor (TDF), that triggers male development. In the seventh week, the Sertoli cells and primordial germ cells organize themselves into testis cords. The inner aspect of the developing gonad makes connections with the mesonephric tubules, which become the rete testis. In the eighth week, the interstitial cells of Leydig within the developing gonad begin

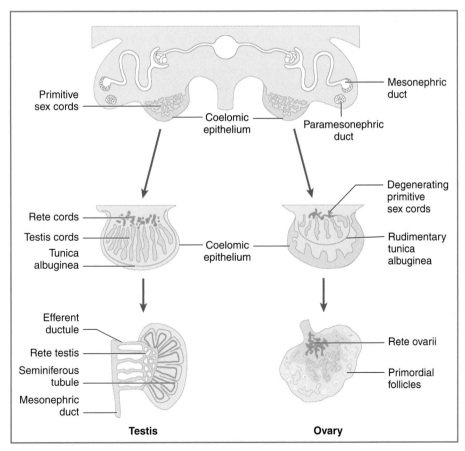

Figure 7-19. Early development of gonads.

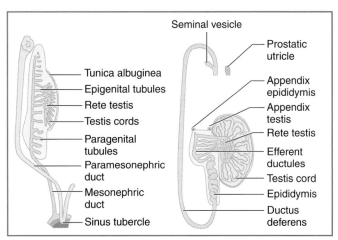

Figure 7-20. Development of male genital ducts.

CLINICAL MEDICINE

Male Pseudohermaphrodite

Pseudohermaphrodites are individuals whose genotype is different from their phenotype. In the case of male pseudohermaphrodites, the genotype is XY yet their external genitalia can be ambiguous or feminized. Typically this can happen in three ways. First, in androgen insensitivity syndrome (AIS), the individual makes normal levels of testosterone but the receptors on the target cells are defective and do not respond to testosterone appropriately. Second, insufficient levels of testosterone may be produced, resulting in ambiguous genitalia as well as incomplete male ductal elements. Lastly, absence of the enzyme 5α-reductase, which converts testosterone to dihydrotestosterone, can cause feminization of the external genitalia.

to produce and secrete testosterone, which further drives the development of the testes and the associated duct system. At the same time, the Sertoli cells produce antimüllerian hormone (AMH; also called müllerian inhibiting substance [MIS]), which causes complete degradation of the paramesonephric duct system except for two vestigial pieces—the appendix of the testis and the prostatic utricle.

The mesonephric tubules differentiate into the different parts of the male duct system (Fig. 7-20). The caudal end of the mesonephric tubules becomes the epididymis. The next portion acquires a smooth muscle coat and becomes the ductus deferens. In the 10th week, the seminal vesicles bud from a region where the mesonephric tubule joins the pelvic urethra. The portion of the mesonephric tubule that is distal to the seminal vesicle bud is then called the ejaculatory duct. The prostate gland develops in the 10th week as an endodermal outgrowth of the pelvic urethra. Its development is dependent on the presence of dihydrotestosterone (DHT), an androgenic hormone whose precursor is testosterone. The testis cords will remain solid until puberty, when there is an increase in the circulating levels of testosterone. This increase

brings about canalization of the testis cords, which will then become the seminiferous tubules.

●●● FEMALE GENITAL SYSTEM

The female genital system comprises the ovaries, uterine tubes, uterus, and vagina.

Ovaries

The ovaries produce the ova, and they secrete estrogen and progesterone. They are almond-shaped bodies that are smaller than the testes, and their size changes during different stages of a woman's life. They lie in the female pelvis attached to the posterior layer of the broad ligament (of the peritoneum) and are directly attached to the uterus by the ovarian ligament (Fig. 7-21). Since the ovary has a vertical orientation, it has medial (inferior) and lateral (superior) ends, medial and lateral surfaces, and anterior and posterior borders. The lateral end of the ovary is the most superior portion of the gland. It is also the tubal end because it is in proximity to the opening of the uterine tube. The medial end of the ovary is medioinferior in position. It is known as the uterine end because it is attached to the uterus by means of the ovarian ligament. The tubal end of the ovary is attached to the pelvic wall by means of a peritoneal fold known as the *suspensory ligament of the ovary* or the *infundibulopelvic ligament*. The suspensory ligament contains the ovarian neurovascular bundle. The anterior border of the ovary is attached to the broad ligament by means of the mesovarium, while the posterior border is free and faces the rectouterine pouch. In a nulliparous woman (a woman who has never given birth), the lateral surface of the ovary is often found in a depression in the peritoneum called the *ovarian fossa*, bounded by the ureter and internal iliac vessels. The medial surface is covered with the fimbriae of the uterine tube and the coils of the ileum.

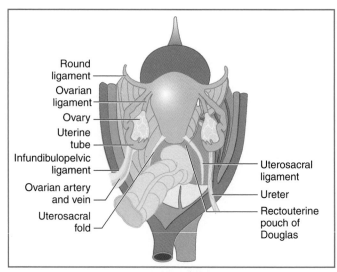

Figure 7-21. Posterior view of female reproductive organs.

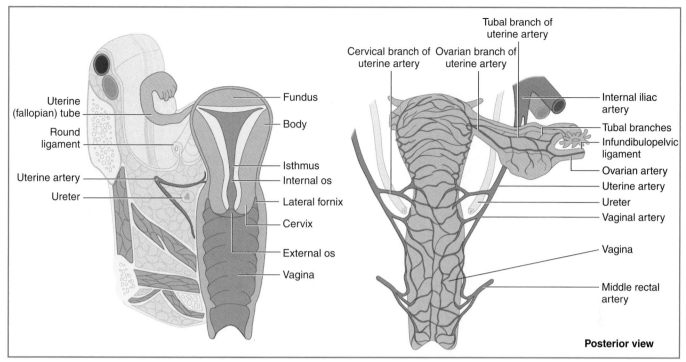

Figure 7-22. Blood supply to female reproductive organs.

The ovaries develop from the intermediate mesoderm behind the peritoneum. The germinal epithelium (cuboidal to columnar cells) that covers the ovary is derived from the same cells that develop into the parietal peritoneum. The germinal epithelium was incorrectly thought to give rise to the primordial germ cells. The germinal epithelium is continuous with the flat mesothelial cells of the parietal peritoneum at the mesovarium. Thus, ovulation is the release of an ovum through the germinal epithelium, which is the mesothelial covering of the ovary. Ovulation occurs into the peritoneal cavity.

The connective tissue supporting the cells of the ovary is the tunica albuginea. Although this term is used for the capsule of both the testis and ovary, it is well developed in the testis and poorly developed in the ovary.

Blood Supply

The hilum of the ovary lies along the mesovarium attachment to the ovary. At this point, the ovary receives the ovarian artery and venous plexus (pampiniform) as well as the ovarian branches of the uterine artery (Fig. 7-22). Each ovarian vein starts as the pampiniform plexus and drains, as do the testicular veins, into the IVC on the right and into the left renal vein on the left.

Lymphatic Drainage

The lymphatic drainage (Fig. 7-23) of the ovary is similar to the drainage of the testis, since it follows the ovarian (gonadal)

vessels. Thus, the right ovary drains into the lumbar nodes adjacent to the IVC and below the right renal vein. The left ovary drains into the lumbar nodes adjacent to and below the point where the left renal vein crosses anterior to the aorta. These nodes also drain the uterine tube and fundus of the uterus.

Innervation

Preganglionic sympathetic fibers have their cell bodies at the T10 to T11 spinal cord levels, run in the lesser and least splanchnic nerves, and synapse in the aorticorenal and renal ganglia. Postganglionic sympathetic fibers reach the ovary by traveling with the ovarian artery. The cell bodies of the afferents traveling from the ovary have their cell bodies in the dorsal root ganglia of T10 to T11.

PHYSIOLOGY

Menstrual Cycle

The menstrual cycle involves the actions of gonadotropin-releasing hormone (GnRH) from the hypothalamus and follicle-stimulating hormone (FSH) and luteinizing hormone (LH) from the pituitary. The release of GnRH from the hypothalamus causes the secretion of FSH and LH from the pituitary. FSH and LH, in turn, stimulate follicle development, ovulation, and the synthesis of the female sex hormones.

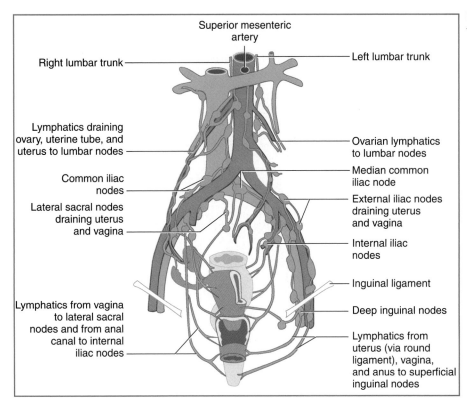

Figure 7-23. Lymphatic drainage of the female pelvis.

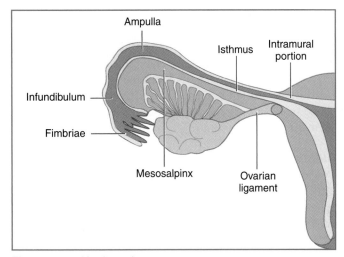

Figure 7-24. Uterine tube.

Uterine (Fallopian) Tubes (Salpinx)

The uterine (fallopian) tubes, or salpinx (Figs. 7-24 and 7-25), allow the peritoneal cavity to communicate with the lumen of the uterus. Thus, the female peritoneal cavity is an open serous cavity (the *only* open serous cavity), and the ovum is initially released into the peritoneal cavity and then swept into the uterine tube. Fertilization usually takes place in the ampulla of the uterine tube, and the fertilized egg stays in the uterine tube for 4 to 5 days. The uterine tube is a partially coiled tube that stretches from the laterally placed ovary to

the medially placed uterus. The uterine tube is found in the superior free surface of the broad ligament above the posteriorly attached ovary. This portion of the broad ligament is the mesosalpinx.

As in any canal or tube-like structure, there are two openings or ends to the uterine tube. In addition, there are several different morphologic parts to the uterine tube as it passes from the peritoneal cavity close to the ovary into the uterus. The lateral aspect of the uterine tube is characterized by numerous finger-like projections (fimbriae), which are responsible for sweeping the ovum into the tube. One of the fimbriae (fimbria ovarica) is often longer than the others and is attached to the ovary to maintain this intimate relationship. The other fimbriae overlie the posterior and lateral aspects of the ovary and surround the pelvic opening of the uterine tube. This ostium opens into the pelvic portion of the peritoneal cavity even though it is called the abdominal opening. The abdominal opening leads to the infundibulum, a funnel-shaped portion of the tube. The next portion of the uterine tube is the ampulla, which has a dilated diameter. The diameter of the uterine tube then narrows as it approaches the uterus. This narrow portion is the isthmus of the uterine tube. The last portion of the tube passes through the wall of the uterus and is the uterine's intramural portion. The intramural portion ends as the uterine opening into the lumen of the uterus.

Blood Supply

The tubal branches of both the ovarian and uterine arteries supply the uterine tubes (see Fig. 7-22). This anastomosis can

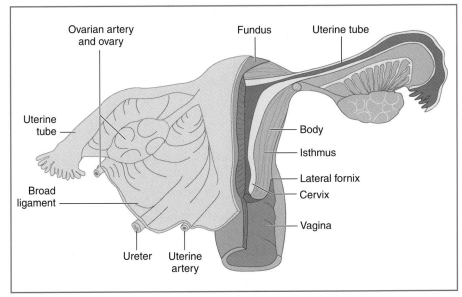

Figure 7-25. Posterior view of the uterus.

HISTOLOGY

Oviducts (Uterine Tubes, Fallopian Tubes)

The oviducts are lined by a simple columnar epithelium, which contains two cell types: ciliated and nonciliated. The ciliated cells are responsible for moving the ovum toward the uterus. The nonciliated cells, known as peg cells, secrete the fluid, which both carries the ovum and helps nourish it. Both cell types undergo changes in response to the hormonal cycle.

CLINICAL MEDICINE

Ectopic Pregnancy

An ectopic pregnancy results when implantation of the fertilized ovum occurs outside the uterus. This can happen at various sites including the outside of the ovary, the inside of the fallopian tube, and the wall of the peritoneal cavity. The most common site of ectopic implantation is within the fallopian tube. As with intrauterine implantations, in the normal lining of the uterus, the trophoblast cells from the conceptus penetrate the tubal wall and connect with blood vessels. Thus, as the embryo grows, it will eventually rupture the uterine tube with concomitant hemorrhage from branches of the uterine artery and the ovarian artery, threatening both mother and fetus.

be a problem if the uterine tube ruptures during an ectopic pregnancy. The venous return follows the arteries, while the lymphatic drainage is into the lumbar nodes that drain the ovaries.

Innervation

Innervation to the uterine tube consists of preganglionic sympathetic fibers that arise from spinal cord segments T10 and T11, which synapse in the aorticorenal ganglia and intermesenteric ganglia. Postganglionic sympathetic fibers run mostly with the ovarian artery. However, some may reach the uterine tube by means of the uterine artery.

Uterus

The uterus is often described as an inverted, pear-shaped organ found shifted slightly to one side of the midline, often the right. The uterus has a fundus, body, isthmus, and cervix (see Figs. 7-22 and 7-25). The size and shape of the uterus are a function of physiology and age. The uterus of a nulliparous woman is different from the uterus of a woman who has had one or more pregnancies.

The fundus is that portion of the uterus above and slightly anterior to the opening of the intramural portion of the uterine tubes (see Fig. 7-25). The body is the major portion of the

uterus and is separated from the cervix by a narrow constriction found on the anterior and posterior surfaces known as the isthmus. The body has anterior and posterior surfaces as well as lateral margins.

The cervix (neck) of the uterus penetrates the anterior wall of the vagina near its superior aspect (see Fig. 7-25). Thus, the cervix has a supravaginal portion that is in the pelvis and an intravaginal portion that protrudes into the vagina. The intravaginal portion of the cervix has an anterior and a posterior labium, or lip. The opening to the lumen of the uterus at the cervix is found between the two lips and is called the external os (ostium of the uterus). The lumen of the cervix is constricted at its external end and at its internal end at the isthmus. Since a potential route exists from the external environment through the vagina, uterus, and uterine tube into the peritoneal cavity, these constrictions plus mucous plugs help isolate and protect the uterine cavity. The consistency of the cervix changes during pregnancy. In the nonpregnant woman, the cervix is as firm as the tip of the nose, while in pregnant females the cervix is usually as soft as the lips.

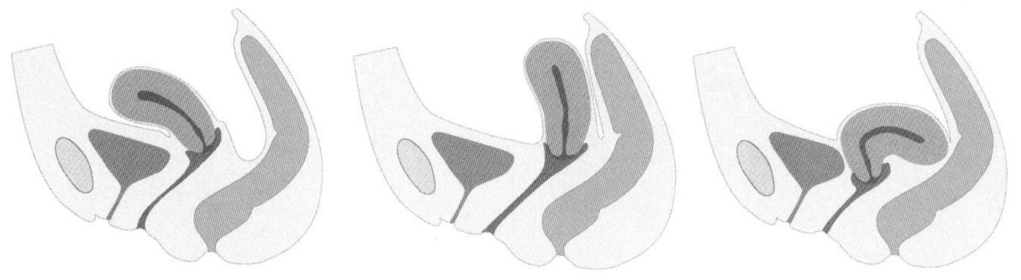

Figure 7-26. Positions of the uterus.

Normal anteverted, anteflexed position   Retroversion   Retroflexion

PATHOLOGY

Uterine Fibroids

Uterine fibroids are benign tumors of the myometrium and are present in about 20% of women over age 30. These tumors are derived from the smooth muscle tissue and vary enormously in their size. The site of the fibroid within the uterus determines the symptomatology. Submucous and intramural fibroids cause extended or heavy menstrual periods (menorrhagia). Fibroids that are subserosal may become pedunculated (attached via a stalk or pedicle) and cause colicky pain as the uterus attempts to expel it. If the fibroid grows very large in size it may put pressure on the bladder or rectum and thereby cause symptoms. Fibroids may also cause miscarriages because they often grow in size during pregnancy. Fibroids that do not cause symptoms are usually not treated. However, in cases of excessive pain or bleeding, there are several possible treatments based on whether preservation of reproductive function is desired. If the woman is of childbearing age, uterine artery embolism involves the injection of polyvinyl particles to reduce the blood supply to the uterus. The ischemia causes the fibroid to shrink. Alternatively, hysterectomy or myomectomy (removal of a myoma, a benign muscular neoplasm) can be performed. However, the rate of recurrence after myomectomy is surprisingly high—40%.

Indeed, Goodell's sign is the softening of the cervix and vagina that can be indicative (but not definitively) of pregnancy.

The labia of the cervix interface with the walls of the vagina to produce a sulcus or arched recess between the cervix and the vaginal wall. This is the *fornix* of the vagina, and it is divided into an anterior part, a posterior part, and lateral parts. The posterior fornix is between the posterior labium and the vaginal wall and is the deepest aspect of the vaginal fornix. The anterior fornix is the arch between the anterior cervical labium and the superior vaginal wall. This usually is the fornix that is observed upon examination. The lateral fornices are very shallow (see Fig. 7-25). The ureters are found just lateral to the lateral fornices. The position and shape of the fornices change under certain conditions.

The uterus is at approximately a 90-degree angle to the vagina; therefore, the cervix penetrates the anterosuperior wall of the vagina (Fig. 7-26). This position is the anteverted position and is the normal position. If the cervix makes a more obtuse angle with the vagina, the position is referred to as retroverted. In the retroverted position, the cervix can approach a position in line with the long axis of the vagina. This may be the result of weakened ligaments that hold the cervix in its proper anatomic position. In this case, the uterus may protrude more and more into the vaginal vault in a condition known as a prolapsed uterus. The body of the uterus can also flex at the isthmus on the cervix. If the body flexes anteriorly at the cervix, the uterus is considered anteflexed. If the body of the uterus flexes posteriorly at the cervix, the uterus is retroflexed. This aspect of the position of the uterine body depends in part on the contents of the anterior bladder or the posterior rectum or on pregnancy.

The peritoneum covers most but not all of the uterus. Obviously, the intravaginal cervix is devoid of peritoneum. However, the lateral margins are also devoid of peritoneum. The peritoneum is reflected from the bladder onto the anterior surface of the uterus (at approximately the isthmus) to produce the vesicouterine pouch (of the peritoneal cavity). The peritoneum is reflected from the posterior wall of the body and cervix as well as the posterior vaginal wall onto the rectum to produce the rectouterine pouch (of the peritoneal cavity). The lower portion of this pouch between the posterior cervix, posterior vaginal wall, and rectum is also termed the cul-de-sac or pouch of Douglas (see Fig. 7-21). An incision in the posterior fornix of the vagina can pass through the vaginal wall, extraperitoneal connective tissue, rectovaginal septum and the peritoneum into the pouch of Douglas.

The peritoneum is reflected off the lateral pelvic wall and passes toward the uterus and is reflected onto its anterior and posterior surfaces. However, the peritoneum does not reach the lateral margins of the uterus, producing a slightly thickened peritoneal ligament between the lateral pelvic wall and the lateral borders of the uterus. This peritoneal ligament is the broad ligament (see Figs. 7-21 and 7-25). The lateral borders of the uterus are covered by extraperitoneal (subserous) fascia that separates the layers of the broad ligament. This extraperitoneal fascia is referred to as the *parametrium*.

The broad ligament (see Figs. 7-21 and 7-25) is subdivided by the presence of the attached ovary to its posterior surface. The portion of the posterior leaf of the broad ligament that attaches the ovary to the broad ligament is the mesovarium. The portion of the broad ligament that is superior to the

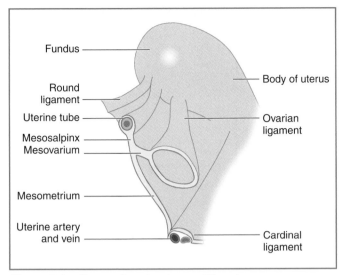

Fundus

Round ligament

Uterine tube

Mesosalpinx
Mesovarium

Mesometrium

Uterine artery and vein

Body of uterus

Ovarian ligament

Cardinal ligament

Figure 7-27. Supporting structures of the uterus.

attachment of the mesovarium to the broad ligament is the mesosalpinx. Finally, the portion of the broad ligament below the mesovarium is the mesometrium. Each of these portions of the broad ligament contains different structures. The mesovarium contains the ovarian artery, pampiniform (ovarian) venous plexus, lymphatics, and nerves as well as ovarian branches of the uterine artery and vein and the ovarian ligament. The mesosalpinx contains the uterine tube and its neurovascular supply, which includes branches from both the uterine and ovarian arteries. The mesometrium contains the uterine neurovascular bundle and the round ligament (Fig. 7-27).

The round ligament and ovarian ligament are remnants of the fetal gubernaculum and are almost continuous with each other. The broad ligament is subdivided by the attachment of the ovary by means of the mesovarium. However, the transverse cervical (cardinal) ligament of the uterus is a specialization of extraperitoneal fascia that contains the uterine vessels that cross above the ureter.

The ligaments (see also Figs. 7-7 and 7-27) that help maintain the position of the uterus are those formed from condensations of extraperitoneal fascia and containing some smooth muscle. These ligaments run from the neck of the uterus to the walls of the pelvis and adjacent organs. The most important of these ligaments are the transverse cervical ligaments that extend from the lateral wall to the cervix. The transverse cervical ligament is also called the *cardinal ligament* (see Fig. 7-27). The other ligaments are the uterosacral and the pubocervical ligaments. Part of the latter ligament is also referred to as the vesicouterine ligament. It should be noted that the levator ani and the round ligament and, to a lesser degree, the urethrovaginal sphincter are also extremely important in maintaining the position of the uterus by supporting the surrounding organs such as the bladder, vagina, and rectum.

Blood Supply

The arterial supply (see Fig. 7-22) to the uterus consists of the uterine artery. This artery is homologous to the artery of the

ductus deferens in the male. It supplies the uterus and part of the vagina and anastomoses with the ovarian artery to help supply the ovary and salpinx. The uterine plexus of veins anastomoses with the adjacent veins to drain into the internal iliac vein. The uterine artery and vein pass through the upper portion of the transverse cervical ligament over the ureter to enter the broad ligament and reach the uterus.

Innervation

Preganglionic sympathetic fibers from thoracic spinal cord segments T11 and T12(L1) synapse in the aorticorenal and intermesenteric ganglia. Postganglionic fibers run from the superior hypogastric plexus via the hypogastric nerve to the uterovaginal portion of the inferior hypogastric plexus where branches follow the uterine artery to the body and fundus of the uterus. The uterovaginal portion of the inferior hypogastric plexus consists of sympathetic fibers and parasympathetic fibers. However, few parasympathetic fibers reach the uterus. Therefore, in contrast to most pelvic organs, the afferents from the fundus and body of the uterus travel with the sympathetics and have their cell bodies located in the dorsal root ganglia of spinal nerves T11 and T12(L1). Thus, pain from the uterus is usually felt in the lower abdomen but may radiate to the sides and back. However, afferents from the cervix travel with the parasympathetics and have their cell bodies in the dorsal root ganglia of spinal nerves S2, S3, and S4 and will be felt in the sacral region. Thus, the afferent supply of the uterus is different from that of most pelvic organs, which travel primarily with the parasympathetics.

Lymphatic Drainage

The lymphatic drainage (see Fig. 7-23) of the uterus varies depending on the specific part in question. The fundus and upper body drain with the ovary and uterine tubes into the lumbar nodes (close to and below the origin of the renal veins). The lower uterine body drains into external iliac nodes, while the cervix drains into the sacral nodes and both internal and external iliac nodes. A few lymphatics from the region of the attached round ligament drain to the superficial inguinal nodes.

Relationships of the Uterus

The uterus has several important relationships with the surrounding organs (Fig. 7-28). Anterior to the fundus and body is the vesicouterine pouch and bladder. However, the anterior surface of the supravaginal cervix is separated from the bladder only by some extraperitoneal fascia, while the anterior labium of the intravaginal portion of the cervix helps form the anterior fornix. Because of the close relationship between the bladder and the anterior surface of the uterus, the peritoneum is often stripped off of the anterior surface of the uterus during a cesarean section in order to ensure that the bladder is not incised along with the anterior wall of the uterus. Posterior to the fundus, body, and extravaginal cervix is the rectouterine pouch, typically containing coils of the ileum, and the rectum. The uterine artery crosses above the ureter,

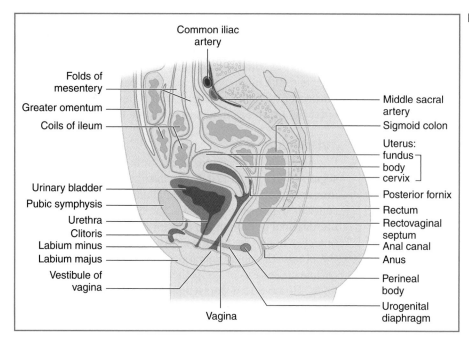

Figure 7-28. Relationships of the uterus.

Labels in figure:

Common iliac artery
Folds of mesentery
Greater omentum
Coils of ileum
Urinary bladder
Pubic symphysis
Urethra
Clitoris
Labium minus
Labium majus
Vestibule of vagina
Vagina
Middle sacral artery
Sigmoid colon
Uterus:
fundus
body
cervix
Posterior fornix
Rectum
Rectovaginal septum
Anal canal
Anus
Perineal body
Urogenital diaphragm

just lateral to the supravaginal cervix on the superior aspect of the transverse cervical ligament. This relationship is important because these vessels have to be ligated during a hysterectomy.

Vagina

The vagina (see Fig. 7-28) is a fibromuscular tubular canal. Although the vagina is usually flat, it can be easily dilated during copulation or physical examination. The vagina is 8 to 12 cm long. Its anterior and posterior walls are usually in contact with each other except in the region of the cervix of the uterus. The arching furrow between the labia of the uterine cervix and the vaginal wall is the fornix of the vagina and has been described with the cervix. Since the cervix penetrates the anterior vaginal wall, the anterior wall is shorter than the posterior vaginal wall (see Fig. 7-28). The vagina passes through the urogenital diaphragm to end in the vestibule of the vagina in the perineum (see Perineum section).

The vagina is held in its proper anatomic position by several supporting structures including the ligaments to the cervix (transverse cervical, uterosacral, and pubocervical ligaments and endopelvic attachments to the arcus tendineus) as well as muscle fibers from the pubococcygeus and urethrovaginal sphincter muscles. Clinically, the uterosacral ligament and its smooth muscle support the cervix and upper vaginal apex posteriorly over the levator ani muscle. The cardinal (transverse cervical) ligament may assist, but it is mostly perivascular fascia surrounding the uterine vessels. When the levator ani pathologically weakens, the urogenital hiatus enlarges, placing stress on the ligaments, especially the uterosacral ligaments, encouraging prolapse.

Blood Supply

The upper portion of the vagina is derived from the müllerian ducts, and the lower portion is derived from the urogenital sinus (Table 7-9). The division of the vaginal wall along embryologic lines (the part derived from ectoderm versus endoderm) is just external to the hymen. Thus, the upper 80% of the vagina receives its supply from visceral neurovascular structures. The arterial supply to the vagina consists of the vaginal branches of the uterine arteries and the vaginal branches that are direct branches from the internal iliac arteries. Only the orifice of the vagina and adjacent walls may also receive an arterial supply from the internal pudendal artery. The venous plexus of the vagina communicates with the venous plexus of the bladder and drains into the internal iliac veins.

PATHOLOGY

Human Papillomavirus (HPV)

Certain types of human papillomavirus are associated with precancerous and cancerous conditions of the cervix. These viruses are identified based on their DNA sequences. Some strains are associated with low-grade cervical intraepithelial neoplasia (CIN), such as types 6 and 11, whereas types 16, 18, 45, and 56 are correlated with carcinoma of the cervix. The direct role of HPV in cellular changes has not yet been definitively established; however, HPV is present in 95% of squamous cell cervical cancers and in 60% of adenocarcinomas. The efficacy of HPV testing in predicting cervical carcinoma has not been established, but the presence of certain strains of HPV may be an indication for more frequent cytologic screening.

TABLE 7-9. Blood Supply and Innervation of Female Reproductive Organs

Organ	Blood Supply	Venous Drainage	Lymphatics	Innervation
Ovary	Ovarian artery and uterine artery	Ovarian vein	Lumbar nodes	Sympathetics from T10 to T11
Uterus—body and fundus	Uterine artery and ovarian artery	Uterine vein	Fundus and upper body to lumbar lymph nodes; lower body to external iliac nodes	Sympathetics from T11 to T12
Uterus—cervix	Uterine artery	Uterine vein	Sacral nodes and external and internal iliac nodes	Sympathetics from T11 to T12(L1); visceral afferents run with pelvic splanchnics
Uterine tube	Uterine and ovarian arteries	Ovarian vein and uterine venous plexus	Lumbar nodes	Sympathetics from T11 to L1
Vagina	Branches of uterine artery superiorly and middle rectal and internal pudendal arteries inferiorly	Uterine venous plexus	Superior: to internal and external iliac nodes Middle: to internal iliac nodes Inferior: to sacral and superficial inguinal nodes	Superior: pelvic splanchnics and sympathetics Inferior: perineal branch of pudendal nerve

Innervation

The innervation of most of the vagina is the uterovaginal plexus derived from the inferior hypogastric plexus with the parasympathetics from spinal cord segments S2, S3, and S4 and the sympathetics derived from the superior hypogastric plexus. Afferents from most of the vagina follow the pelvic splanchnics to spinal cord segments S2–S4 and have their sensory cell bodies in the dorsal root ganglia of these spinal cord segments. Only the innervation to the lowest portion of the vagina, near the vestibule, is somatic via branches of the pudendal nerve.

Lymphatics

The lymphatic drainage of most of the vagina, in the region of the cervix, is into the internal and external iliac nodes and the sacral nodes. However, the lymphatics from the lower portion of the vagina near the vestibule drain into the superficial inguinal nodes (see Fig. 7-23).

Relationships of the Vagina

1. The uterine cervix penetrates the anterior wall of the vagina.
2. The ureters pass about 1 cm lateral to the supravaginal cervix, close to the anterior wall of the vagina to reach the bladder.
3. The bladder is closely related to the anterior vaginal wall, separated only by some extraperitoneal fascia.
4. The urethra is *attached* by means of fascia to the lower aspect of the anterior wall of the vagina.

Posteriorly, the vagina is separated from the rectum by the rectouterine peritoneal pouch, rectouterine septum, and extraperitoneal fascia. In the perineum, the ostium of the vagina is separated from the anus and anal canal by the posterior aspect of the urogenital diaphragm and the perineal body. Intravaginal examination allows for the direct palpation of the cervix. The urethra and bladder can be assessed through the anterior vaginal wall, the rectum, and rectovaginal septum through the posterior wall. Lateral to the vagina is the ischial spine and sacrospinous ligament of the pelvic wall.

During bimanual manipulation, the examiner can determine if the uterus is anteverted and can evaluate the ovaries and uterine tubes.

●●● DEVELOPMENT OF FEMALE REPRODUCTIVE ORGANS

The female embryo has no Y chromosome and therefore no SRY gene and its products. Thus, the indifferent gonads will develop into ovaries. The primitive sex cords of the gonad degenerate, and the mesothelium of the genital ridge forms secondary sex cords (Fig. 7-29). The secondary sex cords in turn surround the germ cells to form the follicular cells of the ovary. The germ cells develop into oogonia and enter the first mitotic division. When they come in close contact with the follicular cells, further development is arrested. They will remain this way until puberty, when circulating gonadotropins will cause individual oocytes to resume gametogenesis on a monthly basis.

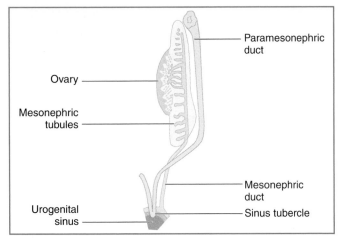

A

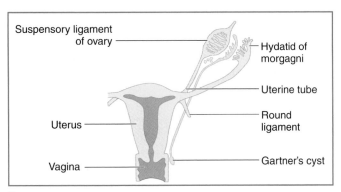

B

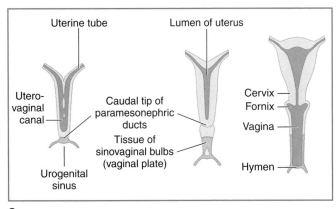

C

Figure 7-29. Development of female reproductive organs.
A, Uterine tubes. **B,** Uterus. **C,** Superior portion of the vagina.

Without the presence of antimüllerian hormone and testosterone, the mesonephric ducts will degenerate, leaving behind two vestigial pieces—the appendix of the ovary and Gartner's cysts—and the paramesonephric ducts will persist (see Fig. 7-29). The paramesonephric ducts will develop into the uterine tubes, uterus, and superior portion of the vagina. The cranial end of the duct, with its funnel-shaped opening into the abdominal cavity, will become the uterine tubes. At the caudal end, the two paramesonephric ducts fuse with the each other to form a tube with a single lumen called the *uterovaginal canal,* which will become the uterus and superior end of the vagina.

If the fusion is not complete, a uterus with two lumens may form. As the paramesonephric tubules fuse, they contact the urogenital sinus forming the sinus tubercle, which in turn induces the formation of two endodermal swellings called the *sinovaginal bulbs.* The sinovaginal bulbs fuse together to become the vaginal plate. As the cells of the vaginal plate proliferate, the distance between the urogenital sinus and the uterus increases, thereby forming the inferior portion of the vagina, which will be completely canalized by the fifth month. The vagina remains separated from the urogenital sinus by a membrane called the *hymen* (see Fig. 7-29C).

PERINEUM

Perineum is Greek for the region between the nates (buttocks). The perineum is a specialized portion of the body wall that contains all the basic components of the body wall (i.e., skin, superficial fascia, deep fascia, and skeletal muscles). As such, it is innervated by spinal nerves that contain general somatic motor and general sensory fibers as well as postganglionic sympathetic fibers. The unusual aspect of this region of the body wall is the interfacing of visceral structures (the GI and urogenital systems derived from endoderm and splanchnic mesoderm) with somatic structures (derived from ectoderm and somatic mesoderm). This is reflected in the innervation of this region, in which different portions of an organ are innervated by either the somatic or autonomic nervous system. In addition, this region includes the erectile tissue of the external genitalia, which is innervated by parasympathetic fibers.

The perineum is usually described in the lithotomy position. In this position, the patient is on the back, knees and hips flexed, thighs abducted and laterally rotated at the hip joint. The peripheral boundaries of the diamond-shaped perineum coincide with the boundaries of the pelvic outlet in this position (Figs. 7-30 and 7-31). They are the inferior surface of the pubic symphysis anteriorly, the ischiopubic rami anterolaterally, the ischial tuberosities laterally, the sacrotuberous ligaments posterolaterally, and the tip of the coccyx posteriorly.

The superficial boundary of the perineum is the skin and superficial fascia. The deep boundary is the inner investing layer of deep fascia on the pelvic diaphragm.

The perineum is separated from the pelvis by the pelvic diaphragm. Since the perineum is external to the pelvic diaphragm, the origins and insertions of the pelvic diaphragm shape the perineum's architecture. The lateral wall of the pelvis is lined by the obturator internus muscle, which courses toward and then through the lesser sciatic foramen. The endopelvic fascia on the medial surface of the obturator internus muscle is thickened into the arcus tendineus between the ischial spine and the superior pubic ramus. The arcus tendineus is the origin of the iliococcygeus portion of the levator ani muscle.

The perineum is subdivided by an imaginary line drawn between the two ischial tuberosities into an anterior or

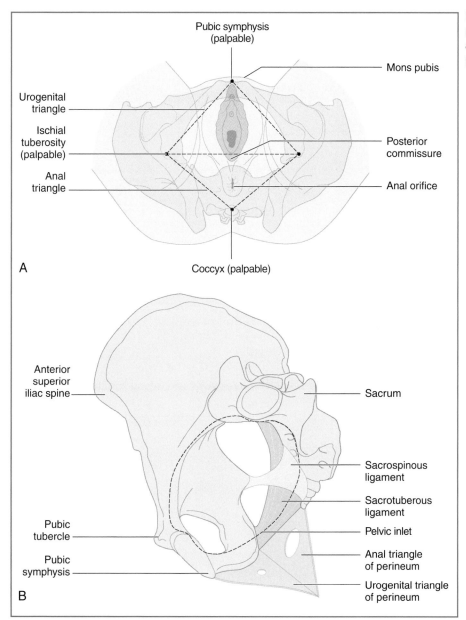

Figure 7-30. A, Boundaries of the perineum. **B,** Note that urogenital triangle and anal triangle are not in the same plane.

urogenital triangle and a posterior or anal triangle (see Fig. 7-30A). However, these two triangles are not planar; they form an obtuse angle with each other (see Fig. 7-30B). The perineal body (central tendon of the perineum) is found approximately in the middle of this line. It is a pyramid-shaped fibromuscular mass in which several muscles insert and is of great importance in obstetrics.

●●● UROGENITAL TRIANGLE

The urogenital triangle is that part of the perineum bounded by the pubic symphysis, the ischiopubic rami, and a line drawn between the ischial tuberosities. The superficial boundary consists of skin and superficial fascia, while the deep boundary consists of the inner investing layer of fascia on the pelvic diaphragm. The urogenital triangle contains the urogenital diaphragm and the superficial pouch.

Urogenital Diaphragm

The urogenital diaphragm is a muscular shelf that passes from one ischiopubic ramus to the contralateral one in such a way that it covers the urogenital hiatus found in the pelvic diaphragm (Fig. 7-32). The urogenital hiatus is necessary to allow the passage of the urethra in both males and females and the vagina in females. However, the opening in the pelvic diaphragm is too large to remain uncovered. Without the presence of the muscles and fascia of the urogenital diaphragm, it would be easy for pelvic structures to collapse through the hiatus (prolapse).

The urogenital diaphragm consists of the sphincter urethrae (in males) or urethrovaginal sphincter muscle (in females), deep transverse perineal muscles, as well as their muscular fasciae. These muscles arise from the ischiopubic rami and insert into the midline. The associated muscular fascia is also attached to

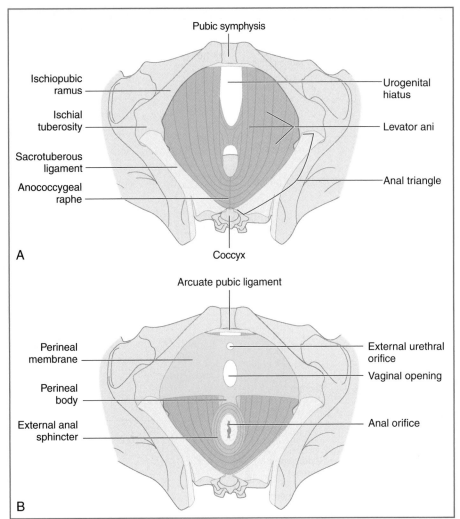

Figure 7-31. Urogenital triangle with urogenital hiatus. Without (**A**) and with (**B**) urogenital diaphragm.

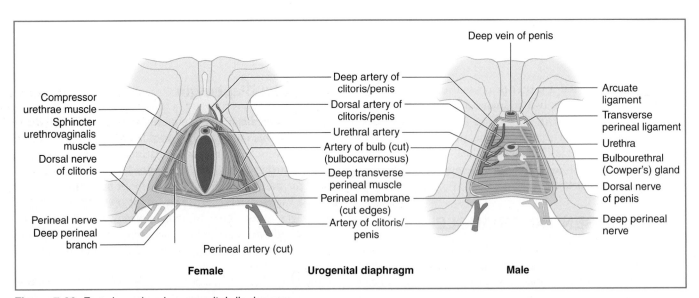

Figure 7-32. Female and male urogenital diaphragms.

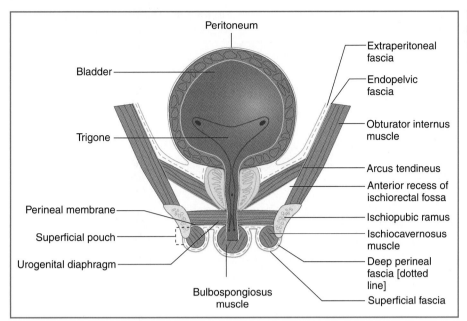

Figure 7-33. Coronal section of the male superficial pouch and urogenital diaphragm, anterior recess of the ischioanal fossa, and fascial planes.

Labels in figure:
Peritoneum
Bladder
Trigone
Perineal membrane
Superficial pouch
Urogenital diaphragm
Bulbospongiosus muscle
Extraperitoneal fascia
Endopelvic fascia
Obturator internus muscle
Arcus tendineus
Anterior recess of ischiorectal fossa
Ischiopubic ramus
Ischiocavernosus muscle
Deep perineal fascia [dotted line]
Superficial fascia

the ischiopubic rami. Different parts of this muscular fascia are given specific names.

The inferior fascia of the muscles of the urogenital diaphragm is located on the inferior (external) surface and is thickened into a strong membrane, which is also referred to as the perineal membrane.

The arcuate pubic ligament strengthens the inferior surface of the pubic symphysis (see Fig. 7-32). The anterior aspect of the perineal membrane does not reach the inferior surface of the pubic symphysis or the arcuate pubic ligament, and forms a thickening called the transverse perineal ligament. Between the arcuate pubic ligament and the transverse perineal ligament is a potential space occupied by the deep dorsal vein of the penis or clitoris.

Male and Female Urogenital Diaphragms

In the male, the urogenital diaphragm contains the second (membranous) portion of the urethra, nerves and vessels, and the bulbourethral (Cowper's) glands (see Fig. 7-32). Although these glands are located on either side of the membranous urethra, their ducts penetrate the perineal membrane to enter the third portion of the urethra, the spongy urethra.

In the female, the urogenital diaphragm is penetrated by the vagina and contains the membranous urethra and neurovascular structures. The vagina is located just posterior to the membranous urethra and is attached to this portion of the urethra by means of connective tissue.

Recent evidence suggests that the urogenital diaphragm is not the planar structure previously described. The current notion is that the sphincter urethrae muscle in both males and females is actually considered to be associated with the membranous urethra and extends superiorly into the visceral region, where it is attached to the prostate in the male and the bladder in the female. This muscle stops the flow of urine, whereas the internal sphincter is the key muscle for continence. The sphincter urethrae in the female is called the

sphincter urethrovaginalis to reflect its interaction with the vagina. In addition, in the female there is an additional muscular component called the compressor urethrae, which arises from each ischiopubic rami and passes around the anterior aspect of the urethra to fuse with the contralateral muscle deep to the sphincter urethrovaginalis (see Fig. 7-32).

The deep transverse perineal muscles lie slightly inferior to the sphincter urethrae and sphincter urethrovaginalis muscles.

Superficial Pouch

The superficial pouch contains the external genitalia in both males and females, and as the name suggests it is found superficial to the urogenital diaphragm. In fact, the superficial pouch and the urogenital diaphragm share a common boundary—the perineal membrane. The perineal membrane, the inferior fascia of the urogenital diaphragm, forms the superior boundary of the superficial pouch. The inferior boundary is formed by the outer investing layer of deep fascia, which in this site is called the *deep perineal fascia* (Fig. 7-33).

Male Superficial Pouch

The superficial pouch in the male contains the root of the penis, the skeletal muscles associated with the root of the penis (ischiocavernosus muscles and bulbospongiosus muscles), plus the superficial transverse perineal muscles (Fig. 7-34).

Erectile Tissues

The penis (see Fig. 7-34) consists of erectile tissue and contains the third portion of the urethra, the spongy urethra. The penis is described anatomically as if it were erect. The urethral surface is the ventral surface, and the opposite (corpus cavernosum) surface is the dorsal surface (see Fig. 7-34).

The penis has a root and a body. The root of the penis (see Fig. 7-34A) is the portion attached to the perineal membrane and ischiopubic rami. It is formed by the two lateral crura and

Erectile Tissues

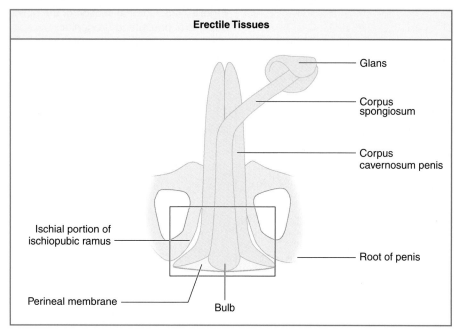

- Glans
- Corpus spongiosum
- Corpus cavernosum penis
- Ischial portion of ischiopubic ramus
- Root of penis
- Perineal membrane
- Bulb

A

Muscles

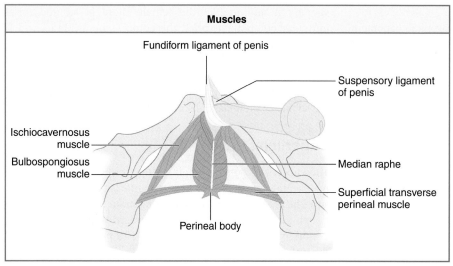

- Fundiform ligament of penis
- Suspensory ligament of penis
- Ischiocavernosus muscle
- Bulbospongiosus muscle
- Median raphe
- Superficial transverse perineal muscle
- Perineal body

B

Figure 7-34. Male superficial pouch. **A,** Erectile tissues. **B,** Skeletal muscles.

the midline bulb of the penis. Each crus of the penis is laterally placed and attached to an ischiopubic ramus. The crus runs forward, enlarging to form the corpus cavernosum penis. The two corpora unite to form the body of the penis. Each corpus cavernosum is represented as a cylinder of erectile tissue (see Fig. 7-34A), which is surrounded by a strong capsule called the tunica albuginea (Fig. 7-35). The septum of the tunica albuginea dips between the two cylinders of erectile tissue to *incompletely* separate these two cylinders. The pendulous encapsulated corpora cavernosa extend distally to end bluntly, where they are covered by the glans penis of the corpus spongiosum (see Fig. 7-34A).

At the root of the penis, the bulb of the penis is found in the midline. It is a dilated, circular enlargement of erectile tissue attached to the perineal membrane between the two crura (see Fig. 7-34A). The bulb of the penis narrows as it forms the corpus spongiosum penis on the ventral (urethral)

surface of the penis. The corpus spongiosum penis also is wrapped by the tunica albuginea, but this portion of the capsule is much thinner and contains more elastic fibers (see Fig. 7-35). The corpus spongiosum ends by expanding into the enlarged glans penis, which covers the free end of the corpora cavernosa. The expanded prominent posterior border of the glans penis is the corona. The constriction behind the glans is called the neck of the glans.

Skeletal Muscles Found in the Superficial Pouch

In the root of the penis, the three masses of erectile tissue are covered by skeletal muscles. An ischiocavernosus muscle covers each crus, and the *two* bulbospongiosus muscles cover the bulb of the penis (see Fig. 7-34B).

Each ischiocavernosus muscle arises from the adjacent ischial ramus and runs anteriorly along the crus to *insert* into the corpus cavernosum penis and the inferior pubic ramus.

Midsagittal Section of the Penis

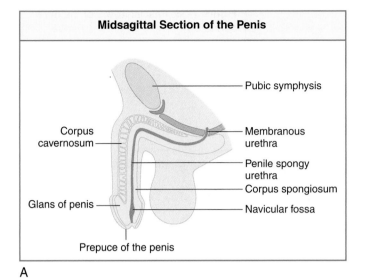

Pubic symphysis

Corpus cavernosum

Membranous urethra

Penile spongy urethra

Corpus spongiosum

Navicular fossa

Glans of penis

Prepuce of the penis

A

Transverse Section of the Penis

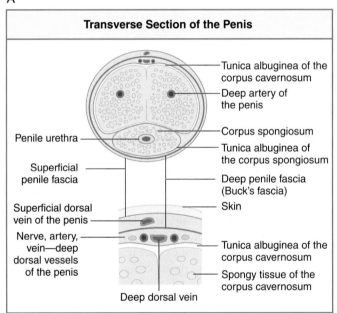

Tunica albuginea of the corpus cavernosum

Deep artery of the penis

Corpus spongiosum

Tunica albuginea of the corpus spongiosum

Penile urethra

Superficial penile fascia

Deep penile fascia (Buck's fascia)

Skin

Superficial dorsal vein of the penis

Nerve, artery, vein—deep dorsal vessels of the penis

Tunica albuginea of the corpus cavernosum

Spongy tissue of the corpus cavernosum

Deep dorsal vein

B

Figure 7-35. Midsagittal (**A**) and transverse (**B**) sections of the penis.

Each bulbospongiosus muscle arises from a midline raphe on the ventral (free) surface of the bulb, which unites these muscles, also arise from the perineal body. The posterior muscle fibers surround the bulb to *insert* into the perineal membrane while the more anterior muscle fibers sweep around the corpus spongiosum and the corpus cavernosum to join with fibers from the contralateral muscle, thereby encircling the root of the penis (see Fig. 7-34B).

In addition, the superficial transverse perineal muscles arise from the ischial tuberosities and *insert* into the perineal body. The superficial transverse perineal muscles do not cover the muscle of the root of the penis, but they arise from the same embryologic cloacal myotome and are covered by the same fascia.

These skeletal muscles are covered externally by the outer investing layer of deep fascia, which is called the *deep*

perineal fascia. This fascia is attached to the perineal body and posterior margin of the perineal membrane posteriorly, the ischiopubic rami laterally, and the pubic symphysis anteriorly.

Spongy (Penile) Urethra

The urethra enters the bulb of the penis, runs through the corpus spongiosum penis, and ends in the glans at the external urethral orifice (meatus) (see Fig. 7-35). The external urethral meatus is the narrowest and least distensible portion of the urethra. The spongy urethra has two dilatations, one just proximal to the external urethral orifice, the fossa navicularis, and one in the bulb of the penis. The fossa navicularis is the approximate site of the ruptured urogenital membrane. Thus, pain due to infection or trauma of the urethra in the fossa navicularis will be carried by general somatic afferent fibers.

The anatomy of the male urethra must be taken into consideration when passing a urethral catheter in a man, so as not to damage the spongy urethra (see Fig. 7-35).
1. The urethra in the bulb is dilated and the membranous urethra is of a smaller diameter.
2. The urethra makes an approximately 90-degree turn as it leaves the perineal membrane and enters the bulb of the penis.
3. The superior aspect of the urethral wall in the bulb is thinner and more distensible than in the membranous urethra, which is rigid in comparison.

Therefore, the bulb is the most likely site of a catheter penetrating the urethra.

Deep Perineal Fascia

The deep perineal fascia (Fig. 7-36; see also Fig. 7-33) is the outer investing layer of deep fascia found in the urogenital triangle. It is the deep fascia of the ischiocavernosus and the bulbospongiosus muscles. The deep perineal fascia attaches to the pubis, the two ischiopubic rami, and the anteroinferior surface of the perineal membrane to produce the superficial pouch. Thus, the superficial pouch will be defined by the distribution and attachment of the deep perineal fascia and is also a *closed pouch*. The deep (superior) boundary of the superficial pouch is the perineal membrane (see Fig. 7-36).

The deep perineal fascia that forms the superficial boundary of the superficial pouch is continuous with the deep (Buck's) fascia of the penis. This fascia is extended out over the penis to the end of the corpora cavernosa, just behind the corona of the glans at the neck of the glans (see Fig. 7-35). Thus, the superficial pouch is continuous with the potential cleft (fissure-like space) between the capsule of the penis (tunica albuginea) and the deep fascia of the penis. This cleft normally contains the dorsal arteries, the dorsal nerves, and the single midline deep dorsal vein of the penis.

Scrotum and Superficial Fascia

Recall that in most portions of the body superficial fascia has two layers: an outer fatty layer, and an inner membranous layer. The inner membranous layer does not vary from

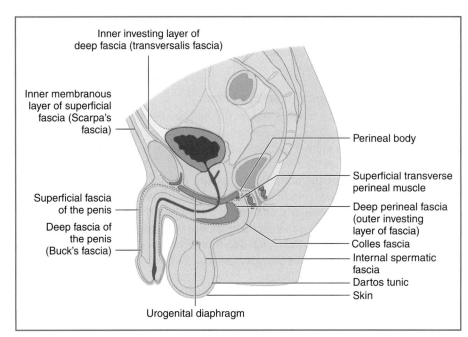

Inner investing layer of
deep fascia (transversalis fascia)

Inner membranous
layer of superficial
fascia (Scarpa's
fascia)

Superficial fascia
of the penis

Deep fascia of
the penis
(Buck's fascia)

Perineal body

Superficial transverse
perineal muscle

Deep perineal fascia
(outer investing
layer of fascia)

Colles fascia

Internal spermatic
fascia

Dartos tunic

Skin

Urogenital diaphragm

Figure 7-36. Fascial layers of the male perineum.

anatomic region to anatomic region; however, the outer fatty layer contains different amounts of fat in different regions. In addition, the inner membranous layer sometimes attaches to bone but usually is only loosely attached to the underlying deep fascia.

The superficial fascia (see Fig. 7-36) of the male urogenital triangle has several specializations. The outer layer loses its fat over the penis and in the scrotum. Over the penis, the outer layer has scant smooth muscle fibers, while the inner membranous layer is only loosely applied to the underlying deep (Buck's) fascia.

The penile superficial fascia is firmly attached at the neck of the penis, where it and the overlying skin are folded over to form the prepuce, or foreskin. The skin of the prepuce is continuous with the skin of the glans at the neck of the glans. The prepuce is often surgically excised (circumcision).

The scrotum is a cutaneous pouch that contains the testes and the spermatic cords. As such, it is composed of superficial fascia and skin. However, the superficial fascia is highly specialized. The outer fatty layer is replaced by a layer of smooth muscle and is referred to as the dartos or dartos tunic. The inner membranous layer associated with the dartos does not change and is continuous with the inner membranous layer of the penile superficial fascia and the superficial fascia of the remaining urogenital triangle. However, immediately posterior to the scrotum as the superficial fascia approaches the area of the perineal body, an outer fatty layer returns. The inner membranous layer of this fascia when it has an adjacent outer fatty layer is referred to as Colles' fascia.

The superficial fascia is attached to the perineal body and posterior margin of the perineal membrane as well as the ischiopubic rami (see Fig. 7-36). Anteriorly this superficial fascia is continuous with Scarpa's fascia. These relationships become important during any event that results in extravasation of urine. Extravasation of urine can occur upon erosion of the spongy urethra without concurrent erosion of the deep fascia of the penis and/or the deep perineal fascia. Urine will make a tract between the capsule of the penis (tunica albuginea) and the next external fascial layer. This fascial layer is the deep perineal fascia and/or the deep fascia of the penis. Urine will be confined to the superficial pouch and/or the penis. It will not involve the scrotum or anal triangle.

However, if the deep perineal fascia or penis is also compromised by disease or trauma, then urine can run between the deep fascia of the perineum and/or penis and the next external layer, which is the inner membranous layer of superficial fascia. This layer is continuous as Colles' fascia, dartos tunic, and the superficial fascia of the penis. Again, urine can engorge the penis. It cannot reach the anal triangle because of the attachment of the inner membranous layer of superficial fascia to the posterior margin of the perineal membrane. It cannot move directly into the thigh because the inner membranous layer is also attached to the ischiopubic rami. However, it *can* flow into the anterior abdominal wall, since the inner membranous layer of perineal superficial fascia is directly continuous with Scarpa's fascia and is not attached to the pubis (see Fig. 7-36).

Female Superficial Pouch

The female superficial pouch (Fig. 7-37) is substantially different from that of the male. The female external genitalia are known as the vulva (covering). The perineal membrane is not so well developed as in the male. In addition, the female urethrovaginal sphincter is penetrated by both the urethra and the vagina.

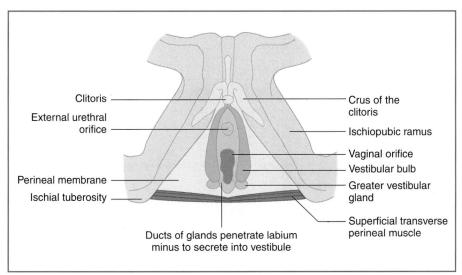

Figure 7-37. Contents of the female superficial pouch.

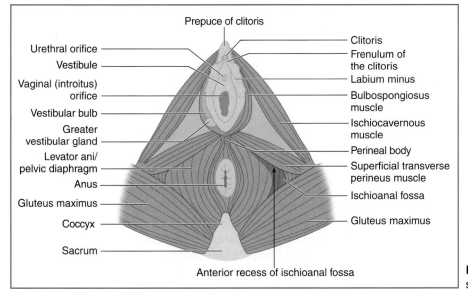

Figure 7-38. Muscles of the female superficial pouch.

Clitoris

The clitoris is homologous to the penis. The clitoris is not penetrated by the spongy urethra. The clitoris has a root composed of two crura of erectile tissue attached to the pubic rami (see Fig. 7-37). Each of the two crura runs forward to unite with the contralateral corpus to form the corpora cavernosa clitoridis. The corpora cavernosa clitoridis ends as the glans clitoris of the female corpus spongiosum, which is continuous with the tapered ends of the two vestibular bulbs. Each crus is covered by an ischiocavernosus muscle (Fig. 7-38).

Vestibule Bulb

The bulbs of the vaginal vestibule (see Figs. 7-38 and 7-39) are homologous to the bulb of the penis. However, the bulbs of the vestibule consist of two separate masses of erectile tissue that are attached to the perineal membrane. The vestibular bulbs are found just lateral to the plane of the labia minora (minor lips of the perineum) and therefore are not in the vaginal vestibule (see Fig. 7-38). The bulbs narrow anteriorly and unite as a narrow commissure, the female corpus spongiosum, which extends to the glans clitoridis as a slender extension of erectile tissue. The vestibular bulbs are covered by the two bulbospongiosus muscles, which arise from the perineal body and insert into the inferior pubic rami and the dorsal surface of the clitoris (see Fig. 7-38). These muscles, like the vestibular bulbs, are just lateral to the labia minora and therefore are separated by the vaginal vestibule.

Labia Minora

The labia minora (*labium minus*, singular) are two folds of skin and fascia that are homologous to the ventral surface of the spongy urethra (see Figs. 7-39 and 7-40). They do not have a fatty layer. Each labium minus continues forward toward the clitoris and splits into two extensions that meet the corresponding folds of the contralateral labium above and below the clitoris. The extensions above form the prepuce of the

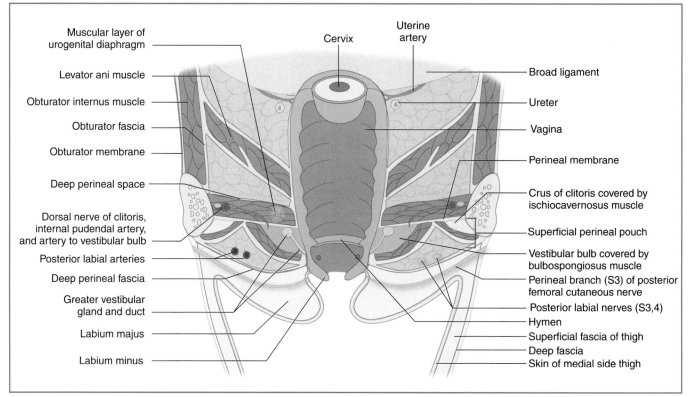

Figure 7-39. Coronal section of female perineum.

clitoris (see Fig. 7-38), while the two folds that meet below form the frenulum of the clitoris that often cover the very sensitive skin of the glans clitoridis. The two labia minora meet posteriorly as the frenulum of the labia (also referred to as the fourchette).

Vaginal Vestibule

The vestibule of the vagina or vaginal introitus (entrance) is the region bounded by the labia minora laterally, the frenulum of the clitoris anteriorly and the frenulum of the labia (fourchette) posteriorly (see Fig. 7-40). The vestibule of the vagina contains the external urethra orifice, the orifice of the vagina, and the ducts of the greater vestibular glands. Directly posterior to the clitoris (approximately 2.5 cm) is the external urethral orifice. The female urethra is firmly attached to the anterior vaginal wall; therefore, the opening of the vagina is directly behind the external urethral opening.

Greater Vestibular and Paraurethral Glands

The greater vestibular (Bartholin's) glands (see Figs. 7-39 and 7-40) are located directly posterior to the bulbs of the vestibule, where they are attached to the perineal membrane. They secrete a mucus product that lubricates the vulva. They are homologous to the male bulbourethral glands, which are located in the urogenital diaphragm. The greater vestibular glands are not located in the vestibule (they are found just lateral to the labia minora). However, the greater vestibular gland's ducts empty into the vestibule between the labia minora and the lower portion of the vagina (see Fig. 7-40). In the male, bulbourethral glands empty into the spongy urethra in the bulb, a homologous point to where the greater vestibular (Bartholin's) glands open in the female.

The paraurethral (Skene's) glands have numerous ducts that empty just lateral to the external urethral orifice. The paraurethral glands are homologous to the prostatic ducts that empty into the membranous urethra.

The part of the vestibule between the vaginal orifice (introitus [opening of any canal-like structure]) and the posterior frenulum of the labia is the fossa navicularis of the vestibule.

Mons Pubis and Labia Majora

The largest structures of the female urogenital triangle are the mons pubis and labia majora (*labium majus pudendi*) (see Fig. 7-40). The mons pubis consists of the fatty connective tissue that covers the female pubic symphysis. These structures surround the clitoris, the labia minora, and the vestibule. The labia majora are the two lateral folds of skin and superficial fascia that are homologous to the fused scrotum. The superficial fascia of the labia majora contains an outer fatty layer that also contains some smooth muscle. A thin, poorly developed layer of smooth muscle, the dartos *muliebris* (Latin, "pertaining to women") is homologous to the dartos layer of the scrotum.

The labia majora are also characterized by a considerable amount of hair except on their medial surfaces. The labia majora enlarge anteriorly (and appear to meet as the anterior

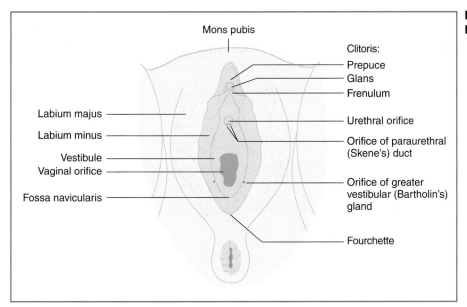

A

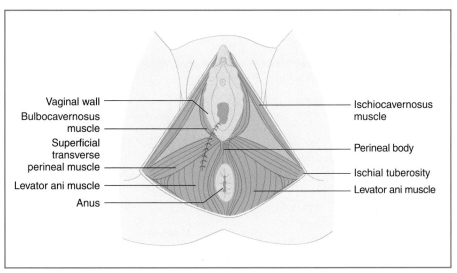

B

Figure 7-40. A, Female external genitalia. **B,** Posterolateral episiotomy.

commissure that expands over the pubic symphysis) at the mons pubis. The labia also decrease in size and meet posteriorly over the perineal body, close to the anus, as the posterior commissure of the labia majora. The two labia are usually in contact with each other. Between them is the pudendal cleft that contains the labia minora and the vestibule of the vagina.

The vaginal introitus is often torn during childbirth. To limit the degree of laceration and the unpredictable nature of these tears, an episiotomy is sometimes performed (see Fig. 7-40). A midline episiotomy is an incision in the posterior vaginal wall, labial frenulum, and perineal body. This procedure results in less bleeding and is easier to repair than the posterolateral episiotomy. However, it also increases the risk of harm to the rectum.

●●● DEVELOPMENT OF EXTERNAL GENITALIA

The external genitalia in males and females develop from common precursors (Fig. 7-41 and Table 7-10). In fact, until the seventh week, they are morphologically indistinguishable. In week 6, cloacal folds form on either side of the cloacal membrane and a swelling called the genital tubercle develops at the anterior end. When the urogenital septum divides the cloaca and fuses with the cloacal membrane, these folds are then called *urogenital folds* and folds lateral to these become known as the *labioscrotal folds*. At this point, the development of male and female genitalia diverges. In response to testosterone and a by-product of testosterone—dihydrotestosterone—the genital tubercle in the male elongates to form the shaft and

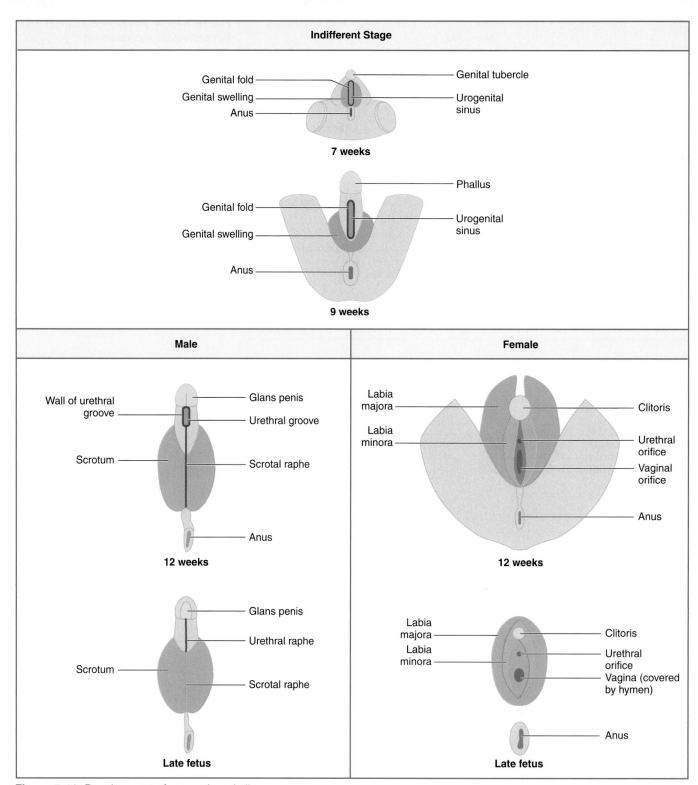

Figure 7-41. Development of external genitalia.

glans of the penis, the urogenital folds fuse and contribute to the shaft of the penis and the penile urethra, and the labioscrotal folds fuse to form the scrotum. In the female, where there is an absence of high levels of testosterone, the genital tubercle folds over to form the clitoris without enlarging, the urogenital folds form the labia minora, and the labioscrotal folds form the labia majora. The importance of appropriate levels of sex hormones can be appreciated by virtue of the fact that the external genitalia are ambiguous in newborns who are exposed to abnormal levels of sex hormones.

<table>
<tr><td colspan="3">TABLE 7-10. Homologous Structures in Males and Females</td></tr>
<tr><td>Embryologic Structure</td><td>Adult Male Structure</td><td>Adult Female Structure</td></tr>
<tr><td>Primitive urogenital sinus</td><td>Bladder</td><td>Bladder</td></tr>
<tr><td>Definitive urogenital sinus</td><td>Penile urethra</td><td>Lower vagina and vestibule</td></tr>
<tr><td>Mesonephric ducts</td><td>Epididymis, ductus deferens, and ejaculatory duct</td><td>Appendix of ovary and Gartner's cyst</td></tr>
<tr><td>Paramesonephric ducts</td><td>Appendix of testis and prostatic utricle</td><td>Uterine tube, uterus, and superior portion of vagina</td></tr>
<tr><td>Genital tubercle</td><td>Glans penis</td><td>Clitoris</td></tr>
<tr><td>Urogenital folds</td><td>Shaft of penis and spongy urethra</td><td>Labia minora</td></tr>
<tr><td>Labioscrotal folds</td><td>Scrotum</td><td>Labia majora</td></tr>
</table>

●●● ANAL TRIANGLE

The anal triangle is subdivided into right and left halves at the midline, where the anus and perineal body are found (see Fig. 7-30). Laterally, the anal triangle has a wedge-shaped configuration called the *ischioanal fossa* (Fig. 7-42).

Ischioanal Fossa

The lateral wall of the ischioanal fossa, formed by the obturator internus muscle and fascia, has a vertical configuration. The superomedial wall of the ischioanal fossa is formed by

PATHOLOGY

Ischioanal Abscess

Abscess of the ischioanal fossa can be caused by inflammation of the anal mucosa, which causes release of intestinal flora into the fossa, which in turn causes an infection in the ischioanal fossa. Abscesses are typically associated with obstruction of the anal crypts, which produces stasis of the secretion of the 4 to 10 anal glands associated with the crypts. Since both sides of the fossa communicate with each other, the infection can spread to the contralateral side via the posterior rectal space, producing a horseshoe-shaped abscess. The abscesses can be quite painful. Treatment includes stool softeners to prevent further inflammation of the anal canal and antibiotics to clear the infection. Surgery may be necessary.

the levator ani muscle and its fascia. It slopes from its origins (including the arcus tendineus) downward toward the midline to its insertions (see Fig. 7-42). The inferior (superficial) boundary of the ischioanal fossa consists of skin and superficial fascia. The ischioanal fossa is filled with fat and fascial septa that make the dissection especially difficult.

Posterior Recess of the Ischioanal Fossa

The ischioanal fossa extends posteriorly to the lesser sciatic foramen and gluteal region. This aspect of the ischioanal fossa is covered externally or deepened by the gluteus maximus muscle arising from the sacrotuberous ligament and is called the *posterior recess of the ischioanal fossa* (Fig. 7-43). The gluteal region communicates with the posterior recess by means of the lesser sciatic foramen.

Anterior Recess of the Ischioanal Fossa

Anteriorly, the boundary of the ischioanal fossa changes to now include the lateral origin of the deep transverse perineal

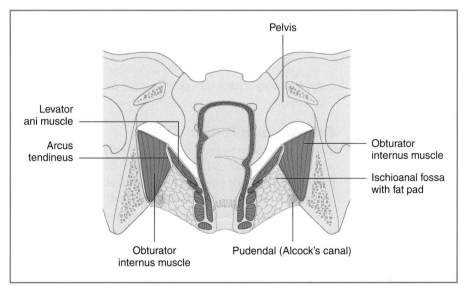

Figure 7-42. Coronal section through ischioanal fossa of the anal triangle.

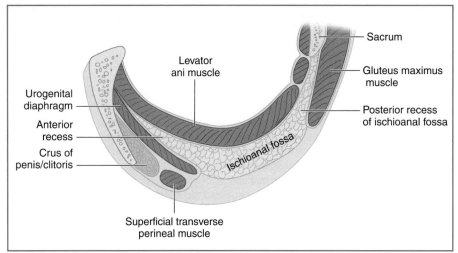

Figure 7-43. Parasagittal section through ischioanal fossa.

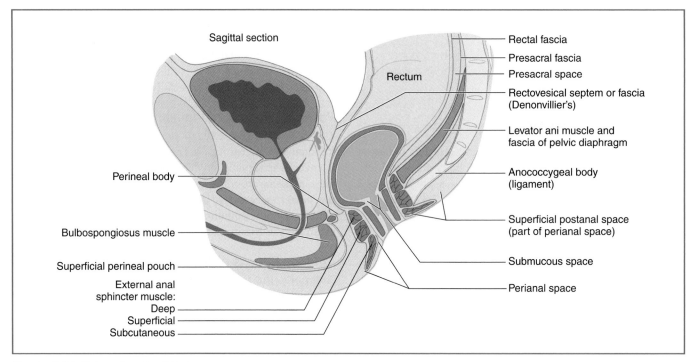

Figure 7-44. External anal sphincter.

and sphincter urethrae muscles. Close to the ischiopubic rami, the muscles of the deep pouch are found positioned *between* the superficial fascia and the levator ani muscle. Thus, the boundaries of the anterior portion of the ischioanal fossa are the obturator internus muscle, the levator ani muscle and the muscles of the urogenital diaphragm (which replaces the superficial fascia as the base of the fossa). This is the anterior recess of the ischioanal fossa (see Fig. 7-43).

External Anal Sphincter Muscle

The external anal sphincter muscle has three portions, which are not easily distinguishable (subcutaneous, superficial, and deep), moving from the skin to the puborectalis muscle (Fig. 7-44).

Subcutaneous Portion

The subcutaneous portion is found directly beneath the skin and is not attached to bone. Anteriorly, it is attached to the perineal body, while posteriorly it may decussate (cross), since it is attached to the anococcygeal ligament. The subcutaneous portion of the external anal sphincter is separated from the rest of the external sphincter by the fascial prolongation of the longitudinal smooth muscle layer of the anal canal (see Fig. 7-11). This fascial extension of the longitudinal smooth muscle layer attaches to the mucosa of the anal canal to form the intersphincteric line. This longitudinal layer also has lateral fibers that separate the subcutaneous portion of the external anal sphincter from the rest of the external sphincter. The longitudinal layer of smooth muscle also has medial fibers (as described above) that separate the external sphincter from the internal anal sphincter muscle.

Superficial Portion

The superficial portion of the external anal sphincter muscle is the largest portion and consists of two parallel bundles of skeletal muscle. Posteriorly, they attach to the tip of the coccyx and the anococcygeal raphe, and anteriorly to the perineal body.

Deep Portion

The deep portion of the external anal sphincter muscle, like the subcutaneous portion, is without bony attachments. It is annular in nature, attached anteriorly to the perineal body, and laterally and posteriorly merges with the puborectalis muscle. The puborectalis muscle surrounds the lateral and posterior aspects of the rectum but not the anterior surface of the rectum. Anteriorly, only the deep portion of the external anal sphincter muscle is present to maintain continence. The deep portion of the external anal sphincter and the puborectalis muscle overlap the internal anal sphincter and are important in maintaining anal continence. The external anal sphincter is supplied by the perineal branch of S4 and the inferior rectal branch of the pudendal nerve (S2–S4).

●●● NEUROVASCULAR BUNDLES OF THE PERINEUM

Pudendal Nerve

The pudendal nerve (Figs. 7-45 and 7-46) and the internal pudendal vessels are the major neurovascular supply to the perineum. The pudendal nerve is a typical mixed nerve in that it contains general somatic motor, general somatic sensory, and postganglionic sympathetic fibers. It arises from the ventral rami of sacral spinal nerves 2, 3, and 4.

Other neurovascular structures also help supply the perineum. Branches of the ilioinguinal, genital branch of the genitofemoral, and perineal branch of the posterior femoral cutaneous nerves are also found in the perineum. The ilioinguinal nerve follows the spermatic cord and round ligament through the superficial inguinal ring into the scrotum or labia majus. It provides anterior scrotal/labial branches that are sensory to the scrotum, the labia majus, and the adjacent thigh. The genital branch of the genitofemoral nerve passes through both the deep and superficial rings into the scrotum and labium majus. It has sensory branches that also supply the anterior aspect of the scrotum and labium majus. The genital branch also supplies general somatic motor and sensory fibers to the cremaster muscle in the male. Sensory branches from the perineal branch of the posterior femoral cutaneous nerves provide posterior scrotal or labial nerves to the scrotum or labia majora, respectively. Finally, the perineal

branch of the pudendal nerve also supplies posterior cutaneous nerves to the posterior scrotum/labia majora.

The pudendal nerve leaves the pelvis through the greater sciatic foramen with the internal pudendal vessels to enter the gluteal region. This neurovascular bundle then winds around the ischial spine and the attached sacrospinous ligament and enters the lesser sciatic foramen to reach the posterior recess of the ischioanal fossa. The pudendal nerve is the most medial of the structures on the ischial spine and adjacent sacrospinous ligament, followed by the internal pudendal artery and vein. The nerve to the obturator internus muscle is the most lateral structure to enter the lesser sciatic foramen.

The pudendal neurovascular bundle immediately enters the pudendal (Alcock's) canal. This fascial canal runs along the lateral wall of the ischioanal fossa from its posterior recess to its anterior recess. The pudendal nerve (see Figs. 7-45 and 7-46) has many branches that penetrate the fascial walls of the pudendal canal. The major branches of the pudendal nerve are the inferior rectal, the perineal, and the dorsal nerve to the penis or clitoris.

The first branches of the pudendal nerve are the inferior rectal (hemorrhoidal) nerves (S3 and S4) to the skin around the anus, external anal sphincter, and anal canal below the pectinate line, and the adjacent structures, but not the rectum (see Figs. 7-45 and 7-46).

The pudendal nerve continues forward in the pudendal canal to divide into the perineal nerve and the dorsal nerve to the penis or clitoris. The perineal nerve leaves the pudendal canal and separates into superficial and deep divisions.

The superficial division of the perineal nerve is cutaneous, runs either inferiorly or through the posterior margin of the perineal membrane, and passes onto the posterior aspect of the scrotum or labia majora to become the medial and lateral posterior scrotal nerves in males and the medial and lateral posterior labial nerves to the labia majora in females. It is one of four nerves that supplies these structures. Additional supply to this area is also derived from the perineal branch of the posterior femoral cutaneous nerve.

The deep division of the perineal nerve travels inferior to the perineal membrane. Branches of the deep division reach the bulbospongiosus and ischiocavernosus muscles while other branches penetrate the perineal membrane to enter the urogenital diaphragm and innervate the ureteral sphincter and deep transverse perineal muscles. It innervates all the skeletal muscles found in the urogenital triangle, since they are all derived from the cloacal sphincter. The deep division of the perineal nerve also sends branches to the mucous membranes of the spongy urethra.

The other terminal branch of the pudendal nerve is the dorsal nerve to the penis or clitoris. It passes through the deep pouch with the internal pudendal artery (see Figs. 7-45 and 7-46). The dorsal nerve runs forward for several centimeters *in* the muscles of the urogenital diaphragm to reach a point beyond the attachment of the crus. The dorsal nerve then penetrates the perineal membrane to run forward on the dorsal surface of the corpus cavernosum penis between the tunica albuginea and the deep penile (Buck's)

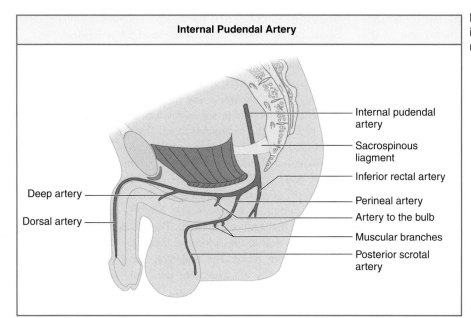

Internal Pudendal Artery

Internal pudendal artery

Sacrospinous liagment

Inferior rectal artery

Perineal artery

Artery to the bulb

Muscular branches

Posterior scrotal artery

Deep artery

Dorsal artery

A

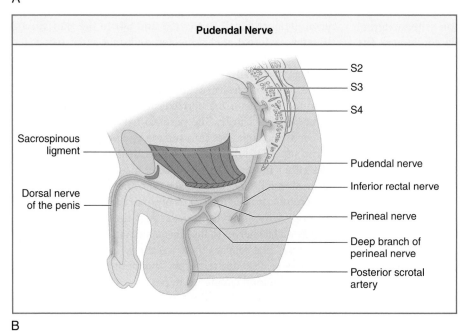

Pudendal Nerve

S2

S3

S4

Pudendal nerve

Inferior rectal nerve

Perineal nerve

Deep branch of perineal nerve

Posterior scrotal artery

Sacrospinous ligment

Dorsal nerve of the penis

B

Figure 7-45. **A,** Internal pudendal artery in the male. **B,** Pudendal nerve in the male.

fascia. Here, it is found lateral to the dorsal artery. The dorsal nerve conveys sensory fibers to the distal portion of the penis. The dorsal nerve to the clitoris has a similar course but is considerably smaller.

Parasympathetic Nerves

Preganglionic parasympathetic fibers (pelvic splanchnics or nervi erigentes) have their cell bodies located in sacral spinal cord segments 2–4. These fibers synapse in the ganglia found in the prostatic portion of the inferior hypogastric plexus. The postganglionic parasympathetic nerves to the erectile tissue are found in the cavernous nerve. The cavernous nerves pene-

trate the urogenital diaphragm and are distributed with the branches of the pudendal nerve.

Internal Pudendal Artery

The internal pudendal artery (see Figs. 7-45 and 7-46) is a branch of the anterior division of the internal iliac artery. The internal pudendal artery and the accompanying two veins leave the pelvis by passing through the greater sciatic foramen close to the coccygeus muscle. These vessels follow the pudendal nerve as they immediately leave the gluteal region by passing through the lesser sciatic foramen into the pudendal canal. The internal pudendal artery has inferior rectal,

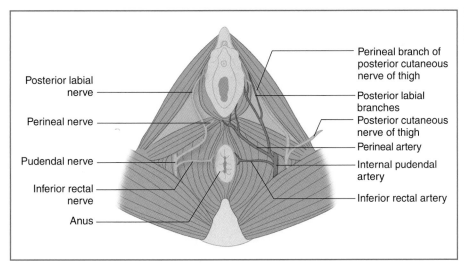

Figure 7-46. Course of pudendal nerve and internal pudendal artery in the female.

muscular, perineal, bulbar, and urethral branches. The internal pudendal artery terminates as the dorsal artery and the deep artery to the penis or clitoris (see Figs. 7-45 and 7-46).

The inferior rectal arteries supply the anus and anal canal below the pectinate line. The inferior rectal veins drain the external hemorrhoidal plexus, which is the site of external hemorrhoids into the internal pudendal vein (see Fig. 7-12).

The internal pudendal artery continues forward in the pudendal canal and gives off the perineal branches close to the posterior margin of the perineal membrane. The perineal artery passes either over or through the posterior margin of the perineal membrane. It ends as the posterior scrotal (posterior labial in females) arteries and the transverse perineal artery (see Figs. 7-45 and 7-46). This latter artery is directed toward the perineal body.

The internal pudendal artery enters the posteroinferior margin of the urogenital diaphragm by way of the anterior recess with the dorsal nerve to the penis to run forward together. The internal pudendal artery gives off the artery to the bulb as it passes forward in the urogenital diaphragm. The artery to the bulb runs through the deep transverse perineal muscle and is distributed to the bulb and corpus spongiosum.

The internal pudendal artery passes forward in the urogenital diaphragm close to the inferior ramus of the pubis to reach the suspensory ligament of the penis/clitoris. In this manner, the artery can reach the dorsal surface of the penis or clitoris.

In the male deep pouch, the internal pudendal artery ends as the deep artery of the penis and the dorsal artery of the penis. The deep artery of the penis enters the crus and runs in the corpus cavernosum while the dorsal artery of the penis passes onto the dorsal surface of the penis just medial to the dorsal nerve of the penis. These neurovascular structures are located between the tunica albuginea and the deep penile fascia (see Fig. 7-35). The dorsal artery of the penis and the deep artery of the penis communicate with each other by way of highly coiled arteries called helicine arteries.

The dorsal artery and the deep artery of the clitoris have a similar course but are significantly smaller than the homologous arteries in the male.

Additional Blood Supply

The femoral artery also helps supply the skin over the penis and scrotum (or clitoris and labia majora). It gives rise to the external pudendal arteries that help supply the scrotum (or labia majora). The scrotal branches of the deep external pudendal artery help supply the layers of spermatic fascia and can anastomose with branches of the testicular artery that also supply these layers of the spermatic cord.

Internal Pudendal Vein

The internal pudendal vein drains most, but not all, of the perineum. It has inferior rectal and perineal branches. However, the vein that drains most of the penis or clitoris does not drain into the internal pudendal vein. The unpaired deep dorsal vein of the penis or clitoris is found in the midline between the paired dorsal arteries and dorsal nerves. The deep dorsal vein passes directly into the pelvis between the arcuate pubic ligament and the transverse perineal ligament. In the pelvis, the deep dorsal vein of the penis drains into the prostatic plexus of veins while the deep dorsal vein of the clitoris drains into the vesical plexus.

Lymphatics of the Perineum

Since the perineum is part of the body wall, most of the lymphatic drainage is similar to that of the superficial body wall below the umbilicus (i.e., to the inguinal nodes).

As would be expected, some deep structures drain by means of lymphatics that run with the internal pudendal vessels to the internal iliac nodes. These structures include the urogenital diaphragm, membranous urethra, anal canal, and part of the vagina just above the level of the hymen.

The testes and ovaries have lymphatics that drain to the lumbar nodes found just below the renal vessels alongside the IVC or abdominal aorta (see Figs. 7-13 and 7-23). Thus, enlarged lymph nodes, due to disease of the testis, are not palpable.

Lower Limb

8

CONTENTS

OVERVIEW

DEVELOPMENT OF THE LIMBS

GLUTEAL REGION AND HIP JOINT
Bones
Muscles
Fascia
Hip Joint
Nerves of the Gluteal Region and Hip Joint
Blood Supply to the Gluteal Region and Hip Joint

THIGH AND KNEE JOINT
Fascia
Bones
Anterior Compartment of the Thigh
Medial Compartment of the Thigh
Posterior Compartment of the Thigh
Knee Joint
Femoral Triangle
Femoral Sheath
Adductor Canal
Nerves of the Thigh and Knee Joint
Blood Supply to the Thigh and Knee Joint
Lymphatic Drainage of the Thigh and Knee Joint

LEG AND ANKLE JOINT
Bones
Fascia
Posterior Compartment of the Leg
Lateral Compartment of the Leg
Anterior Compartment of the Leg
Popliteal Fossa
Ankle Joint
Nerves of the Leg and Ankle Joint
Blood Supply to the Leg and Ankle Joint
Lymphatic Drainage of the Leg and Ankle Joint

FOOT
Arches of the Foot
Ligaments
Intrinsic Muscles of the Foot
Innervation of the Foot
Blood Supply to the Foot

SUMMARY

OVERVIEW

The lower limb is specialized for supporting the body's weight when standing and for bipedal locomotion. Therefore, the joints, bones, and muscles are organized to optimize this role. This is illustrated by the lower limb joints, which are much better fitted than those in the upper limbs, where stability is sacrificed for mobility.

The weight of the upper portion of the body is transmitted to the lower limbs through the bony pelvis. The pelvis is connected to the axial skeleton through the sacroiliac joint, which is a very stable and unmovable joint. The two lower limbs are connected to the bony pelvis at the acetabulum.

The lower limb can be divided into four main regions: gluteal, thigh, leg, and foot (Fig. 8-1). The gluteal region is found between the iliac crest and the gluteal fold. The thigh begins at the inguinal ligament anteriorly and the gluteal fold posteriorly and ends at the knee joint. The leg is the portion of the lower limb between the knee and the ankle joint. Lastly, the foot is the region distal to the ankle.

The entire lower limb is encased in a layer of deep fascia, which is dense and unyielding and has different names depending on the region. In the thigh, it is called the *fascia lata*, and in the leg it is called *crural fascia*. Its dense and unyielding nature restricts muscles from bulging upon contraction, thereby facilitating venous return from the distal portion of the limb. It also serves as the origin for some of the muscles. The fascia lata attaches superiorly to components and ligaments of the bony pelvis. It attaches to the inguinal ligament, the body of the pubis, and the pubic tubercle, and it fuses with the membranous layer of superficial fascia in the abdomen just below the inguinal ligament.

The blood supply to the lower limb is via branches of the internal and external iliac arteries, gluteal arteries, with the major contribution from the femoral artery, the continuation of the external iliac artery. The innervation to the lower limb is derived from the lumbosacral plexus, which is composed of the ventral rami of spinal nerves (T12)L1–S4. The neurovascular supply will be described in greater detail in each region.

DEVELOPMENT OF THE LIMBS

The upper and lower limbs develop in the same way except that the development of the upper limb precedes that of the lower limb by a few days, and the final rotation of the limbs

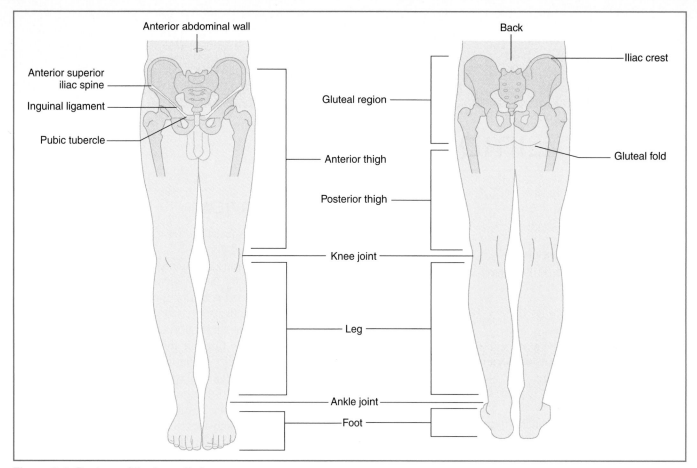

Figure 8-1. Regions of the lower limb.

is different. Limb buds first appear as outgrowths of the ventrolateral body wall. The lower limb buds appear in the lumbar and sacral region of the embryo and the upper limbs develop in the cervical and upper thoracic region (Fig. 8-2). The limb buds consist of mesenchyme, derived from the somatic layer of lateral mesoderm, with an overlying layer of ectoderm. The proliferation of the mesenchymal cells brings about growth of the limb bud.

Differentiation of the limb buds occurs in three different axes—proximal-distal, cranial-caudal, and dorsal-ventral (see Fig. 8-2). At the distal end of the limb buds, the ectoderm forms an apical ectodermal ridge (AER). The AER secretes fibroblast growth factors (FGFs), which interact with the mesodermal core to induce growth of the mesodermal cells in the proximal-distal axis. On the posterior aspect of the limb bud, mesenchymal cells form a region called the zone of polarizing activity (ZPA). The FGFs from the AER induce the cells of the ZPA to produce sonic hedgehog (Shh), which induces the growth of the limb bud in the cranial-caudal axis. This determines the position of the big toe (cranial) versus the smaller toes (caudal) and the thumb (cranial) versus the fingers (caudal). The ectodermal cells determine the dorsal-ventral axis. The ectoderm of the dorsal and ventral surfaces of the limb buds each secrete a different growth factor, which programs the development of the unique features of the dorsal versus ventral regions of the adult limb. The skin on the plantar

(ventral) surface is quite different from the skin on the dorsal surface of the limbs.

The distal ends of the limb buds flatten out to form foot and hand plates, which in turn give rise to digital rays and toe buds by the seventh week. Individual digits form through a process of programmed cell death of the mesenchymal cells between the developing digital rays. Interference with this step can result in webbing of digits.

In the fifth week, somitic mesoderm migrates into the growing limb bud and forms two masses of tissue—one dorsal to the axial mesenchymal column and one ventral to it. The

GENETICS

HOX Genes

HOX genes regulate the proper positioning of the limb buds along the craniocaudal axis. *HOX* genes code for transcription factors, which contain a homeodomain of 60 amino acids that bind to certain regions of DNA. They were first identified in Drosophila and shown to regulate a cascade of genes that specify the properties of each segment of the fly. They have now been identified in humans and play a similar role whereby they activate a cascade of genes that regulate segmentation and axis formation.

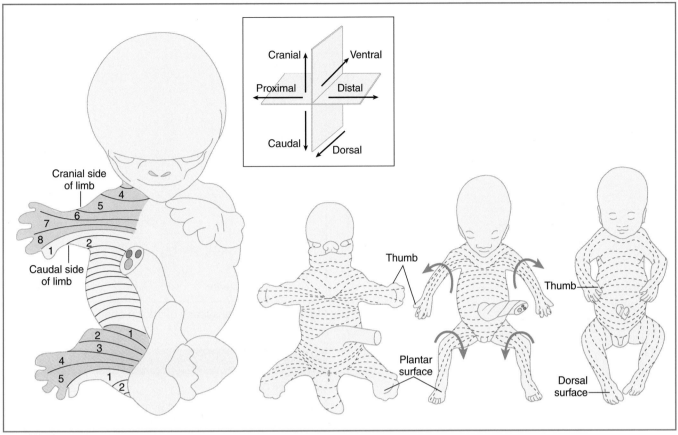

Figure 8-2. Limb buds and axes of development of the limbs.

dorsal mass will form the extensors and abductors of the upper and lower limb, and the ventral mass will form the flexors and adductors of the limbs with a few exceptions. The spinal nerves organize themselves along dorsal and ventral lines as well. All the muscles in the limbs are innervated by the ventral rami of spinal nerves; however, the dorsal branches of the ventral rami innervate the muscles, which are derived from the dorsal masses, and the ventral branches innervate the ventral muscles. Keeping this information in mind is useful in understanding muscle function and innervation. The lower limb undergoes a 90-degree medial rotation along its long axis, thus bringing the extensors of the lower limb into the anterior aspect of the limb. In contrast, the upper limb rotates 90 degrees laterally. Therefore, the extensors of the upper limb are on the opposite side of the limb from the extensors in the lower limb.

●●● GLUTEAL REGION AND HIP JOINT

The muscles of the gluteal region act at the hip joint; therefore, most of them originate from the bony pelvis and insert on the proximal portion of the femur. The hip joint is a synovial ball-and-socket joint between the head of the femur and the acetabulum of the hip bone.

The muscles of the gluteal region are covered by adipose tissue, which gives the region its characteristic shape.

The neurovascular bundles that supply this region originate in the pelvis from the lumbosacral plexus and the internal iliac artery and exit the pelvis posteriorly through the greater sciatic foramen. Movements in this region include extension and flexion of the hip, medial and lateral rotation of the femur, and abduction and adduction of the hip (Fig. 8-3).

Bones

Hip Bones

The internal aspect of the bony pelvis was described in Chapter 7. The external surface of the hip bones has pertinent features for the gluteal region. The acetabulum of the hip bone is a cup-shaped depression on the lateral side of the hip bone, where the head of the femur articulates to form the hip joint (Fig. 8-4). It is formed by the articulation of the pubis, ischium, and ilium. The inferior aspect of the acetabulum is incomplete, and this area is called the *acetabular notch*. The inner surface of the acetabulum is separated into the articular surface, called the *lunate surface*, and the central *acetabular fossa*. There is a fibrocartilaginous lip, called the *acetabular labrum*, which surrounds the acetabulum, thereby deepening it and increasing the stability of the joint.

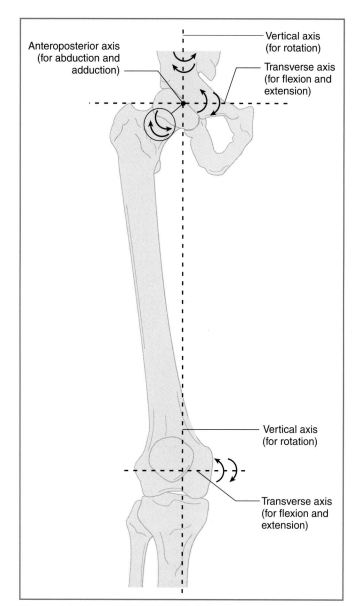

Figure 8-3. Movements at the hip joint.

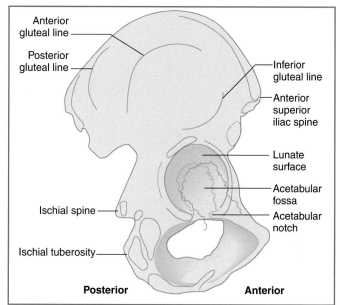

Figure 8-4. External surface of the hip bone.

HISTOLOGY

Articular Cartilage

Articular cartilage is composed of hyaline cartilage and is located at the end of long bones. It differs from hyaline cartilage found in other regions in two ways: articular cartilage has no perichondrium and it contains two types of collagen fibers—type I and type II. Type I collagen is found in bone and so this reflects the articular cartilage's association with bone. It is avascular and capable only of interstitial growth. Wear and tear of the articular cartilage results in osteoarthritis.

On the external surface of the ilium there are three bony landmarks (see Fig. 8-4). Superiorly along the external surface of the iliac crest is the posterior gluteal line. Approximately halfway down is the anterior gluteal line, and just superior to the acetabulum is the inferior gluteal line.

Femur

The femur is the only bone of the thigh and connects the hip region to the knee region and therefore must transmit all the upper body weight to the knee. Its proximal end consists of a rounded ball-like head followed by a narrower neck region (Fig. 8-5). The neck region connects to the long shaft of the femur at an angle of about 125 degrees, which is called the *angle of inclination*. The head of the femur is entirely covered by articular cartilage except for a region on the medial side called the *fovea capitis*, where the ligament of the head attaches. At the junction of the neck and the shaft there are two large bony extensions—the greater and lesser trochanters. The greater trochanter extends superiorly and laterally while the lesser trochanter extends posteriorly and medially. The two trochanters are connected posteriorly by a bony ridge called the *intertrochanteric crest* and anteriorly by a bony line called the *intertrochanteric line*. The intertrochanteric crest has a tubercle on its superior half called the *quadrate tubercle*.

Muscles

The muscles of the gluteal region (Table 8-1) are not compartmentalized as they are in the rest of the lower limb. Therefore, they will be described from a superficial to deep position. The most superficial muscles of the gluteal region are the gluteus maximus and the tensor fasciae latae muscles (Fig. 8-6). The *gluteus maximus* is a large muscle that has an extensive origin on the posterior surface of the bony pelvis and inserts on the gluteal tuberosity of the proximal femur and the iliotibial tract. Its fibers cross the hip joint posteriorly, and thus it functions as a hip extensor and lateral rotator. It is the primary muscle used in standing from a seated position or in

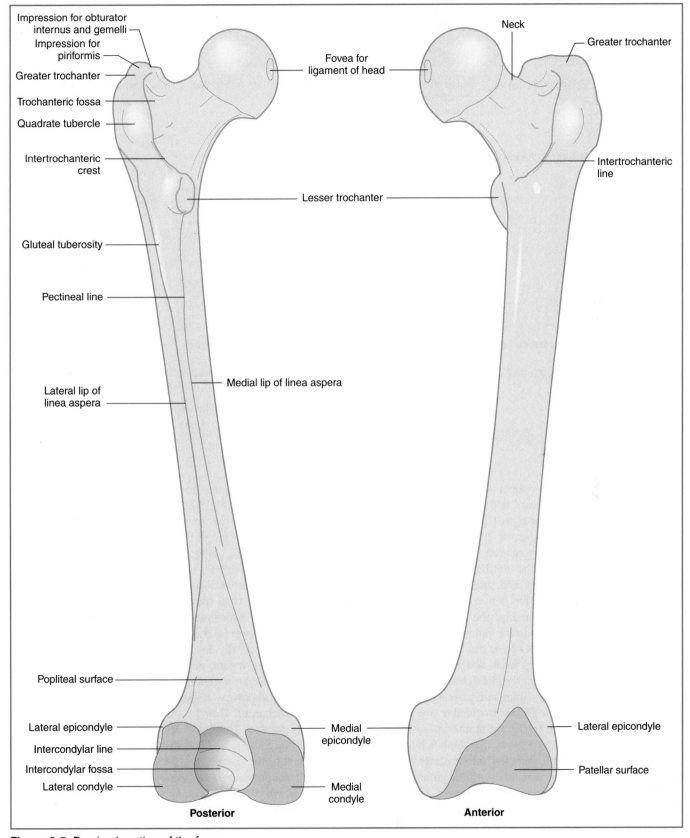

Impression for obturator internus and gemelli
Impression for piriformis
Greater trochanter
Trochanteric fossa
Quadrate tubercle
Intertrochanteric crest
Gluteal tuberosity
Pectineal line
Lateral lip of linea aspera
Popliteal surface
Lateral epicondyle
Intercondylar line
Intercondylar fossa
Lateral condyle

Fovea for ligament of head
Lesser trochanter
Medial lip of linea aspera
Medial epicondyle
Medial condyle

Neck
Greater trochanter
Intertrochanteric line
Lateral epicondyle
Patellar surface

Posterior

Anterior

Figure 8-5. Proximal portion of the femur.

TABLE 8-1. Muscles of the Gluteal Region

Muscle	Principal Function	Origin	Insertion	Innervation
Gluteus maximus	Extension of the hip	Superomedial aspect of dorsal surface of ilium, dorsal surface of sacrum and coccyx, and sacrotuberous ligament	Iliotibial tract and gluteal tuberosity of femur	Inferior gluteal nerve (L5, S1, S2)
Tensor fasciae latae	Flexion of the hip	Anterior superior iliac spine	Iliotibial tract	Superior gluteal nerve (L5, S1)
Gluteus medius	Abduction of the hip	External surface of ilium between posterior and anterior gluteal lines	Superior aspect of greater trochanter	
Gluteus minimus		External surface of ilium between anterior and inferior gluteal lines	Superior aspect of greater trochanter anterior to gluteus medius insertion	
Piriformis	Lateral rotation of the hip	Anterior surface of sacrum and sacrotuberous ligament	Superior border of greater trochanter of femur	Ventral rami of S1 and S2
Superior gemellus		Ischial spine	Medial surface of greater trochanter	Nerve to the obturator internus (L5, S1)
Obturator internus		Internal surface of obturator membrane		
Inferior gemellus		Ischial tuberosity		Nerve to the quadratus femoris (L5, S1)
Quadratus femoris		Lateral aspect of ischial tuberosity	Quadrate tubercle and area inferior to it	

climbing stairs. The gluteus maximus is also called into action when the trunk is bent forward at the pelvis and will remain active until the body returns to the vertical position. The *tensor fasciae latae* originates on the anterior aspect of the bony pelvis, and then its tendon travels inferiorly and posteriorly to form part of the iliotibial tract (see Table 8-1). Since it originates anteriorly and inserts posteriorly, it will flex and medially rotate the hip joint.

The two abductors of the hip, the gluteus medius and gluteus minimus, lie just deep to the gluteus maximus (Fig. 8-7). The *gluteus medius* originates from the lateral aspect of the ilium as well as from the deep fascia and inserts on the upper portion of the greater trochanter (see Table 8-1). The *gluteus minimus* also arises from the ilium and inserts just anterior to the gluteus medius on the greater trochanter (see Table 8-1). These two abductors are important stabilizers of the pelvis when a person is walking. As the leading limb is lifted to take a step, the abductors of the standing limb contract to keep the pelvis from sagging to the side that is off the ground; i.e., they abduct the pelvis over the standing leg. In this way the abductors of each side take turns contracting. Fractures of the intertrochanteric region often involve avulsion of the greater trochanter and therefore detachment of the abductors of the hip. After treatment of such a fracture, the physician must assess the strength of these muscles. This can be done by asking the patient to stand on one leg and then observing whether the anterior superior iliac spines remain at the same level with no sagging to one side. This is called the Trendelenburg test (Fig. 8-8).

The deepest muscles of the gluteal region laterally rotate the hip and include the piriformis, obturator internus, superior and inferior gemelli, and quadratus femoris (see Table 8-1 and Fig. 8-9). The *piriformis*, described in Chapter 7, originates inside the pelvis and passes through the greater sciatic foramen to insert on the greater trochanter. The *obturator internus* bends 90 degrees around the lesser sciatic notch to insert slightly lower on the greater trochanter. In addition, the piriformis muscle divides the greater sciatic foramen into a suprapiriformis region and an infrapiriformis region. The *superior and inferior gemelli* muscles originate on the ischial spine and tuberosity respectively and then insert on the greater trochanter. They lie on either side of the obturator internus tendon. The *quadratus femoris* muscle, a square-shaped muscle, originates on the ischial tuberosity and inserts just distal to the greater trochanter. These muscles are five of the six lateral rotators of the hip, the sixth being the obturator externus, which will be discussed with the adductor muscles of the thigh.

Fascia

The fascia lata in the gluteal region splits around the gluteus maximus muscle and contributes to the formation of the iliotibial tract in the area of the greater trochanter. The iliotibial

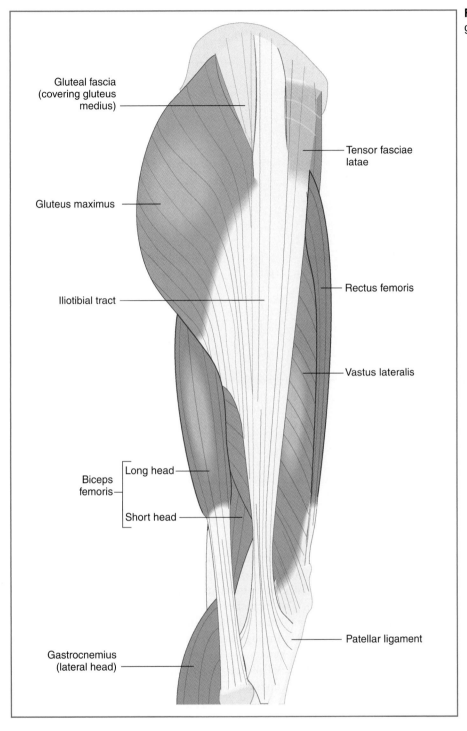

Figure 8-6. Superficial muscles of the gluteal region.

Gluteal fascia (covering gluteus medius)

Tensor fasciae latae

Gluteus maximus

Iliotibial tract

Rectus femoris

Vastus lateralis

Biceps femoris
Long head
Short head

Patellar ligament

Gastrocnemius (lateral head)

tract continues down the lateral side of the thigh to insert on the proximal end of the tibia.

Hip Joint

The hip is a stable ball-and-socket joint. The stability is the result of how well the femur fits into the acetabulum and the ligaments. The muscles play a secondary role. The acetabulum almost entirely surrounds the head of the femur. Thus, the neck of the femur is long. The articular capsule of the hip joint

is very strong and attaches to the femur and the acetabulum. It is reinforced by three ligaments, which wrap around the joint in a spiral fashion (Fig. 8-10).

The iliofemoral ligament (Y ligament of Bigelow) passes from the anterior inferior iliac spine to the intertrochanteric line and helps prevent excessive lateral rotation of the hip and hyperextension. The pubofemoral ligament passes from superior pubic ramus to the inferior aspect of the intertrochanteric line, where it prevents excessive medial rotation. The ischiofemoral ligament is the thinnest of the three

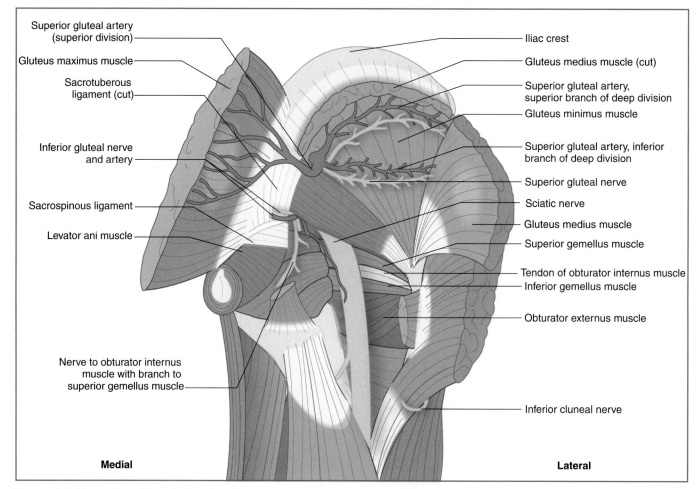

Superior gluteal artery
(superior division)

Gluteus maximus muscle

Sacrotuberous
ligament (cut)

Inferior gluteal nerve
and artery

Sacrospinous ligament

Levator ani muscle

Nerve to obturator internus
muscle with branch to
superior gemellus muscle

Iliac crest

Gluteus medius muscle (cut)

Superior gluteal artery,
superior branch of deep division

Gluteus minimus muscle

Superior gluteal artery, inferior
branch of deep division

Superior gluteal nerve

Sciatic nerve

Gluteus medius muscle

Superior gemellus muscle

Tendon of obturator internus muscle

Inferior gemellus muscle

Obturator externus muscle

Inferior cluneal nerve

Medial

Lateral

Figure 8-7. Deep dissection of gluteal region.

ligaments and attaches to the greater trochanter and the posterior aspect of the acetabulum. When a person is standing, the line of gravity passes posteriorly to the center of the head of the femur, and therefore the weight of the body would tend to push the hip joint into extension. These ligaments resist this movement and allow the hip to maintain its extended weight-bearing position with little or no muscle action necessary. Since theses ligaments spiral around the hip joint, they also limit medial rotation, which would tighten them. Lateral rotation loosens them, as does flexion. Therefore, hip dislocation most often occurs during these movements. There is a fourth ligament of the hip joint, the ligamentum teres, which offers little support to the joint but in some cases does carry the artery of the ligamentum teres.

Nerves of the Gluteal Region and Hip Joint

The nerves to the gluteal region are all branches of the sacral plexus, which consists of the ventral rami of S1–S3, part of S4, and the lumbosacral trunk, which is formed by a small contribution from the ventral ramus of L4 and all of the fifth lumbar ventral ramus (Fig. 8-11). The lumbosacral trunk passes over the brim of the pelvis medial to the psoas major to join

the ventral ramus of the first sacral nerve. The roots of the sacral plexus lie on the piriformis muscle and posterior to the internal iliac vessels, ureters, and on the left, the sigmoid colon. The branches of the internal iliac vessels become intermingled with the branches of the plexus as they leave the pelvis through the greater sciatic foramen to pass into the gluteal region.

The sacral plexus divides into an anterior division and a posterior division. The anterior division gives rise to the

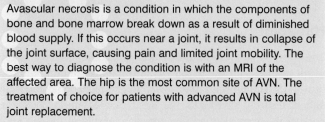

CLINICAL MEDICINE

Avascular Necrosis (AVN)

Avascular necrosis is a condition in which the components of bone and bone marrow break down as a result of diminished blood supply. If this occurs near a joint, it results in collapse of the joint surface, causing pain and limited joint mobility. The best way to diagnose the condition is with an MRI of the affected area. The hip is the most common site of AVN. The treatment of choice for patients with advanced AVN is total joint replacement.

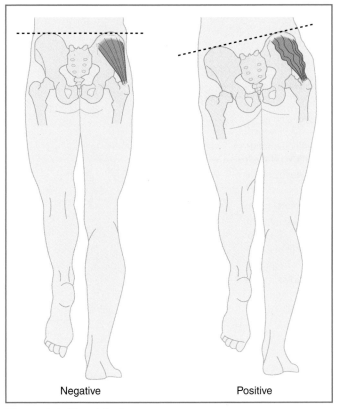

Negative   Positive

Figure 8-8. Trendelenburg test.

nerve to the quadratus femoris and the nerve to the obturator internus before it gives rise to the tibial nerve portion of the sciatic nerve (Fig. 8-12). The nerve to the quadratus femoris (L4, L5, S1) also innervates the inferior gemellus muscle while the nerve to the obturator internus (L5, S1, S2) also innervates the superior gemellus. The nerve to the obturator internus passes over the ischial spine and enters the lesser sciatic foramen lateral to the pudendal nerve.

The posterior division of the sacral plexus gives rise to the nerve to the piriformis, superior gluteal nerve, and the inferior gluteal nerve before it terminates in the common fibular (peroneal) nerve portion of the sciatic nerve (see Fig. 8-12). The superior gluteal nerve (L4, L5, S1) exits the greater sciatic foramen above the piriformis (suprapiriformis recess) and then passes between the gluteus medius and minimus to supply these muscles and the tensor fasciae latae. The remaining branches of the sacral plexus exit below the piriformis (infrapiriformis recess). The inferior gluteal nerve (L5, S1, S2) innervates the gluteus maximus (see Fig. 8-12).

Both divisions contribute to the posterior femoral cutaneous nerve, which runs on the deep surface of the gluteus maximus, medially to the sciatic nerve. It supplies cutaneous innervation to parts of the urogenital triangle and gluteal region (cluneal branches) before continuing down into the thigh and knee region (see Fig. 8-12).

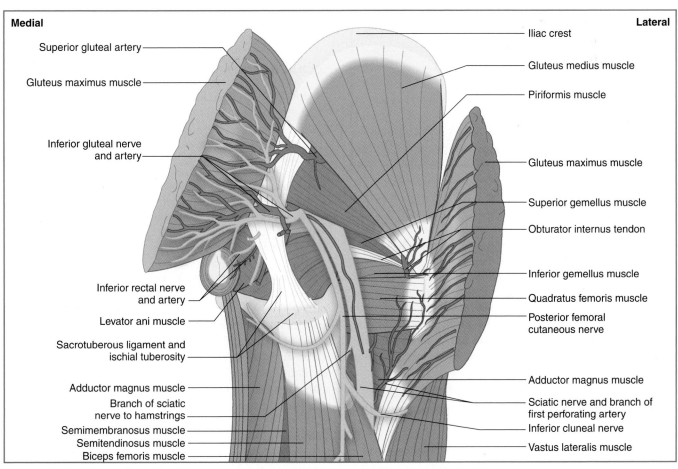

Figure 8-9. Lateral rotators of the hip.

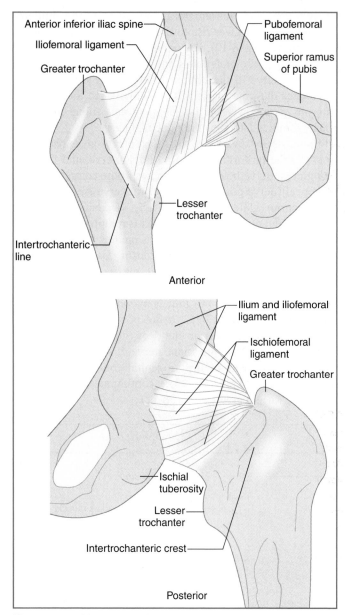

Anterior inferior iliac spine
Iliofemoral ligament
Greater trochanter
Intertrochanteric line
Pubofemoral ligament
Superior ramus of pubis
Lesser trochanter

Anterior

Ilium and iliofemoral ligament
Ischiofemoral ligament
Greater trochanter
Ischial tuberosity
Lesser trochanter
Intertrochanteric crest

Posterior

Figure 8-10. Ligaments of the hip.

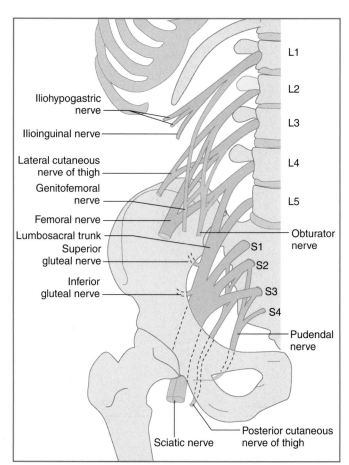

Iliohypogastric nerve
Ilioinguinal nerve
Lateral cutaneous nerve of thigh
Genitofemoral nerve
Femoral nerve
Lumbosacral trunk
Superior gluteal nerve
Inferior gluteal nerve
Sciatic nerve

L1
L2
L3
L4
L5
Obturator nerve
S1
S2
S3
S4
Pudendal nerve
Posterior cutaneous nerve of thigh

Figure 8-11. Sacral plexus in situ.

CLINICAL MEDICINE

Injection to the Gluteal Region

The gluteal region is one of the areas of choice for intramuscular injections because of its large mass of muscles. However, care must be taken in selecting the area to inject because of the danger of injuring the sciatic nerve. The safest place to inject is the upper lateral quadrant. This can be determined by drawing a line between the posterior superior iliac spine and the superior border of the greater trochanter of the femur. Injection should be done above this line to avoid hitting the sciatic nerve.

The sciatic nerve is the thickest nerve in the body (see Fig. 8-12). It is actually composed of two nerves—the common fibular (peroneal) and tibial nerves—which typically separate in the distal thigh but can separate higher or even be arranged so that the common fibular (peroneal) nerve passes through the piriformis muscle and rejoins the tibial nerve. When the common fibular (peroneal) nerve does pass through the piriformis, it is vulnerable to compression when the piriformis contracts.

Blood Supply to the Gluteal Region and Hip Joint

The muscles of the gluteal region receive blood from two branches of the internal iliac artery, the superior and inferior

gluteal arteries. Their origin in the pelvis is described in Chapter 7. After entering the gluteal region above the piriformis, the superior gluteal artery travels between—and supplies both—the gluteus medius and minimus muscles and tensor fascia latae. The inferior gluteal artery enters the gluteal region inferior to the piriformis and supplies the gluteus maximus muscle. Both vessels participate in the cruciate anastomosis of the hip (described below). The venous drainage follows the arteries.

Cruciate Anastomosis

In both the upper and lower limbs where one major artery supplies all the blood to the limb, it is important to have

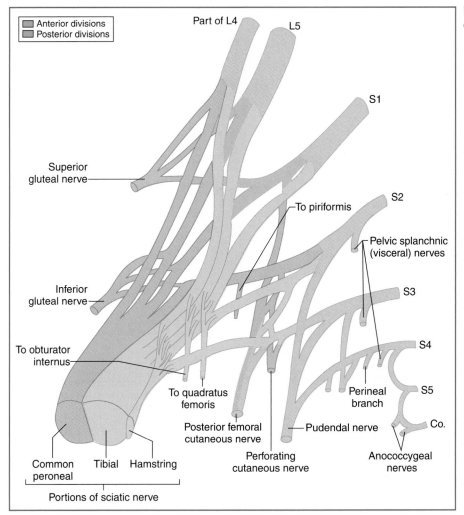

Figure 8-12. Sacral plexus and its divisions.

Legend: Anterior divisions / Posterior divisions

Part of L4 — L5 — S1 — S2 — S3 — S4 — S5 — Co.

Superior gluteal nerve
Inferior gluteal nerve
To obturator internus
To piriformis
Pelvic splanchnic (visceral) nerves
Perineal branch
Pudendal nerve
Anococcygeal nerves
To quadratus femoris
Posterior femoral cutaneous nerve
Perforating cutaneous nerve
Common peroneal   Tibial   Hamstring
Portions of sciatic nerve

collateral networks around the joint regions. In the region of the hip, the anastomosis is the cruciate anastomosis (Fig. 8-13). It is an anastomotic network connecting branches of the internal iliac with the branches of the femoral artery. Branches of the inferior and superior gluteal arteries anastomose with the first perforating branch of the femoral artery as well as the medial and lateral femoral circumflex arteries. This anastomosis is important for both the thigh and the pelvis, especially in women.

●●● THIGH AND KNEE JOINT

The thigh is the region between the hip joint and the knee joint. The muscles of the thigh include flexors and adductors of the hip joint as well as extensors and flexors of the knee joint. Some muscles in the thigh region cross both joints and therefore act on both joints, whereas the majority of the muscles act on only one joint. They are divided into three compartments—anterior, medial, and posterior—by the fascia lata and intermuscular septa. Each compartment shares common functions, nerve supply, and blood supply and will be described separately.

Fascia

As mentioned above, the deep fascia of the lower limb is called the fascia lata in the thigh. There is an opening in the fascia lata slightly inferior to the medial end of the inguinal ligament called the *saphenous opening*. The lateral side of the opening is shaped like a crescent and is known as the falciform margin. A thin layer of fascia derived from the overlying superficial fascia, the cribriform fascia, covers the saphenous opening. The cribriform fascia is sieve-like to allow lymphatics and the great saphenous vein to pass through and join the femoral vein (Fig. 8-14).

Bones

Shaft and Distal End of the Femur

On the posterior surface of the femur, there is a long ridge of bone called the *linea aspera* that has a medial and lateral lip. The medial lip is continuous superiorly with the pectineal line, which is found extending below the lesser trochanter. The lateral lip is continuous superiorly with the gluteal

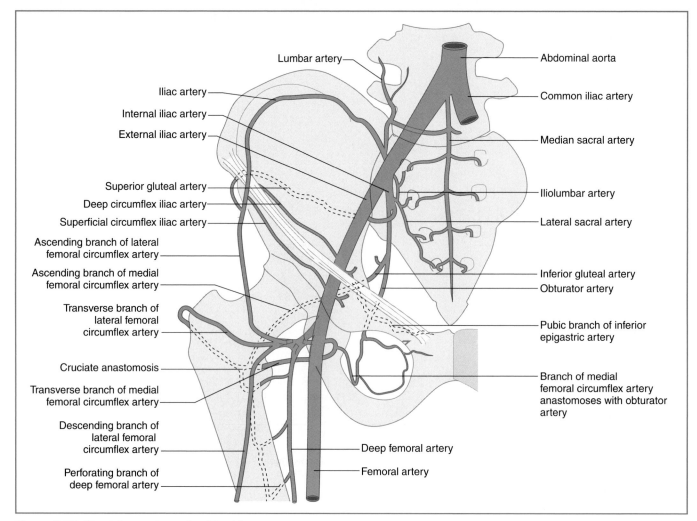

Figure 8-13. Cruciate anastomosis of the hip.

tuberosity (see Fig. 8-5). Toward the distal end of the femur, the medial and lateral lips form the medial and lateral supracondylar lines, which terminate in the medial and lateral epicondyles. Just superior to the medial epicondyle is a protrusion called the *adductor tubercle*. The articular surface of the distal end of the femur consists of two rounded condyles, medial and lateral. They are separated posteriorly by a deep indentation called the *intercondylar fossa*, and anteriorly they blend to form the patellar articular surface.

Patella

The patella is the largest sesamoid bone in the body. Sesamoid bones are bones that develop within tendons or ligaments. The patella is pyramidal in shape with its base directed superiorly and its apex toward the leg. The quadriceps tendon inserts onto its base with some of its fibers continuing over the anterior surface and joining the patellar

ligament, which connects the apex of the patella to the tibial tuberosity (Fig. 8-15A).

Proximal End of the Tibia and Fibula

The proximal ends of the tibia and fibula are considered here, since they participate in the knee joint and provide the areas of insertion for the thigh muscles that act on the knee. The tibia is the large, medially placed weight-bearing bone of the leg (Fig. 8-15B). The proximal end has a medial and lateral condyle separated by anterior and posterior intercondylar areas. The medial and lateral condyles receive the medial and lateral condyles of the femur. In the center there is an intercondylar eminence. The entire proximal surface of the tibia is also called the *tibial plateau*. The fibula is a slender long bone whose proximal end (head) articulates with the tibia on the inferior surface of the lateral condyle. The portion of the fibula inferior to the head narrows and is called the neck of the fibula.

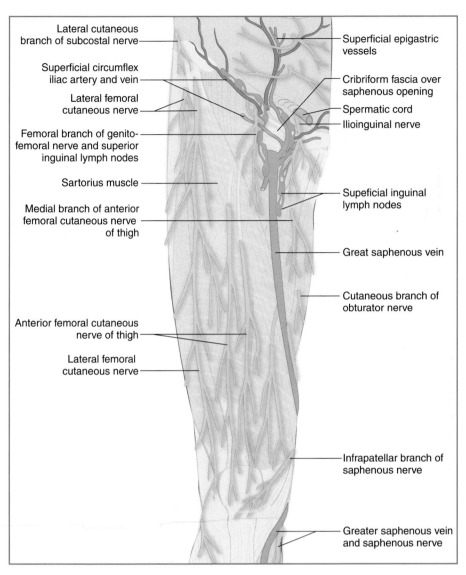

Figure 8-14. Saphenous opening.

Lateral cutaneous branch of subcostal nerve

Superficial circumflex iliac artery and vein

Lateral femoral cutaneous nerve

Femoral branch of genito-femoral nerve and superior inguinal lymph nodes

Sartorius muscle

Medial branch of anterior femoral cutaneous nerve of thigh

Anterior femoral cutaneous nerve of thigh

Lateral femoral cutaneous nerve

Superficial epigastric vessels

Cribriform fascia over saphenous opening

Spermatic cord

Ilioinguinal nerve

Supeficial inguinal lymph nodes

Great saphenous vein

Cutaneous branch of obturator nerve

Infrapatellar branch of saphenous nerve

Greater saphenous vein and saphenous nerve

Anterior Compartment of the Thigh

Muscles

There are four muscles in the anterior compartment of the thigh (Table 8-2). The femoral neurovascular bundle supplies most of these muscles, and this compartment contains the principal extensors of the knee joint and the strongest flexor of the hip joint. The most superficial muscle in the compartment is the *sartorius* (Fig. 8-16). This slender, strap-like muscle crosses both the hip and knee joints. It originates on the anterior superior iliac spine just medial to the origin of the tensor fasciae latae and then travels inferiorly and medially across the thigh to insert on the medial side of the knee. It assists in flexing the hip and knee and can assist in abduction of the femur. It gets its name from the fact that all the movements it can assist with are used when one sits cross-legged, as tailors used to do.

The largest muscle in this compartment is the quadriceps femoris, which is the principal extensor of the knee (see Fig. 8-16 and Table 8-2). The *quadriceps femoris* has four heads that join together to form the quadriceps tendon, which inserts on the patella. The rectus femoris portion of the muscle is the only head that also crosses the hip joint. It originates on the anterior inferior iliac spine and the ilium above the acetabulum and then passes inferiorly to join the other three portions. Therefore, this part of the quadriceps helps flex the hip joint. The vastus lateralis is found deep to the rectus femoris on the lateral side of the thigh. However, it originates on the posterior side of the femur from the greater trochanter—the lateral linea aspera—and in part from the deep fascial septae. The vastus medialis is found medial and deep to the rectus femoris. It originates from the intertrochanteric line and linea aspera. Lastly, the vastus intermedius lies deep to all parts of the quadriceps femoris arising from

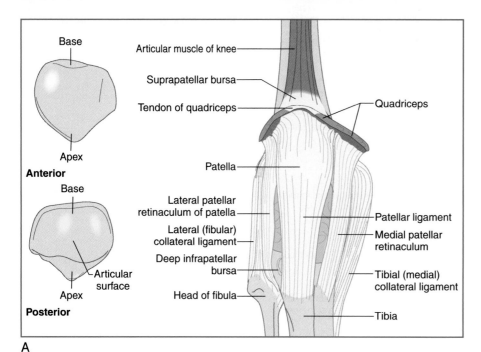

Figure 8-15. A, Patella. **B,** Proximal portions of tibia and fibula.

the anterior and lateral aspects of the femor's shaft and is covered by the vastus lateralis. The quadriceps femoris is the only muscle in the leg that actively extends the leg.

Deep to these muscles is the *iliopsoas muscle*, which is the principal flexor of the hip joint (Fig. 8-17; see also Table 8-2). It is a combination of the iliacus and psoas major and

minor muscles. Its components originate in the pelvis from the ilium and the lumbar vertebrae and pass deep to the inguinal ligament to reach the anterior thigh.

The *pectineus muscle* lies just medial to the iliopsoas (see Fig. 8-17). It arises on the superior ramus of the pubis and inserts on the pectineal line of the femur. Since it crosses the

TABLE 8-2. Muscles of the Anterior Compartment of the Thigh

Muscle	Origin	Insertion	Main Functions	Innervation
Sartorius	Anterior superior iliac spine	Proximal part of medial tibia	Flexes, abducts, and laterally rotates thigh at hip joint and flexes knee joint	Femoral nerve
Quadriceps femoris—rectus femoris	Anterior superior iliac spine	Tibial tuberosity through patellar tendon	Flexes hip joint and extends knee joint	Femoral nerve
Quadriceps femoris—vastus lateralis	Greater trochanter and linea aspera		Extends knee joint	
Quadriceps femoris—vastus intermedius	Intertrochanteric line and linea aspera			
Quadriceps femoris—vastus medialis	Anterior and lateral surfaces of the femur			
Iliopsoas—psoas major	Sides of T12–L5 vertebrae and intervertebral disks	Lesser trochanter	Strongest flexor of the hip	Ventral rami of L1, L2, and L3
Psoas minor	Sides of T12–L1 vertebrae and intervertebral disks	Iliopectineal eminence		Ventral rami L1
Iliopsoas—iliacus	Iliac fossa, ala of sacrum, and sacroiliac joint	Psoas major and lesser trochanter		Femoral nerve
Pectineus	Pecten of the pubis	Posterior aspect of the femur below the lesser trochanter	Hip flexion, thigh adduction	Femoral nerve and obturator nerve

hip joint anteriorly, it assists in flexion, but it also assists the adductors and is sometimes considered a member of the adductor compartment. The iliopsoas and the pectineus muscles form the floor of the femoral triangle, which is the area in which the femoral neurovascular bundles enter the thigh from the pelvis (Fig. 8-18).

Medial Compartment of the Thigh

Most muscles of the medial compartment of the thigh adduct the hip so the medial compartment is also called the adductor compartment (Table 8-3; see also Fig. 8-18B). Most of them also medially rotate and flex the hip joint. The obturator neurovascular bundle supplies all the muscles in this compartment.

Adductor longus is the most superficial muscle (see Fig. 8-18A and B). It lies just medial to the pectineus muscle and originates on the body of the pubis and inserts on the linea aspera on the posterior surface of the femur. Lying just deep to it is the adductor brevis, which also originates on the pubis and inserts above the adductor longus on the linea aspera and

the pectineal line. Deep to the adductor brevis is the adductor magnus, the largest and most posterior muscle in the group. It has a hamstring portion and an adductor portion. The adductor portion of the muscle originates like its companions on the pubis and inserts along the linea aspera. Although not a true hamstring, the hamstring portion's origin on the ischial tuberosity reflects its similarity to the posterior compartment muscles and its participation in extending the thigh. The adductor magnus also has dual innervation. The obturator

CLINICAL MEDICINE

Psoas Sign

One of the tests used to determine if a patient has appendicitis is called the psoas sign. The physician places his or her hand on the patient's thigh just superior to the knee and asks the patient to flex the hip joint. Pain elicited by this maneuver is one sign of potential appendicitis.

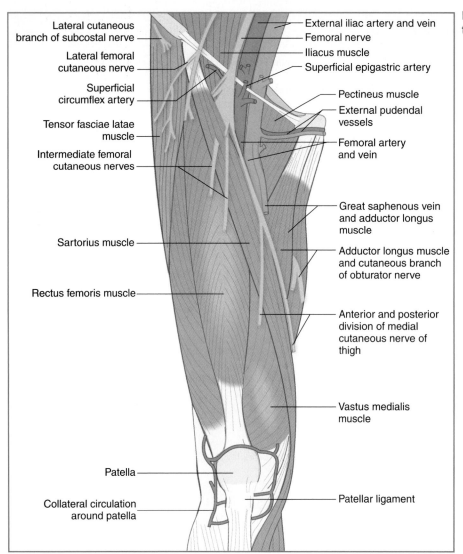

Lateral cutaneous branch of subcostal nerve

Lateral femoral cutaneous nerve

Superficial circumflex artery

Tensor fasciae latae muscle

Intermediate femoral cutaneous nerves

Sartorius muscle

Rectus femoris muscle

Patella

Collateral circulation around patella

External iliac artery and vein

Femoral nerve

Iliacus muscle

Superficial epigastric artery

Pectineus muscle

External pudendal vessels

Femoral artery and vein

Great saphenous vein and adductor longus muscle

Adductor longus muscle and cutaneous branch of obturator nerve

Anterior and posterior division of medial cutaneous nerve of thigh

Vastus medialis muscle

Patellar ligament

Figure 8-16. Anterior compartment of the thigh, superficial view.

nerve innervates the adductor portion, whereas the tibial nerve innervates the hamstring portion. At the distal end of the muscle just superior to its insertion on the adductor tubercle, there is an opening in the tendon called the *adductor hiatus* (see Fig. 8-18B). The femoral artery and vein pass through this opening to reach the popliteal fossa, where they are called the popliteal vessels, and the distal end of the lower limb.

The *gracilis muscle* is a long, strap-like muscle along the medial side of the thigh (see Fig. 8-18B). It arises from the pubis and crosses the knee joint to insert on the medial surface of the tibia inferior to the medial condyle. Since it crosses the knee joint, it flexes the knee in addition to adducting the hip. Its insertion expands and blends with those of the sartorius and semitendinosus to form a structure called the *pes anserinus* (Fig. 8-19).

The deepest muscle of the medial compartment is the *obturator externus* (see Fig. 8-18B). It originates on the external surface of the obturator membrane and inserts on the trochanteric fossa of the femur. Since it passes posteriorly to the hip joint, the obturator externus is not an adductor of the hip but rather assists in lateral rotation.

Posterior Compartment of the Thigh

The posterior compartment comprises three muscles that extend the hip and flex the knee (Fig. 8-20 and Table 8-4). They are called the hamstring muscles, and all have at least one origin on the ischial tuberosity. The tibial nerve provides the innervation to all the hamstring muscles. A true hamstring muscle crosses both the hip and knee joints posteriorly.

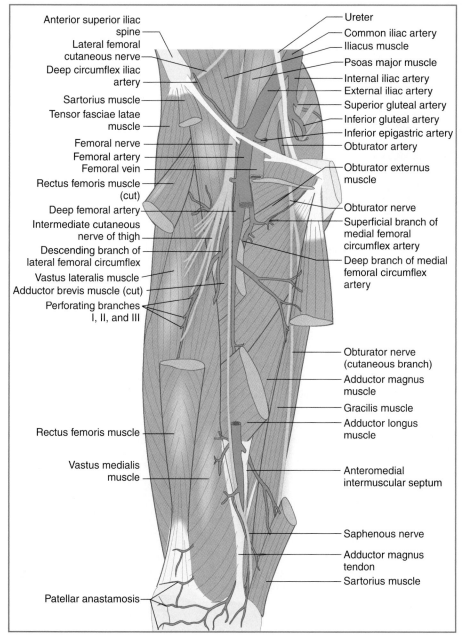

Anterior superior iliac spine
Lateral femoral cutaneous nerve
Deep circumflex iliac artery
Sartorius muscle
Tensor fasciae latae muscle
Femoral nerve
Femoral artery
Femoral vein
Rectus femoris muscle (cut)
Deep femoral artery
Intermediate cutaneous nerve of thigh
Descending branch of lateral femoral circumflex
Vastus lateralis muscle
Adductor brevis muscle (cut)
Perforating branches I, II, and III
Rectus femoris muscle
Vastus medialis muscle
Patellar anastamosis

Ureter
Common iliac artery
Iliacus muscle
Psoas major muscle
Internal iliac artery
External iliac artery
Superior gluteal artery
Inferior gluteal artery
Inferior epigastric artery
Obturator artery
Obturator externus muscle
Obturator nerve
Superficial branch of medial femoral circumflex artery
Deep branch of medial femoral circumflex artery
Obturator nerve (cutaneous branch)
Adductor magnus muscle
Gracilis muscle
Adductor longus muscle
Anteromedial intermuscular septum
Saphenous nerve
Adductor magnus tendon
Sartorius muscle

Figure 8-17. Deep dissection of the anterior compartment of the thigh.

Of the three muscles, the *biceps femoris* is the only one to pass down on the lateral side of the thigh (see Fig. 8-20). The biceps femoris has two heads: a long head and a short head. The short head originates on the linea aspera, and the long head originates with the other hamstrings from the ischial tuberosity. Its tendon crosses the knee joint to insert on the proximal part of the fibula. In addition to having two heads, it has dual innervation.

The semimembranosus and semitendinosus are found on the medial side of the thigh. Their names describe their appearances. The *semitendinosus muscle* has a fusiform muscle belly and a long tendon that crosses the knee joint to insert on the medial side of the proximal tibia near the insertion of the gracilis and sartorius. The *semimembranosus muscle* is deep to the semitendinosus muscle and is broader. Its tendon inserts into the medial condyle of the tibia (see Fig. 8-20). The hamstring portion of the adductor magnus is anterior to the semimembranosus and semitendinosus in the anatomic position as it inserts into the adductor tubercle or the femur's medial condyle.

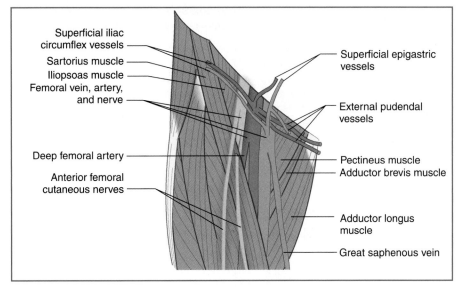

A

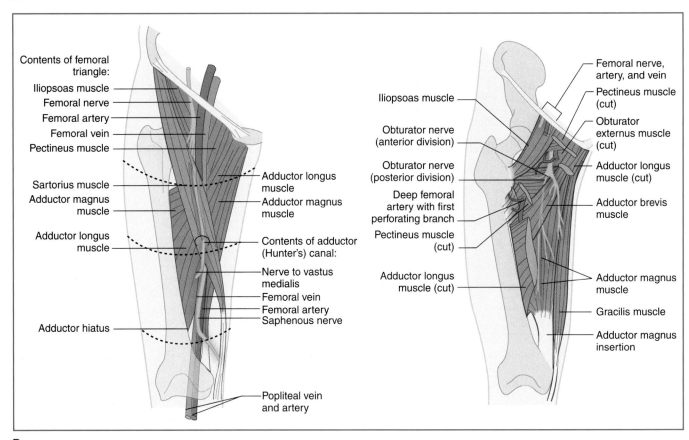

B

Figure 8-18. A, Femoral triangle. **B,** Medial compartment of the thigh.

TABLE 8-3. Muscles of the Medial Compartment of the Thigh

Muscle	Origin	Insertion	Principal Function	Innervation
Adductor longus	Pubic tubercle and body	Medial lip of linea aspera	Adduction and flexion of hip	Obturator nerve (L2–L4)
Adductor brevis	Inferior ramus of pubis	Pectineal line of femur, proximal portion of linea aspera		
Adductor magnus, adductor portion	Ischiopubic ramus	Linea aspera		
Adductor magnus, hamstring portion	Ischial tuberosity	Adductor tubercle	Extension of hip	Tibial nerve portion of sciatic nerve (L4)
Gracilis	Inferior ramus of pubis, ramus of ischium	Medial surface of proximal tibia	Adduction of hip and flexion of leg	
Obturator externus	External surface of obturator membrane, external surface of pelvis	Trochanteric fossa of femur	Lateral rotation of thigh	Obturator nerve (L2–L4)

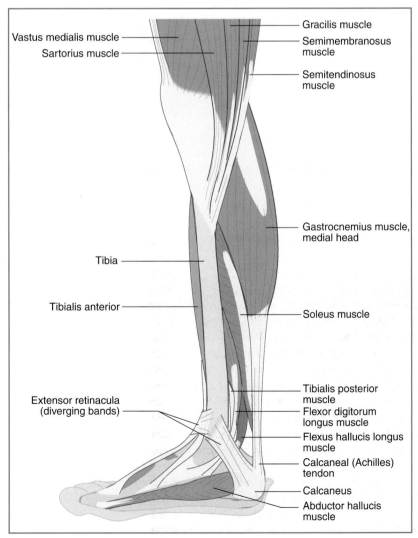

Figure 8-19. Pes anserinus.

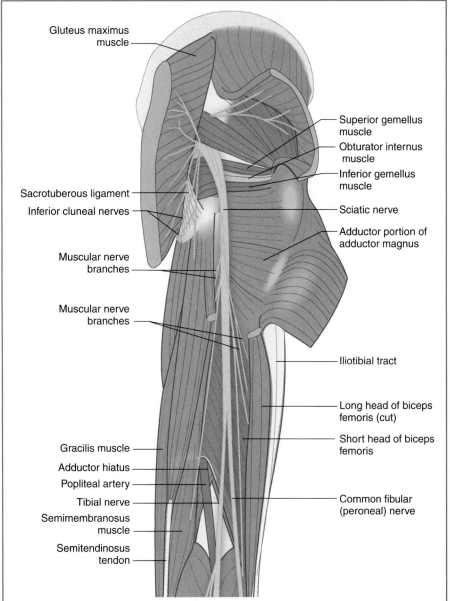

Figure 8-20. Posterior compartment of the thigh.

Gluteus maximus muscle

Superior gemellus muscle

Obturator internus muscle

Inferior gemellus muscle

Sacrotuberous ligament

Inferior cluneal nerves

Sciatic nerve

Adductor portion of adductor magnus

Muscular nerve branches

Muscular nerve branches

Iliotibial tract

Long head of biceps femoris (cut)

Short head of biceps femoris

Gracilis muscle

Adductor hiatus

Popliteal artery

Tibial nerve

Semimembranosus muscle

Semitendinosus tendon

Common fibular (peroneal) nerve

TABLE 8-4. Muscles of the Posterior Compartment of the Thigh

Muscle	Origin	Insertion	Principal Function	Innervation
Biceps femoris, short head	Linea aspera of femur	Head of the fibula	Flexion of the knee	Common fibular (peroneal) nerve portion of sciatic nerve (L5, S1, S2)
Biceps femoris, long head	Ischial tuberosity	Head of the fibula		Tibial nerve portion of sciatic nerve (L5, S1, S2)
Semitendinosus		Medial surface of proximal end of tibia	Extension of the hip joint	
Semimembranosus		Medial condyle of tibia and forms oblique popliteal ligament, which runs superolaterally to lateral femoral condyle		

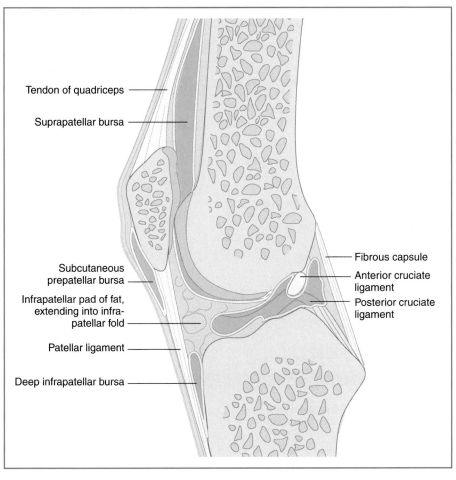

Figure 8-21. Sagittal view of knee joint.

Tendon of quadriceps

Suprapatellar bursa

Subcutaneous prepatellar bursa

Infrapatellar pad of fat, extending into infra-patellar fold

Patellar ligament

Deep infrapatellar bursa

Fibrous capsule

Anterior cruciate ligament

Posterior cruciate ligament

CLINICAL MEDICINE

The Unhappy Triad

The medial collateral ligament (MCL) of the knee is the most commonly torn ligament of the knee when playing contact sports. It typically happens when the foot is planted, the knee is extended, and force is exerted from the posterior lateral direction. This produces a twisting movement above the fixed leg, which causes the MCL and anterior cruciate ligament (ACL) to rupture. Since the medial meniscus is attached to the MCL, it also is usually injured at the same time. Injury to the MCL, ACL, and medial meniscus is known as the "unhappy triad."

Knee Joint

The knee joint is a synovial hinge joint. Movement involves articulations between the femur and the tibia as well as between the patella and the femur (Fig. 8-21). The knee joint receives forces that approach five times the body's weight. The stability of the knee joint is dependent on muscle action and supporting ligaments. Because it is a weight-bearing joint,

it also has a locking mechanism when the knee is fully extended to reduce the amount of energy needed to maintain the standing position.

The articular surfaces of the medial and lateral condyles of the tibia are deepened by the presence of two fibrocartilaginous menisci (Fig. 8-22). The medial meniscus is C-shaped and is attached to the medial collateral ligament of the knee. The lateral meniscus is rounder and is *not* attached to the lateral collateral ligaments.

The joint is surrounded by a fibrous capsule that is reinforced laterally by the iliotibial tract and medially by the patellar retinaculum (Fig. 8-23). The patellar ligament forms the anterior aspect of the fibrous capsule. The lateral (fibular) collateral ligament (LCL) runs from the lateral epicondyle of the femur to the head of the fibula (see Fig. 8-23). It is external to the joint capsule and does not attach to the lateral meniscus. The medial (tibial) collateral ligament (MCL) runs from the medial epicondyle of the femur to medial condyle and shaft of the tibia. In contrast to the lateral collateral ligament, the medial collateral ligament does blend with the joint capsule and attaches to the medial meniscus.

Inside the joint capsule are two other ligaments: the anterior and posterior cruciate ligaments (see Fig. 8-23). They stabilize the joint when the knee is fully extended. The anterior cruciate ligament (ACL) runs from the anterior

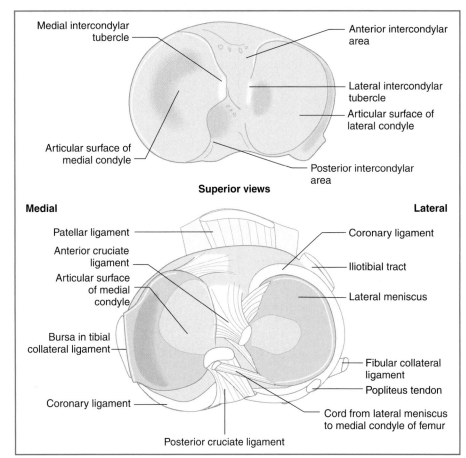

Medial intercondylar tubercle

Anterior intercondylar area

Lateral intercondylar tubercle

Articular surface of lateral condyle

Articular surface of medial condyle

Posterior intercondylar area

Superior views

Medial

Lateral

Patellar ligament

Coronary ligament

Anterior cruciate ligament

Iliotibial tract

Articular surface of medial condyle

Lateral meniscus

Bursa in tibial collateral ligament

Fibular collateral ligament

Popliteus tendon

Coronary ligament

Cord from lateral meniscus to medial condyle of femur

Posterior cruciate ligament

Figure 8-22. Medial and lateral menisci.

intercondylar area on the tibia to the intercondylar fossa of the femur. It limits the anterior movement of the tibia on the femur. The posterior cruciate ligament (PCL) arises on the posterior intercondylar area of the tibia and passes posteriorly to the anterior cruciate ligament to insert on the lateral surface of the medial femoral condyle. The posterior cruciate ligament limits posterior movement of the tibia on the femur (see Fig. 8-23).

Femoral Triangle

The femoral triangle is the area of the upper thigh where the femoral neurovascular bundle, the major neurovascular supply to the lower limb, enters from the trunk. The borders of the femoral triangle are the inguinal ligament superiorly, the lateral border of the adductor longus medially, and the sartorius laterally (see Fig. 8-18A). The posterior wall of the femoral triangle is formed by the iliopsoas, the pectineus, and the adductor longus while the anterior border of the femoral triangle is the fascia lata. The femoral triangle is bisected by the femoral artery and vein, and the femoral nerve is the most lateral component in the triangle.

Femoral Sheath

The femoral artery and vein are enclosed in a funnel-shaped fascial sheath, the femoral sheath, as they enter the femoral

triangle. The femoral sheath is formed by an extension of the inner investing layer of deep fascia in the lower abdomen deep to the inguinal ligament. The femoral sheath is divided into three compartments (Fig. 8-24). The lateral portion encloses the femoral artery, the intermediate compartment encloses the femoral vein, and the medial compartment contains lymphatics and is also known as the *femoral canal*. The entrance to the femoral canal is known as the *femoral ring*. The borders of the femoral ring are the femoral vein laterally, the superior ramus of the pubis posteriorly, the lacunar ligament medially, and the inguinal ligament anteriorly. The femoral canal is the main route for lower limb lymphatics to reach the abdominal lymphatics. It is also the site of femoral hernias.

Adductor Canal

The femoral neurovascular bundle leaves the femoral triangle and enters the adductor canal in the middle of the thigh between the vastus medialis and the adductor muscles. The adductor canal, a fibromuscular passageway, leads to the deficit in the tendon of the adductor magnus called the *adductor hiatus* (see Fig. 8-18B). In the adductor canal, the femoral artery and vein are accompanied by the saphenous nerve. However, the saphenous nerve leaves the canal by penetrating its fascial anterior border, the subsartorial fascia, before the adductor hiatus, passing between the sartorius and gracilis

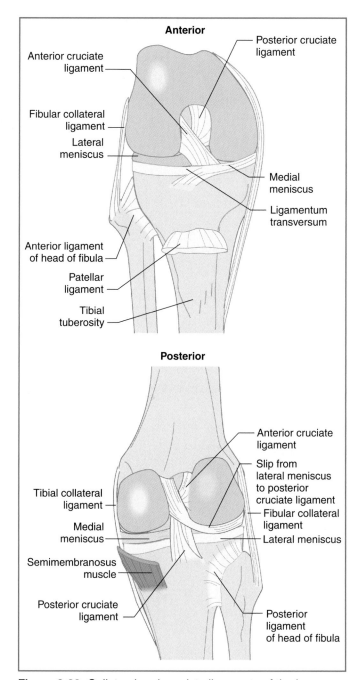

Figure 8-23. Collateral and cruciate ligaments of the knee.

muscles to meet and run with the greater saphenous vein. These structures descend together on the medial side of the leg and foot, thereby extending the L4 dermatome to the medial aspect of the foot. The femoral artery and vein continue through the adductor hiatus into the popliteal fossa as the popliteal artery and vein.

Nerves of the Thigh and Knee Joint

Branches of the lumbosacral plexus innervate the thigh muscles. The lumbosacral plexus is formed by the ventral rami of the lumbar plexus (L1–L4) and the sacral plexus (L4–S4). The lumbosacral plexus then separates into an anterior division and a posterior division (see Fig. 8-11). The anterior divisions typically innervate flexors and adductors while posterior divisions typically innervate extensors and abductors. Owing to the medial rotation of the lower limb during development, the extensors of the knee—quadriceps femoris, sartorius, and pectineus—end up in the anterior compartment of the thigh. Thus, these muscles are supplied by the femoral nerve, which is derived from the posterior divisions of the ventral rami of L2, L3, and L4. It also supplies the hip flexors.

Femoral Nerve

The femoral nerve emerges from the lateral border of the psoas major in the iliac fossa close to the inguinal ligament. The femoral nerve gives branches to the iliacus and pectineus muscles. It then passes deep to the inguinal ligament, lateral to the femoral artery and outside the femoral sheath. Then it separates into anterior and posterior divisions. The anterior division has anterior cutaneous branches that supply the anterior and medial aspect of the thigh to the knee. The anterior division of the femoral nerve also supplies the sartorius muscle (Fig. 8-25).

The femoral nerve's posterior division gives rise to the saphenous nerve, which follows the femoral vessels into the adductor canal (see Fig. 8-25). It also supplies the quadriceps femoris muscle. Occasionally the saphenous nerve can be entrapped as it penetrates the roof of the adductor canal. The femoral nerve is not commonly susceptible to entrapment distally. However, retroperitoneal hemorrhage, especially as it associates with the psoas major muscles, tumors, and fractures of the pelvis or femur can damage this nerve with weakness or wasting of the quadriceps femoris. If the injury involves both the iliopsoas and quadriceps femoris, then walking forward becomes difficult owing to the loss of both hip flexion and knee extension.

Obturator Nerve

The anterior division of the lumbar plexus forms the obturator nerve in the psoas major (see Fig. 8-11). At the pelvic brim and pelvis, the obturator nerve passes along the medial side of the psoas, along the lateral pelvic wall, lateral to the internal iliac artery. The obturator nerve runs to the obturator foramen, where it separates into anterior and posterior divisions. As these nerves emerge from the obturator canal, the anterior division runs over the obturator externus, posteriorly to the pectineus, and then between the adductor longus and brevis to innervate the pectineus, gracilis, and adductor longus and brevis muscles (Fig. 8-26). The femoral nerve typically innervates the pectineus, but the obturator nerve can also innervate this muscle. The obturator nerve's posterior division passes through the obturator externus, innervates it, and then passes between the abductor brevis and magnus to innervate the adductor portion of the magnus and sometimes the adductor brevis. The hamstring portion of the adductor magnus, which arises from the ischial tuberosity and passes posteriorly to the hip joint to insert into the medial epicondyle's adductor tubercle, is innervated by the tibial

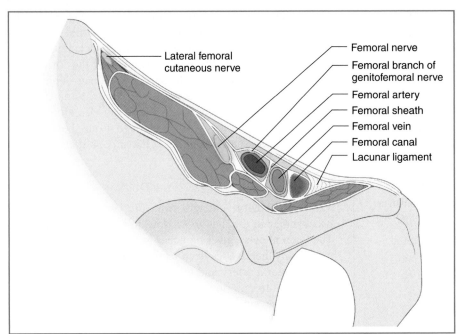

Lateral femoral cutaneous nerve

Femoral nerve

Femoral branch of genitofemoral nerve

Femoral artery

Femoral sheath

Femoral vein

Femoral canal

Lacunar ligament

Figure 8-24. Femoral sheath.

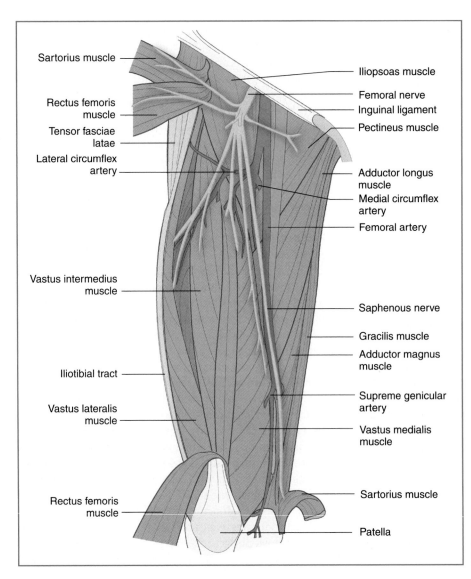

Sartorius muscle

Rectus femoris muscle

Tensor fasciae latae

Lateral circumflex artery

Vastus intermedius muscle

Iliotibial tract

Vastus lateralis muscle

Rectus femoris muscle

Iliopsoas muscle

Femoral nerve

Inguinal ligament

Pectineus muscle

Adductor longus muscle

Medial circumflex artery

Femoral artery

Saphenous nerve

Gracilis muscle

Adductor magnus muscle

Supreme genicular artery

Vastus medialis muscle

Sartorius muscle

Patella

Figure 8-25. Femoral nerve and branches and adductor canal.

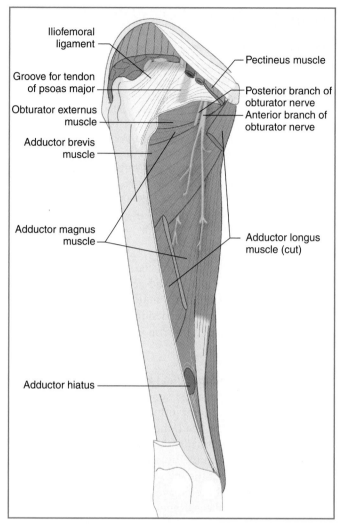

Figure 8-26. Obturator nerve in the thigh.

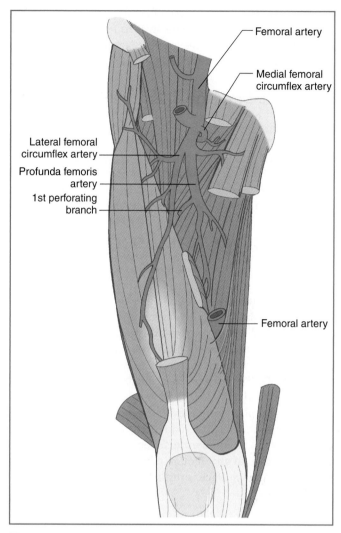

Figure 8-27. Femoral artery and its deep branches.

nerve. The obturator nerve has a cutaneous supply to the inferior medial aspect of the thigh, especially just above the knee.

Injuries to the obturator nerve are rare. Pressure from trauma, a difficult delivery, hysterectomy, obturator hernia, and carcinoma of the cervix, rectum, or bladder may injure the obturator nerve. In these cases, the patient has difficulty walking and a tendency to abduct the thigh. The patient also has difficulty with medial rotation and pain or decreased sensation to the inferomedial thigh.

Sciatic Nerve

The sciatic nerve is the largest nerve in the body. It forms from the ventral rami of L4–S3 (see Fig. 8-12). It is actually two nerves, the common fibular (peroneal) and tibial nerves that typically separate in the lower thigh. The tibial portion arises from the anterior divisions and innervates the hamstring muscles of the thigh, whereas the common fibular (peroneal) nerve arises from the posterior divisions and innervates the short head of the biceps femoris.

Blood Supply to the Thigh and Knee Joint

The thigh receives its blood from the femoral artery. The femoral artery is the direct continuation of the external iliac artery. It enters the thigh deep to the inguinal ligament and into the femoral triangle. In the femoral triangle the femoral artery gives off numerous small cutaneous branches that supply the upper thigh and perineum: superficial epigastric artery, superficial circumflex iliac artery, superficial external pudendal artery, and deep external pudendal artery. The largest branch it gives off is the deep femoral (profundus femoris) artery, which gives rise to three or four perforating branches that penetrate the adductor magnus muscle near its attachment to the linea aspera to supply the posterior compartment (see Fig. 8-27). The first perforating branch also participates in the cruciate anastomosis of the hip (see Fig. 8-13). The deep femoral artery usually also gives rise to the medial and lateral circumflex femoral arteries. The medial circumflex femoral artery typically passes between the iliopsoas and pectineus muscles to pass medially around the proximal end of the femur. As it does so, it gives off a branch that joins the cruciate anastomosis. The lateral circumflex femoral artery passes deep to the sartorius and rectus femoris to supply the lateral thigh and participate in the cruciate anastomosis. The deep veins of the thigh follow the arteries and have similar names.

Lymphatic Drainage of the Thigh and Knee Joint

Lymphatic drainage of the thigh is via superficial and deep lymph vessels. The superficial lymph vessels travel with the great saphenous vein and ultimately drain into the superficial inguinal nodes (see Fig. 8-14). Deep lymphatic vessels from the thigh drain into the deep inguinal nodes.

●●● LEG AND ANKLE JOINT

The leg is the region between the knee and the ankle. The majority of the muscles in this region are responsible for movement at the ankle. Therefore, most of them cross the ankle joint to insert on the bones of the ankle and foot. The leg is similar to the forearm in that there are two bones. The two leg bones are attached via an interosseous membrane, as they are in the forearm, but they move as a unit instead of independently. The primary movement at the ankle is flexion and extension (Fig. 8-28). The movements of inversion and eversion take place primarily through the transverse tarsal joint. Inversion and eversion are particularly important when a person walks on an uneven surface. Inversion is when the plantar surface of the foot is turned medially; eversion is when the plantar surface is turned laterally.

Bones

Tibia

The tibia is the medially placed, weight-bearing bone of the leg. Its proximal portion was described above with the knee joint. The tibial shaft is triangular in shape and therefore can be described as having anterior, medial, and lateral borders (Fig. 8-29). The lateral border is the site of attachment of the interosseus membrane that connects the tibia to the fibula. The anterior border is a sharp, palpable ridge that begins at the tibial tuberosity and extends inferiorly for about two thirds of the shaft. The anterior border also separates the medial surface and lateral surfaces of the tibia. The medial surface is devoid of muscle attachments and is subcutaneous. For this reason, fractures of the tibia are commonly compound (having bone fragments that penetrate the skin). On the posterior surface of the upper end of the tibia is an oblique line running from lateral to medial called the *soleal line*. Distally the tibia expands to end with a flat surface laterally and an extended portion medially called the *medial malleolus*. The medial malleolus is palpable on the medial side of the ankle.

Fibula

The fibula is a thin, needle-like bone that is non-weight-bearing but serves as the attachment site for the majority of

CLINICAL MEDICINE

Intermittent Claudication

Atherosclerosis can cause blockage of many different arteries, one of which is the femoral artery and its branches. When the femoral artery becomes blocked, the muscles it supplies become ischemic, particularly during exertion such as walking, causing the individual pain. When the pain disappears after a period of rest, this is called intermittent claudication (Latin, limping). Since the femoral artery supplies blood to the entire lower limb, the area of pain indicates the approximate location of the blockage. For example, if the profunda femoris is blocked, pain will develop in the posterior thigh upon walking, whereas pain localized to the calf would indicate a blockage of femoral artery branches more distally.

the muscles in the leg. Therefore, the only parts of the fibula that are palpable are the head and neck region and the distal end, which is called the *lateral malleolus*. The lateral malleolus articulates with the lateral side of the distal tibia such that the two bones form a mortise joint (see Fig. 8-29).

Tarsal Bones

There are seven tarsal bones that make up the ankle (see Fig. 8-28A). The talus is the most superior tarsal bone and articulates with the mortise joint formed by the tibia and fibula. It has three portions: the head, the body, and the trochlea tali (see Fig. 8-28B). The trochlea is the saddle-shaped superior portion that inserts into the tibiofibular joint. The trochlea is superior to the body of the talus and posterior to the head of the talus. The body of the talus articulates inferiorly with the largest tarsal bone, the calcaneus. The calcaneus forms the heel of the foot. On its medial surface is a rather deep shelf called the *sustentaculum tali*. There is a groove in the posterior talus and at the base of the sustentaculum tali for the flexor hallucis longus tendon. The head of the talus articulates anteriorly with the concave surface of the boat-shaped navicular bone. The navicular bone in turn articulates with the three cuneiform bones, so-called because of their wedge shape. They are designated medial, intermediate, and lateral based on their position relative to each other. The last tarsal bone is the cuboid bone, which as the name implies is cube-shaped. It articulates with the calcaneus posteriorly and the lateral cuneiform bone.

Metatarsal Bones

There are five metatarsal bones (see Fig. 8-28A). The first three each articulate with one of the cuneiform bones, and the fourth and fifth both articulate with the cuboid bone. Their proximal ends are referred to as their bases, and their distal ends as the heads. There is a clinically important protrusion, the tubercle of the base of the fifth metatarsal, on the base of the fifth metatarsal bone, which is the insertion site of the peroneus brevis. The head of the first metatarsal articulates inferiorly with two sesamoid bones, which aid in transmitting the body's weight to the ground. These three bones also form what is called the "ball of the foot."

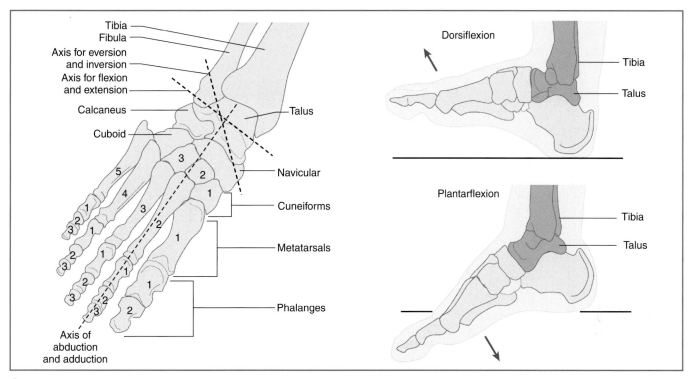

A

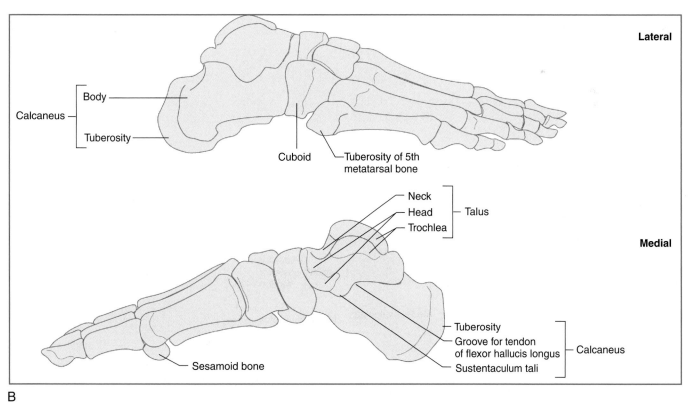

B

Figure 8-28. A, Movements at the ankle joint. **B,** Medial and lateral views of the foot.

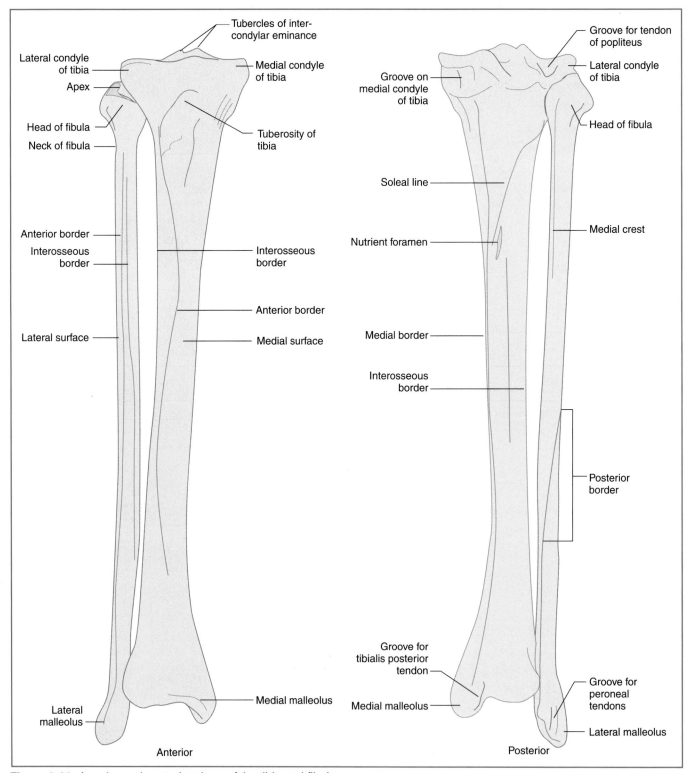

Figure 8-29. Anterior and posterior views of the tibia and fibula.

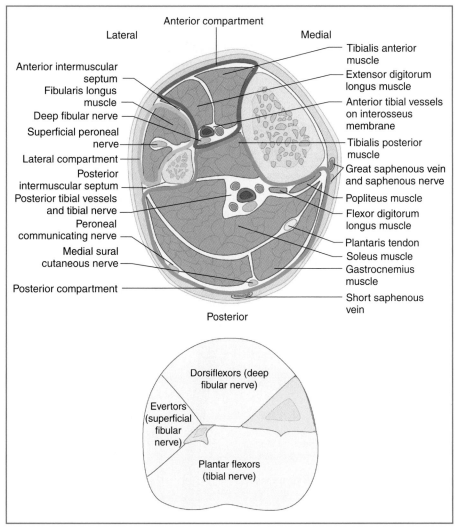

Figure 8-30. Cross-section of the leg.

Phalanges

The phalanges are the distal bones in the foot. There are fourteen phalanges in the foot; three—proximal, intermediate, and distal—are associated with each of the second to fifth metatarsals and two with the first metatarsal. The joints, starting at the head of metatarsals, are metatarsal phalangeal, proximal interphalangeal, and distal interphalangeal. The long flexors and extensors of the toes will insert on these bones. The big toe is referred to as the hallux.

Fascia

The crural fascia is dense and unyielding and has been referred to as the exoskeleton. It serves as the origin of some of the muscles of the leg. It blends with the periosteum of the subcutaneous anterior surface of the tibia and then as it passes laterally, it forms two septae: the anterior and posterior intermuscular septae that attach to the fibula (Fig. 8-30). The

CLINICAL MEDICINE

Gout

Gout is a metabolic disease in which circulating levels of uric acid are elevated (hyperuricemia) and uric acid crystals are deposited in the joints, particularly the metatarsophalangeal joint of the big toe. Joints become red, hot, and extremely tender. This inflammation is a result of the interaction of monosodium urate crystals with mononuclear phagocytes, which in turn release interleukin-1, which initiates the inflammatory reaction. The crystals also lyse neutrophils, which release lysosomal enzymes that contribute to the inflammation. Levels can be elevated because of the kidneys' inability to clear uric acid or from overproduction. Alcohol consumption can bring on an attack because beer and wine contain high concentrations of purines, which are metabolized to uric acid. Gout is diagnosed by the presence of uric acid (monosodium urate) crystals in the joint fluid.

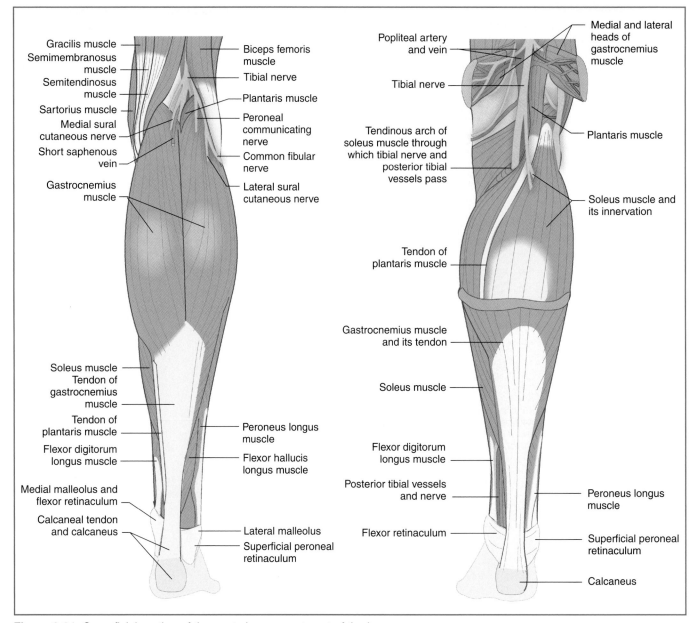

Figure 8-31. Superficial portion of the posterior compartment of the leg.

crural fascia continues around the posterior aspect of the leg, splitting to form superficial and deep posterior compartments of the leg. Thus, the interosseous membrane and the tibia form the anterior, lateral, and posterior compartments of the leg (see Fig. 8-30).

Distally the fascia thickens to form retinacula in the ankle region. These thickenings help maintain the muscle tendons in the proper position to maximize their efficiency. There are two retinacula over the extensor muscles and tendons: a wide, superior extensor retinaculum and a Y-shaped inferior extensor retinaculum. On the lateral side of the ankle are two more retinacula that cover the muscle tendons of the lateral compartment.

Posterior Compartment of the Leg

The posterior compartment of the leg has a superficial and a deep portion. All the muscles in this compartment plantar-flex the ankle except one, the poplitens. They are all inner-vated by the tibial nerve and receive their blood supply from the posterior tibial artery. The superficial compartment is composed of three muscles that all contribute to the formation of the Achilles tendon.

Most superficial is the *gastrocnemius muscle*, which has a medial and lateral head that originate on the medial and lateral distal end of the femur (Fig. 8-31). The two muscle heads blend together to form a tendon, which inserts on the

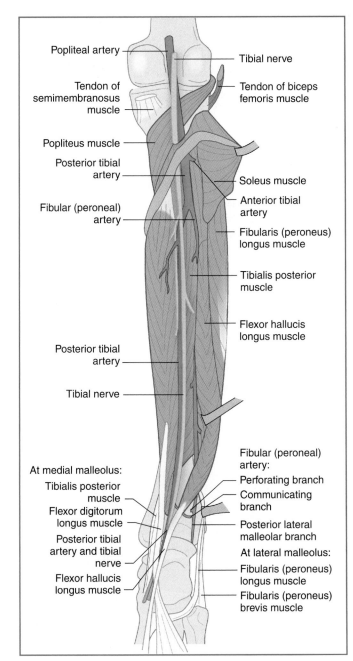

Popliteal artery

Tendon of semimembranosus muscle

Popliteus muscle

Posterior tibial artery

Fibular (peroneal) artery

Posterior tibial artery

Tibial nerve

At medial malleolus:
Tibialis posterior muscle
Flexor digitorum longus muscle
Posterior tibial artery and tibial nerve
Flexor hallucis longus muscle

Tibial nerve

Tendon of biceps femoris muscle

Soleus muscle

Anterior tibial artery

Fibularis (peroneus) longus muscle

Tibialis posterior muscle

Flexor hallucis longus muscle

Fibular (peroneal) artery:
Perforating branch
Communicating branch
Posterior lateral malleolar branch
At lateral malleolus:
Fibularis (peroneus) longus muscle
Fibularis (peroneus) brevis muscle

Figure 8-32. Deep portion of the posterior compartment of the leg.

calcaneal tuberosity. The two heads form the inferior borders of the popliteal fossa. The gastrocnemius muscle forms the bulge on the surface of the back of the calf. Since it arises from the distal femur, it assists in flexion of the knee joint in addition to plantar-flexing the ankle. Deep to the gastrocnemius muscle lies the *soleus muscle*, which originates on the soleal line of the tibia as well as from the fibula (see Fig. 8-31). Therefore, it does not cross the knee joint. Its tendon joins the gastrocnemius muscle. It is a strong plantar flexor of the ankle. The third muscle is the *plantaris*, which has a very short muscle belly that originates on the lateral side of the distal femur and a very long tendon, which joins the other two tendons on their medial side to form the Achilles tendon. Together these three muscles are sometimes called the *triceps surae*.

The deep portion of the posterior compartment has four muscles, three of which act on the ankle and foot and one that acts only on the knee (Fig. 8-32 and Table 8-5). The *popliteus* is a short muscle that attaches to the lateral side of the distal femur and inserts on the posterior surface of the tibia. Since it crosses posterior to the knee joint, it flexes the knee joint. It is also believed to unlock the knee when a person takes a step. The knee joint locks when the knee is fully extended, and the action of the popliteus is believed to unlock the knee by slightly rotating the femur laterally. This allows flexion to take place. The popliteus also serves as a landmark for the name change of the popliteal artery to anterior and posterior tibial artery. This takes place at the inferior boundary of the muscle.

The *tibialis posterior* is the deepest muscle in the compartment. It originates from the interosseus membrane and the posterior surfaces of both bones (see Fig. 8-32). Its tendon passes behind the medial malleolus to insert on the medial side of the foot. Since it passes behind the medial malleolus, it plantar-flexes the ankle. In addition, since the tibialis posterior inserts on the medial side of the foot, it also inverts the foot. On either side of the tibialis posterior lie the long flexors of the toes. They originate from the opposite side of the leg than the side of the foot they are inserting on. The *flexor digitorum longus muscle* originates on the medial side of the tibialis posterior, and then after it passes posterior to the medial malleolus it must cross laterally on the plantar surface of the foot to insert on the distal phalanges of toes two to five (see Fig. 8-32). In contrast, the *flexor hallucis longus* originates from the fibula on the lateral side of the tibialis posterior, passes in the groove on the posterior surface of the talus and inferior surface of the sustentaculum tali, and crosses deep to the flexor digitorum longus to reach the distal phalanx of the big toe (see Fig. 8-32).

Lateral Compartment of the Leg

The lateral compartment contains only two muscles, both of which plantar-flex the ankle and evert the foot (Table 8-6 and Fig. 8-33). They are innervated by the superficial fibular (peroneal) nerve and receive their blood supply via perforating branches from the fibular (peroneal) artery. The *fibularis (peroneus) longus muscle* is superficially placed and arises from the proximal end of the fibula and passes inferiorly and posteriorly around the lateral malleolus to insert in multiple locations on the medial side of the plantar surface of the foot. Deep to the fibularis longus muscle lies the *fibularis (peroneus) brevis muscle*, which arises more distally on the fibula and inserts on the tubercle at the base of the fifth metatarsal. Its tendon is deep to the fibularis longus. It also everts the foot and plantar-flexes the ankle.

Anterior Compartment of the Leg

The anterior compartment contains the only dorsiflexors of the foot and ankle (Table 8-7 and Fig. 8-34). These muscles receive their innervation from the deep fibular (peroneal) nerve and their blood supply from the anterior tibial artery.

TABLE 8-5. Muscles of the Posterior Compartment of the Leg

Muscle	Origin	Insertion	Function	Innervation
Gastrocnemius	Medial and lateral epicondyles of femur	Calcaneal tuberosity via Achilles tendon	Plantar-flexion of ankle joint and flexion of the knee	Tibial nerve (L4–S3)
Soleus	Soleal line on posterior tibia, posterior proximal end of fibula, and medial border of tibia		Plantar-flexion of ankle joint	
Plantaris	Lateral epicondyle of femur			
Popliteus	Lateral condyle of femur	Proximal end of tibia superior to soleal line	Lateral rotation of femur to unlock knee	
Tibialis posterior	Proximal two thirds of fibula and tibia and interosseous membrane	Navicular, medial cuneiform, cuboid bones, and bases of second, third, and fourth metatarsals	Plantar-flexion of ankle and inversion of foot	
Flexor digitorum longus	Medial part of posterior surface of tibia inferior to soleal line	Bases of distal phalanges of lateral four toes	Plantar-flexion of ankle and flexion of lateral four toes	
Flexor hallucis longus	Distal two thirds of fibula and interosseous membrane	Base of distal phalanx of big toe	Flexion of big toe and plantar-flexion of ankle	

TABLE 8-6. Muscles of the Lateral Compartment of the Leg

Muscle	Origin	Insertion	Principal Function	Innervation
Fibularis longus	Head and lateral surface of fibula and adjacent deep fascia	Lateral side of medial cuneiform and base of first metatarsal	Eversion and plantar-flexion	Superficial fibular (peroneal) nerve (L5, S1, S2)
Fibularis brevis	Lower lateral surface and adjacent fascia	Dorsolateral surface of the base of fifth metatarsal	Eversion and plantar-flexion	Superficial fibular (peroneal) nerve (L5, S1, S2)

The most medial muscle in this compartment is the *tibialis anterior*. It arises from the lateral surface of the tibia, the interosseous membrane, and deep fascia and inserts on the medial side of the dorsum of the foot. Therefore, this muscle inverts in addition to dorsiflexing the ankle. Lying lateral to this muscle is the *extensor hallucis longus*, which originates on the anterior surface of the fibula and inserts on the distal phalanx of the big toe. The last two muscles in the compartment are the extensor digitorum longus and fibularis (peroneus) tertius, which are continuous at their origin from the anterior surface of the fibula. The *extensor digitorum longus* inserts on the distant phalanges of the four lateral toes and the *fibularis (peroneus) tertius* tendon inserts on the tubercle of the fifth metatarsal near the insertion of the fibularis (peroneus) brevis, which explains its name.

Popliteal Fossa

The popliteal fossa is the transition zone between the posterior thigh and leg. The neurovascular supply to the leg and foot is found in this fossa. It is a diamond-shaped region and therefore has four borders (Fig. 8-35A). The biceps femoris muscle forms the superolateral border, and the semitendinosus and semimembranosus muscles form the superomedial border. Inferiorly the two heads of the gastrocnemius form the borders. As the sciatic nerve travels down the posterior

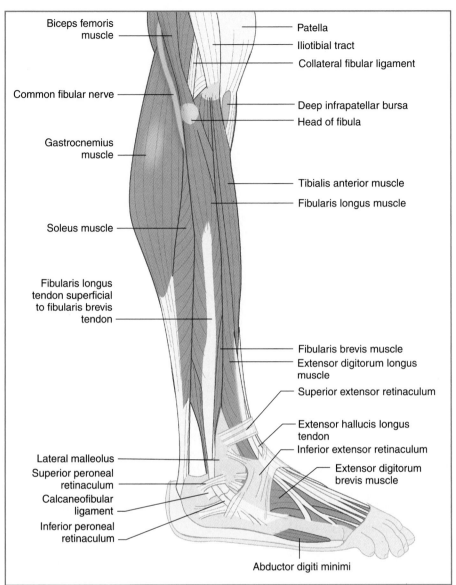

Figure 8-33. Lateral compartment of the leg.

Labels (top to bottom, left side):
- Biceps femoris muscle
- Common fibular nerve
- Gastrocnemius muscle
- Soleus muscle
- Fibularis longus tendon superficial to fibularis brevis tendon
- Lateral malleolus
- Superior peroneal retinaculum
- Calcaneofibular ligament
- Inferior peroneal retinaculum

Labels (right side):
- Patella
- Iliotibial tract
- Collateral fibular ligament
- Deep infrapatellar bursa
- Head of fibula
- Tibialis anterior muscle
- Fibularis longus muscle
- Fibularis brevis muscle
- Extensor digitorum longus muscle
- Superior extensor retinaculum
- Extensor hallucis longus tendon
- Inferior extensor retinaculum
- Extensor digitorum brevis muscle
- Abductor digiti minimi

TABLE 8-7. Muscles of the Anterior Compartment of the Leg

Muscle	Origin	Insertion	Principal Function	Innervation
Tibialis anterior	Lateral condyle and proximal portion of tibia, interosseus membrane	Medial and inferior surfaces of medial cuneiform bone	Dorsiflexion of the ankle and inversion	Deep fibular (peroneal) nerve (L4, L5, S1)
Extensor hallucis longus	Middle portion of anterior surface of fibula, interosseus membrane	Dorsal aspect of base of distal phalanx of big toe		
Extensor digitorum longus	Lateral condyle of tibia, proximal portion of fibula, interosseus membrane	Middle and distal phalanges of lateral four digits	Dorsiflexion of the ankle	
Fibularis (peroneus) tertius	Distal third of anterior surface of fibula, interosseous membrane	Dorsal surface of tuberosity of base of fifth metatarsal		

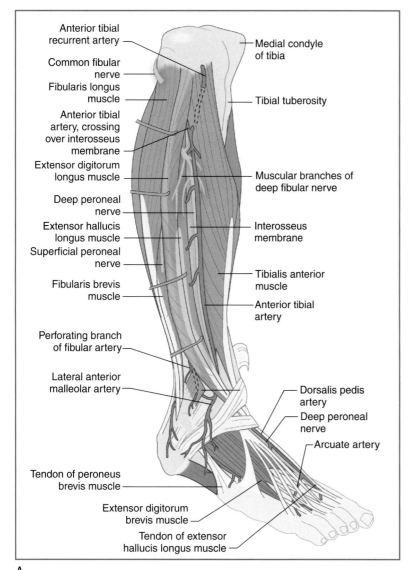

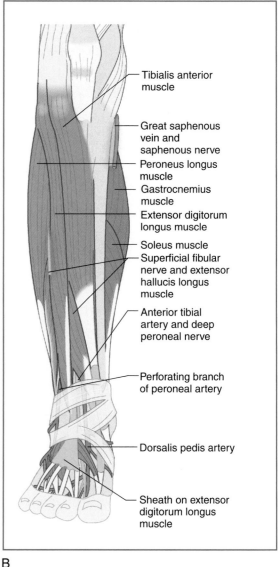

Figure 8-34. Deep (**A**) and superficial (**B**) views of the anterior compartment of the leg.

thigh, it typically divides at the superior border of the fossa. The common fibular (peroneal) nerve travels down along the medial side of the biceps femoris tendon and then runs superficially and medially to the head and neck of the fibula—where it is highly vulnerable to injury—to supply the anterior and lateral compartments of the leg. The tibial portion of the sciatic nerve travels down the middle of the fossa with the popliteal artery and vein. The tibial nerve is the most posterior (superficial when approached from the posterior surface) structure of this neurovascular bundle, since the femoral vessels become the popliteal vessels at the adductor hiatus. Here, the femoral vein is posterior to the

femoral artery as they enter in the popliteal fossa. Thus, the popliteal artery is closest to the knee joint, the popliteal vein is in the middle, and the tibial nerve is the most posterior member of this neurovascular bundle (see Fig. 8-35B).

While in the popliteal fossa, the tibial nerve gives rise to the sural nerve, a cutaneous branch, which passes between the two heads of the gastrocnemius and joins a contribution from the common fibular (peroneal) nerve to supply the lateral and posterior aspect of the leg (see Fig. 8-35A). The sural nerve continues down and passes around the lateral aspect of the ankle. At this point it gives rise to calcaneal branches to the heel's lateral and plantar surfaces and

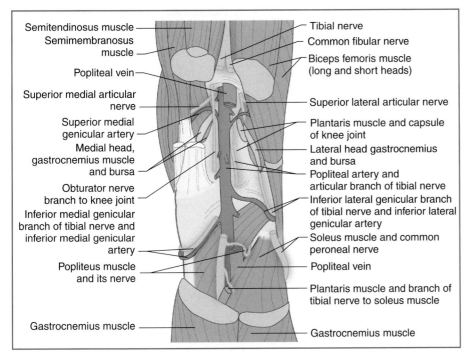

Semitendinosus muscle
Semimembranosus muscle
Popliteal vein
Superior medial articular nerve
Superior medial genicular artery
Medial head, gastrocnemius muscle and bursa
Obturator nerve branch to knee joint
Inferior medial genicular branch of tibial nerve and inferior medial genicular artery
Popliteus muscle and its nerve
Gastrocnemius muscle

Tibial nerve
Common fibular nerve
Biceps femoris muscle (long and short heads)
Superior lateral articular nerve
Plantaris muscle and capsule of knee joint
Lateral head gastrocnemius and bursa
Popliteal artery and articular branch of tibial nerve
Inferior lateral genicular branch of tibial nerve and inferior lateral genicular artery
Soleus muscle and common peroneal nerve
Popliteal vein
Plantaris muscle and branch of tibial nerve to soleus muscle
Gastrocnemius muscle

A

Figure 8-35. Deep (**A**) and superficial (**B**) views of the popliteal fossa.

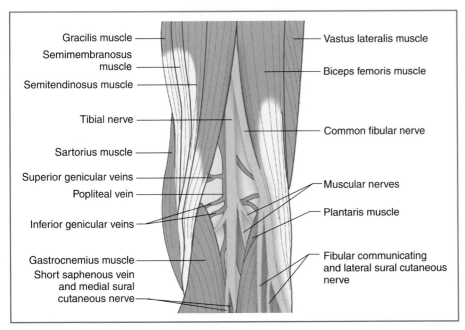

Gracilis muscle
Semimembranosus muscle
Semitendinosus muscle
Tibial nerve
Sartorius muscle
Superior genicular veins
Popliteal vein
Inferior genicular veins
Gastrocnemius muscle
Short saphenous vein and medial sural cutaneous nerve

Vastus lateralis muscle
Biceps femoris muscle
Common fibular nerve
Muscular nerves
Plantaris muscle
Fibular communicating and lateral sural cutaneous nerve

B

continues down the lateral side of the foot to the little toe. This allows the S1 dermatome to reach the lateral side of the heel and foot.

Ankle Joint

The ankle joint is formed by the articulation of the distal ends of the tibia and fibula with the talus of the ankle. As men-

tioned above, the primary movements that take place at the ankle joint are flexion (plantar flexion) and extension (dorsiflexion), whereas inversion and eversion are limited at the ankle joint, especially when the ankle is dorsiflexed. Although inversion and eversion are important when a person walks on uneven terrain, when they occur forcibly at the ankle joint, the result can be an ankle sprain or fracture, often requiring surgical repair. Therefore, the ankle joint is reinforced with

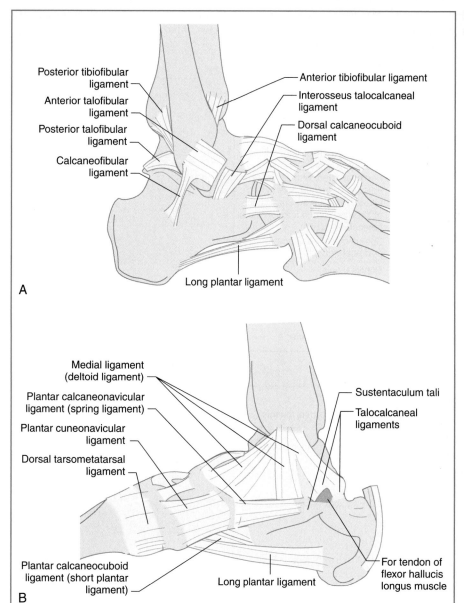

Figure 8-36. Collateral ligaments of the ankle. **A,** Lateral view. **B,** Medial view.

A

Posterior tibiofibular ligament
Anterior talofibular ligament
Posterior talofibular ligament
Calcaneofibular ligament

Anterior tibiofibular ligament
Interosseus talocalcaneal ligament
Dorsal calcaneocuboid ligament

Long plantar ligament

B

Medial ligament (deltoid ligament)
Plantar calcaneonavicular ligament (spring ligament)
Plantar cuneonavicular ligament
Dorsal tarsometatarsal ligament
Plantar calcaneocuboid ligament (short plantar ligament)

Sustentaculum tali
Talocalcaneal ligaments

Long plantar ligament

For tendon of flexor hallucis longus muscle

collateral ligaments that stabilize it and limit inversion and eversion at this joint (Fig. 8-36). On the medial side is a group of ligaments that together form the *deltoid ligament*, named for its triangular shape. The deltoid ligament protects against over-eversion. The lateral side of the ankle has *lateral collateral ligaments* that protect against over-inversion. Sprains of the ankle joint (tearing of the collateral ligaments) usually are of the inversion type and therefore involve tearing of the lateral collateral ligaments. In the assessment of an inversion injury, it is important that the radiograph include the base of the fifth metatarsal because in some cases over-inversion of

the ankle causes the peroneus brevis to avulse the tuberosity of the base of the fifth metatarsal. Most of the normal movements of inversion and eversion occur through the transverse tarsal joint, a joint consisting of the talonavicular and the calcaneocuboid joints, which are aligned transversely across the foot.

Nerves of the Leg and Ankle Joint

The tibial nerve (L4–S3) supplies all the muscles in the posterior compartment of the leg. The tibial nerve descends between the superficial and deep compartments (see Fig. 8-31). As it reaches the ankle joint, it passes posteriorly around the medial malleolus, with the long tendons from the posterior compartment deep to the flexor retinaculum, to supply the muscles and cutaneous innervation to the plantar aspect of the foot. Thus, injury to the tibial nerve results in loss of plantar flexion of the ankle as well as loss of sensation and motor innervation to the plantar and distal surfaces of the foot.

The common fibular (peroneal) nerve splits into a superficial and a deep branch after it passes around the neck of the fibula and passes deep to the fibularis longus. The superficial fibular (peroneal) nerve (L5, S1, S2) passes between and supplies both muscles of the lateral compartment and then becomes superficial to supply cutaneous innervation to the lateral side of the leg and the entire dorsal surface of the foot except for the first dorsal web space and the distal phalanges and nail beds of the toes. Cutaneous innervation of the toes is analogous to that of the fingers; thus, it is shared by the medial and lateral plantar nerves. The deep fibular (peroneal) nerve (L4, L5, S1) passes between the fibularis longus and the fibula to reach the anterior compartment, where it runs along the interosseous membrane supplying all the muscles of this compartment. It passes into the foot, where it supplies the extensor hallucis brevis and extensor digitorum brevis before it ends as a cutaneous nerve that supplies the first dorsal web space (see Fig. 8-33).

The common fibular (peroneal) nerve is superficial and therefore vulnerable to injury as it wraps around the neck of the fibula (see Fig. 8-33). Here, the nerve can be injured by compression from direct trauma, a poorly fitted cast, and even prolonged sitting with crossed knees. If the knee is injured, the patient has weakness or paralysis of the muscles of the anterior or lateral compartments of the leg. Loss of the use of the anterior compartment muscles results in weakness or loss of the dorsiflexors of the foot and extensors of the toes. This condition is known as foot drop. When walking, the patient must lift the leg at the knee to compensate for the inability to dorsiflex the foot. The patient also loses sensation on the lateral calf and the dorsal surface of the foot with loss of the common fibular (peroneal) nerve or just to the first dorsal web space if only the deep fibular (peroneal) nerve is involved.

Blood Supply to the Leg and Ankle Joint

The blood supply to the leg is from the popliteal artery. As the popliteal artery passes the inferior border of the popliteus muscle, it divides into two arteries, the anterior and posterior tibial arteries. The posterior tibial artery continues inferiorly and gives rise to a fibular branch, which travels down the lateral side of the posterior aspect of the leg close to the fibula, deep to the flexor hallucis longus (see Fig. 8-32). The fibular artery sends branches into the lateral compartment to supply the fibularis longus and brevis muscles and terminates in a network of vessels around the lateral malleolus after giving off a perforating branch, which passes through the distal end of the interosseous membrane to anastomose with branches from the anterior tibial artery and the dorsalis pedis artery.

As soon as the anterior tibial artery arises in the proximal leg, it passes through a gap in the interosseus membrane to reach the anterior compartment of the leg (see Fig. 8-34). It travels inferiorly along the interosseus membrane within the deep fibular nerves. In the distal part of the compartment, the anterior tibial artery is found between the extensor hallucis longus and the tibialis anterior tendons. At the distal end, it gives rise to an anterior lateral and an anterior medial malleolar artery, both of which pass around the distal ends of the leg bones and anastomose with branches from the posterior tibial and fibular arteries, providing a collateral network around the ankle joint. Finally, the anterior tibial artery becomes superficial on the dorsal aspect of the foot, and its name changes to the dorsalis pedis artery (see Fig. 8-34). The veins of the leg follow the arteries.

Lymphatic Drainage of the Leg and Ankle Joint

The lymphatic drainage of the leg takes place through deep and superficial lymphatic vessels. Both types of vessels drain into nodes located in the popliteal fossa. From the popliteal fossa, lymph will follow deep lymphatic vessels through the thigh and drain into the deep inguinal nodes.

●●● FOOT

The foot is the platform on which the lower limb contacts the ground. It is designed and organized for proper weight bearing and for bipedal locomotion. The foot is arranged so that when a person is standing, the foot contacts the ground only at the calcaneus and the heads of the metatarsals. This is accomplished with the arches of the foot, which are the curved plantar surfaces of the foot (Fig. 8-37). The arches are important for two additional reasons: shock absorption and initiation of walking. The muscles of the foot are described in two groups: a dorsal group and a plantar group. They are very similar to the muscles of the hand and have potentially the same actions. However, given the fact that the foot is used as a platform and not as a tool for fine movement and manipulation, their main function is to support the arches and in so doing ensure proper weight distribution within the foot.

Arches of the Foot

There are two arches, a longitudinal arch and a transverse arch. The longitudinal arch has a medial and a lateral portion. The medial portion of the longitudinal arch is higher than the lateral portion. When a person is walking, the lateral portion flattens out to touch the walked-on surface; however, the medial portion stays off the surface under normal circumstances. This explains the typical footprint. The transverse arch passes through four of the tarsal bones: talus, navicular, calcaneus, and cuboid (see Fig. 8-37), and the heads of metatarsals. The arches are maintained in three ways. First, the

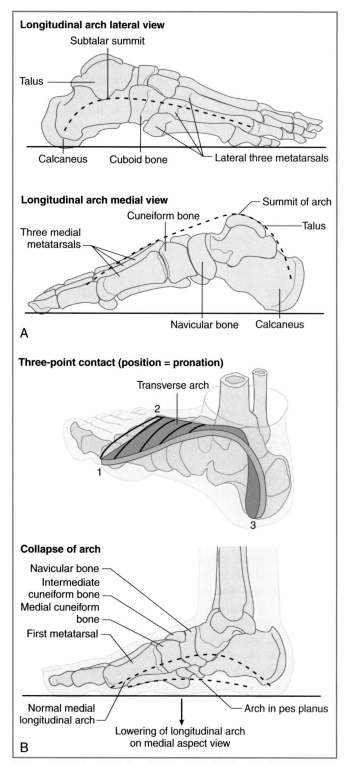

Figure 8-37. A, Medial and lateral longitudinal arches. **B,** Comparison of normal and collapsed (fallen) arches.

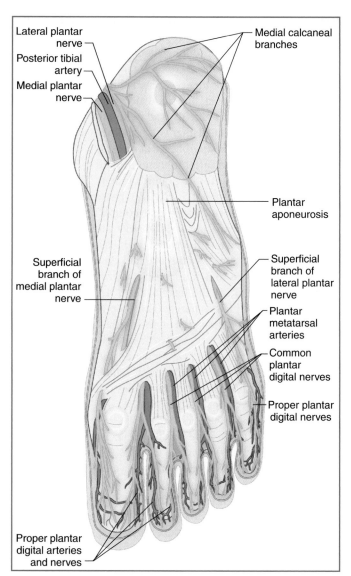

Figure 8-38. Plantar aponeurosis.

intrinsic shape of the tarsal and metatarsal bones helps shape the foot into arches. Second, there are a number of important ligaments, which offer support. Third, the intrinsic muscles of the foot as well as some tendons from the leg muscles also assist.

Ligaments of the Foot

The most superficial and strongest ligamentous structure in the foot is the plantar aponeurosis, which is similar to the palmar aponeurosis in the hand. It extends from the calcaneus to the toes (Fig. 8-38). It is thickest medially, with longitudinally placed bands of tissue covering the digital tendon sheaths. It is thinner on the medial and lateral sides of the foot.

The spring (plantar calcaneonavicular) ligament runs from the sustentaculum tali to the navicular bone (Fig. 8-39). It acts as a hammock-like structure to support the head of the talus and the medial side of the longitudinal arch. As the weight passes from the tibia to the talus, it ideally should be transferred posteriorly to the calcaneus and anteriorly to the heads

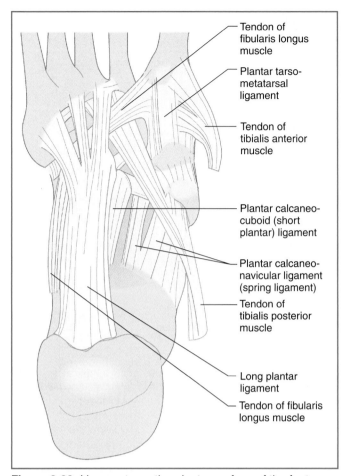

Figure 8-39. Ligaments on the plantar surface of the foot.

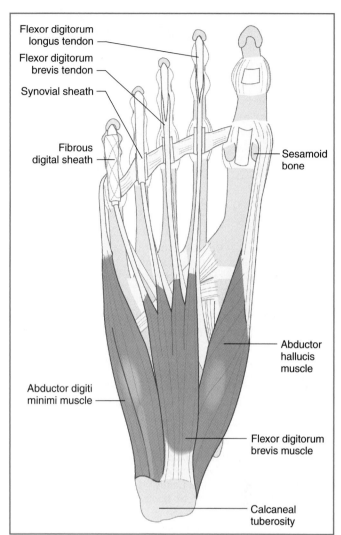

Figure 8-40. First layer of the intrinsic muscles of the foot.

of the metatarsals. However, gravity exerts force directly inferiorly. The spring ligament resists this downward pull. Damage or stretching of the spring ligament can result in pes planus, or flat feet. This is a painful condition that can be treated by placing orthotics in the shoes, thereby imposing an arch on the foot.

The long and short plantar ligaments are also instrumental in maintaining the longitudinal arches of the foot (see Fig. 8-39). The long plantar ligament attaches to the calcaneus and the cuboid bone. A portion of the long plantar ligament's fibers extends to the bases of the metatarsals, forming a tunnel for the tendon of the fibularis longus. The short plantar ligament (plantar calcaneocuboid) is deep to the long plantar ligament and arises distal to the long plantar ligament on the calcaneus and also inserts on the cuboid bone.

Intrinsic Muscles of the Foot

The intrinsic muscles of the foot are divided into plantar and dorsal groups. The plantar muscles are arranged in four layers from superficial to deep. The first layer includes three muscles: the short flexor of the toes, *flexor digitorum brevis*, and two abductors, one for the big toe and one for the little toe, *abductor hallucis* and *abductor digiti minimi*, respectively (Fig. 8-40 and Tables 8-8 and 8-9).

The second layer of muscles contains only two intrinsic muscles of the foot (Fig. 8-41). However, both muscles attach to the long tendons of the flexor digitorum longus, which arises in the posterior compartment of the leg. The *quadratus plantae* has two heads both of which arise from the calcaneus and together insert on the lateral side of the flexor digitorum longus tendon. The quadratus plantae muscle assists in flexion of the toes. Since the flexor digitorum longus muscle enters the sole of the foot from the medial side, the lateral attachment of the quadratus plantae assists in flexion by straightening out the tendon for more efficient flexion of the toes.

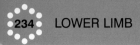

TABLE 8-8. Intrinsic Muscles of the Plantar Surface of the Foot

Muscle	Origin	Insertion	Main Function	Innervation
First Layer of Plantar Surface				
Flexor digitorum brevis	Calcaneal tuberosity, plantar aponeurosis	Four tendons insert into the middle phalanges of toes 2–5 after dividing to allow flexor digitorum longus tendons to reach distal phalanges	Flexes the proximal interphalangeal joints of toes 2–5	Medial plantar nerve
Abductor hallucis	Medial side of calcaneal tuberosity, flexor retinaculum	Medial side of base of great toe's proximal phalanx	Abducts and flexes the great toe	Medial plantar nerves
Abductor digiti minimi	Both sides of calcaneal tuberosity, plantar aponeurosis	Lateral side of base of fifth toe's proximal phalanx	Abducts and flexes the fifth toe	Lateral plantar nerve
Second Layer of Plantar Surface				
Quadratus plantae (flexor digitorum accessorius)	Two heads from the calcaneus	Lateral side of tendon of flexor digitorum longus	Assists in toe flexion by straightening out the tendon of insertion	Lateral plantar nerve
Four lumbrical muscles	Tendons of flexor digitorum longus	Medial side of extensor hoods of toes 2–5 over their proximal phalanges	Flex the metatarsophalangeal joints and extend the interphalangeal joints	First lumbrical is innervated by medial plantar nerve, remaining lumbricals by lateral plantar nerve
Third Layer of Plantar Surface				
Flexor hallucis brevis	Two heads from cuboid bone, cuneiform bones, and tendon of tibialis posterior	Lateral and medial sides of large toe's proximal phalanx	Flexes the first metatarsophalangeal joints	Medial plantar nerve
Flexor digiti minimi	Base of the fifth metatarsal	Base of proximal phalanx of the fifth toe	Flexes the fifth metatarsophalangeal joints	Lateral plantar nerve
Adductor hallucis	Transverse head from plantar surface of metatarsophalangeal ligaments 2-4, oblique heads from base of metatarsal bones 2-4	Two heads blend to insert into lateral side of large toe's proximal phalanx	Adducts big toe	Lateral plantar nerve
Fourth Layer of Plantar Surface				
Four dorsal interossei	Shafts of adjacent metatarsal bones	Muscles 1 and 2 insert into both sides of the proximal phalanx of digit 2; muscles 3 and 4 insert into lateral side of proximal phalanx of digits 3 and 4	Moves second toe toward first, third, and fourth toes; abducts toes from plane of second toe	Lateral plantar nerve
Three plantar interossei	Base and medial sides of metatarsal bones 3–5	Medial side and base of proximal phalanges of toes 3–5	Adduct the third, fourth, and fifth toes toward the second toe, which is the plane of adduction and abduction	Lateral plantar nerve

TABLE 8-9. Intrinsic Muscles of the Dorsal Surface of the Foot

Muscle	Origin	Insertion	Main Function	Innervation
Extensor digitorum brevis	Anterior superior calcaneal surface	Dorsal aspect of big toe's proximal phalanx	Assists in extension of the proximal phalanx	Deep fibular (peroneal) nerve
Extensor hallucis brevis	Anterior superior calcaneal surface	Dorsal aspect of proximal phalanx of toes 2–4	Assists in extending phalanges of toes 2–4	Deep fibular (peroneal) nerve

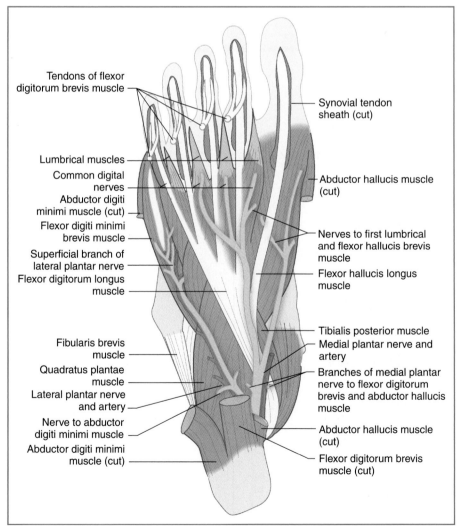

Figure 8-41. Second layer of the intrinsic muscles of the foot.

The second group of muscles, the four worm-like *lumbrical muscles* of the foot each attach to the medial side of the extensor hoods of toes two to five. They flex the metatarsophalangeal joints and extend the interphalangeal joints.

The third layer contains the two short flexors—flexor hallucis brevis and flexor digiti minimi—and the adductor of the big toe, adductor hallucis (Fig. 8-42). *Flexor hallucis brevis* has two heads. The lateral head arises from the cuboid bone, and the medial head arises from the tibialis posterior tendon. The two heads blend together near the base of the first metatarsal and then diverge to each insert on the lateral and medial side of the proximal phalanx. The two sesamoid bones found at the head of the first metatarsal are embedded in their tendons of insertion. The *flexor digiti minimi* is a short muscle, which arises from the base of the fifth metatarsal and inserts on the lateral side of the proximal phalanx of the fifth toe. It flexes the little toe at the metatarsophalangeal joint. The *adductor hallucis* has two heads, transverse and oblique, which blend together before they insert on the lateral side of the proximal phalanx to adduct the big toe at the metatarsal phalangeal joint.

The fourth and final layer contains the dorsal and plantar interossei (Fig. 8-43). There are three *plantar interossei* and four *dorsal interossei*. The plantar interossei adduct the toes, and the dorsal ones abduct. The abduction/adduction axis is through the second toe in the foot. Therefore, the three plantar

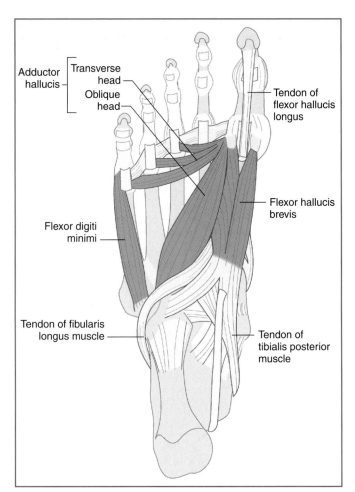

Figure 8-42. Third layer of the intrinsic muscles of the foot.

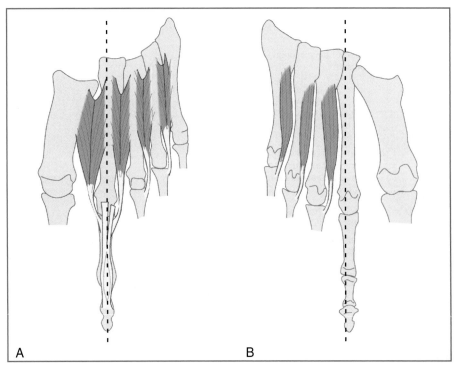

Figure 8-43. Dorsal (**A**) and plantar (**B**) interosseous muscles. *Dotted line* indicates abduction/adduction axis.

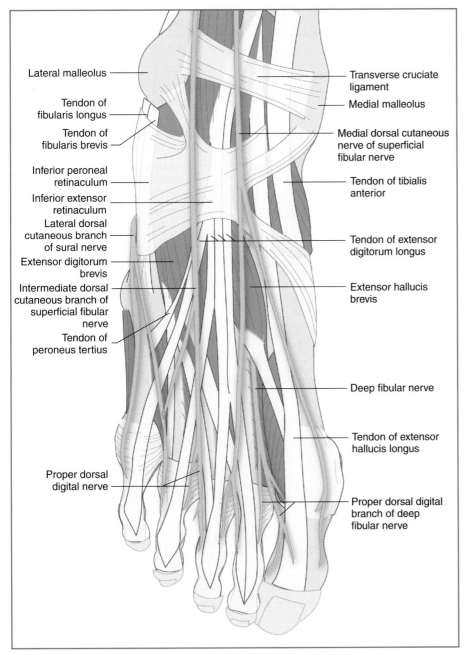

Figure 8-44. Dorsal muscles of the foot.

Lateral malleolus

Tendon of fibularis longus

Tendon of fibularis brevis

Inferior peroneal retinaculum

Inferior extensor retinaculum

Lateral dorsal cutaneous branch of sural nerve

Extensor digitorum brevis

Intermediate dorsal cutaneous branch of superficial fibular nerve

Tendon of peroneus tertius

Proper dorsal digital nerve

Transverse cruciate ligament

Medial malleolus

Medial dorsal cutaneous nerve of superficial fibular nerve

Tendon of tibialis anterior

Tendon of extensor digitorum longus

Extensor hallucis brevis

Deep fibular nerve

Tendon of extensor hallucis longus

Proper dorsal digital branch of deep fibular nerve

interossei only need to adduct the third, fourth, and fifth toes toward the second toe. The big toe has its own adductor. The second toe has two dorsal interossei, one on each side, reflecting its role as the longitudinal axis. Then the third and fourth toes each have a dorsal interosseous muscle on their lateral sides. These muscles abduct the toes.

There are two intrinsic muscles on the dorsum of the foot. They are the *extensor digitorum brevis* and the *extensor hallucis brevis* (Fig. 8-44). There is no extensor digitorum brevis muscle to the fifth toe. These muscles assist the long muscles of the anterior compartment of the leg and have the same innervation—the deep fibular (peroneal) nerve.

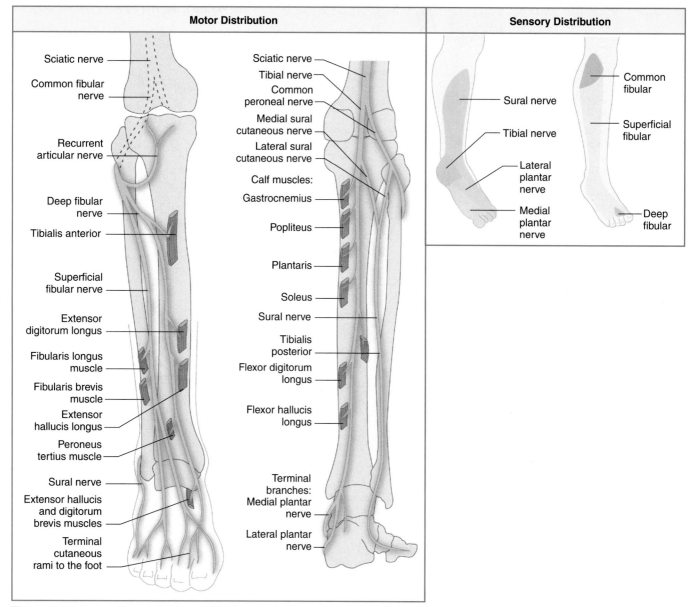

Figure 8-45. Innervation of the leg and foot.

Innervation of the Foot

The innervation to the plantar surface of the foot is from the tibial nerve (Figs. 8-45 and 8-46). The tibial nerve reaches the foot by passing around the medial malleolus with the long tendons from the posterior compartment of the leg. As the nerve passes through the tunnel, it gives rise to medial calcaneal branches, which supply the heel. The tibial nerve then separates into a medial plantar nerve and a lateral plantar nerve.

The medial plantar nerve supplies all the muscles that move the big toe, except the adductor hallucis, as well as the flexor digitorum brevis and the first lumbrical muscle. Its cutaneous supply is analogous to that of the median nerve in the pronated hand. Thus, it supplies the medial three and one-half toes starting with the great toe. This supply is also extended to the dorsal surface over the distal and middle phalanges (see Fig. 8-46).

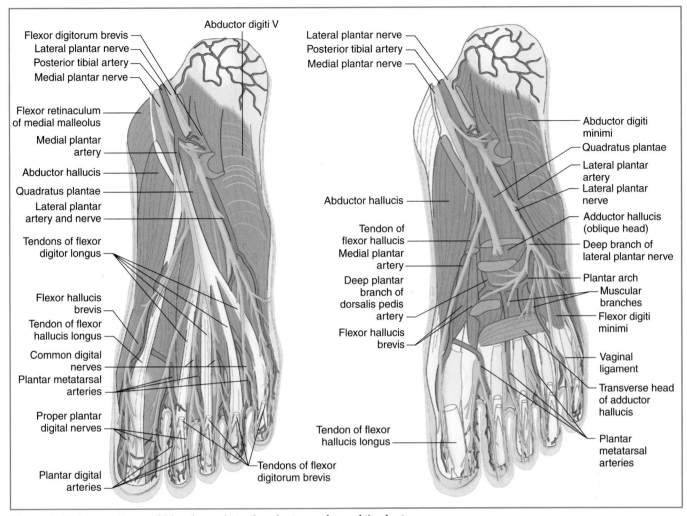

Figure 8-46. Innervation and blood supply to the plantar surface of the foot.

The lateral plantar nerve supplies motor innervation to the rest of the intrinsic muscles. Its cutaneous distribution is analogous to that of the ulnar nerve in the pronated hand. Thus, it supplies the lateral one-half of the fourth toe and the little toe along with the adjacent plantar surface of the foot. Both nerves travel in the plane of the second layer of muscles.

Blood Supply to the Foot

The blood supply to the foot is from the posterior tibial artery and dorsal pedis arteries (Fig. 8-47; see also Fig. 8-46). The posterior tibial artery runs with the tibial nerve posteriorly to the medial malleolus. It is possible to find the pulse of the posterior tibial artery by palpating midway between the medial malleolus and the heel. Then the posterior tibial artery gives rise to a small medial and a larger lateral plantar artery, which will run with the medial and plantar nerves in

the second layer of intrinsic muscles (see Figs. 8-41 and 8-46). The lateral plantar artery traverses the sole of the foot between the flexor digitorum brevis and quadratus plantae muscles to the lateral aspect where it then forms the plantar arch, which runs along the bases of the metatarsals to join the deep branch of the dorsalis pedis artery that reaches the sole of the foot between the first and second metatarsal. The plantar arch gives rise to plantar metatarsal arteries, which in turn give rise to digital branches on the sides of the toes. The medial plantar artery supplies the medial side of the plantar surface of the foot and anastomoses with dorsal metatarsal artery from the dorsalis pedis.

●●● SUMMARY

The lower limb receives most of its innervation from branches of the lumbar and sacral plexuses. The typical pattern of

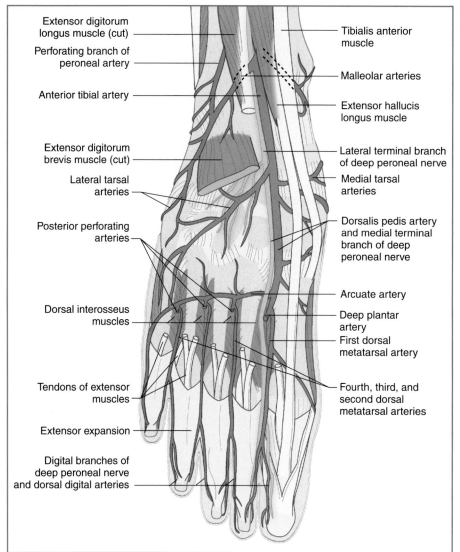

Extensor digitorum longus muscle (cut)

Perforating branch of peroneal artery

Anterior tibial artery

Extensor digitorum brevis muscle (cut)

Lateral tarsal arteries

Posterior perforating arteries

Dorsal interosseus muscles

Tendons of extensor muscles

Extensor expansion

Digital branches of deep peroneal nerve and dorsal digital arteries

Tibialis anterior muscle

Malleolar arteries

Extensor hallucis longus muscle

Lateral terminal branch of deep peroneal nerve

Medial tarsal arteries

Dorsalis pedis artery and medial terminal branch of deep peroneal nerve

Arcuate artery

Deep plantar artery

First dorsal metatarsal artery

Fourth, third, and second dorsal metatarsal arteries

Figure 8-47. Blood supply to the dorsal surface of the foot.

innervation of the skin of the lower extremity has been determined from studies of spinal nerve injuries. In addition, it is possible to assign spinal cord levels to various movements of the lower limb from similar studies. However, it is important to keep in mind that most of the limb muscles have two or more spinal cord segments represented in their innervation. Therefore, complete loss of movement occurs only if multiple spinal nerves are affected or there is a spinal cord injury. If the roots of one spinal nerve are involved, then the motor deficit may be only weakness. However, a single spinal nerve can be the major innervation to a muscle, and its loss can result in paralysis. If a nerve is damaged, then the weakness and paralysis can be followed by atrophy.

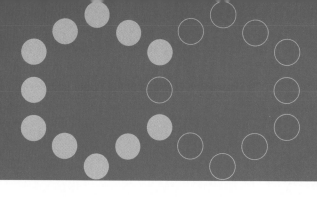

Upper Limb

9

CONTENTS

OVERVIEW

BRACHIAL PLEXUS
Branches from the Roots
Branches of the Trunks
Branches from the Cords

SHOULDER REGION
Bones
Sternoclavicular Joint
Acromioclavicular Joint
Glenohumeral Joint
Axilla
Chest Muscles That Move the Shoulder
Back Muscles That Move the Shoulder
Intrinsic Muscles of the Shoulder
Innervation to the Shoulder Region
Blood Supply to the Shoulder Region

ARM, ELBOW JOINT, AND CUBITAL FOSSA
Bones
Movements at the Elbow Joint
Muscles of the Arm
Innervation of the Arm
Blood Supply to the Arm
Cubital Fossa

FOREARM
Bones of the Forearm and Hand
Flexor Compartment of the Forearm
Extensor Compartment of the Forearm
Innervation of the Forearm
Blood Supply to the Forearm
Carpal Tunnel
Anatomic Snuffbox
Wrist Joint

HAND
Overview of the Hand
Fascia of the Hand
Muscles of the Hand
Innervation of the Hand
Blood Supply to the Hand

●●● OVERVIEW

The upper limb can be divided into the following regions: shoulder and axilla, arm (between the shoulder and elbow joint) and elbow joint, forearm (between the elbow and wrist) and wrist, and hand (Fig. 9-1). All the upper limb innervation is derived from the brachial plexus, which is formed from the ventral rami of cervical spinal nerves 5, 6, 7, and 8 (C5–C8) and the first thoracic spinal nerve (T1). In contrast to the lower limb, where mobility is sacrificed for stability, the upper limb is organized to promote mobility. Therefore, the joints in the upper limb involve bones that do not fit as well together as those in the lower limb. The integrity of the upper limb joints is dependent on the supporting ligaments and most importantly the actions of the muscles. The blood supply for the upper limb is derived from the subclavian artery. As the subclavian artery passes laterally to the first rib, its name changes to the axillary artery.

●●● BRACHIAL PLEXUS

The brachial plexus originates from the ventral rami of cervical spinal nerves 5, 6, 7, and 8 and the first thoracic spinal nerve (C5–C8 and T1). The functional fibers in these nerves are general somatic afferent (GSA), general somatic efferent (GSE), and postganglionic sympathetic fibers. The cell bodies of the GSE fibers are located in the ventral horn nuclei of spinal cord segments C5–C8 and T1. The cell bodies of the GSA fibers are located in the dorsal root ganglia associated with these spinal cord segments (see Chapter 2). GSA fibers provide cutaneous sensations such as pain, touch, temperature from the skin and dermis, as well as deep sensation (proprioception) from the skeletal muscle, tendons, and joints.

The cell bodies of the preganglionic sympathetic fibers for the upper limb are located in the lateral horn of spinal cord levels T3–T6. The cell bodies of the postganglionic sympathetic fibers for the brachial plexus are found in the middle and inferior cervical and the first thoracic sympathetic ganglia. Often the inferior cervical and first thoracic sympathetic ganglia are joined into the cervicothoracic (stellate) ganglion. Each ventral ramus that contributes to the roots of the brachial plexus receives postganglionic sympathetic fibers from the middle cervical or cervicothoracic ganglia via gray

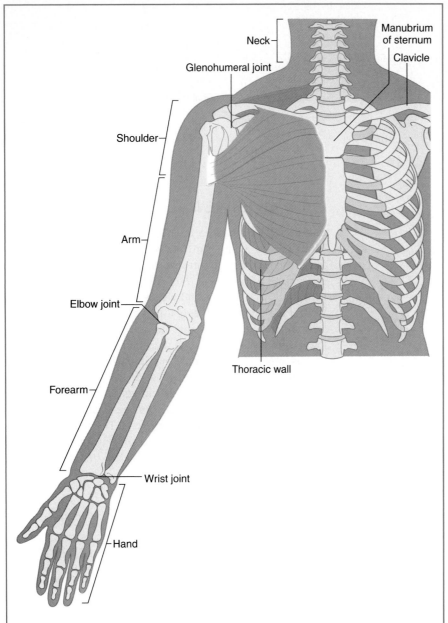

Figure 9-1. Regions of the upper limb.

rami communicantes. There are no parasympathetic fibers in the limbs.

The basic scheme of the brachial plexus (Fig. 9-2) consists of roots (ventral rami) that form trunks that divide into anterior and posterior divisions, which in turn form cords that end as terminal branches. Other branches arise directly from the roots, trunks, and cords.

The ventral rami of C5–C8 and T1 spinal nerves form the roots of the brachial plexus. This terminology can be confusing, since the term root can describe two different structures. The spinal cord's dorsal and ventral roots carry sensory and motor fibers, respectively. These roots come together to form a spinal nerve, which then divides into ventral and dorsal rami. On the other hand, the roots of the brachial plexus are the ventral rami of the C5–C8 and T1

spinal nerves. Here, the term root means the beginning portion of the plexus.

Because of the curvature of the cervical vertebral column, the spinal canal and the roots of the brachial plexus are located anteriorly in the neck. The transverse processes are palpable in the anterior neck and can be used as landmarks in locating the respective intervertebral foramina and spinal nerves. The trunks emerge between the anterior and middle scalene muscles. These muscles along with the first rib form the interscalene (scalene) triangle.

The trunks (see Fig. 9-2) are arranged from superior to inferior and are named accordingly upper, middle, and lower (superior, middle, and inferior) trunks. The ventral rami of the fifth and sixth cervical spinal nerves are the roots that unite to form the upper, or superior, trunk. The ventral ramus of the

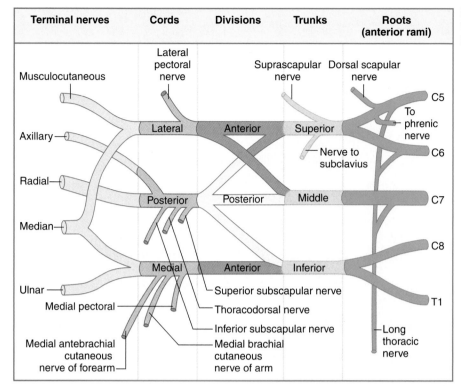

Terminal nerves	Cords	Divisions	Trunks	Roots (anterior rami)

Musculocutaneous

Lateral pectoral nerve

Suprascapular nerve

Dorsal scapular nerve

C5

To phrenic nerve

Lateral — Anterior — Superior

Axillary

Nerve to subclavius

C6

Radial

Posterior — Posterior — Middle

C7

Median

C8

Medial — Anterior — Inferior

Ulnar

Superior subscapular nerve

Thoracodorsal nerve

Medial pectoral

Inferior subscapular nerve

T1

Medial antebrachial cutaneous nerve of forearm

Medial brachial cutaneous nerve of arm

Long thoracic nerve

A

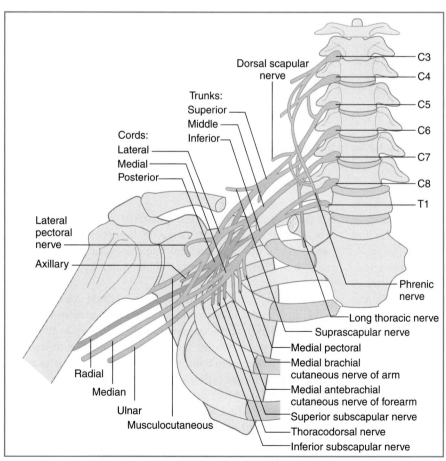

Dorsal scapular nerve

C3
C4
C5
C6
C7
C8
T1

Trunks:
Superior
Middle
Inferior

Cords:
Lateral
Medial
Posterior

Lateral pectoral nerve

Axillary

Phrenic nerve

Long thoracic nerve
Suprascapular nerve
Medial pectoral
Medial brachial cutaneous nerve of arm
Medial antebrachial cutaneous nerve of forearm
Superior subscapular nerve
Thoracodorsal nerve
Inferior subscapular nerve

Radial

Median

Ulnar

Musculocutaneous

B

Figure 9-2. A, Schematic representation of the brachial plexus. **B,** The brachial plexus in situ.

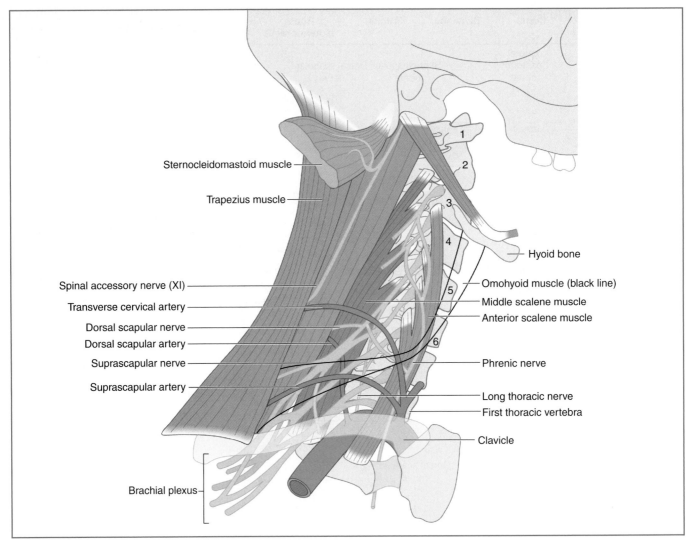

Figure 9-3. Posterior triangle of the neck demonstrating trunks of the brachial plexus emerging from the interscalene (scalene) triangle.

seventh cervical nerve continues as the root of the middle trunk, and the ventral rami of the eighth cervical and the first thoracic spinal nerves are the roots that form the lower, or inferior, trunk. Not all of the first thoracic spinal nerve's ventral ramus participates in the formation of the lower trunk. A small branch of the first thoracic nerve's ventral ramus forms the first intercostal nerve. The first thoracic ventral ramus must run superiorly to cross the first rib to help form the inferior trunk. As it does so, this ventral ramus is vulnerable to compression or avulsion (tearing away) injuries.

In a small percentage of the population there is some variation in the formation of the brachial plexus. A prefixed plexus has a significant contribution from the fourth cervical spinal nerve and a postfixed plexus has a significant contribution from the T2 spinal nerve.

Each trunk has anterior and posterior divisions. The anterior divisions of the upper and middle trunk unite to produce the lateral cord. The anterior division of the lower trunk continues as the medial cord, and all three posterior

divisions contribute to the posterior cord (see Fig. 9-2). Functionally, the anterior division branches supply flexors, whereas the posterior division branches usually supply extensors. However, some muscles innervated by the posterior divisions can be flexors.

The upper trunk is formed at the lateral margin of the anterior scalene muscle while the middle and lower trunks are formed in the interscalene triangle (Fig. 9-3). In the posterior triangle of the neck, the trunks lie posterior to the inferior belly of the omohyoid muscle. The divisions arise in the neck and then pass through the cervicoaxillary canal (or costoclavicular space) into the axilla. The boundaries of the cervicoaxillary canal are the superior margin of the scapula, the middle third of the clavicle, and the first rib. The middle third of the clavicle lies just medial to the coracoid process of the scapula. Therefore, the divisions and cords of the plexus are in jeopardy when there is a fracture of the clavicle.

As the cords initially enter the upper axilla, the lateral cord lies lateral to the axillary artery while the medial and posterior cords are deep (posterior) to the artery. As the artery and cords descend posteriorly to the pectoralis minor muscle, the cords take positions that correspond to their names.

Branches from the plexus can be described as either supraclavicular or infraclavicular based on their relation to the clavicle. The supraclavicular branches arise from the roots and trunks, while infraclavicular branches include the cords and their branches.

Branches from the Roots

Two nerves arise directly from the roots: the dorsal scapular nerve and the long thoracic nerve (nerve to the serratus anterior; see Fig. 9-2). The dorsal scapular nerve is the only brachial plexus nerve derived from a single root, C5. It emerges from the middle scalene muscle and passes along the deep (anterior) surface of the levator scapulae to supply the rhomboid muscles and often the levator scapulae.

The long thoracic nerve arises from the roots C5, C6, and C7. It runs deep (posteriorly) to the plexus within the middle scalene muscle to reach the superficial surface of the serratus anterior, which it supplies. This is unusual because nerves typically innervate muscles from their deep surface.

Branches of the Trunks

The upper trunk has two branches: the nerve to the subclavius and the suprascapular nerve. The other trunks do *not* have branches except for their terminal branches, the anterior and posterior divisions.

The nerve to the subclavius (C5 and C6) runs anteriorly to the plexus to supply the subclavius muscle. The suprascapular nerve arises at the union of C5 and C6. This nerve innervates the supraspinatus and infraspinatus muscles.

Branches from the Cords

Lateral Cord

The lateral cord receives fibers from the anterior divisions of the upper and middle trunks and contains fibers from C5, C6, and C7 (see Fig. 9-2). The lateral cord gives rise to the lateral pectoral nerve, which supplies the clavicular head of the pectoralis major. A nerve loop crosses the axillary vessels to connect the lateral pectoral nerve with the medial pectoral nerve.

The terminal branches of the lateral cord include the musculocutaneous nerve (C5, C6, and C7) and the lateral root of the median nerve (C6 and C7). The musculocutaneous nerve pierces the coracobrachialis muscle about an inch and a half below the muscle's origin on the coracoid process. This nerve passes between the biceps brachii and the brachialis muscles to end as the lateral antebrachial cutaneous nerve. The musculocutaneous nerve innervates all the muscles of the anterior compartment of the arm: biceps brachii, coracobrachialis muscle, and most of the brachialis muscle.

The lateral antebrachial cutaneous nerve penetrates the deep fascia just lateral to the biceps tendon. It continues down the radial (lateral) side of the forearm to supply cutaneous innervation to the anterolateral and posterolateral aspects of the forearm. Injury to the musculocutaneous nerve produces marked weakness or loss of elbow flexion, weakness of shoulder flexion, weakness of forearm supination, and sensory deficits in the distribution of the lateral antebrachial cutaneous nerve (C6 dermatome).

Medial Cord

The medial cord receives fibers only from the anterior division of the lower trunk and contains fibers from C8 and T1 (see Fig. 9-2). Sometimes the lateral cord sends a branch with fibers from C7 to join the ulnar nerve in some individuals. High in the axilla, the medial cord gives rise to the medial pectoral nerve, which receives fibers from C8 and T1. This nerve passes between the axillary vessels to reach the deep surface of the pectoralis minor and joins with a branch from the lateral pectoral nerve to supply this muscle. Some fibers pass through or along the lateral border of the pectoralis minor to reach the pectoralis major's sternal portion.

The terminal branches of the medial cord from lateral to medial are the medial head of the median nerve, ulnar nerve, medial antebrachial cutaneous nerve, and medial brachial cutaneous nerve (see Fig. 9-2). The median nerve arises from branches from both lateral and medial cords and therefore receives fibers from (C5)C6–T1.

Posterior Cord

The posterior cord is formed by the three posterior divisions and contains contributions from all of the roots of the brachial plexus. The three branches that arise from the posterior cord are the upper subscapular nerve (C5 and C6) to the

CLINICAL MEDICINE

Lower Brachial Plexus Injury

A lower brachial plexus injury (Klumpke's palsy) involves ventral rami C8–T1 and results from a forceful abduction of the shoulder that places undue traction on the roots of the lower trunk. The T1 root (ventral ramus) is especially vulnerable because of the angle that it makes as it passes superiorly to the first rib to help form the lower (inferior) trunk. A lower plexus injury involves the distribution of C8 and T1 fibers in the lower trunk to both the medial and posterior cords. Therefore, all muscles that receive innervation from C8 and T1 would be affected regardless of the nerve that carries these fibers. The resulting loss would include an adductor of the shoulder, all of the finger flexors including all of the deep flexors, wrist flexors, and all the intrinsic muscles in the hand. Therefore, both the medial and lateral portions of the flexor digitorum profundus would be affected, as would all the lumbricals. These muscles all receive C8 and T1 fibers that run in both ulnar and median nerves. For the same reason, all intrinsic hand muscles would be affected. The patient would have sensory losses over the medial side of the forearm and hand.

subscapularis, the thoracodorsal nerve (C5–C7) to the latissimus dorsi, and the lower subscapular nerve (C5 and C6) to the subscapularis and the teres major muscles (see Fig. 9-2).

● ● ● SHOULDER REGION

The shoulder is capable of a wide degree of movement. Movement of the shoulder actually occurs through movement at four separate joints: sternoclavicular, acromioclavicular, glenohumeral, and costoscapular. The muscles that act on the shoulder joint include chest muscles, back muscles, and arm muscles. Actions of the shoulder are flexion and extension, abduction and adduction, and medial and lateral rotation (Fig. 9-4). Most movements of the shoulder involve combinations of these movements.

Bones

Clavicle

The clavicle is a long bone, which is the only bony connection that the upper limb has to the axial skeleton (Fig. 9-5). It is responsible for keeping the arm at the side of the body. The clavicles are S-shaped with their medial end convex and their lateral end concave. They are the first bones to begin ossification in utero and the only bone of the upper limb to form through the process of intramembranous bone formation. The medial end of the clavicle is rounded, and the lateral end is flat. Its superior surface is smooth, and its inferior surface has three roughenings for the attachment of ligaments. The lateral two are called the conoid tubercle and the trapezoid tubercle. Medially there is one for the attachment of the sternoclavicular ligament.

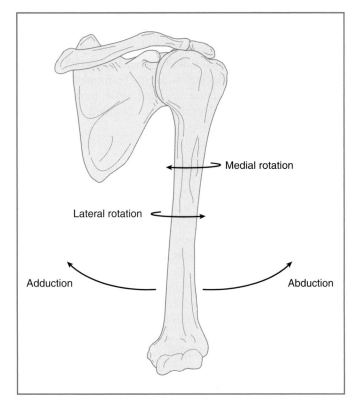

Figure 9-4. Movements of the shoulder.

Scapula

The scapula is a triangular shaped bone that articulates with the clavicle and the humerus (Fig. 9-6). Its anterior surface is concave and is called the *subscapular fossa*. The posterior surface is convex and divided into two unequal parts by the

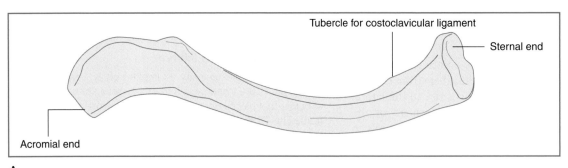

A

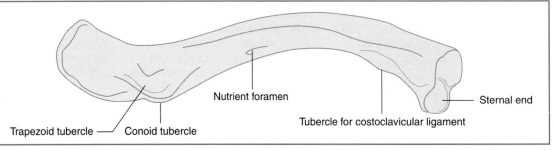

B

Figure 9-5. The right clavicle as seen from above (**A**) and below (**B**).

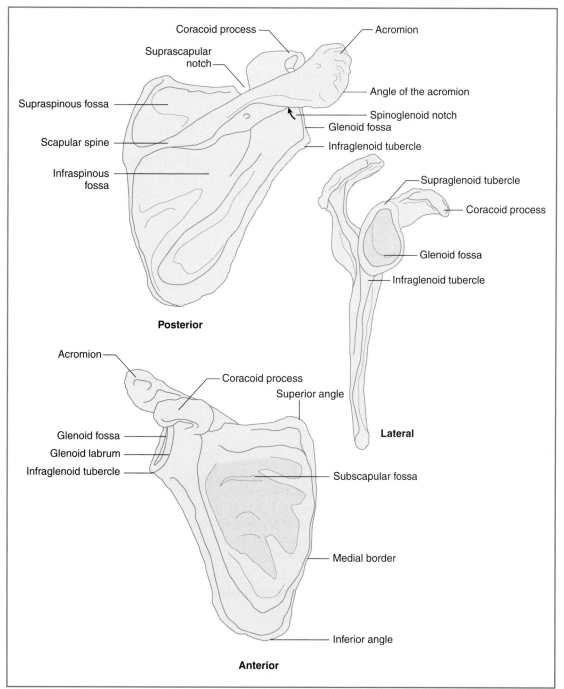

Figure 9-6. Anterior, lateral, and posterior views of the scapula.

HISTOLOGY

Intramembranous Bone Formation

Bones form through either endochondral or intramembranous bone formation. In intramembranous bone formation, mesenchymal cells differentiate into osteoblasts, which synthesize and secrete osteoid, the bone matrix. The osteoblasts become surrounded by the osteoid, which mineralizes, and they are then known as osteocytes. Bone can only grow appositionally. In this way, the bone spicule continues to grow, with concomitant osteoclast activity.

spine of the scapula. The two resulting divisions are called the *supraspinous fossa* and the *infraspinous fossa*, located superior and inferior to the scapular spine, respectively. The scapular spine extends from the medial side of the scapula laterally and makes a sharp turn anteriorly to end as the acromion. The sharp turn anteriorly is called the *angle of the acromion* (tip of shoulder). At the lateral end of the attachment of the scapular spine to the scapula is a connection between the supraspinous fossa and the infraspinous fossa called the *spinoglenoid (great scapular) notch*. It is a passageway for neurovascular structures on the posterior surface of the scapula.

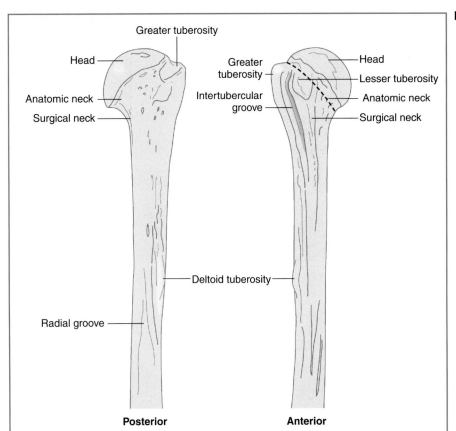

Figure 9-7. Proximal end of the humerus.

The superior border of the scapula has a notch, the *suprascapular notch*, which is converted to a foramen by the addition of the superior transverse scapular ligament. Just lateral to the notch is a bony extension called the coracoid (Latin, "crow's beak") process. The *coracoid process* is palpable just inferior to the lateral end of the clavicle. Three muscles of the arm attach to the coracoid process. Surgeons call it the "lighthouse" of the shoulder because it serves as a landmark to avoid the major neurovascular structures entering the upper limb. Surgical approach to the shoulder region always takes place lateral to the coracoid process.

The superior and inferior angles of the scapula lie at the second and seventh ribs in the anatomic position. The lateral angle is expanded to form the glenoid fossa for articulation of the humerus. The glenoid fossa is slightly deepened by the attachment of a fibrocartilaginous rim called the *glenoid labrum*. There are two bony extensions on the superior and the inferior aspect of the glenoid fossa, called the *supraglenoid and infraglenoid tubercles*.

Proximal Humerus

The proximal humerus has an expanded round end called the *head of the humerus* (Fig. 9-7). The head of the humerus ends at the *anatomic neck*. Then the bone becomes narrower, forming the surgical neck. The *surgical neck* is so-named because many fractures of the humerus occur in this region. The proximal humerus has two bony protuberances. The *lesser tubercle* on the medial side of the anterior surface is separated from the larger laterally placed *greater tubercle* by a groove known as the *intertubercular (bicipital) groove*. There is a tuberosity on the lateral side of the humerus about a third of the way down the humeral shaft called the *deltoid tuberosity*. The posterior surface of the proximal end of the humerus has an oblique depression called the *radial groove*.

Sternoclavicular Joint

The sternoclavicular joint is located between the medial end of the clavicle and the manubrium of the sternum (Fig. 9-8). It is the site of the only bony articulation between the upper limb and the axial skeleton. It is an ill-fitting synovial joint, which is stabilized by a number of ligaments. The *anterior and posterior sternoclavicular ligaments*, which pass from the clavicle to the sternum in an inferomedial direction, resist the upward and lateral movements of the medial end of clavicle. The *costoclavicular ligament*, which connects the clavicle to the first rib, also resists dislocation of this joint. Lastly, the *interclavicular ligament* connects the two medial ends of the clavicles.

Acromioclavicular Joint

The acromioclavicular joint is the articulation between the acromion of the scapula and the lateral end of the clavicle (see Fig. 9-8). It allows the clavicle to override the acromion, thereby giving the shoulder added mobility. The articular

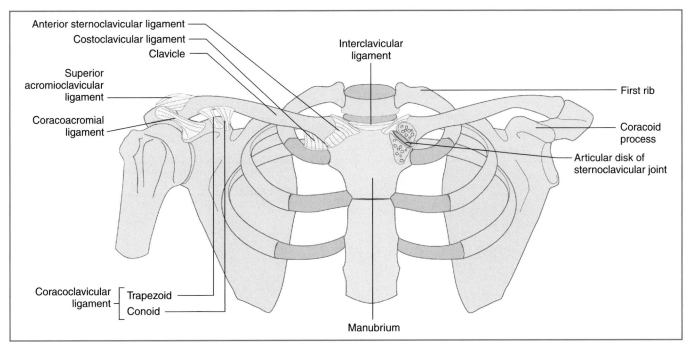

Figure 9-8. Sternoclavicular and acromioclavicular joints (anterior view).

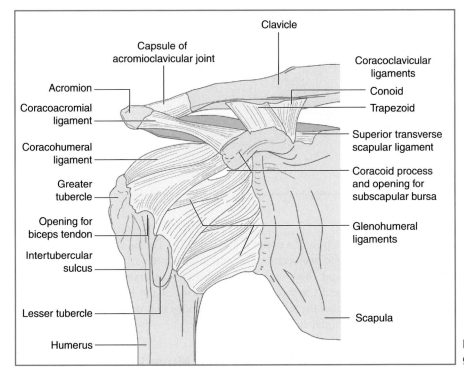

Figure 9-9. Acromioclavicular and glenohumeral joints.

capsule of this joint is quite loose to allow the overriding. To maintain its integrity, it relies on a very strong two-part ligament known as the *coracoclavicular ligament* (see Fig. 9-8). The medial portion is called the conoid ligament, and the lateral portion is the trapezoid ligament. Disruption of this ligament is called a "shoulder separation" and occurs commonly in players of contact sports like ice hockey and football.

Glenohumeral Joint

The glenohumeral joint is the articulation between the head of the humerus and the glenoid fossa of the scapula (Fig. 9-9). In describing this articulation, it would be more accurate to say that the head of the humerus articulates *against* the glenoid fossa, not within it. Although this joint has ligamentous

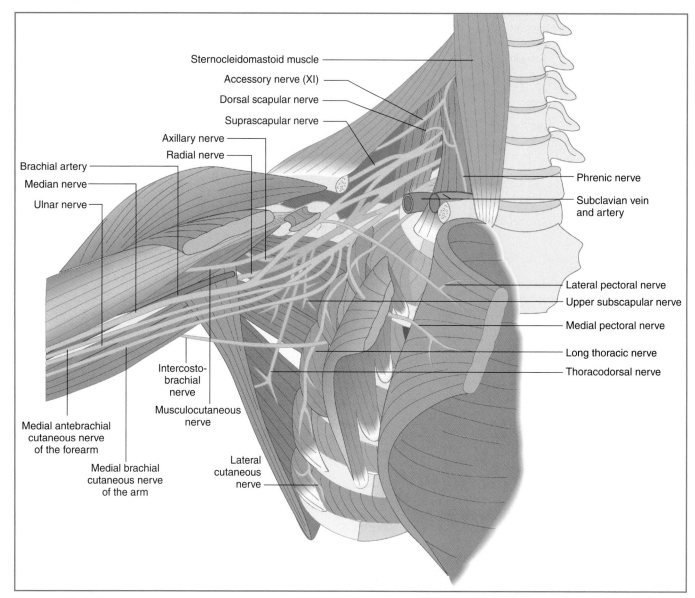

Figure 9-10. Axilla.

support, muscle action is the main force that keeps the joint intact. The articular capsule is approximately three times larger than the joint cavity to ensure maximum mobility. The capsule is reinforced by three glenohumeral ligaments: superior, middle, and inferior. There are two additional ligaments: the coracoacromial and the coracohumeral. The *coracoacromial ligament* attaches to the coracoid process and the acromion, parts of the same bone, and therefore does not hold two bones together but rather acts to resist the upward movement of the head of the humerus. The *coracohumeral ligament* attaches to the head of the humerus and the coracoid process and resists the downward movement of the head of the humerus when the upper limb is hanging at rest.

Axilla

The axilla is the pyramid-shaped passageway between the neck and the upper limb for the neurovascular bundles that supply the upper limb (Fig. 9-10). The borders of the axilla are the pectoralis major and minor anteriorly, the latissimus dorsi and teres major posteriorly, the serratus anterior medially, and the intertubercular groove of the humerus laterally. It is also the site of the lymph nodes that drain the breast and the upper limb.

Chest Muscles That Move the Shoulder

Four muscles arise in the pectoral region and insert on bones of the upper limb: pectoralis minor and major, subclavius, and serratus anterior. The *pectoralis major* is the most superficial muscle of the chest region. It has two heads, a clavicular head and a sternocostal head, which are innervated by two different nerves and have different functions (Fig. 9-11 and Table 9-1). The *pectoralis minor* is found directly deep to the pectoralis major. The pectoralis minor arises from the surface of ribs 3–5 and inserts into the coracoid process.

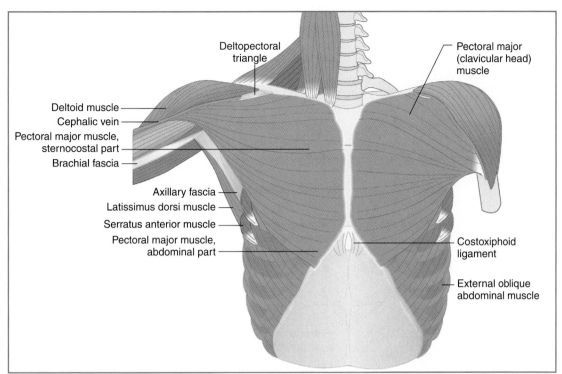

A

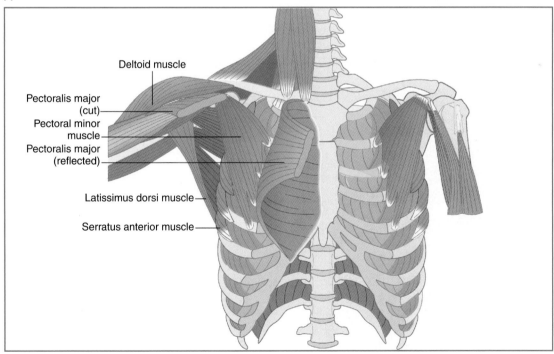

B

Figure 9-11.
Pectoralis major (**A**) and pectoralis minor (**B**).

Labels for A:
- Deltopectoral triangle
- Deltoid muscle
- Cephalic vein
- Pectoral major muscle, sternocostal part
- Brachial fascia
- Axillary fascia
- Latissimus dorsi muscle
- Serratus anterior muscle
- Pectoral major muscle, abdominal part
- Pectoral major (clavicular head) muscle
- Costoxiphoid ligament
- External oblique abdominal muscle

Labels for B:
- Deltoid muscle
- Pectoralis major (cut)
- Pectoral minor muscle
- Pectoralis major (reflected)
- Latissimus dorsi muscle
- Serratus anterior muscle

The pectoralis minor muscle crosses the axillary artery and divides it into three portions.

The *subclavius* is a small muscle found on the undersurface of the clavicle (see Table 9-1). Because it attaches to the first rib and the clavicle, it is able to depress and rotate the clavicle. In a fracture of the clavicle, it may also provide some protection for the subclavian vessels against damage.

The *serratus anterior muscle* is a large muscle that arises from the external surface of the lower ribs and inserts on the medial border of the anterior aspect of the scapula (Fig. 9-12; see also Table 9-1). However, the insertion is not uniform. The larger four inferior segments insert into the inferior angle, and therefore when the muscle contracts, it rotates the scapula laterally, thereby moving the glenoid fossa laterally and superiorly.

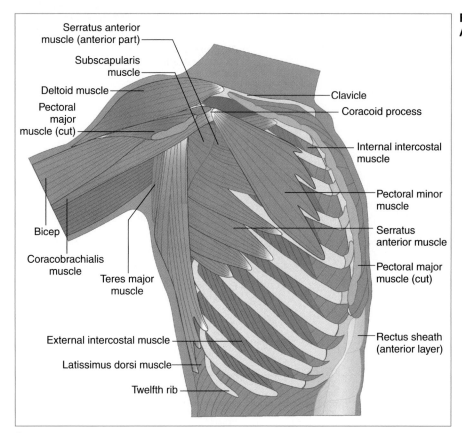

Serratus anterior muscle (anterior part)

Subscapularis muscle

Deltoid muscle

Pectoral major muscle (cut)

Bicep

Coracobrachialis muscle

Teres major muscle

External intercostal muscle

Latissimus dorsi muscle

Twelfth rib

Clavicle

Coracoid process

Internal intercostal muscle

Pectoral minor muscle

Serratus anterior muscle

Pectoral major muscle (cut)

Rectus sheath (anterior layer)

A

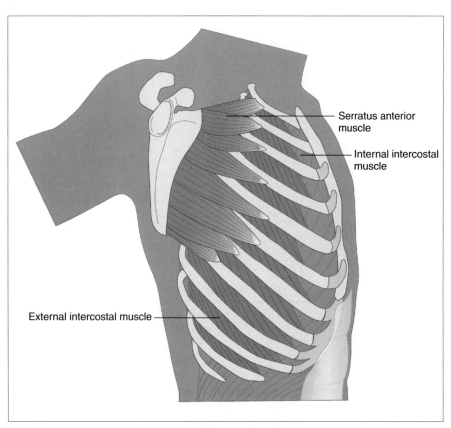

Serratus anterior muscle

Internal intercostal muscle

External intercostal muscle

B

Figure 9-12. Serratus anterior. **A,** Superficial view. **B,** Deep view.

TABLE 9-1. Muscles of the Pectoral Region

Muscle	Origin	Insertion	Principal Function	Innervation
Pectoralis major, clavicular head	Anterior surface of medial end of clavicle	Lateral lip of intertubercular groove	Flexion and adduction of shoulder	Lateral pectoral nerve (C5–C7)
Pectoralis major, sternocostal head	Anterior surface of sternum, superior six costal cartilages, and aponeurosis of external oblique muscle	Lateral lip of intertubercular groove	Extension and adduction of shoulder	Medial pectoral nerve (C8, T1)
Pectoralis minor	Medial end of third to fifth ribs	Coracoid process of scapula	Protraction of depression of scapula	Medial pectoral nerve (C8, T1)
Subclavius	Junction of first rib and its costal cartilage	Inferior surface of middle third of clavicle	Depression of clavicle	Nerve to the subclavius (C5, C6)
Serratus anterior	External surface of first through eighth ribs	Anterior surface of medial border of scapula	Protraction (upper portion) and rotation of scapula (lower portion)	Long thoracic nerve (C5–C7)

TABLE 9-2. Back Muscles That Act on the Shoulder Joint

Muscle	Origin	Insertion	Principal Function	Innervation
Trapezius	External occipital protuberance, ligamentum nuchae, and spinous processes of C7 and all thoracic vertebrae	Lateral third of clavicle, acromion, and scapular spine	Rotation of scapula superiorly, elevation of scapula, depression of scapula, and retraction of scapula	Spinal accessory nerve (XI) and cervical plexus
Rhomboideus major	Spinous processes of T2–T5	Medial border of scapula	Elevation and retraction of scapula and rotation of glenoid cavity downward	Dorsal scapular nerve (C5)
Rhomboideus minor	Ligamentum nuchae and spinous processes of C7 and T1	Medial border of scapula superior to the rhomboideus major	Elevation and retraction of scapula and rotation of glenoid cavity downward	Dorsal scapular nerve (C5)
Levator scapula	Transverse processes of C1–C4	Superior angle and upper portion of medial border of scapula	Elevation of scapula	Dorsal scapular nerve and C3 and C4
Latissimus dorsi	Spinous processes of lower six thoracic vertebrae, all lumbar and all sacral vertebrae, and posterior iliac crest and inferior angle of scapula	Medial lip of intertuburcular groove	Adduction, extension, and medial rotation of humerus	Thoracodorsal nerve (C7, C8, T1)

Thus, this movement is important for allowing the upper limb to be raised above the shoulder. The serratus anterior also stabilizes the scapula against the thoracic wall when a person throws a punch or pushes a heavy object. This muscle, with the help of the back muscles described below, forms the costoscapular joint.

Back Muscles That Move the Shoulder

The trapezius has an extensive origin from the back above and below the shoulder region and also inserts anteriorly, laterally, and posteriorly to the shoulder region (Fig. 9-13 and Table 9-2). Therefore, it has several different actions with respect to the shoulder joint. The superior fibers that insert on the clavicle, the acromion, and the spine of the scapula assist in elevation of the glenoid fossa during abduction. They are assisted by the inferior fibers of the trapezius that insert on the base of the scapular spine. The inferior fibers working alone are able to pull the scapula inferiorly. The superior fibers are the only fibers that can elevate the point of the shoulder. The trapezius typically receives motor innervation from the

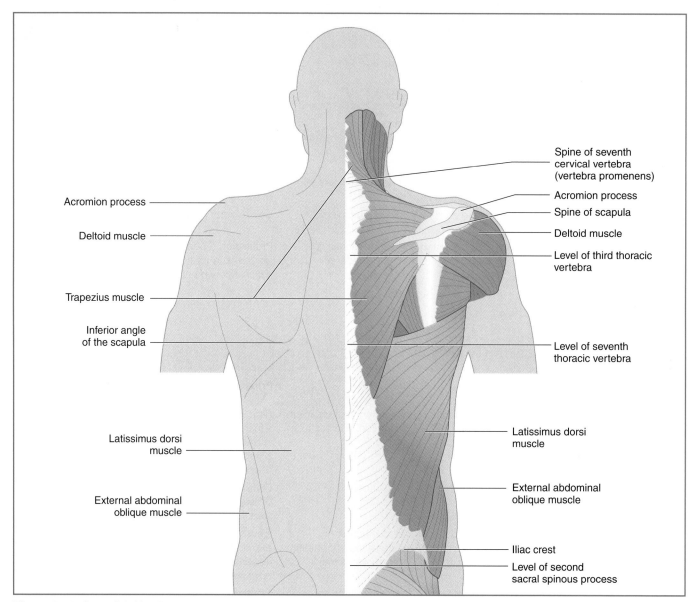

Acromion process

Deltoid muscle

Trapezius muscle

Inferior angle
of the scapula

Latissimus dorsi
muscle

External abdominal
oblique muscle

Spine of seventh
cervical vertebra
(vertebra promenens)

Acromion process

Spine of scapula

Deltoid muscle

Level of third thoracic
vertebra

Level of seventh
thoracic vertebra

Latissimus dorsi
muscle

External abdominal
oblique muscle

Iliac crest

Level of second
sacral spinous process

Figure 9-13. Superficial back muscles.

spinal accessory nerve and sensory innervation from the cervical plexus. However, about 30% of individuals also receive motor innervation from the cervical plexus.

The levator scapulae, rhomboideus minor, and rhomboideus major are back muscles that lie deep to the trapezius, and all insert in a continuous fashion on the medial border of the scapula and therefore participate in movements of the shoulder (Fig. 9-14; see also Table 9-2). They elevate the shoulder, retract the scapula, and assist in rotation of the scapula.

The levator scapulae is the most superior and the one that is most involved in elevating the shoulder. The rhomboideus minor and major are sometimes hard to differentiate from one another. The rhomboideus minor is the superior one of the two. Their major function is to retract the scapula to square the shoulders.

The latissimus dorsi muscle is a large muscle that connects the humerus to the axial skeleton (see Fig. 9-14 and Table 9-2).

It has an extensive origin from the lower six thoracic vertebrae, all the lumbar and the upper sacral vertebrae, and the iliac crest. Its tendon twists 180 degrees anteriorly before inserting on the anterior surface of the humerus. As it passes through the axilla, it forms the posterior axillary fold with the teres major muscle. Since it arises posteriorly and inserts anteriorly, it is a medial rotator of the humerus in addition to being a strong adductor and extensor of the arm.

Intrinsic Muscles of the Shoulder

The deltoid muscle covers the shoulder on three sides (Fig. 9-15 and Table 9-3). It originates approximately where the trapezius inserts. The muscle has three heads—anterior, lateral, and posterior—which each perform different functions owing to their unique relationships to the shoulder joint. The anterior fibers flex the shoulder joint, the lateral fibers

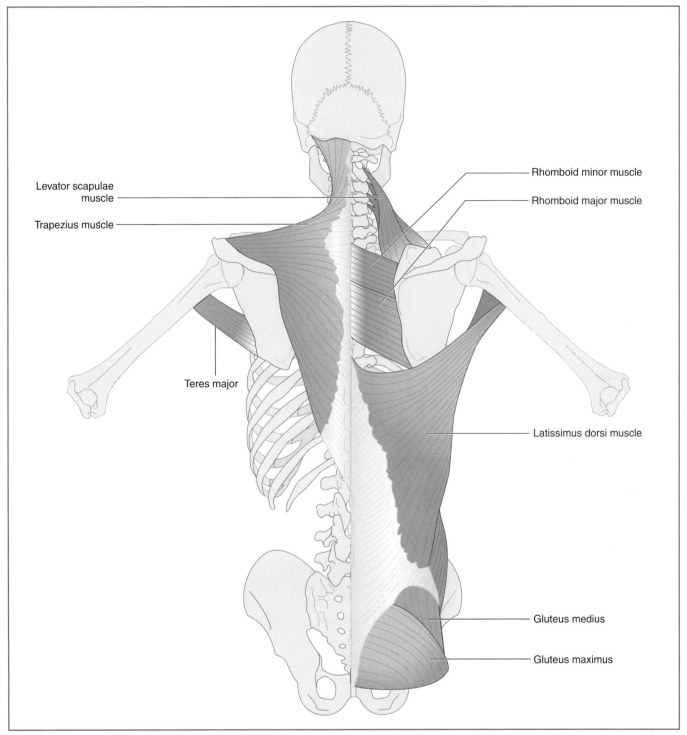

Levator scapulae muscle

Trapezius muscle

Teres major

Rhomboid minor muscle

Rhomboid major muscle

Latissimus dorsi muscle

Gluteus medius

Gluteus maximus

Figure 9-14. Levator scapulae, rhomboideus minor and major, and latissimus dorsi.

participate in abduction of the shoulder, and the posterior fibers extend the shoulder joint. When acting together, the deltoid is an abduction. The anterior head forms one side of the deltopectoral triangle with the clavicle and the clavicular head of the pectoralis major forming the other two borders (see Fig. 9-14). The cephalic vein runs in the deltopectoral triangle to drain into the subclavian vein.

There are four intrinsic muscles, which blend together with the articular capsule of the shoulder, forming a musculo-tendinous cuff. These four muscles—supraspinatus, infra-spinatus, teres minor, and subscapularis—are known as the *rotator cuff muscles* (Fig. 9-16). They are responsible for keeping the head of the humerus in the glenoid fossa during all movements.

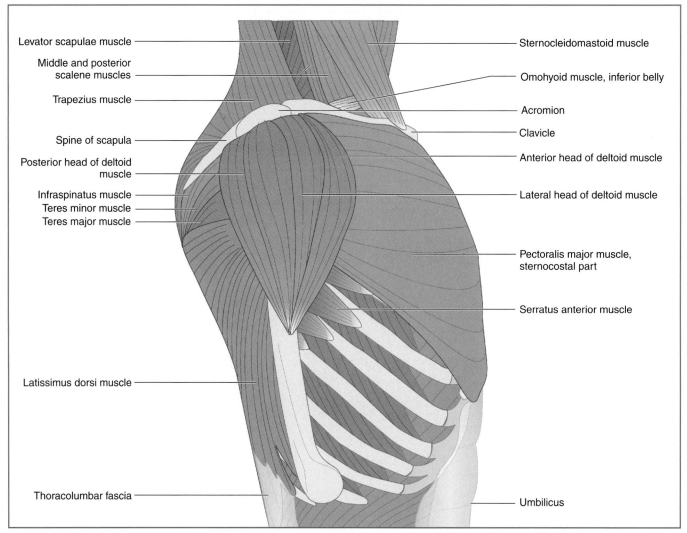

Levator scapulae muscle

Middle and posterior scalene muscles

Trapezius muscle

Spine of scapula

Posterior head of deltoid muscle

Infraspinatus muscle
Teres minor muscle
Teres major muscle

Latissimus dorsi muscle

Thoracolumbar fascia

Sternocleidomastoid muscle

Omohyoid muscle, inferior belly

Acromion

Clavicle

Anterior head of deltoid muscle

Lateral head of deltoid muscle

Pectoralis major muscle, sternocostal part

Serratus anterior muscle

Umbilicus

Figure 9-15. Deltoid muscle.

TABLE 9-3. Intrinsic Muscles of the Shoulder

Muscle	Origin	Insertion	Principal Function	Innervation
Deltoid	Lateral third of the clavicle, acromion, and spine of the scapula	Deltoid tuberosity of the humerus	Anterior portion—flexes shoulder Middle portion—abducts humerus Posterior portion—extends shoulder	Axillary nerve (C5, C6)
Subscapularis	Subscapular fossa	Lesser tubercle humerus	Medial rotation	Upper and lower sub-scapular nerves (C5–C7)
Supraspinatus	Supraspinous fossa	Upper portion of greater tubercle	Abduction of humerus	Suprascapular nerve (C5, C6)
Infraspinatus	Infraspinous fossa	Middle portion of posterior aspect of greater tubercle	Lateral rotation of humerus	Suprascapular nerve (C5, C6)
Teres minor	Lateral border of scapula inferior to glenoid fossa	Inferior portion of posterior aspect of greater tubercle	Lateral rotation of humerus	Axillary nerve (C5, C6)
Teres major	Lateral border of scapula inferior to teres minor	Medial lip of intertubercular groove	Medial rotation	Lower subscapular nerve (C6, C7)

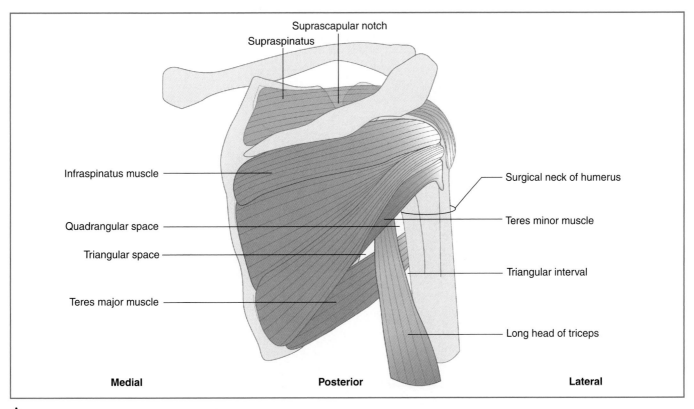

A

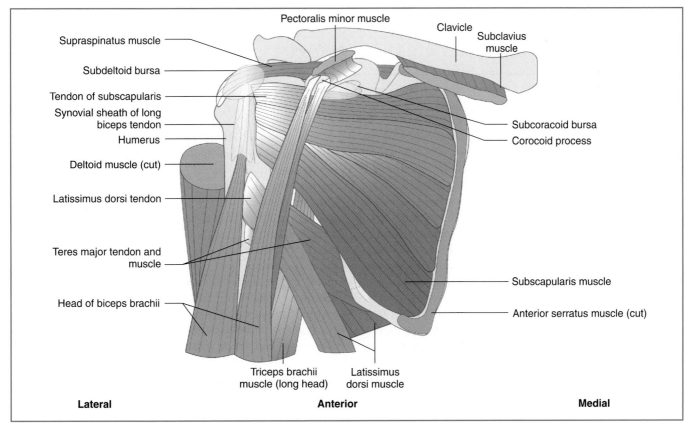

B

Figure 9-16. Rotator cuff muscles. **A,** Posterior view. **B,** Anterior view.

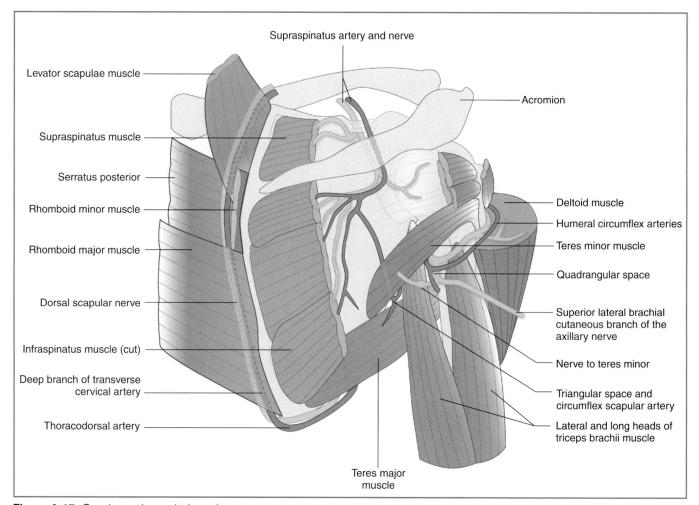

Figure 9-17. Quadrangular and triangular spaces.

The *supraspinatus muscle* arises in the supraspinous fossa of the scapula, and its tendon passes over the top of the head of the humerus to insert on the superior aspect of the greater tubercle of the humerus (see Fig. 10-16). It is responsible for the first 10 to 15 degrees of abduction of the arm. Its tendon is separated from the acromion of the scapula by an extension of the subdeltoid bursa called the *subacromial bursa*. A bursa is a connective tissue sac that is fluid-filled. Bursae are found in areas of potential friction between tendons and bones. They facilitate the smooth movement of the structures past one another.

The *infraspinatus muscle* is a large muscle that arises from the infraspinous fossa and inserts just below the supraspinatus muscle on the greater tubercle. Since it passes behind the humerus to insert, it is a lateral rotator of the humerus.

The *teres minor* is another lateral rotator of the humerus. It originates on the lateral border of the scapula, passes posteriorly to the shoulder, and inserts just below the infraspinatus muscle on the greater tubercle.

The last muscle in the group is the *subscapularis*. It arises on the anterior surface of the scapula and passes anteriorly to the humerus to insert on the lesser tubercle of the humerus; therefore, it is a medial rotator of the humerus.

There is one additional intrinsic muscle that is not considered a rotator cuff muscle—the teres major muscle. The *teres major* arises on the lateral border of the scapula just below the teres minor. It forms part of the posterior axillary fold with the latissimus dorsi, passes anterior to and inserts on the humerus to function as a medial rotator. It has several relationships with surrounding muscles that create anatomic spaces, which are useful in locating important neurovascular structures. It forms the inferior boundary of the quadrangular space and the triangular space (Fig. 9-17). The axillary nerve and the posterior humeral circumflex arteries pass through the quadrangular space. The circumflex scapular artery is associated with the triangular space. The teres major insertion also marks the transition between axilla and arm.

Innervation to the Shoulder Region

The shoulder region receives its innervation predominantly from spinal cord levels C5 and C6. Two nerves that supply the muscles of the shoulder region come directly from the roots of the plexus, the dorsal scapular and long thoracic nerves, which supply the levator scapulae (along with C3 and C4) and rhomboids, and the serratus anterior, respectively.

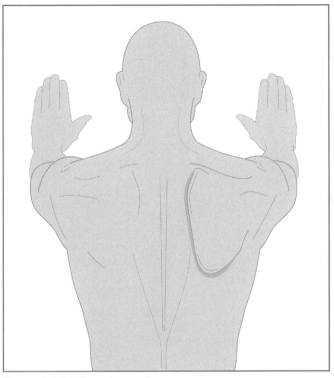

Figure 9-18. Winged scapula.

The nerve to the serratus anterior (long thoracic nerve) can be damaged by several circumstances such as a constant downward pulling on the shoulder produced by carrying a very heavy suitcase or backpack over time. In addition, the long thoracic nerve lies on the medial side of the axilla, where it could be placed in jeopardy during an axillary dissection for breast cancer or melanoma. Injury to the serratus anterior nerve can result in paralysis of the serratus anterior. The injured patient is not be able to abduct the arm above the level of the shoulder. In addition, when the patient pushes on a fixed object (such as a wall), the inferior angle of the scapula protrudes away from the posterior body wall (Fig. 9-18). This condition is referred to as winged scapula.

Two nerves that supply the shoulder region arise from the upper trunk: the suprascapular and the nerve to the subclavius. The suprascapular nerve runs parallel and deep to the clavicle and passes through the enclosed superior scapular notch to reach the supraspinatus muscle and then travels through the spinoglenoid notch to reach the infraspinatus muscle. If there is an injury to the suprascapular nerve due to entrapment in the enclosed suprascapular notch, then only the supraspinatus and infraspinatus muscles are affected. The clinical presentation is difficulty in initiating abduction and weakness of lateral rotation. However, there is no accompanying sensory loss.

The posterior cord gives rise to most of the nerves that supply the shoulder region. The upper and lower subscapular nerves arise on either side of the thoracodorsal nerve from the posterior cord. The upper and lower subscapular nerves both supply the subscapularis, and the lower subscapular nerve goes on to supply the teres major muscle. The thoracodorsal nerve travels with the lower subscapular and then supplies the latissimus dorsi muscle. The axillary nerve, one of the terminal branches of the posterior cord, travels with the posterior humeral circumflex artery through the quadrangular space to the posterior aspect of the shoulder, where they supply the deltoid and the teres minor muscles (see Fig. 9-17). The axillary nerve gives rise to a cutaneous branch before entering the deltoid muscle that supplies the lateral side of the upper arm. Both the axillary nerve and its accompanying artery are in jeopardy from a fracture of the surgical neck of the humerus. Therefore, a test of the cutaneous sensation over the lateral arm is a good clinical test of the axillary nerve's integrity after a fracture. Under normal circumstances, the test for motor function is the ability to abduct, and to a lesser extent, medially rotate the arm.

The medial and lateral cords supply the shoulder region with only one branch each. They are the medial and lateral pectoral nerves, which get their names from the cord they are derived from rather than from their anatomic relationship to one another, which can be a source of confusion. They are the only shoulder nerves that contain fibers from the lower part of the brachial plexus (C8, T1).

Blood Supply to the Shoulder Region

Branches of the axillary artery as well as the subclavian artery supply the shoulder region. The thyrocervical trunk of the subclavian artery typically gives rise to the transverse cervical artery and the suprascapular artery, which both supply muscles of the shoulder region (Fig. 9-19). The suprascapular artery supplies the supraspinatus and infraspinatus muscles. It reaches the supraspinatus muscle by passing over the superior transverse scapular ligament, rather than by passing through the enclosed suprascapular notch, as the suprascapular nerve does, and then continues on passing through the spinoglenoid notch to reach the infraspinatus muscle (see Fig. 9-17). The transverse cervical artery sometimes divides into a superficial branch that supplies the trapezius muscle and a deep branch that supplies the levator scapulae and the rhomboids. More commonly, a dorsal scapular artery branches separately from the last part of the subclavian to supply the rhomboids.

The axillary artery is the direct continuation of the subclavian artery and begins as the subclavian artery passes laterally to the first rib (Fig. 9-20). The axillary artery is divided into three sections by its relationship with the pectoralis minor. The portion of the axillary artery medial to the pectoralis minor is the first part. The portion directly deep to the pectoralis minor tendon is the second part. The third portion begins at the lateral aspect of the pectoralis minor and extends to the inferior border of the insertion of the teres major muscle. The first portion of the axillary artery typically has one branch, the supreme thoracic artery that supplies the first and possibly the second intercostal space. The second portion has two branches: the thoracoacromial and the lateral thoracic arteries. The thoracoacromial trunk typically has four branches: the pectoral, acromial, clavicular, and deltoid branches. The lateral thoracic artery runs along the lateral aspect of the rib

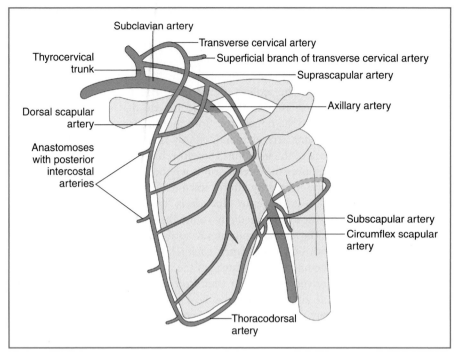

Figure 9-19. Shoulder anastomosis.

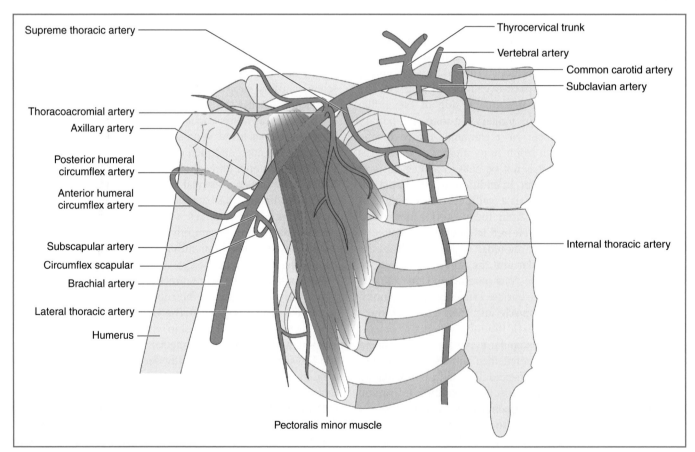

Figure 9-20. Blood supply to the shoulder.

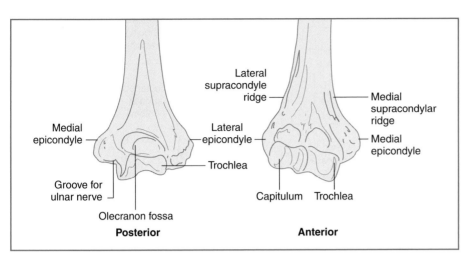

Figure 9-21. Right distal humerus.

cage to supply the serratus anterior muscle and the mammary gland. The third division of the axillary artery gives rise to three branches: the anterior and posterior humeral circumflex arteries and the subscapular artery. The anterior and posterior humeral circumflex arteries pass around the surgical neck of the humerus in opposite directions. The posterior humeral circumflex travels with the axillary nerve. The subscapular artery typically gives rise to the thoracodorsal artery, which supplies the latissimus dorsi muscle, and the circumflex scapular artery, which contributes to an anastomotic network on the posterior surface of the scapula deep to the intraspinatus muscle.

Shoulder Anastomosis

There is an anastomotic network on the posterior surface of the scapula that is important for maintaining the blood supply to the distal upper limb in the event of an obstruction in the axillary artery (see Fig. 9-19). Blood from the subclavian artery, via the transverse cervical and/or dorsal scapular and suprascapular arteries, reaches the posterior surface of the scapula and, in the decreased flow or absence of any flow through the thoracodorsal and circumflex scapular arteries from the axillary artery, will pass from the posterior surface of the scapula into the axillary artery. Thus, the blood can bypass the first and second divisions of the axillary artery.

●●● ARM, ELBOW JOINT, AND CUBITAL FOSSA

The arm is the portion of the upper limb that lies between the shoulder joint and the elbow joint. The principal function of the muscles in this region is movement at the elbow joint although a few muscles cross both the shoulder and the elbow joints. The right and left intermuscular septa divide the arm into two compartments: anterior (flexor) and posterior (extensor). The musculocutaneous nerve innervates the anterior compartment muscles, and the radial nerve innervates the posterior compartment muscles.

Bones

Distal Humerus

The medial and lateral borders of the humerus end distally as the medial and lateral supracondylar ridges, which lead to the medial and lateral epicondyles (Fig. 9-21). There is a deep groove for the ulnar nerve on the inferior surface of the medial epicondyle. The distal end of the humerus has two distinct bony areas for articulation with the ulna and radius. The lateral articulation is rounded and is called the *capitulum* while the medial side is more elongated and is called the *trochlea*. When the elbow is flexed, there is a depression superior to the capitulum—the radial fossa—which receives the head of the radius, and a depression superior to the trochlea—the coronoid fossa, which articulates with the ulna. On the posterior aspect of the humerus there is another fossa, the olecranon fossa, which receives the olecranon process of the ulna when the elbow is flexed.

Proximal Radius

The proximal end of the radius is circular and is slightly expanded and is known as the radial head (Fig. 9-22). It has a slightly concave surface proximally. This is the portion of the radius that articulates with the capitulum of the humerus. The portion of the radius just distal to the head is slightly narrower and is called the neck. Just distal to the neck on the anterior surface is a large bony prominence called the radial tuberosity for the insertion of the biceps brachii muscle.

Proximal Ulna

The ulna is on the medial side of the forearm. The proximal end of the ulna is shaped like the head of a wrench and is called the *olecranon process* (see Fig. 9-22). The concave portion of the olecranon process is called the *trochlear notch*, and it articulates with the trochlea of the humerus allowing flexion and extension. The anterior aspect of the proximal end of the ulna at the inferior aspect of the trochlear notch is called the *coronoid process*. Just distal to the coronoid process is a bony protuberance called the *ulnar tuberosity*

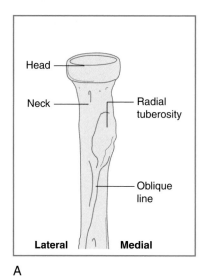

A

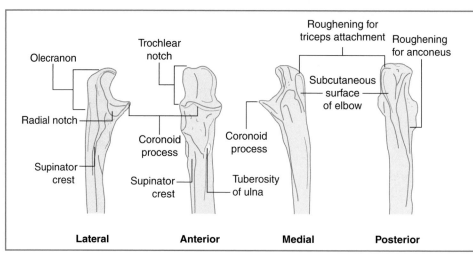

B

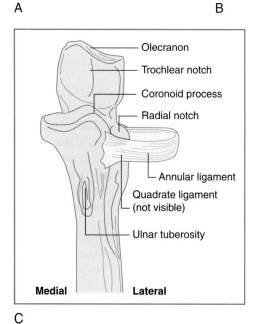

C

Figure 9-22. A, Proximal radius. **B,** Different views of the ulna. **C,** The ulna, showing the annular ligament.

for the attachment of the brachialis muscle. On the lateral side of the coronoid process is a depression called the *radial notch* where the head of the radius articulates.

Movements at the Elbow Joint

There are two sets of movements at the elbow joint: flexion and extension, as well as supination and pronation (Fig. 9-23). Flexion involves articulations between the humerus and the radius and between the humerus and the ulna. Supination and pronation involve the rotation of the radius around the ulna. Despite the presence of three different articulations, there is only one articular capsule at the elbow joint. The articular capsule is rather thin and allows for wide range of movement. The integrity of the elbow joint is reinforced by muscle action and by three important ligaments. The ulnar *collateral ligament* arises from the medial epicondyle and

divides to attach to both the coronoid process and the olecranon process. The *radial collateral ligament* arises from the lateral epicondyle. It has a minor attachment to the radius and a major attachment to the annular ligament. The *annular ligament* arises and inserts into the coronoid process and surrounds the head of the radius (see Fig. 9-22).

Muscles of the Arm

Anterior Compartment

The principal function of the anterior compartment is flexion both at the shoulder joint and the elbow joint. The most superficial muscle of the compartment is the *biceps brachii* (Fig. 9-24 and Table 9-4). It is also the only muscle of the compartment that crosses both the shoulder joint and the elbow joint. The biceps brachii has two heads: a short head and a long head. The long head is unique in that it passes

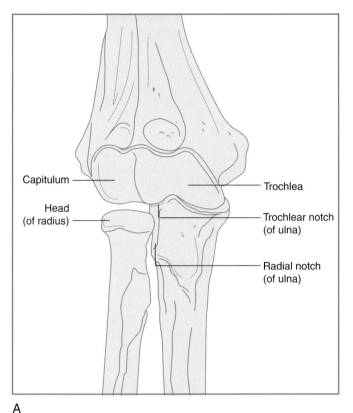

A

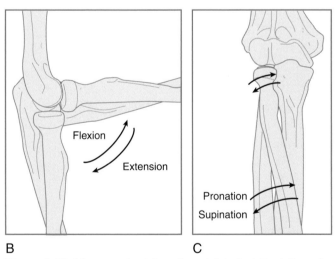

B   C

Figure 9-23. Movements at the elbow joint. **A,** Articulation of the radius and ulna with distal humerus. **B,** Flexion and extension. **C,** Pronation and supination.

through the glenohumeral joint cavity arising from the supraglenoidal tubercle located above the glenoid fossa. Both heads arise from the scapula and therefore cross the shoulder joint, making the biceps brachii muscle a flexor of the shoulder. However, the insertion of the biceps brachii is distal to the elbow joint and therefore it is also able to flex this joint. Its insertion on the radial tuberosity is medial, which allows the biceps brachii to supinate. In fact, its principal function is to supinate the flexed arm.

The other two muscles of the compartment both lie deep to the biceps brachii and each cross only one joint (see Fig. 9-24).

The *coracobrachialis* arises from the coracoid process and inserts on the medial aspect of the humerus. Therefore, it can adduct the arm and assist in flexion of the shoulder. The *brachialis* arises from the humerus just distal to the deltoid tuberosity and inserts on the ulnar tuberosity (see Table 9-4). It is the strongest flexor of the elbow.

Posterior Compartment

The posterior compartment of the arm contains two extensors. The principal muscle of this compartment is the *triceps brachii* (Table 9-5 and Fig. 9-25). As the name denotes, this muscle has three heads. One of the heads, the long head, crosses the shoulder joint so it can assist in shoulder extension. However, its main function is to extend the elbow joint. The other two heads, lateral and medial, arise from the posterior surface of the humerus, above and below the radial groove, respectively, and insert through a common tendon on the olecranon process of the ulna.

The other muscle is the *anconeus*, which is a very short muscle. It arises from the lateral epicondyle of the humerus and inserts on the lateral aspect of the olecranon process (see Fig. 9-25). Because of its small size it is not much of an extensor but rather assists in stabilizing the elbow joint.

Innervation of the Arm

The innervation to the muscles of the arm comes from the lateral and posterior cords of the brachial plexus.

Musculocutaneous Nerve

The lateral cord's musculocutaneous nerve supplies both motor and sensory innervation to the flexor muscles of the arm. It enters the arm by piercing the coracobrachialis muscle to run on the surface of the brachialis muscle deep to the biceps brachii muscle (Fig. 9-26; see also Fig. 9-24). After supplying all the muscles in the anterior arm, the musculocutaneous nerve becomes the lateral antebrachial cutaneous nerve and supplies the lateral aspect of the forearm with cutaneous innervation.

A portion of the brachialis muscle is innervated by the radial nerve. This is due to the fact that this portion migrated anterior to the functional plane of the elbow joint during development.

The medial aspect of the arm receives cutaneous innervation from the medial brachial cutaneous nerve. In the superior medial aspect of the arm, it is joined by the intercostobrachial branch (nerve) of the second intercostal nerve to provide sensory innervation, which represents the second thoracic dermatome.

Radial Nerve

The radial nerve supplies the muscles in the posterior compartment. The radial nerve passes posteriorly to the axillary artery. It runs with the deep brachial artery between the long and medial heads of the triceps muscle and then enters the radial (spiral) groove located between the lateral and medial heads of the triceps (see Fig. 9-25). After the radial nerve innervates the triceps muscle, it runs in the spiral groove to

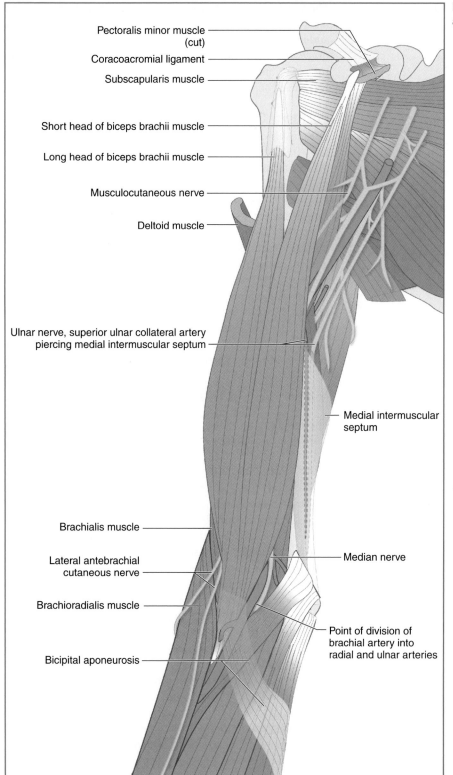

Pectoralis minor muscle (cut)

Coracoacromial ligament

Subscapularis muscle

Short head of biceps brachii muscle

Long head of biceps brachii muscle

Musculocutaneous nerve

Deltoid muscle

Ulnar nerve, superior ulnar collateral artery piercing medial intermuscular septum

Medial intermuscular septum

Brachialis muscle

Median nerve

Lateral antebrachial cutaneous nerve

Brachioradialis muscle

Point of division of brachial artery into radial and ulnar arteries

Bicipital aponeurosis

Figure 9-24. Anterior compartment of the arm. **A,** Superficial. *Continued*

A

Figure 9-24 cont'd. B, Deep.

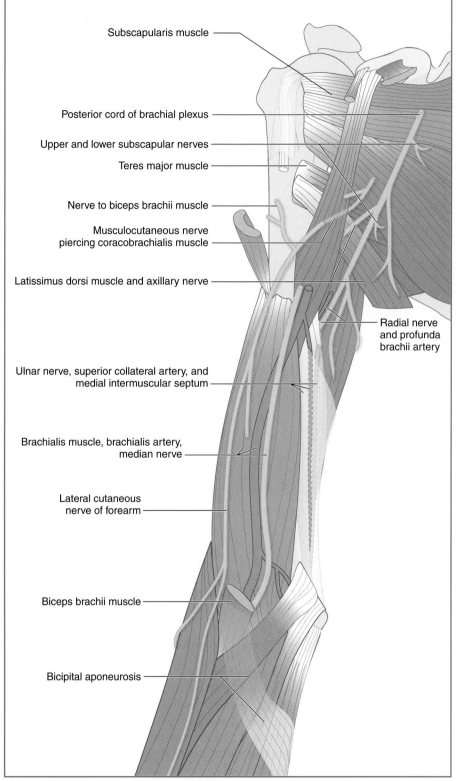

Subscapularis muscle

Posterior cord of brachial plexus

Upper and lower subscapular nerves

Teres major muscle

Nerve to biceps brachii muscle

Musculocutaneous nerve
piercing coracobrachialis muscle

Latissimus dorsi muscle and axillary nerve

Radial nerve
and profunda
brachii artery

Ulnar nerve, superior collateral artery, and
medial intermuscular septum

Brachialis muscle, brachialis artery,
median nerve

Lateral cutaneous
nerve of forearm

Biceps brachii muscle

Bicipital aponeurosis

B

TABLE 9-4. Muscles of the Anterior Compartment of the Arm

Muscle	Origin	Insertion	Principal Function	Innervation
Biceps brachii	Long head from supraglenoid tubercle and short head from coracoid process	Radial tuberosity and fascia of forearm through bicipital aponeurosis	Flexion and supination of forearm	Musculocutaneous nerve (C5, C6)
Coracobrachialis	Coracoid process	Medial side of humerus	Adduction and flexion of arm	Musculocutaneous nerve (C5, C6)
Brachialis	Lower portion of humerus inferior to insertion of deltoid muscle	Ulnar tuberosity	Flexion of forearm	Musculocutaneous nerve (C5, C6)

TABLE 9-5. Muscles of the Posterior Compartment of the Arm

Muscle	Origin	Insertion	Principal Function	Innervation
Triceps brachii, long head	Infraglenoid tubercle	Olecranon process	Extension of arm and forearm	Radial nerve (C6–C8)
Triceps brachii, medial head	Posterior surface of humerus inferior and medial to radial groove	Olecranon process	Extension of forearm	Radial nerve (C6–C8)
Triceps brachii, lateral head	Posterior surface of humerus superior and lateral to radial groove	Olecranon process	Extension of forearm	Radial nerve (C6–C8)
Anconeus	Lateral epicondyle of humerus	Lateral aspect of olecranon process	Extension of forearm	Radial nerve (C6–C8)

the inferolateral aspect of the arm, where it emerges between the brachioradialis and brachialis muscles. Here, the radial nerve supplies the lateral part of the brachialis. It then goes on to supply the extensor muscles of the forearm, which will be discussed below.

The radial nerve can be damaged in the axilla by a dislocation of the head of the humerus, improper use of crutches, or any event or activity that compresses the nerve against the humerus in the lower axilla. Injury will affect extension of the elbow owing to the lack of innervation to the triceps muscle. However, in a fracture of the shaft of the humerus that involves the spiral groove, the triceps are spared because the radial nerve branches to the triceps arise proximal to this point. In both cases, there is a sensory loss to the radial side of the dorsal surface of the hand and loss of wrist extensors (wrist drop).

Although the ulnar and median nerves do not innervate any muscles in the arm, they do pass through and therefore have relationships to structures in the arm. As the ulnar nerve courses inferiorly in the arm, it passes between the axillary vessels and continues medial to the brachial artery. The nerve continues in an inferoposterior direction along the medial side of the arm as it penetrates the medial intermuscular septum to enter the posterior compartment of the arm. Here, the ulnar nerve lies on the medial head of the triceps.

Blood Supply to the Arm

The blood supply to the arm comes from the brachial artery, the continuation of the axillary artery that begins at the inferior aspect of the teres major insertion on the humerus (Fig. 9-27). The deep brachial artery is the first branch off the brachial artery and runs with the radial nerve to supply the extensor muscles of the arm. The brachial artery gives off two additional branches in addition to muscular branches in the arm—the superior and inferior ulnar collateral arteries. These arteries anastomose with ulnar recurrent branches of the ulnar artery to form an anastomotic network around the elbow joint. As the brachial artery proceeds distally in the arm, it runs with the median nerve. The median nerve crosses it from lateral to medial. As the brachial artery reaches the cubital fossa, it lies deep to the bicipital aponeurosis, which protects it during venipuncture.

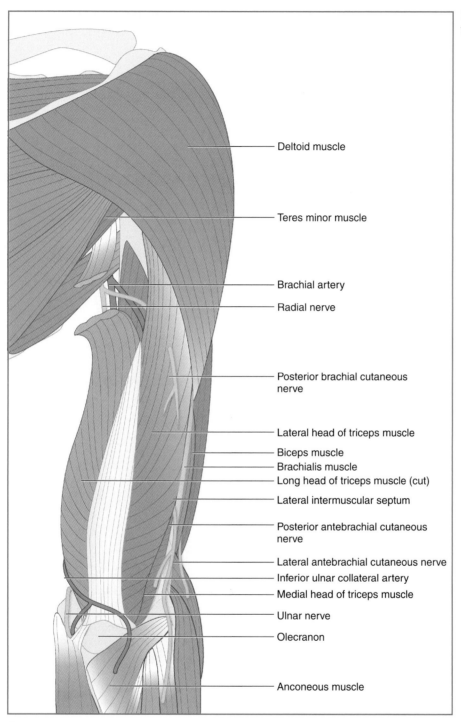

Figure 9-25. Posterior compartment of the arm. **A,** Superficial. *Continued*

Deltoid muscle

Teres minor muscle

Brachial artery

Radial nerve

Posterior brachial cutaneous nerve

Lateral head of triceps muscle

Biceps muscle

Brachialis muscle

Long head of triceps muscle (cut)

Lateral intermuscular septum

Posterior antebrachial cutaneous nerve

Lateral antebrachial cutaneous nerve

Inferior ulnar collateral artery

Medial head of triceps muscle

Ulnar nerve

Olecranon

Anconeous muscle

A

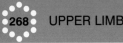

Figure 9-25 cont'd. B, Deep.

Deltoid muscle

Teres minor muscle

Posterior circumflex humeral artery

Axillary nerve

Teres major muscle

Deltoid branch of the deep brachial artery

Posterior brachial cutaneous nerve

Brachial artery

Radial nerve and deep brachial artery

Muscular branches of the radial nerve

Lateral head of triceps muscle

Brachialis muscle

Long head of triceps muscle

Posterior antebrachial cutaneous nerve

Lateral cutaneous nerve of the forearm

Medial head of triceps muscle

Ulnar nerve

Anconeous muscle

B

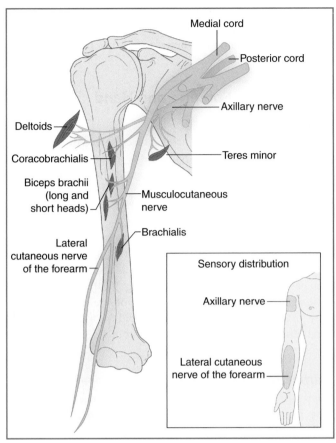

Medial cord

Posterior cord

Axillary nerve

Deltoids

Coracobrachialis

Teres minor

Biceps brachii (long and short heads)

Musculocutaneous nerve

Brachialis

Lateral cutaneous nerve of the forearm

Sensory distribution

Axillary nerve

Lateral cutaneous nerve of the forearm

Figure 9-26. Musculocutaneous and axillary nerves.

The brachial artery is typically used for assessing blood pressure. It can be pressed against the humerus by the blood pressure cuff.

The venous drainage of the arm is through deep and superficial veins (Fig. 9-28). There are typically two brachial veins that accompany the brachial artery (venae comitantes) and become the axillary vein. Superficially there are two veins that run in the arm: the cephalic vein and the basilic vein. These two veins often communicate with each other through the median cubital vein in the cubital fossa. When present, the median cubital vein passes superficially to the bicipital aponeurosis.

Cubital Fossa

The cubital fossa is the depression on the anterior surface of the elbow joint (Fig. 9-29). It is a common region for venipuncture, so the anatomy is clinically important to understand. It is bounded medially by the pronator teres and laterally by the brachioradialis. It extends superiorly to the level of the medial and lateral epicondyles of the humerus. The floor of the cubital fossa is the surface of the brachialis muscle and the supinator muscle, while the roof is the deep fascia of the arm and the bicipital aponeurosis. The contents of the cubital fossa from medial to lateral include the median nerve, brachial artery, tendon of the biceps brachii, and radial nerve. The brachial artery typically gives rise to the radial and ulnar arteries within the cubital fossa. The cephalic vein and

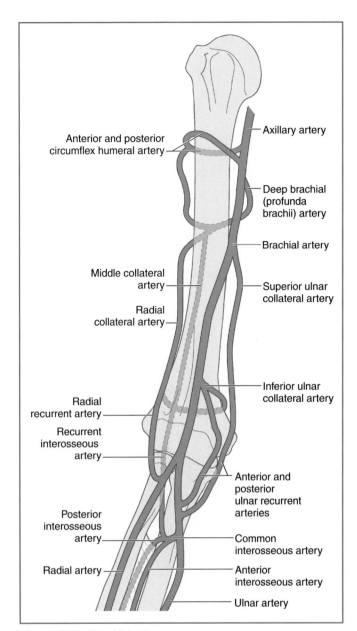

Anterior and posterior circumflex humeral artery

Axillary artery

Deep brachial (profunda brachii) artery

Brachial artery

Middle collateral artery

Superior ulnar collateral artery

Radial collateral artery

Inferior ulnar collateral artery

Radial recurrent artery

Recurrent interosseous artery

Anterior and posterior ulnar recurrent arteries

Posterior interosseous artery

Common interosseous artery

Radial artery

Anterior interosseous artery

Ulnar artery

Figure 9-27. Brachial artery.

CLINICAL MEDICINE

Cardiac Catheterization

Cardiac catheterization is widely used to assess the functioning of the heart. It can provide intracardiac pressure measurements as well as levels of oxygen saturation and cardiac output. The procedure involves placing a catheter in one of the peripheral arteries. Popular choices include the radial, brachial, and axillary arteries. Once inserted, the catheter is directed to the heart by passing through the subclavian artery, brachiocephalic artery, and into the ascending aorta. The axillary artery has an advantage over the brachial artery because it does not have as close a relationship with the median nerve as does the brachial, so potential injury is avoided. The radial artery is increasingly popular because there is a lower instance of vascular complications.

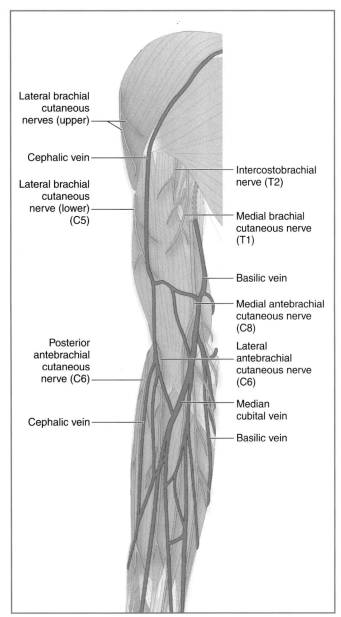

Figure 9-28. Venous drainage and cutaneous innervation of the arm.

the median cubital vein pass superficially to the cubital fossa. One of these two vessels is typically chosen for venipuncture.

●●● FOREARM

The main function of the muscles in the forearm is flexion and extension of the wrist and digits. Therefore, most of the muscles insert distal to the wrist joint. The forearm is also capable of pronation and supination. The forearm has two compartments, flexor and extensor, which spiral around it. The flexor compartment is anteromedial while the extensor compartment is posterolateral. In the anatomic position, the palm faces anteriorly and the thumb laterally. Anatomically and clinically the forearm bones are used to describe medial and lateral sides at the wrist and hand. The ulna is on the medial side of the forearm, and the radius is on the lateral

side. Therefore, the lateral side of the wrist and hand can be referred to as the radial side of the hand, and the medial side of the wrist and hand can be referred to as the ulnar side of the hand.

Bones of the Forearm and Hand

Distal Ulna
The distal ulna does not articulate closely with the carpal bones as it did with the humerus at the elbow joint (Fig. 9-30). The distal ulna is called the *head*, and it has a small projection called the *styloid process*.

Distal Radius
In contrast to the ulna, the radius does have a close articulation with the carpal bones. It has an articular surface known as the *carpal articular surface* as well as a small bony projection called the *styloid process* (see Fig. 9-30). The radioulnar articular disk maintains the integrity of the radioulnar joint that extends from the wrist's styloid process to a ridge separating the radius' ulnar notch from its carpal articular surface.

Carpal Bones
There are eight carpal bones, which are arranged in two rows (see Fig. 9-30). The proximal row from lateral to medial includes the scaphoid, lunate, and triquetrum, and the pisiform bone lies on the anterior surface of the triquetrum.

The distal row from lateral to medial includes the trapezium, trapezoid, capitate, and hamate.

Scaphoid
The scaphoid is the largest of the proximal bones and the most frequently fractured carpal bone. It has a prominent, laterally located tubercle, which can be palpated. The proximal and distal ends of this bone are connected by a narrow waist, which is in jeopardy upon forced abduction and extension. The waist comes into contact with the radial styloid process and can be fractured. The proximal fragment may have a diminished or no blood supply, resulting in a slowly or nonhealing fracture or aseptic necrosis.

Lunate
The lunate has a larger anterior than posterior surface. It is the only carpal bone that usually dislocates anteriorly. The blood supply of the lunate passes through its anterior and posterior ligaments. Anterior dislocation may damage one or both of these ligaments, resulting in either a slowly healing fracture or aseptic necrosis. The lunate articulates with the radius in the adducted wrist. It articulates with both radius and the radioulnar articular disk in the resting position and in the abducted wrist.

Triquetrum
Triangular in shape, the triquetrum articulates with the articular disc. The pisiform bone lies anterior to it, with only a small medial margin observable from behind.

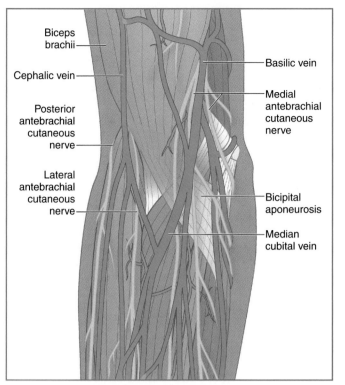

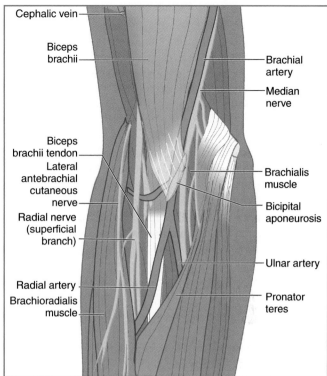

A

B

Figure 9-29. Cubital fossa. **A,** Superficial. **B,** Deep.

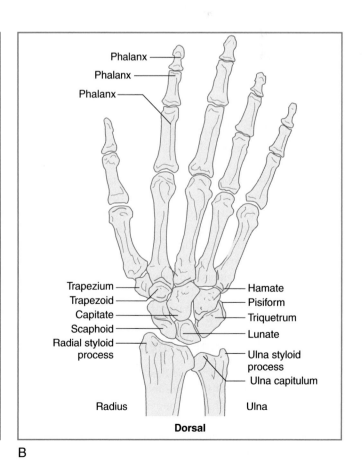

A

B

Figure 9-30. Bones of the wrist and hand. **A,** Palmar view. **B,** Dorsal view.

Pisiform

The pisiform is the smallest carpal bone and the easiest to palpate. It articulates with only the triquetrum and lies just distal to the distal wrist crease. The pisiform is a sesamoid bone within the tendon of flexor carpi ulnaris, and the ulnar nerve and artery pass just laterally to it. The pisiform does not participate in the radiocarpal or midcarpal joints.

Trapezium

The trapezium has a lateral tubercle for the flexor retinaculum and a medial groove for the tendon of the flexor carpi radialis tendon. Distally the trapezium has a saddle-shaped facet for the saddle joint. This facet is concave in one direction and convex in the other direction. It articulates with the reciprocal facet on the first metacarpal's base.

Trapezoid

A wedge-shaped bone, the trapezoid articulates with the base of the second metacarpal bone.

Capitate

The largest of the carpal bones, the capitate has a rounded head that articulates with the concave surface of the lunate bone.

Hamate

The hamate has the medially placed hamulus (hook) that participates in the carpal sulcus and is an attachment site for the flexor retinaculum. It is about 2 cm distal and slightly lateral to the pisiform bone.

There may be extra carpal bones (e.g., the rarely ossified centrale found dorsally between the scaphoid, capitate, and trapezoid). Carpal bones may fuse; e.g., the lunate and triquetrum produce one lunate-triquetrum.

Metacarpal and Phalangeal Bones

There are five metacarpal bones in the hand (see Fig. 9-30). As was true in the foot, the distal ends of the metacarpals are known as the heads the middle portion as the shaft, and the proximal ends as the bases. The bases of the first three metacarpal bones each articulate with a carpal bone: trapezium, trapezoid, and capitate (see Fig. 9-30). The bases of the fourth and fifth metacarpals both articulate with the hamate bone. The heads of the metacarpal bones articulate with the proximal phalanges to form the knuckles of the fist. There are two phalanges for the first metacarpal (pollicis) and three for the remaining four metacarpals.

Flexor Compartment of the Forearm

The muscles of the anterior or flexor compartment of the forearm will be considered from superficial to deep. The first layer of muscles one sees after removing the skin from medial to lateral are flexor carpi ulnaris, palmaris longus (if present), flexor carpi radialis, and pronator teres (Fig. 9-31 and Table 9-6; see also Table 9-5). The muscles have a common origin from the medial epicondyle of the humerus.

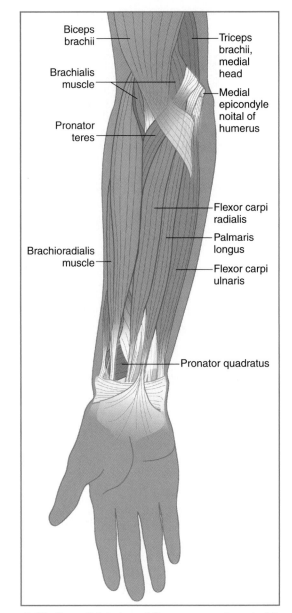

Figure 9-31. Superficial view of flexor compartment of the forearm.

The *flexor carpi ulnaris muscle* has two heads, one from the common flexor tendon and the other from the posterior surface of the ulna. The ulnar nerve, which innervates this muscle, passes between the two heads of the muscle before they join. Since it inserts on the medial side of the wrist, it can adduct (ulnar-deviate) the wrist in addition to flexing the wrist (see Table 9-6).

The *palmaris longus muscle* is a vestigial muscle in humans and is lacking in about 20% of the population. Since it does not add appreciably to any action at the wrist joint, it can be used as a replacement tendon (see Table 9-6).

The *flexor carpi radialis muscle* arises from the common flexor tendon and passes deep to the flexor retinaculum in a fascial compartment distinct from the carpal tunnel. In addition to flexing the wrist, it can abduct (radial-deviate) the wrist.

TABLE 9-6. Muscles of the Flexor Compartment of the Forearm

Muscle	Origin	Insertion	Principal Function	Innervation
Pronator teres	Medial epicondyle of humerus and coracoid process of ulna	Lateral aspect of radius	Pronation	Median nerve (C6, C7)
Palmaris longus	Medial epicondyle of humerus	Palmar aponeurosis	Flexion of wrist	Median nerve (C7, C8)
Flexor carpi radialis	Medial epicondyle of humerus	Base of second and third metacarpals	Flexion and lateral deviation (abduction) of wrist	Median nerve (C6, C7)
Flexor carpi ulnaris	Medial epicondyle of humerus	Base of fifth metacarpal	Flexion and medial deviation (adduction) of wrist	Ulnar nerve (C8, T1)
Flexor digitorum superficialis	Medial epicondyle of humerus	Intermediate phalanx of fingers 2–5	Flexion of middle phalanx of fingers 2–5 proximal interphalangeal joint	Median nerve (C6–C8)
Flexor digitorum profundus	Proximal three quarters of medial and anterior portions of ulna and interosseous membrane	Distal phalanx of fingers 2–5	Flexion of distal phalanx of fingers 2–5 flexes distal interphalangeal joint	Anterior interosseous nerve—fingers 2 and 3 Ulnar nerve—fingers 4 and 5
Flexor pollicis longus	Anterior surface of radius and interosseous membrane	Distal phalanx of thumb	Flexion of distal phalanx of thumb	Anterior interosseous branch of median nerve
Pronator quadratus	Distal portion of ulna	Distal portion of radius	Pronation	Anterior interosseous branch of median nerve

The *pronator teres muscle* has two unequal heads, a large one from the medial epicondyle near the common flexor tendon and a smaller one from the coronoid process of the ulna. The median nerve passes between the two heads before they join and the muscle tendon inserts deep to the brachioradialis muscle on the radius. The pronator teres is capable of strong, quick pronation.

Deep to these muscles lies the *flexor digitorum superficialis*, which arises by two heads and inserts on the middle phalanx of digits two to five (Fig. 9-32; see also Table 9-6). Its principal function is to flex the digits, especially the proximal interphalangeal joint, although it passes all the joints of the upper limb from the elbow on down and therefore assists in flexion at all these joints. As the tendons approach the hand, they enter the carpal tunnel in a unique arrangement. Tendons for the third and fourth digits lie anterior (more superficial) to the tendons for the second and fifth digits.

The deepest layer of the anterior compartment contains three muscles, the flexor digitorum profundus, flexor pollicis longus, and pronator quadratus (Fig. 9-33; see also Table 9-6). The *flexor digitorum profundus* arises from the anterior surface of the ulna and interosseous membrane. Its four tendons pass through the carpal tunnel and the divided insertion of the flexor digitorum superficialis tendons to insert on the distal phalanx of digits two to five. The ulnar half of the muscle is innervated by the ulnar nerve, and the

radial half receives innervation from the median nerve. The *flexor pollicis longus muscle* lies just lateral to the flexor digitorum profundus, and its tendon also passes through the carpal tunnel to insert on the distal phalanx of the thumb. The deepest muscle in this compartment is the quadrangular-shaped *pronator quadratus*, which attaches to the anterior surface of both forearm bones (see Table 9-6).

Extensor Compartment of the Forearm

The extensor (posterior) compartment of the forearm contains muscles that extend the wrist joint, extend the digits, and extend and abduct the thumb. The radial nerve and its branches provide innervation to all of them. Most of these muscles arise from the lateral side of the forearm. They can be separated into a superficial group and a deep group (Tables 9-7 and 9-8).

The brachioradialis is the most anterior member of the compartment. Although it looks like it belongs to the flexor compartment, it is a member of the posterior compartment based on its innervation by the radial nerve and its origin on the lateral epicondyle. It does, however, function as a flexor of the elbow joint (Fig. 9-34; see also Fig. 9-31 and Table 9-6).

The *extensor carpi radialis longus and brevis* lie just medial to the brachioradialis (see Fig. 9-34). They arise in part from the lateral supracondylar ridge and the lateral epicondyle. As

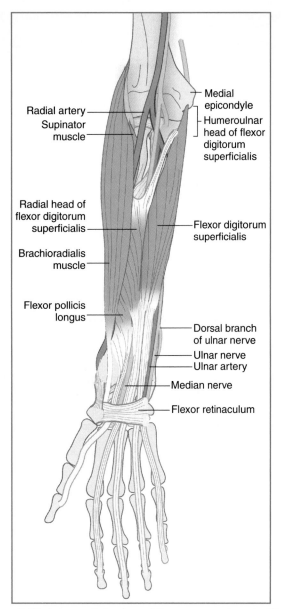

Figure 9-32. Intermediate view of flexor compartment of the forearm.

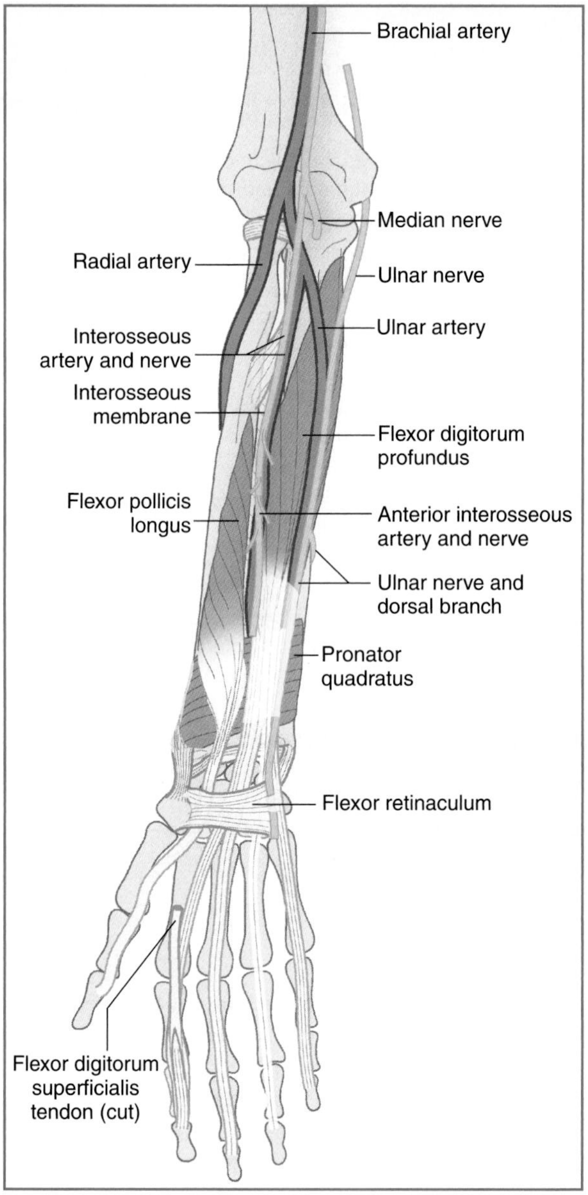

Figure 9-33. Deep view of flexor compartment of the forearm.

they approach the hand, they pass deep to the abductor pollicis longus and extensor pollicis brevis muscles to reach the base of the metacarpals. The brachioradialis and extensor carpi radialis longus and brevis are sometimes referred to as the lateral compartment of the forearm.

The *extensor digitorum* forms most of the superficial aspect of the extensor compartment (see Fig. 9-34 and Table 9-7). It arises like its companions from the lateral epicondyle, and its tendons pass deep to the extensor retinaculum in a common tendon sheath with the extensor indicis to insert on the extensor (dorsal) expansion of digits two to five. In the hand it participates in the formation of the extensor expansion.

The *extensor digiti minimi* appears to be a subdivision of the extensor digitorum, but it is in fact a separate muscle (see Fig. 9-34 and Table 9-7).

The *extensor carpi ulnaris* also arises in part from the lateral epicondyle and passes deep to the extensor retinaculum to its insertion on the base of the fifth metacarpal (see Fig. 9-34 and Table 9-7).

The most proximal deep muscle is the supinator (Fig. 9-35; see also Table 9-8). It wraps itself around the radius so it can be seen from both sides of the deep forearm. The deep branch of the radial nerve pierces its fibers to pass from the anterior side to the posterior side while the posterior interosseous artery passes deep to the supinator. This muscle supinates the forearm and the hand.

The *abductor pollicis longus* and the *extensor pollicis brevis* and longus muscles wrap around the extensor carpi radialis longus and brevis. They also form the boundaries of the anatomic snuffbox (see Fig. 9-35 and Table 9-8).

TABLE 9-7. Superficial Muscles of the Extensor Compartment of the Forearm

Muscle	Origin	Insertion	Principal Function	Innervation
Extensor carpi radialis longus	Lateral supracondylar ridge of humerus and common extensor tendon from lateral humeral epicondyle, intermuscular septum	Base of second metacarpal	Extension and abduction of wrist	Radial nerve (C6, C7)
Extensor carpi radialis brevis	Common extensor tendon, intermuscular septum, and antebrachial fascia	Base of third metacarpal	Extension of wrist	Posterior interosseous nerve C6, C7
Extensor digitorum	Common extensor tendon, intermuscular septum, and antebrachial fascia	Extensor (dorsal) expansion of fingers 2–5 to middle and distal phalynges	Extension of fingers 2–5, mostly at metacarphalangeal joint	Posterior interosseous nerve (C6–C8)
Extensor digiti minimi	Common extensor tendon	Middle and distal phalanx of little finger	Extension of little finger	Posterior interosseous nerve (C6–C8)
Extensor carpi ulnaris	Common extensor tendon and proximal portion of ulna	Base of fifth metacarpal	Extension and adduction of wrist	Posterior interosseous nerve (C7, C8)

TABLE 9-8. Deep Muscles of the Extensor Compartment of the Forearm

Muscle	Origin	Insertion	Principal Function	Innervation
Supinator	Lateral epicondyle of humerus, radial collateral and annular ligaments, supinator fossa, and crest of ulna	Lateral, posterior, and anterior surfaces of proximal third of radius	Supination of forearm and hand	Deep radial nerve (C6–C8)
Abductor pollicis longus	Posterior interosseous membrane and ulna	Lateral aspect of base of first metacarpal	Abduction of thumb and wrist	Posterior interosseous nerve (C6–C8)
Extensor pollicis brevis	Posterior aspect of mid-radius, and interosseous membrane	Base of first phalanx of thumb	Extension of thumb and abduction of wrist	Posterior interosseous nerve (C7, C8)
Extensor pollicis longus	Posterior aspect of interosseous membrane and midshaft of ulna	Base of second phalanx of thumb	Extension of thumb and abduction of wrist	Posterior interosseous nerve (C7, C8)
Extensor indicis	Interosseous membrane and ulna	Middle and distal phalanges of index finger	Extension of index finger and wrist	Posterior interosseous nerve (C7, C8)

Innervation of the Forearm

Median Nerve

The median nerve and its anterior interosseus branch supply all the muscles of the flexor (anterior) compartment of the forearm except the flexor carpi ulnaris and the ulnar (medial) portion of the flexor digitorum profundus (to fingers four and five) (Fig. 9-36). The anterior interosseus nerve supplies the flexor pollicis longus, pronator quadratus, and flexor digitorum profundus to the second and third fingers.

The median nerve can be injured in the cubital fossa by trauma or entrapment. Symptoms would include sensory loss over the radial side of the palm and fingers 1–3 and half of 4 and thenar eminence and muscular involvement of most of the anterior forearm compartment. Pronator function would be weak, and wrist flexion would be weak, with the flexor carpi ulnaris flexing and adducting the wrist. Weakness of the long finger flexors can be discerned by weakness in pinch between the thumb and index fingers produced by the flexor pollicis longus and flexor digitorum profundus to the thumb and index finger, respectively. Fingers two and three would become hyperextended and the thumb abducted by the intact radial and ulnar innervated forearm and hand muscles.

As the median nerve enters the anterior compartment of the forearm, it passes deep to the bicipital aponeurosis, between the two heads of the pronator teres, with the deep head

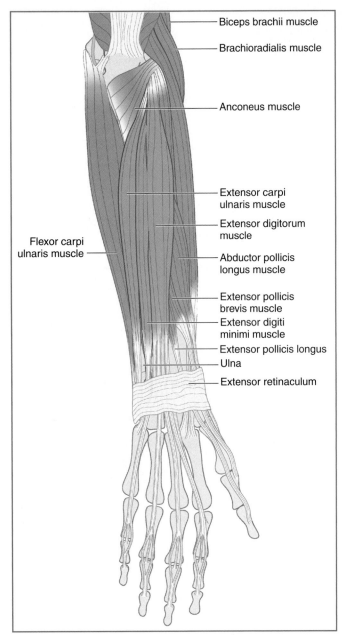

Figure 9-34. Superficial view of extensor compartment of the forearm.

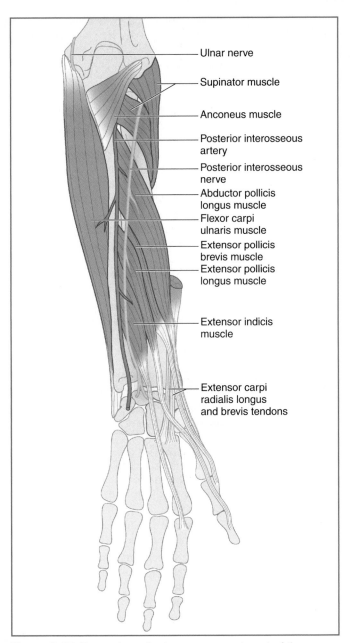

Figure 9-35. Deep view of extensor compartment of the forearm.

separating it from the ulnar artery. The median nerve gives rise to its anterior interosseus branch as it emerges from the pronator teres. The median nerve continues between the ulnar and radial heads of the flexor digitorum superficialis. The nerve is held to the deep surface of the flexor digitorum superficialis by fascia as they pass through the forearm together.

Ulnar Nerve

The ulnar nerve passes through a notch in the posterior surface of the medial epicondyle of the humerus to enter the medial side of the forearm between the two heads of the flexor carpi ulnaris. In the superior aspect of the forearm, the ulnar nerve is sandwiched between the flexor carpi ulnaris

and the ulnar half of flexor digitorum profundus, and it innervates these "one and one-half" muscles. In the distal forearm, the ulnar nerve gives rise to a dorsal cutaneous branch to the ulnar side of the dorsal surface of the hand. A palmar cutaneous branch arises closer to the hand. It supplies the medial surface of the palm.

Radial Nerve

The radial nerve supplies all the muscles in the posterior compartment of the forearm and also provides cutaneous innervation to the radial and dorsal sides of the thumb (Fig. 9-37).

The superficial radial nerve descends laterally to the radial artery and deep to the brachioradialis. This nerve winds between the distal radius and the tendon of the brachioradialis,

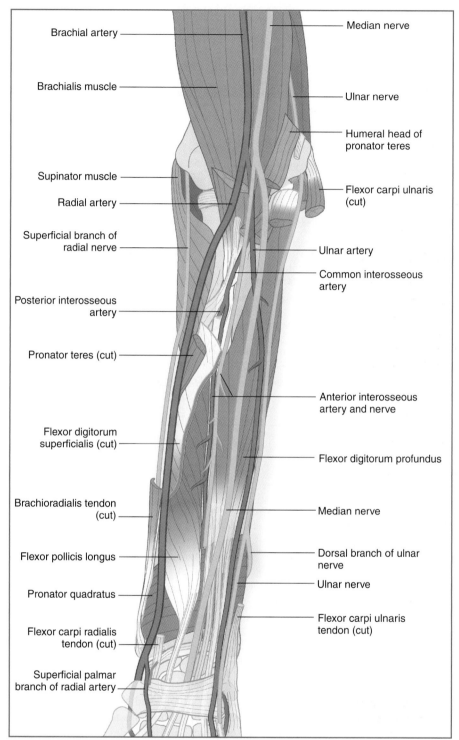

Figure 9-36. Median nerve.

Brachial artery

Brachialis muscle

Supinator muscle

Radial artery

Superficial branch of radial nerve

Posterior interosseous artery

Pronator teres (cut)

Flexor digitorum superficialis (cut)

Brachioradialis tendon (cut)

Flexor pollicis longus

Pronator quadratus

Flexor carpi radialis tendon (cut)

Superficial palmar branch of radial artery

Median nerve

Ulnar nerve

Humeral head of pronator teres

Flexor carpi ulnaris (cut)

Ulnar artery

Common interosseous artery

Anterior interosseous artery and nerve

Flexor digitorum profundus

Median nerve

Dorsal branch of ulnar nerve

Ulnar nerve

Flexor carpi ulnaris tendon (cut)

over the anatomic snuffbox, to reach the radial side of the dorsum of the hand. The superficial radial nerve is the cutaneous nerve to the radial and dorsal sides of the thumb with the area of isolated supply located over the first dorsal interosseous space. It is also cutaneous to the radial side of the hand from the dorsum of the thenar eminence to the middle of the third metacarpal (the middle finger) and distal to the middle of the middle phalanx of these fingers (see Fig. 9-37). However, in some individuals, the superficial radial

nerve may supply cutaneous innervation to the middle of the fourth metacarpal (ring finger).

The deep branch of the radial nerve passes through the supinator muscle, and when it emerges in the posterior compartment, it is called the posterior interosseous nerve. The deep branch can be compressed as it passes between the heads of the supinator. In this case, there is weakness of supination and extension of the wrist. The deficit in wrist extension is not so severe, because the extensor carpi radialis longus

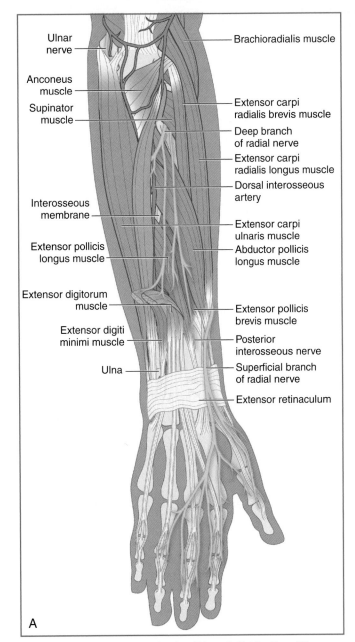

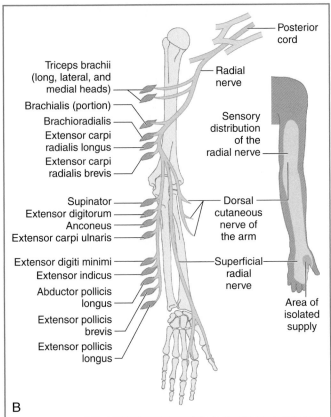

Figure 9-37. Radial nerve in situ (**A**) and distribution (**B**).

is innervated by the radial nerve prior to its division into superficial and deep branches. The superficial radial nerve is not involved. However, if the radial nerve is injured in the arm, the patient cannot extend the wrist and also demonstrates weakness of supination owing to the loss of the brachioradialis and supinator. The wrist will be flaccid. The patient cannot extend the hand against resistance or gravity owing to the loss of the wrist extensors and the extensors on the metacarpophalangeal joints. This condition is called wrist drop.

Blood Supply to the Forearm

The brachial artery splits into the radial artery and the ulnar artery in the cubital fossa (Fig. 9-38). The radial artery runs

deep to brachioradialis initially and then lies between the flexor carpi radialis and brachioradialis tendons at the wrist, where a pulse can be taken anterior to the head of the radius. The ulnar artery gives rise to a short branch called the *common interosseus artery*, which divides into an anterior and a posterior interosseous artery that supply the flexor and extensor compartments, respectively. After giving rise to the common interosseous artery, the ulnar artery runs deep to the flexor carpi ulnaris and is joined by the ulnar nerve. They travel together toward the wrist and pass laterally to the pisiform bone and superficially to the flexor retinaculum in a space called Guyon's canal. This canal is bounded by the pisihamate ligament, pisiform and hamate bones.

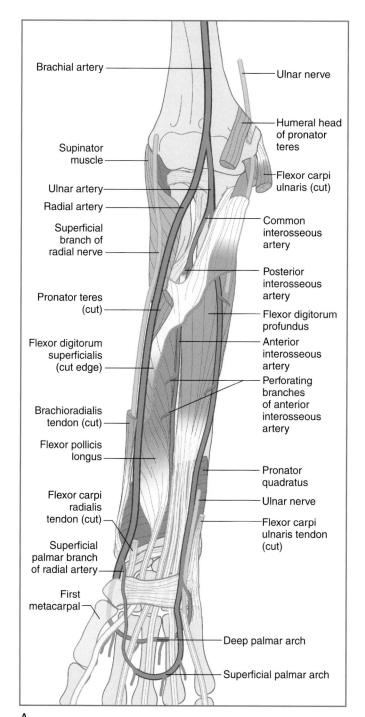

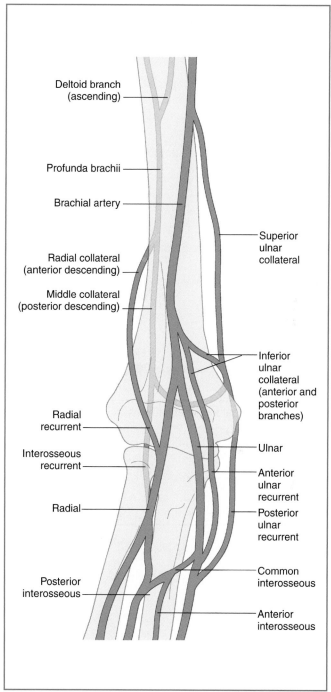

Figure 9-38. A, Blood supply in the forearm. **B,** Collateral circulation around the elbow joint.

Collateral Circulation Around the Elbow

Branches from the brachial artery connect to the radial and ulnar arteries such that an obstruction in the elbow region can be circumvented (see Fig. 9-38). The superior and inferior ulnar collateral arteries arise from the brachial artery proximal to the elbow and join the ulnar recurrent branches of the ulnar artery distal to the elbow joint. On the radial side of the arm, the profunda brachii artery gives rise to a radial collateral and middle collateral that each rejoin the radial recurrent and interosseous recurrent arteries, respectively.

Carpal Tunnel

The carpal tunnel is the passageway of the wrist formed by the flexor retinaculum (transverse carpal ligament) and the eight carpal bones (Fig. 9-39). At the carpal tunnel, the median nerve is lateral to the tendon of the flexor digitorum superficialis to the third finger, medial to the tendon of the flexor carpi radialis, and partly covered by the tendon of the palmaris longus if present (Fig. 9-40).

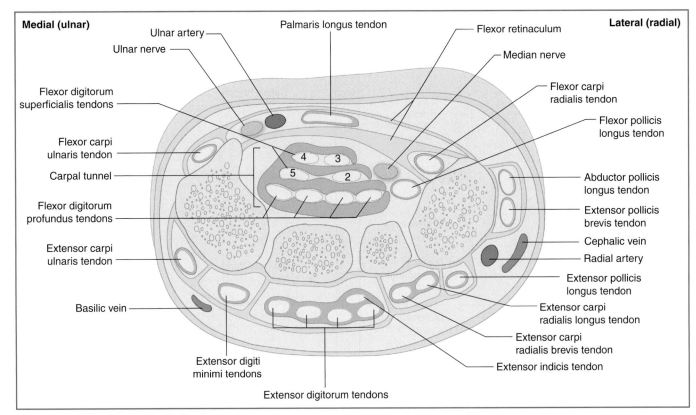

Figure 9-39. Carpal tunnel of left wrist.

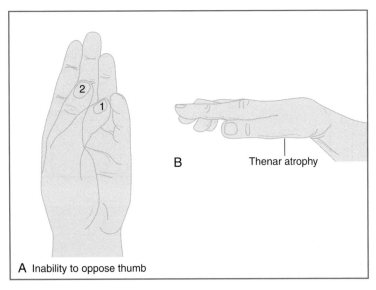

Figure 9-40. Carpal tunnel syndrome. **A,** Normal (1) and inability to oppose thumb (2). **B,** Thenar atrophy.

CLINICAL MEDICINE

Carpal Tunnel Syndrome

The most common entrapment syndrome is carpal tunnel syndrome. The median nerve is entrapped in the carpal tunnel by any condition that decreases the size of the space between the carpal bones that form the carpal sulcus and the flexor retinaculum, which converts the sulcus into a tunnel. The median is the only nerve in the carpal tunnel. Rheumatoid arthritis, dislocation, edema, and tumors are only a few of the conditions associated with carpal tunnel syndrome. The incidence of this condition has greatly increased owing to repetitive activities such as computer use. The patient complains of sensory deficits, such as numbness, paresthesias (burning, pricking, tickling, or tingling) and pain in the thumb, index, middle, and radial half of the ring fingers, which receive cutaneous median nerve innervation.

The fourth finger can be used in electromyogram (EMG) studies to compare median and ulnar nerve cutaneous sensory innervation, since the radial (lateral) side of this finger is supplied by the median nerve and the ulnar side (medial) by the superficial ulnar nerve. In addition, the cutaneous palmar branch of the median nerve, which supplies the radial side of the palm, is not affected because it arises before the median nerve enters the carpal tunnel. This cutaneous nerve is spared because it passes over the flexor retinaculum.

Anatomic Snuffbox

The anatomic snuffbox is a triangular space bordered by the abductor pollicis longus and extensor pollicis brevis radially, and the extensor pollicis longus is the ulnar boundary (Fig. 9-41). The floor of the anatomic snuffbox is the scaphoid bone. Therefore, tenderness over this region after a fall on the outstretched hand can indicate a scaphoid fracture. The radial artery passes through the anatomic snuffbox, and while difficult, a pulse can be palpated in this region as well.

Wrist Joint

The wrist joint encompasses movement at three different locations within the wrist. Proximally there is the articulation between the distal end of the radius and the articular disk of the radioulnar joint and the proximal row of the carpal bones. The articulation between the two rows of carpal bones is the midcarpal joint, and the articulation between the distal row of carpal bones and the metacarpal bones is the carpometacarpal joint. Taken together, these joints account for almost 90 degrees of flexion at the wrist. The distal end of the radius articulates mostly with the scaphoid and lunate bones (Fig. 9-42). This is why these two carpal bones are the most frequently fractured bones after a fall on an outstretched hand. The distal ulna articulates only with the distal radius and not the carpal bones.

●●● HAND

Overview of the Hand

The hand is specialized for interaction with the environment. Therefore, it is organized for manipulation and as a sensory organ. In addition to the familiar movements of the limbs that we have encountered before, the fingers of the hand are capable of opposition. Abduction and adduction of the fingers are described, with the axis for abduction or adduction through the middle finger at rest. The actions of the thumb include flexion and extension, abduction and adduction, and opposition (Fig. 9-43). There is a high concentration of touch receptors on the palm of the hand, particularly at the fingertips.

Fascia of the Hand

The superficial fascia over the palmar aspect of the hand contains lobules of fat separated by fibrous septa. The morphology allows for compression and retention of the skin in place during flexion, which allows for efficient grasp. Traveling through the superficial fascia are cutaneous nerves,

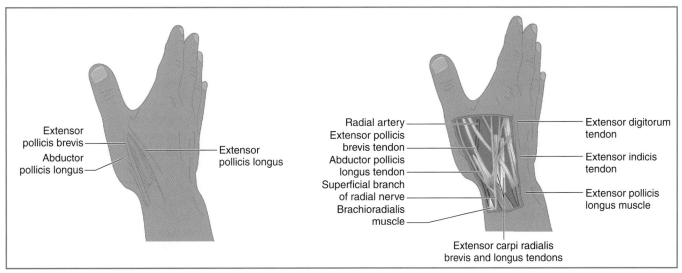

Extensor pollicis brevis
Abductor pollicis longus
Extensor pollicis longus

Radial artery
Extensor pollicis brevis tendon
Abductor pollicis longus tendon
Superficial branch of radial nerve
Brachioradialis muscle
Extensor carpi radialis brevis and longus tendons
Extensor digitorum tendon
Extensor indicis tendon
Extensor pollicis longus muscle

Figure 9-41. Anatomic snuffbox.

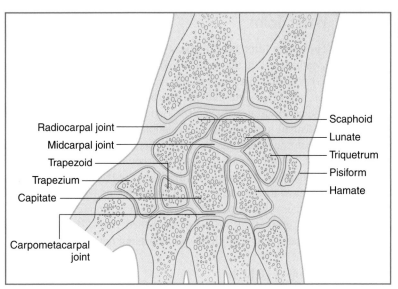

Figure 9-42. Wrist, midcarpal, and carpometacarpal joints.

Radiocarpal joint

Midcarpal joint

Trapezoid

Trapezium

Capitate

Carpometacarpal joint

Scaphoid

Lunate

Triquetrum

Pisiform

Hamate

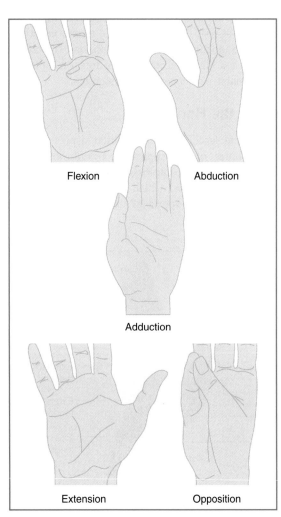

Flexion

Abduction

Adduction

Extension

Opposition

Figure 9-43. Movements of the thumb.

blood vessels, and lymphatics. The *palmaris brevis muscle* is also found within the superficial fascia over the hypothenar eminence. This muscle assists in forming a cupped palm.

The palmar aponeurosis is the strong triangular extension of the deep fascia (Fig. 9-44). Its apex is continuous with the tendon of the palmaris longus. It is attached at the flexor retinaculum and is continuous with the fibrous flexor sheaths and the fascia over the thenar and hypothenar eminences. The central compartment is formed anteriorly by the palmar aponeurosis, medially and laterally by the fascia over the thenar and hypothenar eminences, and posteriorly by the muscular fascia of the interossei and the adductor pollicis muscles. This compartment is subdivided by several septa that extend from the palmar aponeurosis to the posterior fascia. These septa form well-defined fascial canals that extend proximally from the angle between the lumbricals and flexor tendons and distally to the deep transverse metacarpal ligament.

Muscles of the Hand

The intrinsic muscles of the hand can be divided into three groups: the thenar muscles associated with the thumb, the hypothenar muscles associated with the little finger, and the lumbricals and interossei that are found in the center and deep portions of the hand.

Thenar Muscles

The *abductor pollicis brevis* is the superficial muscle on the radial side of the thenar eminence and forms most of the anterolateral surface of this eminence (Fig. 9-45 and Table 9-9). It originates from the tubercles of the scaphoid, the trapezium,

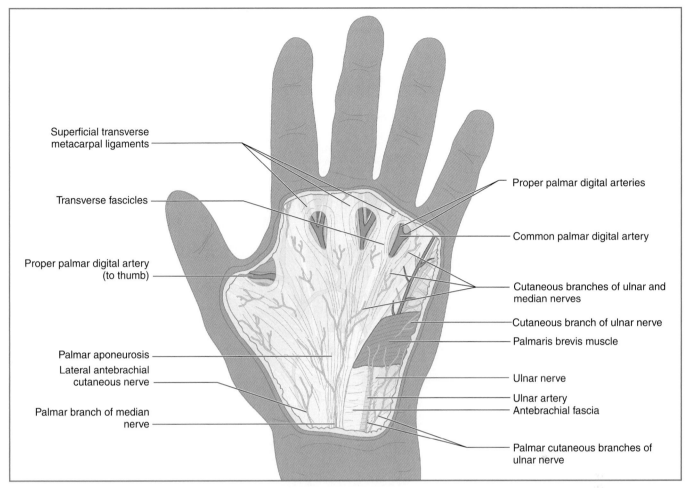

Superficial transverse metacarpal ligaments

Transverse fascicles

Proper palmar digital artery (to thumb)

Palmar aponeurosis
Lateral antebrachial cutaneous nerve

Palmar branch of median nerve

Proper palmar digital arteries

Common palmar digital artery

Cutaneous branches of ulnar and median nerves

Cutaneous branch of ulnar nerve
Palmaris brevis muscle

Ulnar nerve

Ulnar artery
Antebrachial fascia

Palmar cutaneous branches of ulnar nerve

Figure 9-44. Palmar aponeurosis.

and the flexor retinaculum and inserts onto the radial side of the base of the proximal phalanx of the thumb. It crosses both the carpometacarpal and the metacarpal phalangeal (MP) joints. The *abductor pollicis longus* inserts into the base of the first metacarpal. Abduction is produced by a combination of both muscles.

Flexor pollicis brevis is the superficial muscle on the ulnar side of the thenar eminence (see Fig. 9-45 and Table 9-9). It is often fused with the abductor pollicis brevis. The flexor pollicis brevis arises from two heads: a superficial head from the tubercle of the trapezium and the flexor retinaculum and a deep head from the base of the first metacarpal. It inserts into the radial side of the proximal phalanx in a common tendon with the abductor pollicis brevis, and it acts in flexion of the thumb. The tendon of the flexor pollicis longus passes between the two heads of the flexor pollicis brevis.

The *opponens pollicis* is deep to the flexor and abductor pollicis brevis muscles of the thenar eminence (Fig. 9-46; see also Table 9-9). It arises from the trapezium and flexor retinaculum and inserts along the radial border of the first metacarpal. It crosses and functions at the carpal metacarpal (saddle) joint. The opponens pollicis moves the first metacarpal across the surface of the palm and allows for opposition of the thumb with each of the other fingers.

The *adductor pollicis* lies deep in the palm and has two heads of origin: a transverse head from the shaft of the third metacarpal plus an oblique head from the capitate, trapezoid, and trapezium carpal bones and the bases of the first three third metacarpal bones (see Fig. 9-46 and Table 9-9). Both heads insert on the base of the ulnar side of the proximal phalanx of the thumb.

Hypothenar Muscles

The *abductor digiti minimi* is superficially placed on the ulnar side of the hypothenar eminence (Table 9-10; see also Figs. 9-45 and 9-46). This muscle serves to abduct the little finger. It originates from the pisiform bone and flexor retinaculum to insert into the base of the ulnar side of the proximal phalanx of the little finger.

The *flexor digiti minimi* is superficially placed on the radial side of the hypothenar eminence (see Table 9-10 and Figs. 9-45 and 9-46). It takes origin from the hamate bone and the flexor retinaculum. It inserts in the common tendon with the abductor digiti minimi on the base of the ulnar side of the proximal phalanx of the little finger. It acts as a flexor of the little finger.

The *opponens digiti minimi*, like the opponens pollicis, lies deep to the other two muscles (see Fig. 9-46). It arises from

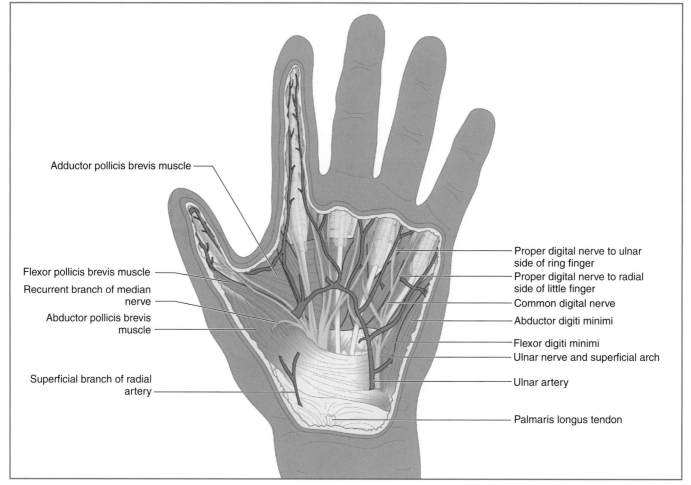

Adductor pollicis brevis muscle

Flexor pollicis brevis muscle

Recurrent branch of median nerve

Abductor pollicis brevis muscle

Superficial branch of radial artery

Proper digital nerve to ulnar side of ring finger

Proper digital nerve to radial side of little finger

Common digital nerve

Abductor digiti minimi

Flexor digiti minimi

Ulnar nerve and superficial arch

Ulnar artery

Palmaris longus tendon

Figure 9-45. Superficial view of thenar and hypothenar muscles.

TABLE 9-9. Thenar Muscles

Muscle	Origin	Insertion	Principal Function	Innervation
Abductor pollicis brevis	Anterior surface of trapezium and scaphoid bones and flexor retinaculum	Lateral aspect of proximal phalanx of thumb	Abduction of thumb	Recurrent branch of median nerve
Flexor pollicis brevis, superficial head	Trapezium and flexor retinaculum	Lateral aspect of base of first phalanx	Flexion of thumb	Recurrent branch of median nerve
Flexor pollicis brevis, deep head	Lateral side of first metacarpal	Lateral aspect of base of first phalanx	Flexion of thumb	Deep branch of ulnar nerve
Opponens pollicis	Trapezium	Radial side of first metacarpal	Opposition	Recurrent branch of median nerve
Adductor pollicis, oblique head	Capitate and bases of first three metacarpals	Medial side of base of first phalanx of thumb	Adduction of thumb	Deep branch of ulnar nerve
Adductor pollicis, transverse head	Shaft of third metacarpal			

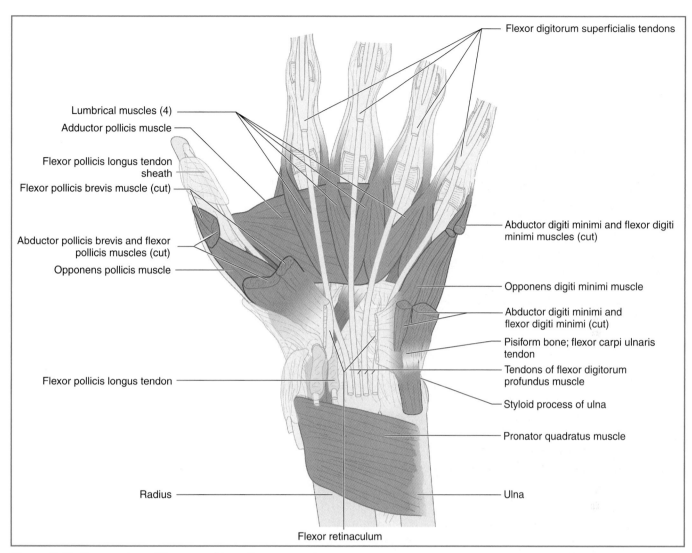

Figure 9-46. Deeper view of thenar and hypothenar muscles.

TABLE 9-10. Hypothenar Muscles				
Muscle	**Origin**	**Insertion**	**Principal Function**	**Innervation**
Abductor digiti minimi	Pisiform bone and flexor retinaculum	Ulnar side of base of fifth proximal phalanx	Abduction of little finger	Deep branch of ulnar nerve
Flexor digiti minimi	Flexor retinaculum and hamulus	Ulnar side of base of fifth proximal phalanx	Flexion of little finger	Deep branch of ulnar nerve
Opponens digiti minimi	Flexor retinaculum and hook of the hamulus	Ulnar side of fifth metacarpal	Flexion and opposition of little finger	Deep branch of ulnar nerve

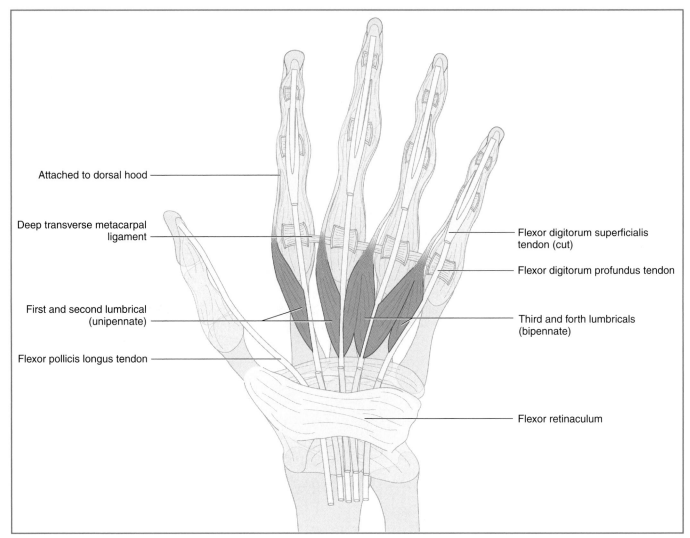

Attached to dorsal hood

Deep transverse metacarpal ligament

First and second lumbrical (unipennate)

Flexor pollicis longus tendon

Flexor digitorum superficialis tendon (cut)

Flexor digitorum profundus tendon

Third and forth lumbricals (bipennate)

Flexor retinaculum

Figure 9-47. Lumbrical muscles of the hand.

the hook of the hamate and flexor retinaculum and inserts into the ulnar border of the fifth metacarpal. The opponens digiti minimi functions in opposition of the little finger at the metacarpophalangeal (MP) joint.

Deep Muscles of the Hand

The lumbricals and the interossei are the two groups of deep muscles of the hand.

The lumbricals are the four worm-like, intrinsic midpalmar muscles of the hand (Fig. 9-47). They arise from the radial sides of the four tendons of the flexor digitorum profundus. The first and second each have one head of origin from the radial side of the profundus tendons to the index and middle fingers. The third and fourth lumbricals arise from adjacent profundus tendons to the middle, ring, and little fingers. Each lumbrical passes on the radial side anteriorly to the deep transverse palmar ligaments to insert into the respective extensor expansions. The lumbricals flex the MP joints and extend the interphalangeal joints.

The interossei are located between the metacarpal bones and are divided into two groups: four dorsal and three palmar (Fig. 9-48). In general, the interossei arise from the sides of the adjacent metacarpal bones and insert into the bases of the proximal phalanges and appropriate extensor expansions. Thus, as a group, these muscles assist the lumbricals in flexion of the MP joints and extension of the interphalangeal joints. The palmar interossei adduct and the dorsal interossei abduct, with the plane of abduction/adduction through the middle finger. Thus, the third finger has two dorsal interossei that abduct this finger to either the radial or the ulnar side.

Innervation of the Hand

Ulnar Nerve

The ulnar nerve enters the hand just lateral to the pisiform bone between the two ligaments, the flexor retinaculum, and the palmar carpal ligament (Fig. 9-49). It passes laterally to the

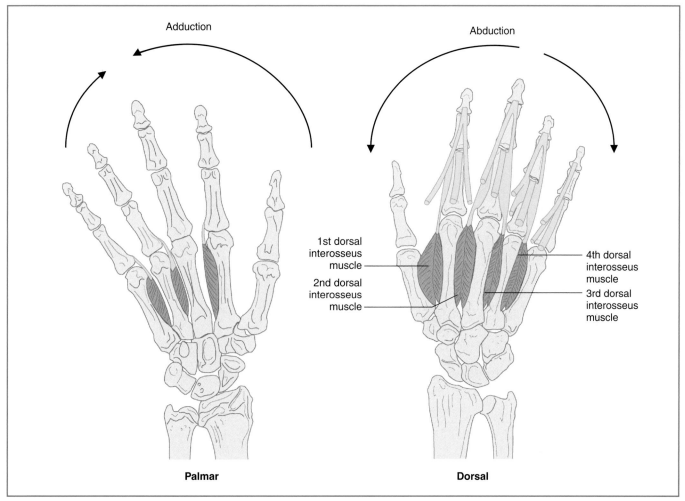

Figure 9-48. Dorsal and palmar interossei.

pisiform bone, lies under the pisohamate ligament, and then lies medial to the hook of the hamate. The palmar carpal ligament and often the palmaris brevis cover it. Here, it lies in the ulnar (Guyon's) canal, where it can be entrapped. The ulnar nerve separates into superficial and deep branches.

Superficial branches are two in number: a proper digital branch that supplies one side of the little finger and a common digital branch that supplies the adjacent sides of the little and ring fingers. The proper digital branch provides innervation to the palmaris brevis and sensation to the ulnar side of the little finger, and the common digital branch divides into adjacent proper digital nerves that supply sensation to the radial half of the little finger and the ulnar half of the ring finger.

The deep branch first passes through a cleft between the flexor digiti minimi and the abductor digiti minimi and then passes through the origins of the opponens digiti minimi, innervating these muscles (the muscles of the hypothenar eminence). It passes medially (ulnar) to the hook of the hamate and turns laterally to continue across the hand by following the deep palmar arch. The deep ulnar nerve supplies all seven interossei, the two ulnar lumbricals (numbers 3 and 4), and

CLINICAL MEDICINE

Claw Hand

Loss of ulnar nerve function results in severe disability in the hand referred to as claw hand. The losses include inability to adduct the thumb (adductor pollicis), to abduct fingers two to five, to adduct fingers two, four, and five, or to extend the interphalangeal joints of fingers two to five. This last observation results from the loss of the functions of the seven interosseous muscles. Extension of the interphalangeal joints for fingers four and five is more greatly affected than for fingers two and three, since the median nerve innervates the lumbricals for fingers two and three.

The loss also includes flexion of the metacarpophalangeal (MCP) joints of fingers four and five by the third and fourth lumbricals, flexion of the MCP joints, and extension of the interphalangeal joints. Without the normal balance between flexion and extension at these joints, the hand will assume a "clawed" position with hyperextension of the MCP joints and hyperflexion of the interphalangeal joints of fingers four and five. Final clawing results from atrophy of the dorsal interossei with abduction of fingers two, three, and four.

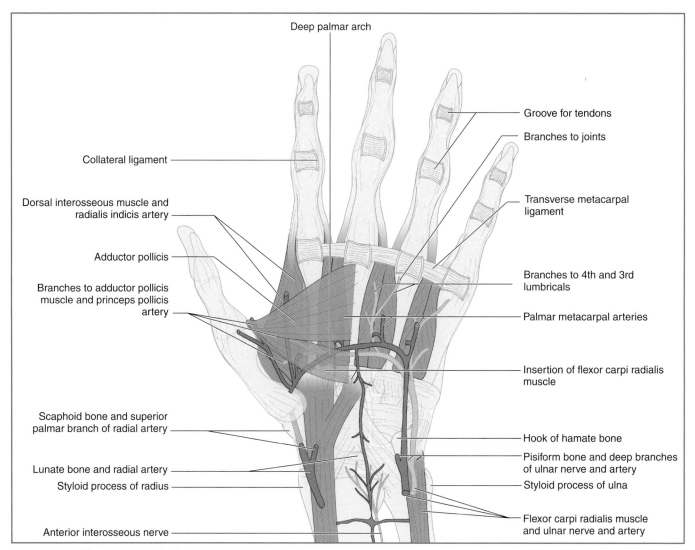

Deep palmar arch

Groove for tendons

Branches to joints

Collateral ligament

Dorsal interosseous muscle and
radialis indicis artery

Transverse metacarpal
ligament

Adductor pollicis

Branches to adductor pollicis
muscle and princeps pollicis
artery

Branches to 4th and 3rd
lumbricals

Palmar metacarpal arteries

Insertion of flexor carpi radialis
muscle

Scaphoid bone and superior
palmar branch of radial artery

Hook of hamate bone

Pisiform bone and deep branches
of ulnar nerve and artery

Lunate bone and radial artery

Styloid process of ulna

Styloid process of radius

Flexor carpi radialis muscle
and ulnar nerve and artery

Anterior interosseous nerve

Figure 9-49. Ulnar nerve in the hand.

the adductor pollicis. Finally, it innervates the deep head of the flexor pollicis brevis.

Median Nerve

The median nerve enters the hand through the carpal tunnel along lateral margin of the tendon of the flexor digitorum superficialis to the middle finger and medial to the tendon flexor carpi radialis. The median nerve splits into a lateral and a medial division.

The lateral division has a recurrent branch that hooks back toward the thenar eminence to innervate the following: abductor pollicis brevis, superficial head of the flexor pollicis brevis, and opponens pollicis. The remainder of the lateral division sends motor innervation to the first (most radial) lumbrical. It is also provides sensory innervation by means of proper digital branches to the radial side of the thumb. A common digital branch divides into proper digital branches to the ulnar sides of the thumb and the radial side of the adjacent index finger.

The recurrent branch takes a very superficial course in the palm as it hooks around to innervate most of the musculature of the thenar eminence. A significant cut at the radial longitudinal crease made by the thenar eminence could sever the nerve. This would result in lose of opposition of the thumb and thus most of the fine movements of the hand. Some of the functions of the other two thenar muscles innervated by this nerve would be retained because of the existence of extrinsic muscles innervated by the radial nerve, which produce some of the same actions (e.g., abductor pollicis longus and flexor pollicis longus).

The medial division supplies motor innervation to the second lumbrical. It also has two common digital branches to supply sensation to the ulnar side of the index finger and the radial side of the middle finger as well as the ulnar side of the middle finger and the radial side of the ring finger.

The median nerve branches provide cutaneous innervation to most of the lateral (radial) side of the palm (Fig. 9-50). Its sensory distribution includes the palmar surface of the

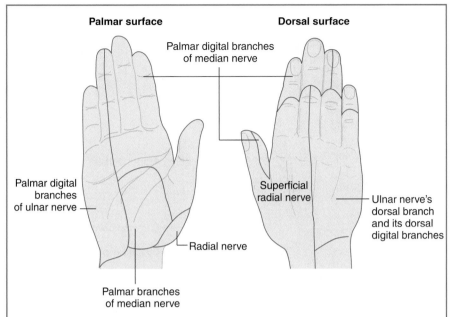

Figure 9-50. Cutaneous supply to the hand.

thumb, except the radial side of the thenar eminence, and the second, third, and lateral half of the fourth finger. This area of cutaneous supply includes the dorsal surface of the distal phalanges and part of the middle phalanges of fingers two to four because the dorsal digital neurovascular branches extend only to the level of the middle phalanges while the palmar neurovascular branches extend to the level of the distal phalanx to supply both palmar and dorsal surfaces. The median nerve's palmar cutaneous branch passes over the transverse palmar ligament (thus, it is not in the carpal tunnel). It supplies cutaneous innervation to the thenar eminence and the palmar surface to the level of the lateral (radial) surface to the middle of the ring finger. The ulnar nerve (a branch of the medial cord with fibers from C8–T1) supplies the flexor carpi ulnaris, the medial (ulnar) portion of the flexor digitorum profundus with tendons to fingers four and five, the remaining intrinsic muscles, and the sensory supply of the hand (see Fig. 9-50).

Loss of the median nerve results in atrophy of the thenar eminence. Fine function and pinch are affected. There is complete loss of ability to oppose the thumb. Sensory loss is highly debilitating.

Radial Nerve

The radial nerve does not supply motor innervation to any intrinsic muscles of the hand. It provides sensory innervation to the dorsum of the hand by means of its superficial branch (see Fig. 9-50).

Blood Supply to the Hand

The radial artery enters the hand on the dorsal side, passing through the floor of the anatomic snuffbox. It then passes between the two heads of the first dorsal interosseous muscle to enter the palm of the hand. Here, it gives off the princeps pollicis and radialis indicis branches before anastomosing with the deep branch of the ulnar artery to form the deep palmar arch (Fig. 9-51). The deep palmar arch lies on the interosseous muscles and gives rise to the palmar metacarpal arteries.

The ulnar artery enters the hand through Guyon's canal, gives rise to the deep ulnar artery that contributes to the deep palmar arch (as described above), and continues to form the superficial palmar arch with contribution from the superficial palmar branch of the radial artery. The superficial palmar arch lies just deep to the palmar aponeurosis and gives rise to the common and proper digital branches. The superficial and deep palmar arches anastomose with each other via the palmar metacarpal arteries.

There is a dorsal carpal arch to which both radial and ulnar arteries contribute, which gives rise to the dorsal digital arteries.

CLINICAL MEDICINE & PATHOLOGY

Raynaud's Syndrome

Raynaud's syndrome is an insufficiency of arterial supply to the digital branches of the hand and feet elicited by exposure to cold or stress. Raynaud's syndrome may occur secondary to other conditions such as systemic lupus erythematosus or progressive systemic sclerosis. Exposure to cold temperatures or stress causes brief contractions or vasospasms of these small vessels. The condition is more prevalent in women than in men.

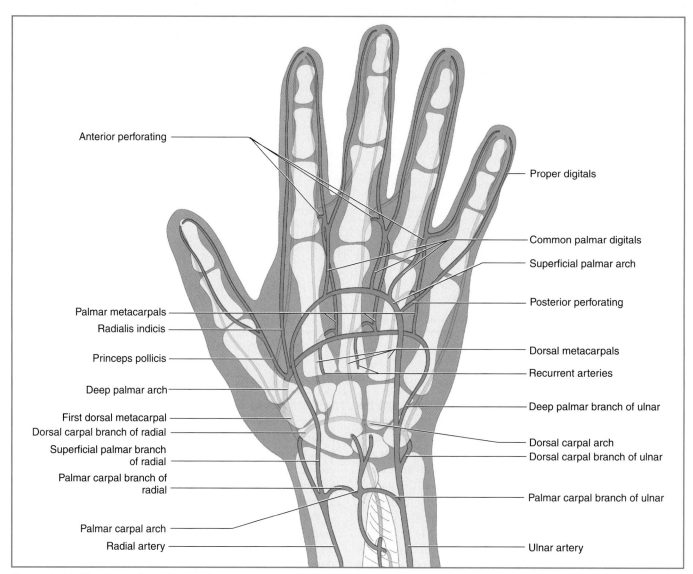

Figure 9-51. Blood supply to the hand.

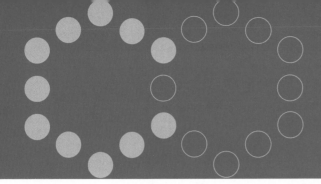

Head and Neck

10

CONTENTS

SKULL
  Morphology
  Embryology
  Cranial Fossae
SCALP
  Muscles of the Scalp
  Innervation of the Scalp
  Blood Supply to the Scalp
FACE
  Bones of the Face
  Muscles of the Face
  Innervation of the Face
  Blood Supply to the Face
  Venous Drainage of the Face and Scalp
  Lymphatic Drainage of the Face and Scalp
  Development of the Face
MENINGES AND DURAL VENOUS SINUSES
  Meningeal Layers
  Dural Venous Sinuses
  Relationships Between the Cranial Nerves and the
  Cavernous Sinus
CRANIAL NERVES
  General Terminology
  Cranial Nerves According to Function
DEVELOPMENT OF PHARYNGEAL ARCHES
NECK
  Overview of the Neck
  Visceral Column
  Vertebral Column
  Fascia of the Neck
  Carotid Sheath
TRIANGLES OF THE NECK
  Posterior and Anterior Triangles
  Digastric (Submandibular) Triangle

  Carotid Triangle
  Muscular Triangle
  Submental Triangle
VENOUS DRAINAGE OF THE NECK
  Superficial Veins
  Deep Veins
LYMPHATIC DRAINAGE OF THE NECK
  Horizontal Chain of Cervical Lymph Nodes
  Deep Cervical Nodes: Superior and Inferior Components
ORBIT
  Orbital Fascia
  Extraocular Muscles
  Superior and Inferior Oblique Muscles
  Innervation of the Orbit
  Circulation
TEMPORAL, INFRATEMPORAL, AND PAROTID REGIONS
  Temporal Fossa
  Infratemporal Fossa
  Parotid Space (Parotid Bed)
PTERYGOPALATINE FOSSA
  Bony Architecture
  Neurovascular Bundles
  Circulation
ORAL CAVITY (MOUTH)
  Vestibule
  Palate
  Tongue
  Blood Supply to the Oral Cavity
  Paralingual or Sublingual Space
  Development of the Palate
NASAL CAVITY AND PHARYNX
  Innervation of the Nasal Cavity
  Blood Supply to the Nasal Cavity
  Pharynx
LARYNX
  Innervation and Blood Supply of the Larynx

●●● SKULL

The skull (Fig. 10-1) can be divided into different regions on the basis of either morphology or embryology.

Morphology

The neurocranium, or cranium vault of the skull, encloses and protects the brain, and the viscerocranium consists of the facial bones that surround the mouth, nose, and part of the orbits. Thus, the viscerocranium encloses the visceral spaces, which house regions designed for vegetative functions such as the beginning of the respiratory system (nasal cavity) and the digestive system (mouth).

In many respects, the orbit is a transitional area between the face and neurocranium. Most of the *bones* of the orbit are by definition part of the viscerocranium. However, the frontal bone is part of the neurocranium. It contains the eye, which

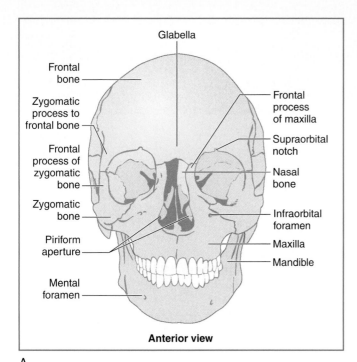

Anterior view

A

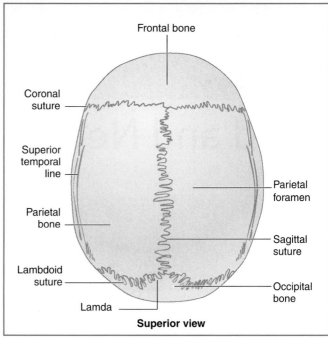

Superior view

B

Continued on page 293

Figure 10-1. Anterior (**A**) and superior (**B**) detailed views of the skull.

developmentally is an extension of the central nervous system (CNS).

Embryology

Membranocranium

The membranocranium is the part of the skull produced by intramembranous bone formation. The outer layer of the primitive mesenchyme that surrounds the embryonic brain is referred to as the ectomeninx. It gives rise to two layers: the membranous bone that forms the calvaria and the adjacent dura mater. This portion of the neurocranium is composed of the squamous portion of the frontal bone, the two parietal bones, and the squamous portion of the occipital bone (see Fig. 10-1C). The squamous frontal initially consists of two halves separated by the frontal suture (Fig. 10-2), which usually obliterates by the sixth year. When it remains open, it is referred to as a metopic suture.

Calvaria

The calvaria is the portion of the cranial vault consisting of the thin (scale-like) bones or parts of bones formed by intramembranous bone formation, specifically, one frontal, one occipital, and two parietal bones. Fibrous joints called sutures separate the bones of the calvaria. This type of joint has dense connective tissue separating the bones. In fetal and neonatal life, there are six regions where the fibrous connective tissue membrane has not yet ossified. These are the fontanelles.

They include an anterior fontanelle, a posterior fontanelle, two anterolateral (sphenoidal) fontanelles, and two posterolateral (mastoid) fontanelles (see Fig. 10-2).

The softness of the bones, the loose sutures, and the fontanelles allow the skull to flatten during birth. During this process, called molding, the parietal bones overlap while the frontal bone flattens and the occipital bone is drawn posteriorly. The bones reposition themselves during the first week after birth.

The bones of the calvaria have an outer and inner table of compact bone. Diploë bone is the layer of spongy bone located between the two layers of compact bone. The diploë bone is hematopoietic marrow throughout life and is a potential site of secondary metastases.

Chondrocranium

The chondrocranium is the part of the skull formed by endochondral bone formation (that is, a bone that develops from cartilage) and consists of the floor of the neurocranium. The bones include most of the occipital bone; the body, lesser wing, and greater wing of the sphenoid bone; the ethmoid bone; and the petrous portion of the temporal bone. In addition, the inferior conchae of the nasal cavity are formed by means of endochondral bone formation. During molding, the chondrocranium is deformed only slightly, if at all. This protects the juncture of the brainstem with the spinal cord. The chondrocranium is derived from the cartilage of the first two branchial arches.

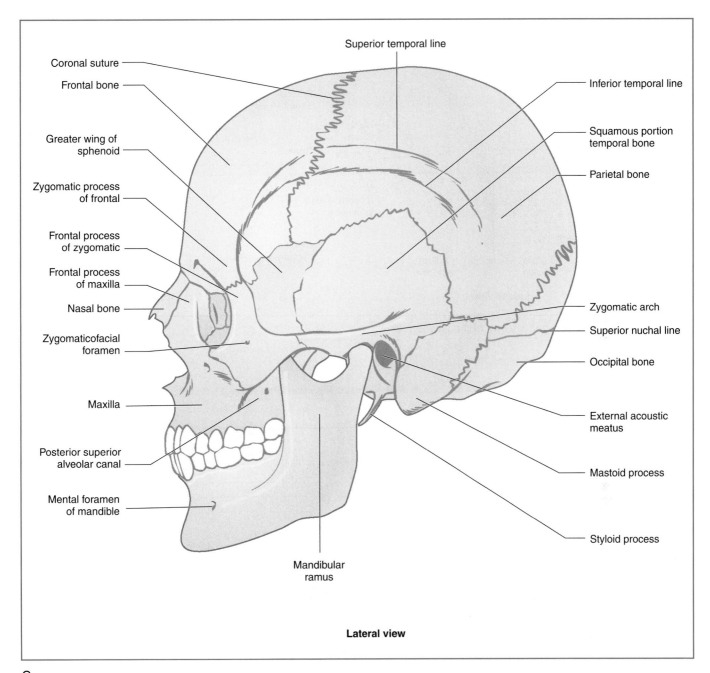

Coronal suture

Frontal bone

Greater wing of sphenoid

Zygomatic process of frontal

Frontal process of zygomatic

Frontal process of maxilla

Nasal bone

Zygomaticofacial foramen

Maxilla

Posterior superior alveolar canal

Mental foramen of mandible

Superior temporal line

Inferior temporal line

Squamous portion temporal bone

Parietal bone

Zygomatic arch

Superior nuchal line

Occipital bone

External acoustic meatus

Mastoid process

Styloid process

Mandibular ramus

Lateral view

C
Figure 10-1 cont'd. C, Lateral detailed views of the skull.

Cranial Fossae

The interior of the bony skull with the brain and meninges removed appears as three successive levels or ditch-like regions termed cranial fossae. The anterior cranial fossa is the highest, and the posterior cranial fossa the lowest (Fig. 10-3).

Anterior Cranial Fossa

The anterior cranial fossa contains the frontal lobes of the brain. The bony floor of this fossa is composed of the following bones: the orbital part of the frontal bone, the cribriform plate of the ethmoid bone, and the lesser wings and part of the body of the sphenoid bone (see Fig. 10-3 and Table 10-1).

The posterior boundary of the anterior cranial fossa consists of the posterior margins of the lesser wings of the sphenoid bone and the anterior margin of the optic chiasmatic groove (sulcus) on the body of the sphenoid bone (see Fig. 10-3).

The frontal bone's orbital parts form much of the floor of this fossa (Fig. 10-4; see also Fig. 10-3). The orbital parts separate the orbits from the anterior cranial fossa, forming a major part of the roof of the orbit (see Fig. 10-4). The anterior

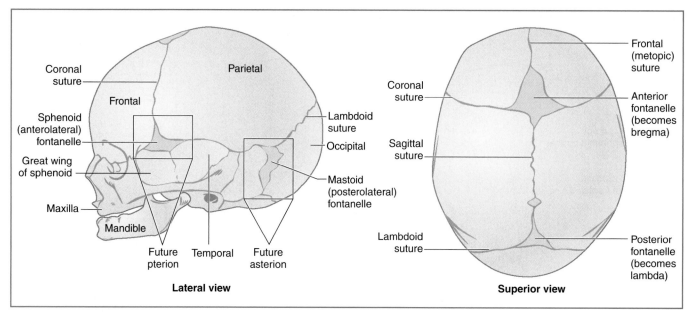

Figure 10-2. Lateral and superior views of the newborn skull.

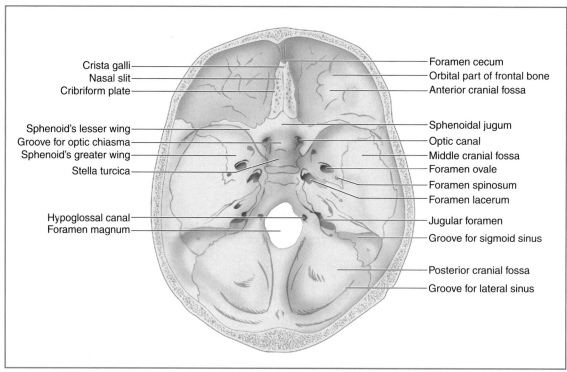

Figure 10-3. The three levels of the cranial fossae.

squamous (thin plate) portion of the frontal bone forms the anterior wall of this fossa (see Figs. 10-1 and 10-4). In the midline, there is a large notch between the orbital parts (the ethmoidal notch of the frontal bone), which articulates with the ethmoid bone. Often, notches and processes are named according to the name of the bone that they will articulate with. The ethmoidal notch of the frontal bone articulates with the superior surface of the ethmoid bone. This portion of the ethmoid bone is called the cribriform plate.

The ethmoid bone's cribriform plate (Fig. 10-5; see also Fig. 10-3) articulates with the frontal bone's ethmoidal notch anteriorly and the sphenoid bone's ethmoid spine to form the median aspect of the floor of the anterior cranial fossa (see Fig. 10-3). The cribriform plate separates the anterior cranial fossa from the nasal cavity.

Projecting superiorly from the cribriform plate is a thick, smooth, triangular process of bone, the crista galli (Latin,

TABLE 10-1. Passageways of the Anterior Cranial Fossa

Passageway	Structures Passing Through
Anterior and posterior ethmoidal canals	Anterior and posterior ethmoidal artery, vein, and nerve
Cribriform plate	Olfactory neuroepithelium (CN I), internal nasal branches of anterior ethmoid nerve, lateral and septal nasal branches of anterior ethmoid vessels

CLINICAL MEDICINE

Meningocele

On occasion, the foramen cecum does not close during development, allowing herniation of meninges and cerebral spinal fluid (a meningocele) or meninges, CSF, and brain tissue (meningoencephaloceles) to protrude into the nasal cavity. This is due to the failure of the small midline nasofrontal fontanelle between the paired frontal and the nasal bones to close.

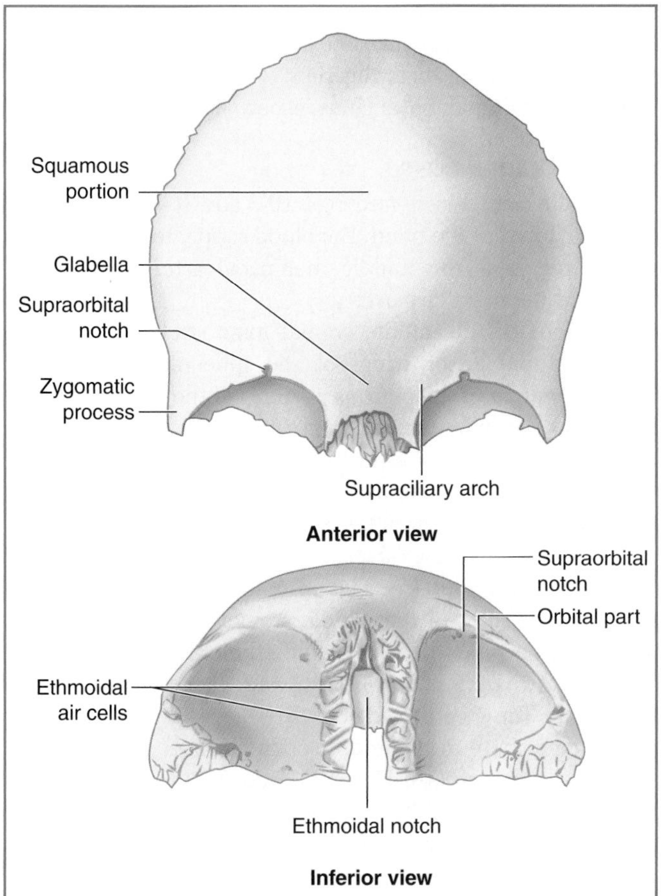

Figure 10-4. Anterior and inferior views of the frontal bone.

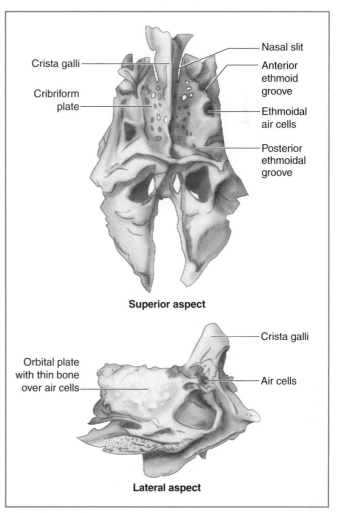

Figure 10-5. Posterosuperior and lateral views of the ethmoid bone.

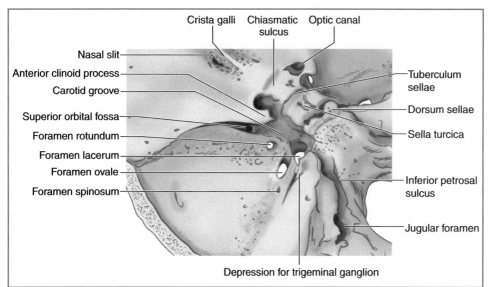

Crista galli Chiasmatic Optic canal
sulcus

Nasal slit
Anterior clinoid process
Carotid groove
Superior orbital fossa
Foramen rotundum
Foramen lacerum
Foramen ovale
Foramen spinosum

Tuberculum sellae
Dorsum sellae
Sella turcica
Inferior petrosal sulcus
Jugular foramen

Depression for trigeminal ganglion

Figure 10-6. Bones and oral passage ways of the middle cranial fossa.

CLINICAL MEDICINE

Anterior Cranial Fossa Fractures

Parts of the floor of the anterior cranial fossa are very delicate. The structures that make up this floor form the shared boundaries between the anterior cranial fossa and the orbits or the nasal cavity. Fracture of the cribriform plate may injure the olfactory nerves, with the resulting hemorrhage and leaking cerebrospinal fluid reaching the nasal cavity (CFS rhinorrhea). Fracture of an orbital part may result in hemorrhage or CSF reaching the orbit. Because the orbital periosteum is loosely attached to the bone except at the fissure and optic canal, hemorrhage, CSF, or both will enter the periorbital spaces and track anteriorly to produce edema in the orbit and eyelids with no involvement of the conjunctiva. This distribution of blood or cerebral spinal fluid in the eyelid is called the raccoon sign.

"cock's comb"), for the attachment of a dural specialization, the falx cerebri (Fig. 10-6; see also Fig. 10-3).

The cribriform plate supports the olfactory bulbs. This plate is pitted to allow the passage of the processes of approximately 20 olfactory neuroepithelial bundles, which constitute cranial nerve I (CN I), the olfactory nerve. These processes pass from the nasal cavity into the anterior cranial fossa through the olfactory foramina (see Fig. 10-5).

The anterior border of the ethmoid bone has thick projections that articulate with reciprocal depressions in the frontal bone, thereby producing the foramen cecum, which is typically a blind pouch. However, this foramen can remain open and transmit an emissary vein from the nasal cavity.

The lesser wings of the sphenoid bone and part of its body contribute to the posterior aspect of the floor of the anterior cranial fossa (see Figs. 10-3 and 10-6). The lesser wings lie posterior to the orbital plates and thus separate the anterior cranial fossa from the orbits. Extending from the lesser wings are the anterior clinoid processes for the attachment of the free margin of the tentorium cerebelli, which will be described with the dural sinuses.

Completing the posterior aspect of the anterior cranial fossa in the midline is the sphenoidal jugum (see Fig. 10-3). This flat surface of the body of the sphenoid bone lies posterior to the cribriform plate and between the two lesser wings, yoking (connecting) them together. It also helps form the roof of the sphenoid paranasal sinus, especially in the aged.

Middle Cranial Fossa

The middle cranial fossa (see Figs. 10-3 and 10-6) contains the temporal lobes of the brain. The blood supply to the meninges in this region is the middle meningeal artery, which is a branch of the maxillary artery.

The floor of the middle cranial fossa stretches from the margin of the lesser wings of the sphenoid bone to the superior margin of the petrous portions of the temporal bone. It includes the sella turcica and greater wings of the sphenoid bone and the superior aspect of the petrous portion of both temporal bones (see Fig. 10-3). Laterally the squamous portion and part of the parietal bones contribute to the lateral wall of the skull (Table 10-2).

The sphenoid bone (see Figs. 5-6 and 10-3) is an unpaired bone in the center of the middle cranial fossa and indeed is wedged in between the frontal and ethmoid bones anteriorly and the two temporal bones and the occipital bone posteriorly. The greater wings of the sphenoid bone and sella turcica contribute to the middle cranial fossa.

The sella turcica (see Figs. 10-3 and 10-6) is a deep fossa located in the midline. Its anterior boundary is the tuberculum (rounded, elevated ridge) sellae, and its posterior boundary is a plate of bone referred to as the dorsum sellae (Fig. 10-7). The posterior clinoid processes extend laterally from the dorsum sellae. The sella turcica houses the hypophysis (pituitary

TABLE 10-2. Passageways of the Middle Cranial Fossa

Passageway	Structures Passing Through
Carotid canal	Internal carotid artery and internal carotid nerve plexus (sympathetics)
Carotid sulcus	Curved groove found lateral to the sella turcica at the articulation of the body and the greater wing of the sphenoid bone Begins at the foramen lacerum and ends at the medial side of the anterior clinoid process and contains the cavernous sinus with its associated cranial nerves and the internal carotid artery
Foramen lacerum	Meningeal branch of ascending pharyngeal artery, meningeal lymph vessels, emissary veins from cavernous sinus to pterygoid plexus of veins
Foramen ovale	Mandibular nerve (V_3), lesser petrosal nerve (sometimes), emissary vein, accessory meningeal artery
Foramen rotundum	Maxillary nerve (V_2) into the pterygopalatine fossa
Foramen spinosum	Middle meningeal artery, recurrent meningeal branch of V_3
Hiatus for the lesser petrosal nerve	Lesser petrosal nerve, in the suture line between the petrous temporal and sphenoid bones
Hiatus for the greater petrosal nerve of the facial canal	Greater petrosal nerve, superior petrosal branch of the middle meningeal artery
Optic canal	Found at the lateral ends of the chiasmatic sulcus CN II, sympathetic nerves from internal carotid plexus, and ophthalmic artery
Optic chiasmatic sulcus	Groove for the optic chiasma found between the jugum of the sphenoid and the tuberculum sellae
Pterygoid canal	Nerve of the pterygoid canal (vidian nerve), which consists of the greater petrosal nerve and deep petrosal nerve, artery, and vein
Superior orbital fissure	Oculomotor nerve (CN III), trochlear nerve (CN IV), ophthalmic division of trigeminal nerve (V_1), abducent nerve (CN VI), postganglionic sympathetics, superior ophthalmic vein, and recurrent branch of lacrimal artery that anastomoses with ophthalmic branch of middle meningeal artery

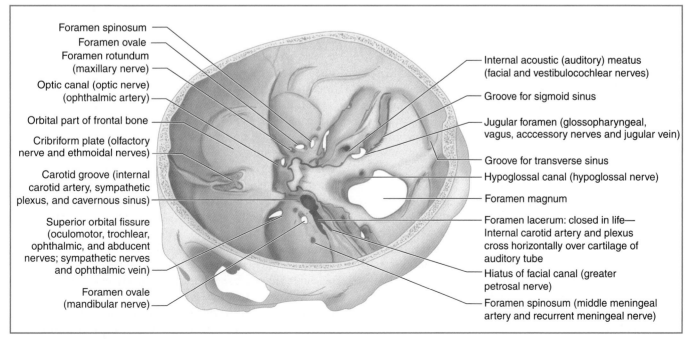

Figure 10-7. Dorsum sellae.

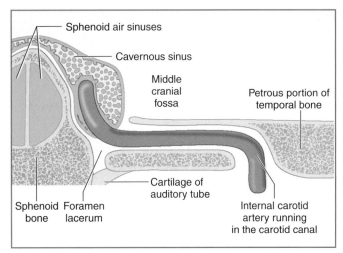

Sphenoid air sinuses

Cavernous sinus

Middle cranial fossa

Petrous portion of temporal bone

Cartilage of auditory tube

Sphenoid bone

Foramen lacerum

Internal carotid artery running in the carotid canal

Figure 10-8. Internal carotid artery passing through the carotid canal and over the foramen lacerum.

gland), the infundibulum, and the intercavernous sinuses. The sella turcica divides the middle cranial fossa into right and left halves.

The superior orbital fissure (see Fig. 10-6) is found between the lesser wing and the greater wing of the sphenoid bone. It allows the middle cranial fossa to communicate with the orbit.

The greater wing of the sphenoid bone (see Fig. 10-3) has three surfaces (orbital, temporal, and infratemporal), which separate the middle cranial fossa from the orbit anteriorly, the temporal region laterally, and the infratemporal fossa inferiorly.

The greater wing of the sphenoid bone has many openings for the passage of structures to or from the middle cranial fossa (see Figs. 10-6 and 10-7):

- *Foramen rotundum* is located medially at the base of the superior orbital fissure.
- *Foramen ovale* is a passageway in the infratemporal portion of the greater wing into the infratemporal region.
- *Foramen spinosum* is the passage in the infratemporal portion of the greater wing posterolateral to the foramen ovale.
- The emissary foramen (of Vesalius) is a passageway that is found posterolateral to the foramen ovale. When present, it transmits an emissary vein between the pterygoid plexus and the cavernous sinus.

The squamous and petrous portions of the temporal bone form the lateral posterior parts of the middle cranial fossa (see Fig. 10-6). The squamous portion is very thin especially superiorly. It forms part of the lateral wall of the skull. The squamous portion articulates with the lateral posterior surface of the greater wing of the sphenoid bone.

The petrous portion of the temporal bone is composed of dense bone that has many anatomic specializations. It is a three-sided pyramid-like structure that extends from the squamous portion medially and anteriorly to articulate with the greater wing of the sphenoid bone. Its apex, which contains the internal opening of the carotid canal, is wedged in between the sphenoid bone's greater wing and the occipital bone, but it does not fully articulate with the body of the sphenoid bone. This incomplete articulation of the apex of the petrous portion of the temporal bone with the body of the sphenoid bone leaves a jagged gap, called the foramen lacerum.

The foramen lacerum (see Figs. 10-6 and 10-7) is an artifact found only in the bony skull. In the living or cadavers, the inferior aspect of the foramen lacerum is closed by fibrocartilage of the pharyngotympanic (auditory) tube (Fig. 10-8), transforming the foramen lacerum into a ditch-like structure. The internal carotid artery and the accompanying internal carotid plexus pass through the carotid canal in the petrous portion of the temporal bone and then horizontally over the top of this fibrocartilage, not through it. Thus, the internal carotid artery and internal carotid plexus do *not* enter the neurocranium by passing vertically through the foramen lacerum from the base of the skull (see Figs. 10-6 and 10-8).

The carotid canal is in the petrous temporal bone. The canal is not linear but has a sharp right angle. It has a short, vertical arm that runs superiorly and a longer horizontal arm that runs anteromedially in the petrous temporal bone (see Fig. 10-8). After the internal carotid artery and nerve plexus pass over the cartilage of the auditory tube, they then pass onto the carotid groove (see Figs. 10-6 and 10-8) to enter the cavernous sinus.

The arcuate eminence is an elevation on the anterior surface of the petrous temporal bone marking the position of the inner ear's anterior semicircular canal. The tegmen tympani (roof of the middle ear) is slightly lateral to this eminence.

The hiatus for the greater petrosal nerve (of the facial canal) is a passageway for the greater petrosal nerve from the facial canal into the middle cranial fossa. It is found on the anterior surface of the petrous temporal bone. A narrow groove, or sulcus, leads from the hiatus to the foramen lacerum. It denotes the course of the greater petrosal nerve and the superficial petrosal artery. The greater petrosal nerve, a branch of the facial nerve (CN VII) exits the middle cranial fossa via the pterygoid canal, which is located in the anterior wall of the foramen lacerum.

The hiatus for the lesser petrosal nerve and the superior tympanic artery are found anterolateral to the groove for the greater petrosal nerve on the anterior surface of the petrous temporal bone. The lesser petrosal nerve, a branch of the tympanic plexus from glossopharyngeal nerve (CN IX), exits the middle cranial fossa in the suture line between the petrous temporal and sphenoid bones or sometimes the foramen ovale.

The trigeminal impression is a depression directly above the anteromedial end of the carotid canal, at the apex of the petrous temporal bone (see Fig. 10-6).

The petrous ridge runs along the superior margin of the petrous temporal bone. It is the site of attachment for the tentorium cerebelli. This ridge is marked by a groove for the superior petrosal sinus (which will be described with the dural sinuses). The petrous ridge, along with the dorsum sellae, forms the boundary between the middle and posterior cranial fossae.

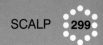

CLINICAL MEDICINE

Skull Fractures Through the Middle Cranial Fossa

The point at which the temporal surface of the greater wing articulates with the temporal, frontal, and parietal bones is called the pterion. This was the site of the sphenoid fontanelle and is a particularly thin part of the adult skull. In addition, the middle meningeal artery usually passes in a groove that runs along the internal aspect of the skull at this point. Trauma at the pterion can cause a hemorrhage of the middle meningeal vessels. *Bleeding of the middle meningeal vessels produces a life-threatening epidural hematoma.* Bleeding of the middle meningeal vessels always flows into a potential epidural space because these vessels are located between the dura mater and the bone.

A fracture may also extend across the body of the sphenoid bone and injure the internal carotid artery. This could result in bleeding into the sphenoid sinus or the nose. A fracture of the tegmen tympani may result in CSF leaking into the middle ear. If the tympanic membrane is also damaged, the CSF can leak out of the external auditory meatus. Therefore, obvious bleeding from the ear, nose, or both after a patient has sustained cranial injuries may be a sign of *severe damage* to the skull.

Posterior Cranial Fossa

The posterior cranial fossa (see Figs. 10-3 and 10-7) contains the brainstem, pons, and cerebellum. Most of the cranial nerves arise from the brainstem in the posterior cranial fossa except CNs I and II (optic nerve). CNs IV (trochlear nerve) to XII (hypoglossal nerve) enter the dura in the posterior cranial fossa. However, although CN III (oculomotor nerve) arises in the posterior cranial fossa, it enters the dura in the middle cranial fossa (see Table 10-2).

The floor and walls of the posterior cranial fossa are formed by the occipital bone, the posterior surfaces of the petrous and mastoid portions of the temporal bones, the dorsum sellae of the sphenoid bone, and laterally a small part of the parietal bones (Table 10-3; see also Fig. 10-7). Included within this fossa is the sloping clivus, which is formed by the posterior surface of the sphenoid bone starting at the dorsum sellae and the basilar portion of the occipital bone to the foramen magnum.

The large foramen magnum allows for the connection between brain and spinal cord and is surrounded by the occipital bone. This is analogous to the vertebral arch surrounding the spinal cord. The basilar, lateral (condylar), and squamous portions of the occipital bone form the foramen magnum.

The internal auditory meatus is found on the posterior surface of the petrous temporal bone. It leads to the inner ear and the facial canal.

The jugular foramen (see Fig. 10-7) is formed by the articulation of the jugular fossa of the petrous temporal bone with the jugular notch and process of the lateral portion of the occipital bone. The jugular foramen is often divided into three compartments. The posterior compartment is for the passage of the sigmoid dural sinus, which is continuous with the

TABLE 10-3. Passageways of the Posterior Cranial Fossa

Passageway	Structures Passing Through
Condyloid (condylar) canal	Emissary veins, meningeal branch of occipital artery
Foramen magnum	Junction of the spinal cord and brainstem, vertebral arteries, anterior and posterior spinal arteries, spinal roots of CN XI, communication of venous plexuses around spinal cord with dural venous sinuses
Hypoglossal canal	Hypoglossal nerve (XII) and its meningeal branch, meningeal branch of ascending pharyngeal artery, emissary vein
Internal auditory (acoustic) meatus	Facial (VII) and vestibulocochlear (VIII) nerves, labyrinthine artery
Jugular foramen	CNs IX, X, and XI; internal jugular vein as formed by sigmoid sinus and inferior petrosal sinus; meningeal branches from occipital and ascending pharyngeal arteries; meningeal branches of CN X
Mastoid canaliculus	Auricular branch of vagus with contributions from CNs IX and VII, emissary vein
Mastoid foramen	Emissary vein, meningeal branch of occipital artery

internal jugular vein (G 650). The middle compartment is for CNs IX, X, and XI (accessory nerve), and the anterior compartment is where the inferior petrosal sinus drains into the internal jugular vein.

The hypoglossal canal (see Fig. 10-7) is found in the lateral portion of the occipital bone that contributes to the lateral wall of the foramen magnum. It is separated from the jugular foramen by a strong ridge of bone (the jugular tuberculum). When viewed from the base of the skull, the hypoglossal canal is just millimeters from the jugular foramen. CNs IX, X, XI, and XII then pass between the internal jugular vein and the internal carotid artery.

●●● SCALP

The bones of the calvaria, or skull cap (see Fig. 10-1B), include the frontal bone's squamous portion, the two parietal bones, and the occipital bone's squamous portion. The tissues overlying the skull cap are referred to as the scalp. It lies between the superior temporal lines laterally, the eyebrows anteriorly, and the superior nuchal line posteriorly.

The five layers to the scalp include skin, often supplied with abundant hair covering a subcutaneous connective tissue layer containing dense connective tissue bundles that

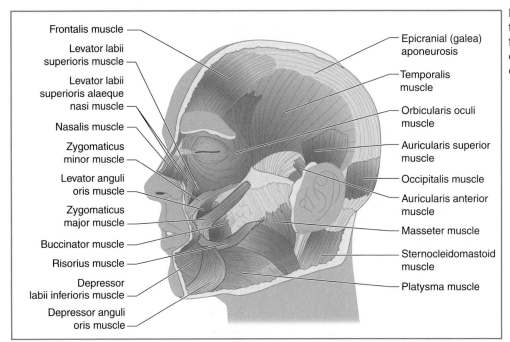

A

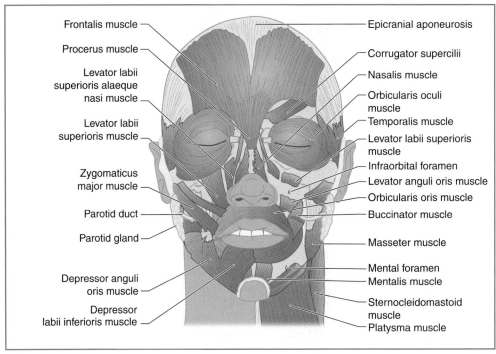

B

Figure 10-9. A, Lateral view of the muscles of the scalp and of facial expression. **B,** Frontal view of the muscles of facial expression.

divide the subcutaneous layer into fat-filled pockets, the epicranial aponeurosis (galea aponeurotica), a layer of loose connective tissue, and the periosteum (pericranium) of the calvaria.

The scalp tends to bleed profusely because the dense connective tissue holds the cut blood vessels open. The neurovascular supply of the scalp is also found in this layer. The epicranial aponeurosis (Fig. 10-9), found deep to the dense connective tissue, is a tough connective tissue sheet whose fibers are oriented in the anteroposterior direction. It connects the two bellies of the paired occipitofrontalis muscles (epicranius; see Fig. 10-9). Underlying the epicranial aponeurosis is a layer of loose connective tissue, allowing for movement of the scalp. The loose connective tissue is a potential plane for the spread of blood or infection and is referred to as the scalp's "danger zone." Injuries of the head can include avulsion of the scalp at the plane of the loose connective tissue, where the scalp is partly or completely torn from the underlying periosteum. Replantation requires retaining or repairing the blood supply.

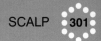

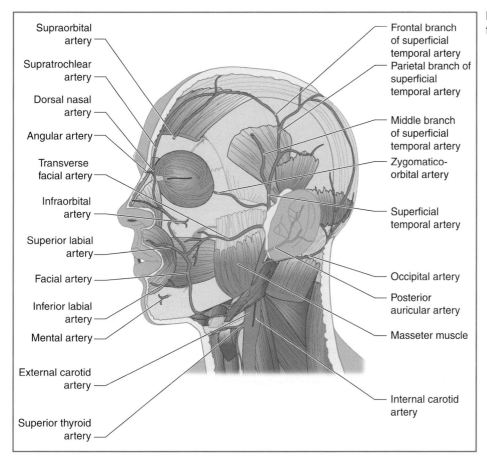

Figure 10-10. Arterial supply to the face and scalp.

Labels (clockwise from top left): Supraorbital artery · Supratrochlear artery · Dorsal nasal artery · Angular artery · Transverse facial artery · Infraorbital artery · Superior labial artery · Facial artery · Inferior labial artery · Mental artery · External carotid artery · Superior thyroid artery · Frontal branch of superficial temporal artery · Parietal branch of superficial temporal artery · Middle branch of superficial temporal artery · Zygomatico-orbital artery · Superficial temporal artery · Occipital artery · Posterior auricular artery · Masseter muscle · Internal carotid artery

Deep to the layer of loose connective tissue is the periosteum of the outer surface of the calvaria. The periosteum on the *external* surface of the calvaria is the pericranium, while the periosteum *internal* to the calvaria is called endosteum, which is the osteogenic layer. These layers are continuous at the sutural ligaments.

Muscles of the Scalp

Each occipitofrontalis (epicranius) muscle has two bellies: a frontal belly in the forehead and an occipital belly that arises from the occipital bone (see Figs. 10-4 and 10-9). The occipital portion of this muscle (occipitalis muscle) is smaller and inserts into the epicranial aponeurosis (galea aponeurotica). The frontal portion (frontalis muscle) arises from the epicranial aponeurosis and inserts into the orbicularis oculi muscle. Thus, the frontalis muscle does not insert into bone. The frontalis muscle produces the horizontal wrinkles in the forehead and slightly raises the eyebrows. The temporal branches of the facial nerve innervate the frontalis, while the posterior auricular branch of the facial nerve innervates the occipitalis.

Innervation of the Scalp

The muscles of facial expression, including occipitofrontalis, are innervated by the branches of the facial nerve.

The sensory innervation can be separated into two components. Anterior to an imaginary interauricular line, innervation is provided by supraorbital and supratrochlear branches of the ophthalmic nerve, while posteriorly innervation is provided by the greater occipital and third occipital (tertius occipitalis) nerves. The latter two nerves are the dorsal rami of C2 and C3, respectively.

Blood Supply to the Scalp

The scalp has an abundant blood supply from branches of both internal and external carotid arteries. The ophthalmic artery arises from the internal carotid artery, and its supraorbital and supratrochlear branches help supply the scalp. The superficial temporal and occipital arteries arise from the external carotid artery and also help supply the scalp. They anastomose with each other.

External Carotid Artery Branches

The superficial temporal artery (Fig. 10-10) is a terminal branch of the external carotid artery that passes over the zygomatic arch into the temporal region. Its branches include anterior auricular, parotid, transverse facial, zygomatico-orbital, and middle temporal to the temporalis muscle. Branches of the superficial temporal's frontal artery anastomose with branches of the supraorbital artery and contralateral superficial temporal artery. Branches of its parietal artery anastomose with branches of the occipital artery and contralateral superficial temporal artery.

The posterior auricular artery is a branch of the external carotid artery that supplies the external ear and the scalp behind the ear.

The occipital artery first follows the inferior border of the posterior belly of the digastric muscle. The artery then passes in a deep groove on the medial aspect of the mastoid notch to eventually follow the greater occipital nerve and supply the posterior scalp. It anastomoses with the superficial temporal artery.

These anastomoses create an overall anastomosis between the internal and external carotid arteries.

●●● FACE

The facial bones surround the visceral spaces of the head: the beginning of the respiratory system (nasal cavity), digestive system (mouth), and part of the orbit. These bones are derived from the first pharyngeal (branchial) arch. The first arch consists of a maxillary process dorsally and a mandibular process ventrally. The pharyngeal arches arise briefly during development to produce specific head and neck structures. The first arch's maxillary process produces the maxilla, lacrimal, nasal, zygomatic, and squamous temporal bones, while the mandibular process produces the mandible (see Figs. 10-1 and 10-2). Although morphologically the bones of the face begin at the superior margin of the orbits, the face is arbitrarily defined as beginning at the hairline.

Bones of the Face

The squamous portion of the frontal bone forms the bony forehead (see Figs. 10-1 and 10-4). The frontal bone is classified as a bone of the neurocranium. It extends from the coronal suture down to the superior aspect of the orbital margin. The frontal bone also forms the roof of the orbit. The supraciliary arches are ridges on the frontal bone just above and paralleling the supraorbital margins. The supraorbital notch or foramen is found in the superior margin of the orbit (see Fig. 10-1A). It is the passageway for the supraorbital neurovascular bundle to pass from the orbit to the face. The frontal bone's nasal part is found between the orbits and articulates with the nasal bones and maxillae (Table 10-4).

The frontal bone also has a process on its lateral aspect that articulates with the zygomatic bone, otherwise known as the zygomatic process of the frontal bone (see Fig. 10-1A). Both of these processes participate in the formation of the margin of the orbit.

The paired nasal bones form the bridge of the nose (see Fig. 10-1A and C). Superiorly, the nasal bones articulate with frontal bones, laterally with the frontal processes of the maxillary bones, and in the midline with each other. The nasal bones are short, rectangular bones that form the superior aspect of the nasal or piriform (pear-shaped) aperture (see Fig. 10-1A). This aperture is the bony opening of the nose. The two maxillary bones (maxillae) form the inferior aspect of this aperture. The interior surface of the nasal bone is often grooved by the external nasal nerve and vessels which then pass between the nasal bone and cartilage.

The maxillary bones form the upper jaw and the middle third of the face (see Fig. 10-1A). The body of the maxilla is found lateral to the nasal cavity and contains the large maxillary air sinus. The frontal process of the maxilla articulates superiorly with the frontal bone and forms the medial aspect of the orbital margin.

The inferior margin of the orbit is formed by both the maxilla and the zygomatic bones. Just inferior to the middle of the inferior orbital margin is the infraorbital foramen. *This foramen is in a vertical line with the supraorbital and mental foramina* (see Fig. 10-1A). The zygomatic process of the maxilla articulates with the zygomatic bone and contributes to the formation of the cheek prominence, which the general public refers to as the cheek bone. Extending inferiorly from the body of the maxilla is the alveolar process, which contains the upper teeth.

The zygomatic bone primarily forms the prominence of the cheek and the lateral aspect of the orbital margin (see Fig. 10-1A). It articulates superiorly with the frontal bone and medially with the maxilla. The anterolateral aspect of the zygomatic bone has small zygomaticofacial foramina on its surface. The anteromedial surface of this bone helps form the lateral aspect of the orbit. The posterior (temporal) aspect of the zygomatic bone may have a zygomaticotemporal foramen.

The mandible develops from two bones connected by a fibrocartilage suture in the midline (see Fig. 10-1A). The two bones fuse at approximately 2 years of age, forming a joint called the mental symphysis.

The mental foramen is found halfway between the upper border of the alveolar process and the inferior margin of the mandible (see Fig. 10-1A). Although it is an opening from the mandibular canal, it is not the canal's terminal end. The mandibular canal extends nearly to the mandible's mental symphysis.

TABLE 10-4. Passageways of the Face

Passageway	Structures Passing Through
Infraorbital foramen	Infraorbital nerve and vessels
Mental foramen	Mental nerve and vessels
Supraorbital foramen	Supraorbital neurovascular bundle
Zygomaticofacial foramina	Zygomaticofacial branches of V_2
Zygomaticotemporal foramen	Zygomaticotemporal branch of V_2

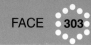

TABLE 10-5. Muscles of Facial Expression

Muscle	Origin	Insertion	Innervation
Muscles Associated with the Orbit			
Occipitofrontalis			CN VII branches
Occipitalis	Superior nuchal line of occipital bone, adjacent temporal bone	Epicranial aponeurosis	Auricular
Frontalis	Epicranial aponeurosis	Orbicularis oculi; skin of eyebrows, forehead, and nose	Temporal
Orbicularis oculi			
Orbital portion	Nasal process of frontal bone and frontal process of maxilla, medial palpebral ligament	Uninterrupted elliptical fibers with the insertion the same as the origin	Temporal and zygomatic
Palpebral portion	Medial palpebral ligament Adjacent parts of frontal and maxillary bones	Lateral palpebrae raphe	Temporal and zygomatic
Lacrimal portion	Posterior lacrimal crest of lacrimal bone	Fascia surrounding the lacrimal sac and the tarsal plates	Temporal and zygomatic
Corrugator supercilii	Nasal portion of the frontal bone	Medial eyebrow muscle interdigitates with orbicularis oculi	Temporal
Procerus muscles	Nasal bones, adjacent nasal cartilage	Skin of eyebrows	Temporal and zygomatic
Muscles of the Nose			
Depressor septi nasi	Maxilla, inferior to the nose	Lowest part of the nasal septum	Buccal
Nasalis			Buccal
Transverse part	Maxilla	Contralateral muscle across bridge of nose	
Alar part	Maxilla	Cartilage of the wing of the nostril	
Muscles of the Mouth			
Buccinator	Pterygomandibular raphe and posterior alveolar processes of both jaws	Angle of the mouth	Buccal
Levator labii superioris alaeque nasi	Frontal process of the maxilla	Upper lip and into the ala of the nose	Buccal
Levator labii superioris	Maxilla *above* the infraorbital foramen	Orbicularis oris upper lip	Buccal
Levator anguli oris	Maxilla *below* the infraorbital foramen	Angle of the lip	Buccal
Zygomaticus major	Zygomatic bone, fascia of the parotid gland	Angle of the mouth, orbicularis oris muscle	Buccal
Risorius	Fascia over the masseter muscle and parotid gland	Angle of the mouth	Zygomatic and buccal
Depressor anguli oris	Oblique line of the mandible	Angle of the mouth	Mandibular
Depressor labii inferioris	Mandible between the mental foramen and symphysis	Orbicularis oris muscle and the lower lip	Mandibular
Mentalis	Mandible inferior to the mouth	Skin of the chin	Mandibular
Platysma	Superficial fascia in the thorax and adjacent deltoid region	Platysma muscle on the opposite side, the facial muscles inferomedial to the mouth	Cervical

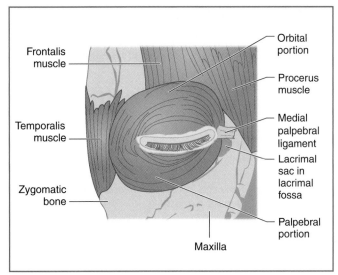

Frontalis
muscle

Temporalis
muscle

Zygomatic
bone

Maxilla

Orbital
portion

Procerus
muscle

Medial
palpebral
ligament

Lacrimal
sac in
lacrimal
fossa

Palpebral
portion

Figure 10-11. Internal view of the orbicularis oculi with its three parts: orbital portion, palpebral portion, and lacrimal portion.

Muscles of the Face

The "muscles of facial expression" have two important functions: to convey emotion and to serve as sphincters or dilators of visceral cavities of the head. The muscles of facial expression usually arise from bone and typically insert into other muscles of facial expression or the skin of the face. Thus, many muscles of facial expression lie in the plane of the superficial fascia. Other skeletal muscles are *not* found in the plane of the superficial fascia. The muscles of facial expression embryologically arise from the second pharyngeal arch.

Muscles of the Orbit and Auricle

The orbicularis oculi (see Fig. 10-9 and Table 10-5) is the sphincter of the orbit that is innervated by temporal and zygomatic branches of the facial nerve. It has three major parts: orbital, palpebral, and lacrimal (Fig. 10-11).

The orbital portion surrounds the orbit in the form of continuous muscular loops that can forcefully close the eye as in squinting.

The palpebral portion is confined to the eyelid. These fibers insert laterally into a delicate connective tissue band (raphe) and produce a sphincter-like action that gently closes the eyelids. The palpebral portion also exerts a medial pull on the eyelid because of its ellipsoidal shape and insertion into the lateral palpebrae raphe. *Contraction of the palpebral portion produces an ongoing blinking of the open eye approximately 6 to 15 times a minute, which spreads the tear film over the eye.* This ongoing blinking proceeds unnoticed.

The lacrimal portion may be responsible for the pressure changes of the lacrimal sac. These changes appear to aid in the drainage of tears via the lacrimal canaliculus, lacrimal sac, and nasolacrimal duct.

The orbicularis oculi muscle is innervated by special visceral efferent (SVE) and general somatic afferent (GSA) fibers of the temporal and zygomatic branches of the facial nerve.

The corrugator supercilii (see Figs. 10-9B and 10-11) penetrates the frontalis muscle and mingles with the orbicularis oculi to insert into the medial end of the eyebrows. These muscles pull the eyebrows medially and inferiorly, producing vertical wrinkles at the root of the nose.

The two procerus muscles (see Fig. 10-9B) act as a single functional unit. The procerus muscles pull the medial eyebrow down, producing transverse (horizontal) wrinkling at the root of the nose.

The anterior, superior, and posterior auricular muscles are the extrinsic muscles of the ear. They are poorly developed in humans.

Muscles of the Nose

The depressor septi draws the nasal septum downward, narrowing the nostril (see Fig. 10-9 and Table 10-5).

The nasalis comprises the transverse and alar parts. The transverse part of the nasalis muscle constricts the nostril. The alar portion of the nasalis flares (dilates) the nostril by pulling it laterally toward the maxilla.

Muscles of the Mouth

The orbicularis oris (see Fig. 10-9) encircles the mouth and forms the muscular component of the lips. The orbicularis oris is a complex of muscle fibers running in different planes and which inserts into external skin and the internal mucous membrane. It serves as the sphincter of the mouth that contracts, compresses, and protrudes the lips. The lips are uniquely developed in humans to help produce speech and whistling. The oral fissure (rima oris) is the line of contact between the lips.

The orbicularis oris also receives elevators and depressors. The levator labii superioris and levator labii superioris alaeque nasi are elevators of the upper lip. The levator labii superioris alaeque nasi also helps the alar portion of the nasalis dilate the nostril. The zygomaticus major and levator anguli oris are elevators of the angle of the mouth. The levator anguli oris arises inferior to the infraorbital foramen and passes deep to the levator labii superioris, which arises superior to the infraorbital foramen.

The buccinator (see Figs. 10-9 and 10-10) forms the muscular aspect of the cheek and lateral wall of the oral cavity. It arises in part from the pterygomandibular raphe that runs from the medial pterygoid plate and its hamulus to the mandible as well as the alveolar processes of both maxilla and mandible. The pterygomandibular raphe is the common attachment of both the buccinator and the superior pharyngeal constrictor muscles.

The buccinator inserts into the angle of the mouth in an unusual manner. The superior and the inferior fibers of this muscle are continuous with the muscle fibers of the upper and lower lips, but the central fibers decussate (cross) before inserting into the orbicularis oris muscle, thereby forming the modiolus (hub) along with many of the muscles that converge on the angle of the mouth. The modiolus strengthens the angle of the mouth and modulates the action of the muscles that insert into the lips. The buccinator forces food and fluid

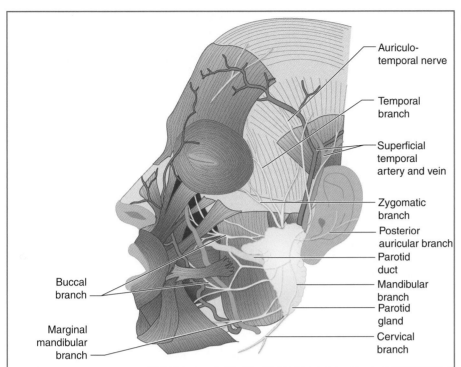

Figure 10-12. Distribution of facial nerve branches.

Labels (clockwise from top): Auriculo-temporal nerve; Temporal branch; Superficial temporal artery and vein; Zygomatic branch; Posterior auricular branch; Parotid duct; Mandibular branch; Parotid gland; Cervical branch; Marginal mandibular branch; Buccal branch

from the oral cavity's vestibule onto the occlusal (contacting) surfaces of the teeth and then into the oral cavity proper. The parotid duct and the buccal branch of mandibular nerve V₃ pierce the buccinator muscle to supply sensory fibers to the oral cavity's lateral wall.

The depressor anguli oris (see Fig. 10-9B) depresses and draws the angle of the mouth laterally, while the depressor labii inferioris depresses the lower lip and also draws it laterally. The depressor labii inferioris is located deep to the depressor anguli oris (see Fig. 10-9B and Table 10-5).

The mentalis inserts into the skin of the chin to wrinkle it and at the same time protrudes the lower lip.

The fibers of the platysma cross the neck to insert into the contralateral platysma muscle as well as other muscles at the angle of the mouth. The platysma tenses the skin of the neck during a grimace.

Innervation of the Face

The face has a dual innervation derived from two different cranial nerves (Figs. 10-12 and 10-13). The facial muscles are derived from the nonsomitic mesoderm of the second pharyngeal (branchial) arch. Efferent fibers innervating the muscles derived from the pharyngeal arch's nonsomitic mesoderm are classified as special visceral efferent. The facial muscles receive SVE fibers from CN VII, the facial nerve. However, the sensory (cutaneous) innervation to the skin of the face overlying these muscles is via branches of the trigeminal nerve (CN V) carrying with GSA fibers.

The facial nerve exits the facial canal through the stylomastoid foramen (see Fig. 10-13). It gives off a posterior

auricular branch supplying the posterior auricular muscle and the occipital belly of the occipitofrontalis muscle. The facial nerve then runs forward, passing *laterally* to the styloid process, and divides into superior and inferior trunks. Upon entering the substance of the parotid gland, the two divisions of the facial nerve divide into five branches: temporal, zygomatic, buccal, marginal mandibular, and cervical. As these branches emerge from the parotid gland, their distribution can be mimicked by placing a hand over the parotid gland with the thumb facing down and spreading the fingers (see Fig. 10-12).

In addition to its SVE fibers, CN VII *may* carry GSA fibers for proprioception, which most likely have their cell bodies in the geniculate ganglion. Distribution of the terminal branches of the facial nerve is listed in Table 10-5.

Sensory Fibers (GSA)

Sensory fibers (GSA) to the face (see Fig. 10-13A) are primarily branches of CN V, the trigeminal nerve. However, some fibers from cervical spinal nerves supply cutaneous innervation to the angle of the mandible.

Fibers from the ophthalmic division of CN V carry sensation from the upper eyelid, eye, the dorsal surface and root of the nose, the forehead, and the scalp as far back as the interauricular line (see Fig. 10-13A). Fibers from the maxillary division of V carry sensation from the lower eyelid, the nose and parts of the cheek and upper lip. Fibers from the mandibular division of V carry sensation from the following: the lower lip, chin, skin of the lower jaw (excluding the angle of the mandible), buccal mucosa, anterior aspect of the lateral ear, external auditory meatus, external surface of tympanic membrane, and adjacent temporal region (see Fig. 10-13).

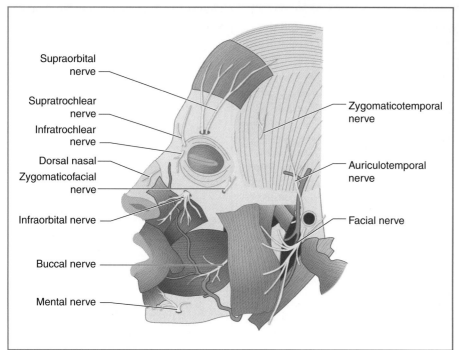

A

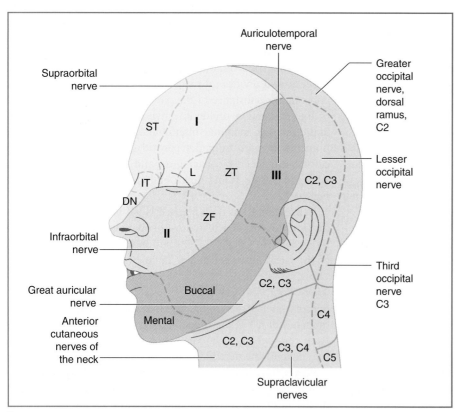

B

Figure 10-13. A, Sensory nerves to the face. **B,** Sensory distribution to the face and scalp. Note that the greater, lesser, and 3rd occipital nerves are supplied by the dorsal rami.

Ophthalmic (V₁) Nerve Branches

- *Supraorbital nerve* exits the orbit through the supraorbital foramen or notch to help supply the upper eyelid and forehead (see Fig. 10-13). It divides into medial and lateral branches that are distributed to the skin of the forehead and scalp as far back as the interauricular line.
- *Supratrochlear nerve* exits the medial aspect of the orbit above the trochlea (pulley for the superior oblique muscle) and innervates a medial portion of the forehead and upper eyelid (see Fig. 10-13).
- *Infratrochlear nerve* emerges from the medial angle of the orbit, below the trochlea. The nerve supplies the lateral side of the bridge of the nose and the medial aspect of *both* eyelids.
- *External (dorsal) nasal nerve* has been described with the skull. It is a branch of the internal nasal nerve, which is in turn a branch of the anterior ethmoidal nerve (of V₁). The external nasal nerve emerges between the nasal bone and the nasal cartilage. Its GSA fibers supply the lower half of the dorsum of the nose to the tip (see Fig. 10-13).
- *Lacrimal nerve* exits the orbit at the lateral superior aspect of the orbit and innervates the lateral aspect of the upper eyelid and adjacent skin.

Maxillary (V₂) Nerve Branches

- *Infraorbital nerve* is the largest branch of the maxillary division. It emerges from the infraorbital foramen and supplies the skin over the lower eyelid, cheek, wing (ala) of the nostril, and upper lip.
- *Zygomaticofacial nerve* (see Fig. 10-13) emerges from the zygomaticofacial foramen in the zygomatic bone. The nerve innervates the skin on the prominence of the cheek and around the lateral angle of the eye.
- *Zygomaticotemporal nerve* emerges from the zygomaticotemporal foramen on the posterior (temporal) surface of the zygomatic bone. This nerve runs between the bone and temporalis muscle and pierces the muscle and deep temporal fascia to supply the skin anterior to the temple just lateral to the orbit.

Mandibular (V₃) Nerve Branches

- *Buccal nerve (long buccal nerve)* (see Fig. 10-13) emerges between the ramus of the mandible and the buccinator muscle onto the cheek. The buccal nerve provides sensory innervation to the skin of the cheek. The nerve also pierces the buccinator muscle with many small branches to provide sensory innervation to the mucous membrane of the lateral wall of the oral cavity and adjacent gingiva.
- *Auriculotemporal nerve* runs with the superficial temporal vessels as they cross the zygomatic arch. It supplies sensory innervation to a small anterolateral part of the auricle and to the skin of the temporal region.
- *Mental nerve* is a branch of the inferior alveolar nerve. It leaves the mandibular canal by means of the mental foramen and supplies the skin of the chin and lower lip (see Fig. 10-13).

Other Sensory Nerves

The great auricular branch of the cervical plexus innervates the skin over the angle of the mandible.

Blood Supply to the Face

The primary arterial supply to the face (see Fig. 10-10) consists of branches of the facial artery, which is a branch of the external carotid artery in the neck. The facial artery emerges between the mandible and the submandibular gland. It passes over the inferior margin of the mandible just antero-inferior to the masseter muscle to reach the face.

On the face, the branches of the facial nerve cross the facial artery superficially. The facial artery has a tortuous course to accommodate the movements of the mandible, lips, and cheeks. It passes deep to many of the superficial muscles of facial expression (platysma, risorius, and zygomaticus major) and in the levator labii superioris alaeque nasi. The facial artery travels superiorly past the angle of the mouth, along-side the nose toward the medial angle of the eye. After its lateral nasal artery branches off, the facial artery continues as the angular artery. This artery helps supply the orbicularis oculi and lacrimal sac and then ends by anastomosing with a terminal branch of the ophthalmic artery, the *dorsal nasal artery*, at the medial angle of the eye. The facial artery is always *anterior* to the more linear facial vein.

The inferior labial artery arises from the facial artery below the angle of the mouth and supplies the lower lip, while the superior labial artery supplies the upper lip and a small portion of the nasal septum. Both superior and inferior labial arteries anastomose with their contralateral superior and inferior labial artery.

The lateral nasal artery supplies the dorsum of the nose and the ala of the nose.

Other Blood Vessels

Many of these arteries freely anastomose with each other to give the face a rich blood supply.

This extensive blood supply allows the surgeon to ligate the facial artery at the margin of the mandible during a radical neck procedure without compromising the face's blood supply.

Ophthalmic Artery Branches

The following branches of the ophthalmic artery, which is a branch of the internal carotid artery, emerge from the orbit to supply surrounding areas of the face (see Fig. 10-10).

- *Dorsal nasal artery* emerges through the upper eyelid and supplies the bridge of the nose. It supplies the lateral aspect of the nose and anastomoses with the angular artery.
- *Supratrochlear artery* follows the course of the supratrochlear nerve and supplies the medial aspect of the forehead to anastomose with the contralateral supratrochlear artery.
- *Supraorbital artery* follows the course of the supraorbital nerve and supplies the lateral forehead and the scalp. The supraorbital artery anastomoses with the frontal branches of

the superficial temporal artery. The two superficial temporal arteries anastomose with each other across the midsagittal line.

Maxillary Artery Branches

- *Maxillary artery* branches anastomose with facial and ophthalmic artery branches (see Fig. 10-10).
- *Infraorbital artery* emerges from the infraorbital foramen and anastomoses with the transverse facial, buccal, and branches of the dorsal nasal arteries.
- *Buccal artery* runs with the buccal nerve of V_3. It anastomoses with the infraorbital and facial arteries.
- *Mental artery* emerges through the mental foramen and anastomoses with the inferior labial artery.

Venous Drainage of the Face and Scalp

The venous drainage of the face and scalp for the most part parallels the arterial supply. However, there are some important differences. Within the parotid gland, the superficial temporal vein joins the maxillary vein to form the retromandibular vein. The latter vein divides into two divisions at the lower pole of the parotid gland. The union of the posterior division of the retromandibular vein and the posterior auricular vein forms the external jugular vein. The anterior division of the retromandibular vein joins the facial vein and drains into the internal jugular vein as the common facial vein. These veins are highly variable.

The facial vein begins as the angular vein and runs parallel and posteriorly to the facial artery. However, the facial vein is not as tortuous as the facial artery.

The deep facial vein arises from the pterygoid venous plexus of the infratemporal region and passes deep to the ramus of the mandible along with the buccal artery and the buccal nerve branch of the mandibular nerve to anastomose with the facial vein. Thus, the facial vein anastomoses with the pterygoid plexus of veins, which in turn can communicate with the cavernous sinus by means of an emissary vein. In addition, the facial vein passes *superficially* to the submandibular gland to reach the internal jugular vein, whereas the facial artery passes *deep* to the submandibular gland in the digastric triangle of the neck.

The anastomoses between the facial veins and the intracranial dural venous sinuses are clinically important. The supratrochlear and supraorbital veins unite to form the angular vein. This is the site of anastomoses of the facial vein with branches of the superior ophthalmic vein. The superior ophthalmic vein drains into the cavernous sinus, creating another anastomotic route between the facial vein and the dural venous sinuses. Infection from the face can spread into the orbit or the infratemporal fossa, eventually reach the cavernous sinus, and subsequently reach the brain.

Lymphatic Drainage of the Face and Scalp

There are a few facial (buccal) nodes along the course of the facial artery, which receive lymph from the external nose, lower face, and medial aspect of the conjunctival sac. The anterior and superficial parotid nodes drain the forehead, temporal region, anterior ear, and lateral aspect of the conjunctival sac. The facial nodes drain into the submandibular nodes of the horizontal lymphatic chain while the parotid nodes drain into the deep cervical nodes such as jugulo-digastric nodes (See Deep Cervical Nodes section).

Development of the Face

The face develops from the fusion of five facial swellings (Fig. 10-14A), which appear by the end of the fourth week. They are the frontonasal process, two maxillary swellings (derived from the dorsal portion of the first pharyngeal arch), and two mandibular swellings (derived from the ventral portion of the first pharyngeal arch). During the fifth week, two nasal placodes develop on the frontonasal process (see Fig. 10-14A). At the same time, the two maxillary swellings increase in size and expand ventrally and medially. In the sixth week, the center of each nasal placode invaginates to form the nasal pit. This creates a lateral and medial nasal process for each nasal

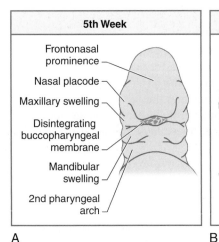
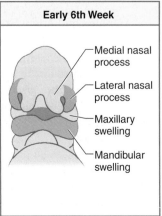
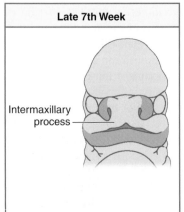
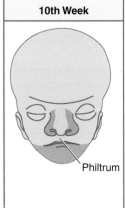

Figure 10-14. Development of the face. **A,** Fifth week. **B,** Early 6th week. **C,** Late 7th week. **D,** Tenth week.

placode (see Fig. 10-14B). The medial nasal processes of each nasal placode fuse to form the intermaxillary process that will become the philtrum (see Fig. 10-14C). As they fuse, they crowd the frontonasal prominence into the midline to form the bridge and septum of the nose. The upper lip forms from the fusion of the lower portion of the medial nasal processes with the maxillary processes. The lower lip forms from proliferation of mesenchyme in the mandibular processes. The mouth is formed by the rupturing of the buccopharyngeal (oropharyngeal) membrane. The cheeks are formed by the fusion of the lateral aspects of the mandibular and maxillary swellings (see Fig. 10-14D).

●●● MENINGES AND DURAL VENOUS SINUSES

Although the cranial meninges are continuous with the spinal meninges (see Chapter 3), there are significant differences.

Meningeal Layers

Dura Mater

The dura mater is the thickest of the three membranes. It is often referred to as the pachymeninx. In the vertebral canal, the dura mater is separated from the periosteum of the vertebrae by the *epidural space*, which is occupied by fat and the internal venous plexus (see Chapter 3). This venous plexus communicates with the external venous plexus that surrounds the vertebral column. The entire vertebral plexus is referred

to as the vertebral venous system or Batson's plexus. It is a potential route for the spread of metastatic carcinoma from the bladder, prostate, or breast to the brain.

The cranial dura is continuous with the spinal dura at the foramen magnum. However, the dura of the neurocranium consists of *two fused layers*: an outer endosteal (periosteal) layer and an inner meningeal layer, whereas the spinal dura has only this one layer (Fig. 10-15). The endosteal layer is analogous to the periosteum of the vertebral canal. This is the osteogenic layer, and it appears rough and thicker than the other layers.

These changes occur at the foramen magnum, thereby eliminating the epidural space in the skull. Thus, the epidural space in the *neurocranium* is produced by trauma (such as head injuries) and is *not* analogous to the epidural space of the vertebral canal, since it is found *outside both layers* of cranial dura. In the head, the endosteal layer of dura is firmly attached to the base of the skull at the foramina, but only loosely attached to the remaining bones of the neurocranium.

The meningeal dura does separate from the outer endosteal layer at certain points to form duplications consisting of only meningeal dura (see Fig. 10-15). These changes produce the dural duplications, which *partially* divide the cranial cavity into spaces that contain the subdivisions of the brain such as the right and left hemispheres of the cerebrum. However, it must be emphasized that these duplications of meningeal dura never isolate any component of the brain (see Fig. 10-15). Separations between endosteal and meningeal dura, or between two layers of meningeal dura, create spaces called dural venous sinuses, through which the blood is drained from the neurocranium.

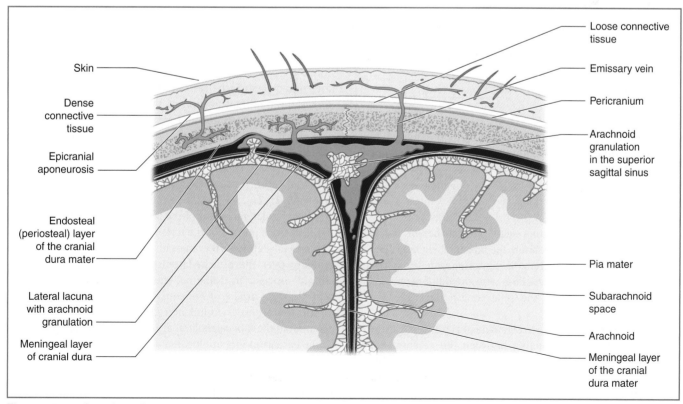

Figure 10-15. Overview of meninges and dural venous sinuses.

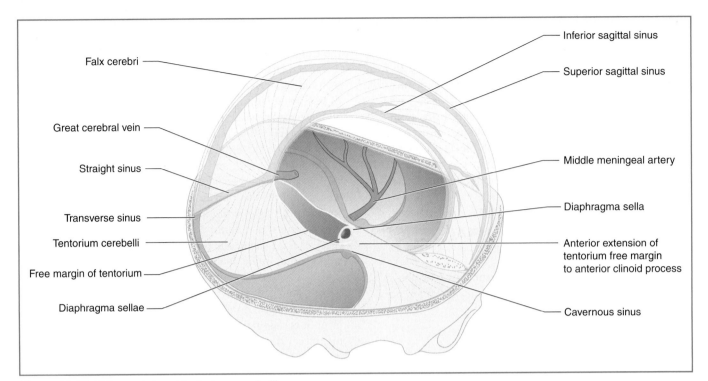

Figure 10-16. Falx cerebri and tentorium cerebelli.

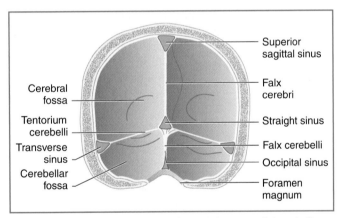

Figure 10-17. Coronal section of posterior part of the skull demonstrating dural sinuses found between endosteum and meningeal dura or between two layers of dura.

The meningeal duplications include the falx cerebri between the hemispheres of the cerebrum, the falx cerebelli between the hemispheres of the cerebellum, the tentorium cerebelli between the cerebrum and the cerebellum, and the diaphragma sellae that incompletely covers the sella turcica (Figs. 10-16 and 10-17).

The falx cerebri is a vertical, sickle-shaped duplication of the meningeal dura projecting between the cerebral hemispheres in the midsagittal plane (see Fig. 10-16). It is attached *anteriorly* to the ethmoid bone's crista galli and the frontal bone's frontal crest. Superiorly, it attaches to the sagittal suture that unites the two parietal bones. The falx cerebri is narrow

anteriorly but expands posteriorly, where it blends into the superior surface of the tentorium cerebelli.

The tentorium cerebelli is a "tent-like" duplication of dura over the cerebellum (see Figs. 10-16 and 10-17). It is attached *posteriorly* to the occipital bone, *laterally* to the groove for the transverse sinus on the occipital and parietal bones, and *anteriorly* to the superior margins of the petrous portion of the temporal bones and the anterior and posterior clinoid processes. This arrangement leaves a deep notch, the tentorial notch or "incisura," located on the tentorium cerebelli's anteromedial surface (see Fig. 10-16). This tentorial notch allows the midbrain portion of the brainstem to connect the cerebrum with the brainstem and cerebellum. The tentorium is elevated in the midline, since it is continuous with the falx cerebri, which is attached to the sagittal suture. This arrangement gives a portion of the falx cerebri that is continuous with the tentorium cerebellum an inverted Y configuration (see Figs. 10-16 and 10-17).

The anterolateral aspect of the tentorium cerebelli is attached to the petrous portion of the temporal bone. The tentorial notch has a well-defined free margin, which continues forward, crossing over the attached tentorium to reach the anterior clinoid process. In doing so, the tentorium helps form the *superolateral aspect of the cavernous sinus* (see Fig. 10-16).

The tentorium is found at right angles to both the falx cerebri and the falx cerebelli. It also separates the occipital lobes of the cerebrum that are located above the tentorium from the cerebellum located below the tentorium (see Fig. 10-17).

The falx cerebelli is a small duplication of dura separating the cerebellar hemispheres and contains the occipital sinus. Superiorly, the falx cerebelli fuses with the tentorium.

The diaphragma sellae (see Fig. 10-16) is a horizontal duplication of meningeal dura, which forms a roof over the sella turcica and covers the hypophysis. The diaphragma sellae is attached anteriorly to the tuberculum sellae and posteriorly to the dorsum sellae. The infundibulum (stalk) passes through the aperture in the diaphragma sellae to allow the hypothalamus to communicate with the hypophysis (pituitary gland). The sella turcica contains the hypophysis (pituitary gland) and the intercavernous sinuses.

Innervation of the Dura Mater

The trigeminal nerve has branches that innervate the dura with GSA fibers. The anterior and posterior ethmoidal branches, which arise from the ophthalmic nerve's nasociliary branch, have meningeal branches that supply the dura of the anterior cranial fossa floor.

A tentorial nerve (recurrent tentorial branch) recurs from CN V_1 in the middle cranial fossa to the superior surface of the tentorium and the adjacent falx cerebri.

Branches of CNs V_2 and V_3 innervate the dura of the middle cranial fossa. The recurrent meningeal nerve of CN V_3 passes from the infratemporal region back into the skull through the foramen spinosum. The meningeal branches of the maxillary nerve (CN V_2) and mandibular nerve (CN V_3) also supply the middle and lateral wall of the anterior cranial fossa. These nerves run with the middle meningeal artery.

The vagus nerve (CN X) has a meningeal ramus whose cell bodies lie in the superior (jugular) ganglion of the vagus nerve. It helps supply the dura of the posterior cranial fossa.

The hypoglossal nerve (CN XII) has a meningeal ramus that is actually a branch of cervical spinal nerves 2 and 3.

The meningeal nerve endings are found near the meningeal arteries and dural sinuses. Stimulation of the nerve endings may be the cause of certain types of headaches. Stimulation of the endings close to the arteries produces well-localized pain, while stimulation of the endings close to the venous sinuses is referred to the temporal regions or forehead.

Arteries That Supply the Dura Mater

The meningeal branches of the ophthalmic artery include branches of the anterior and posterior ethmoidal arteries.

The internal carotid artery's anterior meningeal branch anastomoses with the meningeal branches of the posterior ethmoidal artery.

The middle meningeal artery is a branch of the maxillary artery. Its anterior and posterior branches have the most extensive distribution to the dura of the middle cranial fossa and the lateral aspect of the anterior cranial fossae. The maxillary artery often has an accessory meningeal branch.

The arterial supply of the posterior cranial fossa consists of the following:

- The meningeal branch of the occipital artery passes through the mastoid canal.
- The meningeal branch of the ascending pharyngeal artery passes through the jugular foramen or the foramen lacerum.
- The meningeal branch of the vertebral artery passes through the foramen magnum.

Arachnoid and Pia Mater
Arachnoid

The arachnoid ("spider's web") (see Fig. 10-15) is the meningeal layer found just internal to the dura mater. It is a delicate avascular membrane separated from the dura by the subdural space. This is only a potential space produced by trauma.

The arachnoid is separated from the innermost layer of meninges, the pia mater, by the subarachnoid space that contains cerebrospinal fluid (CSF). The inner two meninges are embryologically derived from a single layer. The CSF produced during development excavates the subarachnoid space between the arachnoid and the pia mater, leaving bands of fibrous tissue lined with cells called trabeculae connecting these two layers. Over the cerebrum and cerebellum, the arachnoid is intimately associated with the pia mater by means of a dense meshwork of processes called arachnoid trabeculae. However, the subarachnoid space is enlarged at other sites into cisterns (cisternae) such as the chiasmatic cistern around the optic chiasm.

The arachnoid has projections that pass through the dura, where they are then covered by the dural endothelium as they now extend into the dural venous sinuses. These projections are arachnoid villi, and aggregations of these villi are called arachnoid granulations (pacchionian granulations). The villi, or granulations, are most numerous in the superior sagittal sinus, where the intrasinus pressure is lowest. They serve as drainage sites for CSF into the venous circulation of specific dural sinuses. It is thought that the capillary-like arachnoid villi are open when the pressure is lower in the sinus than in the subarachnoid space, but if the pressure is greater in the sinus, the capillary-like vessels collapse. This mechanism allows CSF to pass into the venous system but prevents blood from regurgitating from the sinus into the subarachnoid space.

Pressure in the sinuses, especially upon standing, is less than atmospheric. The rigid arrangement of the sinus in the dura holds the sinus open. In the upright position, the CSF pressure is greater in the subarachnoid space than the pressure in the superior sagittal sinus. CSF will pass through arachnoid villi to flow into the dural venous sinuses. It never allows for regurgitation of blood into the subarachnoid space except in cases of trauma or disease.

Pia Mater

The pia mater is the vascular layer that covers the CNS and is adherent to it. The cerebral arteries are associated with the pia in the subarachnoid space. The vessels are found in the trabeculae and are not in direct contact with the CSF. Branches of these vessels travel with extensions of the pia into the brain and the perivascular spaces. The pia mater remains adherent to cranial nerves and spinal nerve roots as they cross the subarachnoid space.

Dural Venous Sinuses

The dural venous sinuses (Figs. 10-18 and 10-19) are the principal venous drainage of the neurocranium. They are often found between the endosteal (periosteal) and meningeal

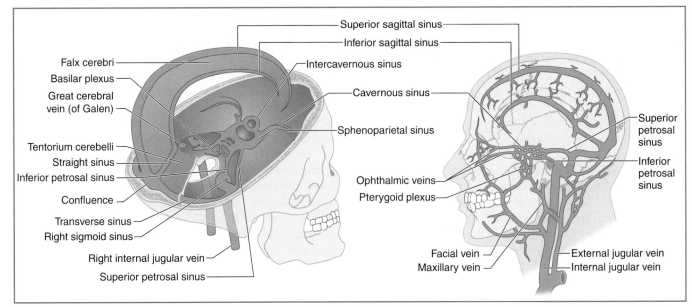

Figure 10-18. Dural venous sinuses.

layers of the dura. However, several sinuses are found between the duplications of meningeal dura (i.e., the falx cerebri, falx cerebelli, and tentorium cerebelli). All dural venous sinuses are lined by endothelium. The dural venous sinuses collect venous blood from the brain, diploë, orbit, and internal ear. They are called dural venous sinuses because they carry blood toward the heart. However, they are quite different from typical veins in that they do not have smooth muscle, valves, or an adventitia. There are two categories of dural venous sinuses: unpaired and paired.

Midline Unpaired Sinuses

The *unpaired* sinuses (see Fig. 10-17) are associated with the duplications of dura matter. They are the superior sagittal sinus, inferior sagittal sinus, straight sinus, and occipital sinus.

The superior sagittal sinus runs along the entire length of the *superior attachment of the falx cerebri*. It extends from the foramen cecum (anterior to the crista galli) to the internal occipital protuberance on the occipital bone (see Fig. 10-18). Occasionally an emissary vein can also drain nasal veins into the superior sagittal sinus through a patent foramen cecum. An emissary vein is a vein that allows the venous sinuses and veins of the head to communicate with each other. The superior sagittal sinus also receives the superior cerebral veins, diploic veins, meningeal veins, and parietal emissary veins when present.

The triangular lumen of this sinus enlarges as it passes posteriorly to accommodate an increase in volume. This increase is due to the venous blood plus the CSF that drains into the sinus through the arachnoid granulations. The superior sagittal sinus communicates with irregular lateral expansions called lateral lacunae, which increase the sinus surface area and also receive arachnoid granulations.

At the internal occipital protuberance, the superior sagittal sinus drains into the confluence of sinuses. This venous blood usually flows into the right transverse sinus.

The inferior sagittal sinus runs in the *inferior free edge of the falx cerebri*. It receives veins from the medial surface of the cerebral hemispheres and from the inferior part of the frontal regions of the cerebral hemispheres. Posteriorly, at the junction of the falx cerebri and the tentorium cerebelli, the inferior sagittal sinus *joins the great cerebral vein* (of Galen) to form the straight sinus (see Fig. 10-18). The two internal cerebral veins that drain the deep structures or inferior surface of the cerebral hemispheres anastomose to form the great cerebral vein (of Galen). The straight sinus runs in the *layers of the tentorium cerebelli* to reach the confluence of sinuses and then typically onto the left transverse sinus (see Figs. 10-18 and 10-19).

The occipital sinus is the smallest of the sinuses. It starts near the foramen magnum from several small sinuses (marginal sinuses) that merge into the occipital sinus in the falx cerebelli to end in the confluence of sinuses.

CLINICAL MEDICINE

Subdural Hematoma

The superior sagittal sinus receives the superior cerebral veins. These veins pass through the subarachnoid space to form approximately six large veins called superficial cortical or "bridging" veins that pass through arachnoid to join the superior sagittal sinus at approximately right angles. This arrangement places the bridging veins in jeopardy during an automobile accident such as whiplash that produces movement of the head and brain in opposite directions. These veins are sheared from the superior sagittal sinus and bleed into the potential subdural space.

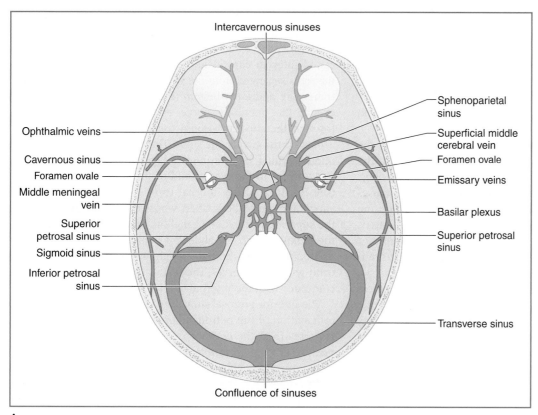

Intercavernous sinuses

Ophthalmic veins

Cavernous sinus

Foramen ovale

Middle meningeal vein

Superior petrosal sinus

Sigmoid sinus

Inferior petrosal sinus

Sphenoparietal sinus

Superficial middle cerebral vein

Foramen ovale

Emissary veins

Basilar plexus

Superior petrosal sinus

Transverse sinus

Confluence of sinuses

A

Figure 10-19. Dural sinuses in base of skull and location of cranial nerves entering the dura.

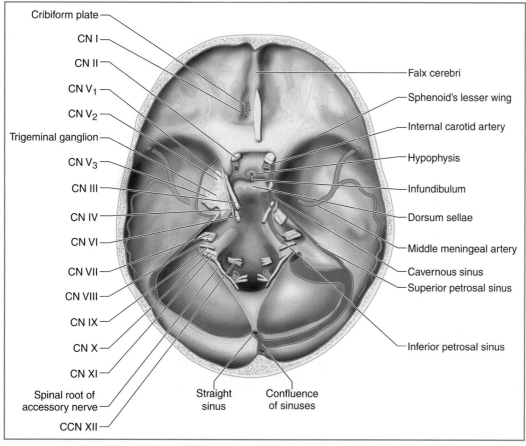

Cribiform plate

CN I

CN II

CN V₁

CN V₂

Trigeminal ganglion

CN V₃

CN III

CN IV

CN VI

CN VII

CN VIII

CN IX

CN X

CN XI

Spinal root of accessory nerve

CCN XII

Straight sinus

Confluence of sinuses

Falx cerebri

Sphenoid's lesser wing

Internal carotid artery

Hypophysis

Infundibulum

Dorsum sellae

Middle meningeal artery

Cavernous sinus

Superior petrosal sinus

Inferior petrosal sinus

B

The confluence of sinuses is located at the internal occipital protuberance. It receives the superior sagittal sinus, straight sinus, and occipital sinus.

Paired Dural Sinuses

The paired dural sinuses are cavernous, intercavernous, superior petrosal, inferior petrosal, transverse, and sigmoid sinuses.

The transverse sinuses (see Figs. 10-18 and 10-19) are the largest of the sinuses. They lie in the grooves located in the attachment of the tentorium cerebelli to the occipital bones. The transverse sinuses begin at the confluence of sinuses usually as continuations of the superior sagittal sinus on the right or straight sinus on the left. Each transverse sinus is continuous with a sigmoid sinus. At this point, the superior petrosal sinus usually joins the transverse sinus just before it becomes continuous with the sigmoid sinus.

The sigmoid sinus (see Figs. 10-18 and 10-19) runs across the mastoid portion of the temporal bone and the occipital bone in the posterior cranial fossa to reach the jugular foramen. The sigmoid sinus passes through the jugular foramen and empties into the superior bulb of the internal jugular vein.

The cavernous sinus occupies a space in the middle cranial fossa just lateral to the sella turcica on the carotid groove (see Fig. 10-19). It extends from the *superior orbital fissure* to the *apex of the petrous temporal bone*. The cavernous sinus is connected to the opposite cavernous sinus by anterior, posterior, and inferior intercavernous (circular) sinuses (see Fig. 10-19). Posterolateral to the cavernous sinus and lateral to the apex of the petrous portion of the temporal bone (petrous temporal) is the trigeminal (Meckel's) cave, which contains the trigeminal ganglion.

The trigeminal cave is a blind extension of the dura mater and arachnoid and the subarachnoid space from the posterior cranial fossa into the middle cranial fossa. This diverticulum is due to a separation of the dura into the endosteum and meningeal dura to produce the trigeminal care as the layers fuse with the connective tissue of the trigeminal ganglion.

Each cavernous sinus is formed by the dura of the tentorium's free margin that reaches the anterior clinoid process and the dura of the floor of the middle cranial fossa. The cavernous sinus receives the superior ophthalmic vein, the sphenoparietal sinus, and emissary veins from the pterygoid venous plexus. It also receives superficial middle cerebral and inferior cerebral veins. The superior and inferior petrosal sinuses, intercavernous sinuses, and the emissary veins can drain it. Since blood moves from high pressure to low pressure, the above pattern could be reversed.

The cavernous sinus (see Fig. 10-19A) is quite small. Its lumen is criss-crossed by connective tissue trabeculae, which resemble cavernous (erectile) tissue. The trabeculae slow the flow of blood through the sinuses. This increases the likelihood of thrombosis of the cavernous sinus. Another view of the cavernous sinus that is gaining favor is that it consists of a venous-like plexus that surrounds the nerves that pass to the superior orbital fissure and foramen rotundum as well as the internal carotid artery.

The lateral wall of the sinus contains the oculomotor, trochlear, ophthalmic, and maxillary nerves. The abducent (abducens) nerve and the internal carotid artery with its associated internal carotid nerve (plexus) pass directly through the sinus separated from the venous blood by connective tissue trabeculae and endothelium (Fig. 10-20). All of these nerves except the maxillary nerve exit the middle cranial fossa through the superior orbital fissure, located at the anterior aspect of the cavernous sinus. The maxillary nerve exits the middle cranial fossa through the foramen rotundum, which is just inferior to the medial end of the superior orbital fissure (see Fig. 10-20). The internal carotid nerve consists of post-ganglionic sympathetic fibers whose cell bodies are located in the superior sympathetic ganglion. Some of these fibers leave the plexus to join the abducent nerve, then pass to both the ophthalmic nerve and the oculomotor nerve to enter the orbit with these nerves. The rest of the internal carotid nerve continues with the internal carotid artery.

The inferior petrosal sinus (see Fig. 10-19A) runs along the articulation of the petrous temporal and the occipital bones. It passes from the *cavernous sinus* to the *anterior compartment of the jugular foramen* and drains into the superior bulb of the internal jugular vein.

The superior petrosal sinus runs along the superior margin of the petrous temporal bone from the *cavernous sinus* to the *transverse sinus* just at its junction with the sigmoid sinus.

The basilar plexus communicates with right and left inferior petrosal sinuses and the vertebral plexus of veins. This connection makes the basilar plexus an important route for potential metastasis between the vertebral venous plexus and the dural sinuses.

The sphenoparietal sinus runs along the posterior margin of the lesser wing of the sphenoid bone to the cavernous sinus.

Venous Drainage into the Dural Sinuses

The diploic veins drain the diploë (the spongy layer of bone sandwiched between the two compact layers).

Emissary veins pass completely through the bone of the skull and connect the veins of the external surfaces of the skull (scalp) or base of the skull with the dural sinuses. An example is the emissary veins that connect the pterygoid venous plexus in the infratemporal fossa with the cavernous sinus. These veins run through either the foramen ovale or an emissary foramen that is just medial to the foramen ovale.

Relationships Between the Cranial Nerves and the Cavernous Sinus

CNs III, IV, V_1, and V_2 all lie in the lateral wall of the cavernous sinus before they enter the orbit (see Fig. 10-20). The oculomotor nerve enters the dura that forms the roof of the cavernous sinus in the middle cranial fossa. CN IV enters the dura on the inferior surface of the tentorium cerebelli in the posterior cranial fossa.

In the posterior aspect of the sinus, the order of the nerves from superior to inferior is as follows: III, IV, V_1, and V_2 (see Fig. 10-20). However, as the nerves travel anteriorly, the

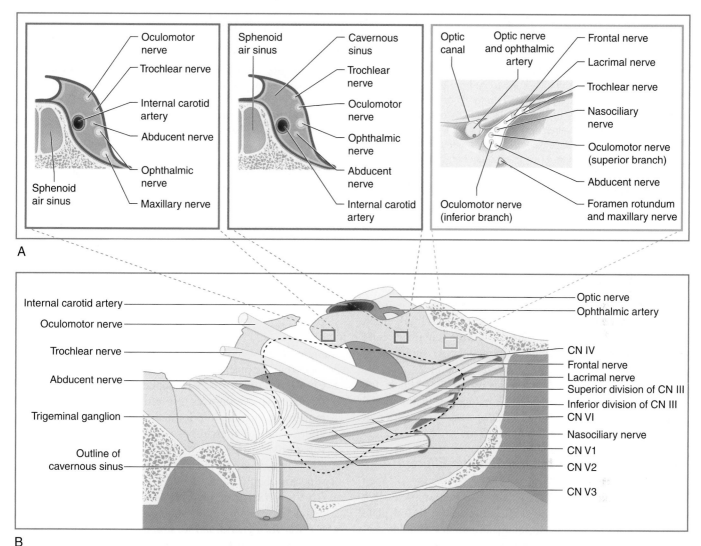

Figure 10-20. A, Relationship of cranial nerves to cavernous sinus. **B,** Change in location of cranial nerves in cavernous sinus.

oculomotor nerve crosses the medial side of the trochlear (CN III) to pass inferiorly. Here CN III divides into superior and inferior divisions, and enters the orbit through the superior orbital fissure inside the anulus formed by the origins of the four rectus muscles. The trochlear nerve runs superiorly to enter the superior orbital fissure above the anulus.

The roots of the trigeminal nerve (CN V) cross the depression on the apex of the petrous temporal bone under the superior petrosal sinus to enter the trigeminal (Meckel's) cave, where the trigeminal ganglion is located (see Figs. 10-19B and 10-20). The trigeminal nerve's ophthalmic, maxillary, and mandibular divisions emerge from the ganglion. The ophthalmic nerve runs anteriorly and superiorly in the lateral wall and splits into its three divisions in the anterior aspect of the sinus wall. The lacrimal and frontal branches run superiorly to enter the superior orbital fissure above the anulus, while the nasociliary nerve passes through the anulus between the divisions of the oculomotor nerve.

The abducent nerve (see Fig. 10-20) enters the dura of the posterior cranial fossa just lateral to the dorsum sellae and

usually passes under the petroclinoid ligament. The petro-clinoid ligament stretches from the posterior clinoid process to the apex of the petrous temporal bone. It forms a canal (of Dorello) for the passage of the abducent nerve (CN VI) and the inferior petrosal sinus. The abducent nerve lies in the cavernous sinus, inferolateral to the internal carotid artery separated from the venous blood by the trabeculae and endothelium. Thus, it is the most susceptible nerve in any disorder involving the sinus, for example, aneurysm or thrombosis.

●●● CRANIAL NERVES

A conceptual approach to the structures of the head and neck should include an understanding of the distribution of the 12 cranial nerves. These cranial nerves provide the functional fibers to large parts of the head and neck that have special terminology due to their development. Thus it is necessary to examine the terminology *and* the development of the head and structures that it represents.

CLINICAL MEDICINE

Spread of Infection to the Cavernous Sinus

The ophthalmic veins drain into the anterior aspect of the cavernous sinus, forming a vascular route from the face to the cavernous sinus. Infections from the upper lip or face near the nose may be carried to the cavernous sinus by means of the facial and ophthalmic veins, and deep infections of the face may be carried to the cavernous sinus by means of the pterygoid plexus of veins. Such infections characteristically result in blockage of the orbital veins, which produces an increase in pressure in the eyeball. Examination of the fundus of the eyeball demonstrates papilledema (optic disc swelling) and venous engorgement.

CLINICAL MEDICINE

Headache

There are many causes of headache, and some headaches are due to many causes, including vascular changes and changes in intracranial pressure, which affect the dura. Vascular changes include vasodilation and subsequent vasoconstriction of intracranial and meningeal arteries and dural venous sinuses. The arteries are innervated up to the point of entry into the neural tissue itself, and the dural sinuses also receive innervation. Any tension on these vessels or increases in arterial or venous pressure can produce a headache. Anteriorly located arteries and sinuses such as the superior sagittal sinus or middle meningeal arteries refer pain to the ophthalmic dermatome. Vertebral or basilar arteries or posterior cranial fossa dural sinuses that are innervated by dorsal rami of cervical spinal nerves refer pain to the occipital and dorsal neck regions.

General Terminology

The following are the four functional categories of neurons found in a typical spinal nerve that innervates the trunk, neck, and limbs: general somatic efferent (GSE), general visceral efferent (GVE), general somatic afferent (GSA), and general visceral afferent (GVA) (as described in Chapter 2).

In addition to these four categories of functional fibers, the cranial nerves have three "special" categories of functional fibers: special visceral efferent (SVE), special visceral afferent (SVA), and special somatic afferent (SSA).

Efferent Fibers and General Somatic Efferent Fibers in Cranial Nerves

Special visceral efferent (SVE) fibers innervate muscles that are embryologically derived from paraxial and lateral plate mesoderm of the pharyngeal (branchial) arches. The designation "special" is to signify that these muscles developed from a special place in the embryo, in other words, any one of the pharyngeal arches. Many authors use the term branchiomeric to describe this type of innervation. Some use the term "branchial motor" for special visceral efferent to emphasize the embryonic origin.

Afferent Fibers and General Somatic Afferent Fibers in Cranial Nerves

Special somatic afferent (SSA) fibers carry sensation from the specialized sensory receptors for smell, sight, and hearing. These receptors are ectodermally derived, and thus the fibers carrying this sensory information are designated as "somatic" sensory.

Special visceral afferent (SVA) fibers carry taste sensation. Taste is the only fiber type in this category. The specialized sensory receptors in this category are derived from endoderm and thus are designated "visceral" afferents.

Cranial Nerves According to Function

General Somatic Efferent Fibers

GSE fibers innervate skeletal muscles derived from the myotomes, which in turn are derived from the somites. In the cranium, these somatic motor fibers innervate structures derived from the prechordal mesenchyme and occipital somites.

- CN III, *oculomotor nerve*, supplies GSE fibers to many of the extrinsic eye muscles responsible for ocular movement (medial, inferior and superior rectus, and the inferior oblique muscles) as well as the levator palpebrae superioris muscle.
- CN IV, *trochlear nerve*, supplies GSE fibers to the superior oblique muscle.
- CN VI, *abducent nerve*, supplies GSE fibers to the lateral rectus muscle.
- CN XII, *hypoglossal nerve*, supplies GSE fibers to all intrinsic and most extrinsic muscles of the tongue. The extrinsic muscles have the suffix "-glossus." All of them are innervated by the XIIth nerve except the palatoglossus, which is innervated by CN X with a contribution from the cranial portion of XI.

General Visceral Efferent Fibers

GVE fibers from the cranial parasympathetic nervous system innervate smooth muscle and glands.

CN III, Oculomotor Nerve
- *Nucleus:* Nucleus of Edinger-Westphal.
- *Ganglion:* The ciliary ganglion receives preganglionic fibers through the motor (short) root, which is a branch of the inferior division of the oculomotor nerve.
- *Effector organs:* Muscles for accommodation (ciliaris) and pupil constriction (sphincter pupillae) receive postganglionic fibers through the short ciliary nerves.

CN VII, Facial Nerve
- *Nucleus:* Superior salivatory nucleus.
- *Two ganglia:* The pterygopalatine (sphenopalatine) ganglion receives the preganglionic fibers of the greater petrosal nerve, which contributes to the nerve of the

pterygoid canal (vidian nerve). The submandibular ganglion receives preganglionic fibers via the chorda tympani, which communicates with the lingual branch of V_3.

- *Effector organs:* The lacrimal, nasal, and palatine glands are innervated by means of postganglionic fibers from the pterygopalatine ganglion. The submandibular and sublingual glands are innervated by postganglionic fibers from the submandibular ganglion.

CN IX, Glossopharyngeal Nerve

- *Nucleus:* Inferior salivatory nucleus.
- *Ganglion:* The otic ganglion receives preganglionic parasympathetic fibers via the lesser petrosal nerve.
- *Effector organ:* The parotid gland receives postganglionic parasympathetic fibers, which communicate with the auriculotemporal branch of V_3.

CN X, Vagus Nerve

- *Nucleus:* Dorsal motor nucleus.
- *Ganglia:* The ganglia are close to or in the organ innervated, for example, myenteric (Auerbach's) and Meissner's plexuses in the intestines and the cardiac ganglia close to the heart.
- *Effector organs:* These are the glands of the larynx, pharynx, and smooth and cardiac muscle and the glands of thorax and abdomen to the proximal two thirds of the transverse colon.

Autonomic (GVE) Nerves

The pelvic splanchnic nerves originate from the lateral horn nuclei of sacral spinal cord segments S2, S3, and S4 as the sacral component of the parasympathetic nervous system. The sympathetic outflow arises from the lateral horn nuclei of spinal cord segments T1–L2.

Special Visceral Efferent Fibers

These SVE fibers innervate muscles derived from the nonsomitic mesoderm of the pharyngeal arches. During development, one cranial nerve invades each arch and innervates all the muscles subsequently derived from that arch.

- CN V, *trigeminal nerve's mandibular division* (V_3), supplies SVE fibers to the mylohyoid, temporalis, masseter, medial pterygoid, lateral pterygoid, anterior belly of the digastric muscle, tensor veli palatini, and tensor tympani muscles. All these muscles are derived from the first arch.
- CN VII, *facial nerve*, supplies SVE fibers to the muscles of facial expression, as well as the stapedius, stylohyoid, and posterior belly of the digastric muscle. All these muscles are derived from the second arch.
- CN IX, *glossopharyngeal nerve*, supplies SVE motor fibers only to the stylopharyngeus muscle. This muscle is the only muscle derived from the third arch.
- CN X, *vagus nerve*, supplies SVE motor fibers to the muscles of the soft palate (except the tensor veli palatini), pharynx (except the stylopharyngeus), and larynx. These muscles are involved with swallowing and

phonation. Many of these fibers actually originate from the cranial portion of CN XI and join the vagus. The above muscles are derived from the fourth and sixth arches. The nucleus ambiguus (wandering nucleus) of CN X and cranial portion of CN XI gives rise to these fibers.

- CN XI, *accessory nerve* (cranial portion), contributes its SVE motor fibers to the vagus nerve. These fibers contribute to the innervation of the muscles for swallowing and phonation. The fibers from the cranial portion of XI contribute to the innervation of the muscles of the palate (except the tensor veli palatini), pharynx, and larynx, which are derived from the fourth and sixth arches. The innervation to these muscles can be referred to as the vagal-accessory (X–XI) complex.

General Somatic Afferent (GSA) Fibers

The GSA fibers supply structures derived from ectoderm with cutaneous sensation, for example, the sensations of pain, touch, and temperature.

CN V, Trigeminal Nerve

- *Ganglion:* Trigeminal ganglion.
- *Sensory distribution:* The trigeminal nerve contributes cutaneous sensation from the face, orbit, nose, mouth, forehead, teeth, meninges and the epithelial covering of the anterior two thirds of the tongue, which is derived from the ectoderm of the first arch.

CN VII, Facial Nerve

- *Ganglion:* Geniculate ganglion.
- *Sensory distribution:* The facial nerve contributes fibers to the auricular nerve (of Arnold) (a branch of X with contributions from VII and IX) to the posterior portions of both the external auditory meatus and the external tympanic membrane.

CN IX and CN X, Glossopharyngeal and Vagus Nerves

- *Ganglia:* Superior (jugular) ganglia of both IX and X and the geniculate ganglion of VII.
- *Sensory distribution:* The auricular nerve (of Arnold) supplies some of the skin on the posterior surface of the external ear, the floor of the external auditory meatus, and the posterior part of the external surface of the tympanic membrane. The external surface of the anterior portion of the tympanic membrane also receives sensory fibers from V_3.

Proprioceptive General Somatic Afferent Fibers

GSA fibers of the trigeminal nerve also carry the sense of proprioception (body position) from the muscles of mastication and the other first arch muscles. These fibers have unipolar cell bodies located in the mesencephalic nucleus of the midbrain. The mesencephalic nucleus is classified as part of the trigeminal nerve.

Typically the neurons for proprioception are derived from neural crest cells (neuroectoderm). Their cell bodies are located in the dorsal root ganglia, and their fibers are classified as

TABLE 10-6. Summary of Fiber Types Distributed to the Head and Neck

Category	Function	Innervated Structure	Cranial Nerve
Afferent Fibers			
General somatic	Pain, touch, temperature, proprioception	Skin, mucous membranes, skeletal muscle	V, VII, IX, X
General visceral	Pain, temperature, interoceptors, chemoceptors, baroceptors, gag and cough reflexes	Pharynx, soft palate, larynx, lining posterior one third of the tongue, gut to transverse colon	VII, IX, X
Special somatic	Smell, vision, hearing, balance	Olfactory epithelium, retina, inner ear	I, II, VIII
Special visceral	Taste	Taste buds	VII, IX, X
Efferent Fibers			
General somatic	Striated muscle	Seven extraocular muscles, tongue muscles except palatoglossus	III, IV, VI, XII
General visceral	Structures innervated by sympathetic and parasympathetic nervous systems, cardiac and smooth muscle glands	Sphincter pupillae, lacrimal, nasal, palatine, sublingual, submandibular parotid glands, glands of the pharynx and larynx	III, VII, IX, X
Special visceral	Striated muscle derived from one of the pharyngeal arches	Muscles of the jaws, face, pharynx, larynx, soft palate, palatoglossus, upper esophagus, and neck (sternomastoid, trapezius, digastric, mylohyoid, stylohyoid)	VII, IX, X, cranial portion of XI

GSA. The mesencephalic nucleus is the only primary sensory group of nerve cell bodies that *lies within the central nervous system*. It is analogous to a dorsal root ganglion but is located in the CNS and therefore called a nucleus.

The proprioception fibers from the first arch muscles and from the temporomandibular joint travel with the mandibular division of V and have their cell bodies in the mesencephalic nucleus. In addition, the periodontal ligaments have GSA fibers in both the mandibular and maxillary nerves (teeth and hard palate).

The extraocular muscles receive sensory fibers, which carry proprioceptive information and eventually travel with the ophthalmic nerve. It is believed that the cell bodies for those proprioceptive fibers are in the trigeminal ganglion. *The trigeminal nerve receives proprioceptive fibers that initially ran with the motor nerves (III, IV, VI) to leave them and join the ophthalmic nerve.* These fibers for proprioception that reach branches of the ophthalmic nerve may have their cell bodies located in the trigeminal ganglion. However, some authors indicate that these cell bodies may be in the mesencephalic nucleus (Table 10-6).

Proprioceptive Fibers from Other Muscle Groups in the Head and Neck

Proprioceptive fibers from many muscle groups in the head are believed to follow the cranial nerve that innervates them with motor fibers.

- CN VII, *facial nerve*, supplies SVE fibers to the muscles of facial expression, as well as the stapedius, stylohyoid, and posterior belly of the digastric muscle. Proprioceptive fibers from these muscles run with the facial nerve and probably have their cell bodies in the geniculate ganglion.
- CN IX, *glossopharyngeal nerve*, supplies SVE motor fibers only to the stylopharyngeus muscle. Proprioceptive fibers from this muscle run with the glossopharyngeal nerve and probably have their cell bodies in its superior ganglion.
- CN X, *vagus nerve*, may run with proprioceptive fibers from the soft palate (except the tensor veli palatini), pharynx (except stylopharyngeus), and larynx; these fibers would have their cell bodies in the superior ganglion of the vagus nerve.
- CN XI, *spinal accessory nerve*, supplies SVE fibers to the trapezius and sternomastoid muscles. Cell bodies for proprioceptive fibers from these muscles are in the dorsal root ganglia of cervical spinal nerves 2–4.

General Visceral Afferent (GVA) Fibers

GVA fibers carry visceral sensation including pain, feeling of fullness for hollow organs, stretching, and distention from structures derived from the splanchnic mesoderm and endoderm. For most of the trunk, pain fibers run with the sympathetic nerve fibers. They have their cell bodies in the dorsal root ganglia of the spinal nerves. Other fibers carrying visceral sensations from the trunk have their cell bodies associated with the parasympathetic system, namely, the inferior ganglion of the vagus as well as the sacral parasympathetics and the dorsal root ganglia associated with sacral spinal nerves 2, 3, and 4.

Listed below are the GVA fibers that are associated with the cranial nerves:

CN VII, Facial Nerve

- *Ganglion:* Geniculate ganglion.
- *Sensory distribution:* Visceral sensation is from the mucous membranes of the soft palate and palatine tonsillar region.

CN IX, Glossopharyngeal Nerve

- *Ganglion:* Inferior (petrous) ganglion.
- *Sensory distribution:* Visceral sensation is from the mucous membranes of the tympanic cavity and middle ear, most of the pharynx, the soft palate, tonsillar region, posterior third of the tongue, chemoreceptors from the carotid body, and baroreceptors from the carotid sinus.

CN X, Vagus Nerve

- *Ganglion:* Inferior (nodose) ganglion.
- *Sensory distribution:* Visceral sensation is from the lower pharynx, larynx, aortic bodies that measure blood gases, and thoracic and abdominal viscera to the proximal two thirds of the transverse colon.

Special Somatic Afferent (SSA) Fibers

These fibers carry signals from specialized sensory receptors derived from ectoderm.

CN I, Olfactory Nerve

- *Ganglion:* Fibers from bipolar cells of olfactory epithelium synapse with neurons of the olfactory bulb.
- *Receptor:* Olfactory neuroepithelium of the superior third of the nasal cavity. These fibers are often described as SVA because of the influence of smell on taste.

CN II, Optic Nerve

- *Ganglion:* Ganglion cells of the retina.
- *Receptors:* Rods and cones of the retina synapse on bipolar cells, which synapse on ganglion cells.

CN VIII, Vestibulocochlear Nerve

- *Ganglion:* The spiral ganglion for hearing and the vestibular ganglion for spatial orientation.
- *Receptors:* Cells of the spiral organ of Corti (for hearing) and the neuroepithelium of the semicircular canals (for spatial orientation).

Special Visceral Afferent (SVA) Fibers

These fibers carry taste from specialized receptors derived from endoderm.

CN VII, Facial Nerve

- *Ganglion:* Geniculate ganglion.
- *Receptors:* Taste buds of the anterior two thirds of the tongue, and some taste buds from the soft palate.

CN IX, Glossopharyngeal Nerve

- *Ganglion:* Inferior (petrous) ganglion.
- *Receptors:* Taste buds of the posterior third of the tongue and the vallate papillae anterior to the sulcus terminalis.

CN X, Vagus Nerve

- *Ganglion:* Inferior (nodose) ganglion.
- *Receptors:* Taste buds of the root of the tongue and the epiglottis.

⬤⬤⬤ DEVELOPMENT OF PHARYNGEAL ARCHES

A series of six paired outpocketings or pharyngeal arches forms on each side of the ventrolateral aspect of the growing embryo at about 4 weeks (Fig. 10-21) although the fifth often never develops or develops and degenerates quickly and the sixth cannot be seen externally. The pharyngeal arches are separated from each other externally by ectodermally lined indentations called pharyngeal clefts. Internally the pharyngeal arches are separated by endodermally lined outpocketings called pharyngeal pouches. Each pharyngeal arch contains an aortic arch, a cartilaginous arch, and a cranial nerve. The cranial nerve associated with each arch will innervate the structures developing from that arch (Table 10-7).

The muscles that arise within the pharyngeal arches are voluntary muscles and therefore skeletal muscle. However, since they do not arise from somites, the innervation of these muscles has been called special visceral efferent (branchiomotor).

The first pharyngeal cleft develops into the external auditory meatus, with the overlying ectoderm contributing to the formation of the tympanic membrane. The second, third, and fourth clefts usually disappear because the second pharyngeal arch enlarges and overlaps them and they form an ectodermally lined cavity called the cervical sinus (see Fig. 10-21B). The cervical sinus usually disappears but occasionally can persist and form what is known as a branchial cyst. The pharyngeal pouches form a number of structures (Table 10-8).

⬤⬤⬤ NECK

Overview of the Neck

The neck is a cylinder that connects the head and trunk. As such, it contains numerous structures that are specialized for communication between the head and trunk and for the support and movement of the head. The neck can be thought of as two compartments or columns contained in a single cylinder of fascia. The two compartments are an anterior one, containing the viscera, and a posterior one, consisting of the vertebral column and associated musculature. The two columns are surrounded by the outer investing layer of deep fascia, superficial fascia, and skin.

Superimposed on these two columns are two large paired muscles—the trapezius and sternocleidomastoid

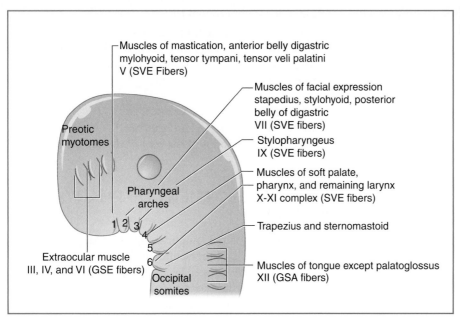

Figure 10-21. Muscles derived from pharyngeal arches and adjacent somites.

A

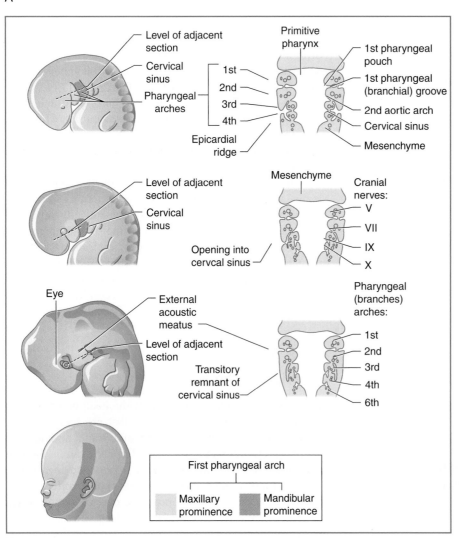

B

TABLE 10-7. Derivatives of the Pharyngeal Arches

Arch	Cranial Nerve	Muscles	Skeletal Elements	Other Structures
First	V, mandibular divisions	Muscles of mastication, tensor tympani, tensor veli palatini	From maxillary cartilage: part of sphenoid, incus From mandibular cartilage: malleus, maxilla, zygomatic, squamous portion of temporal bone, mandible	Mucous membrane of anterior two thirds of the tongue; ectoderm of first arch lines oral cavity and gives rise to anterior pituitary
Second	VII	Muscles of facial expression, posterior belly of the digastric, stylohyoid, stapedius	Stapes, styloid process, stylohyoid ligament, lesser horns of hyoid	
Third	IX	Stylopharyngeus	Greater horns of hyoid	Mucous membrane of posterior third of the tongue
Fourth	X, superior laryngeal nerve, pharyngeal plexus with contributions from the cranial portion of XI	Pharyngeal constrictors, cricothyroid, levator veli palatini	Laryngeal cartilages	
Sixth	X, recurrent laryngeal nerve	Intrinsic muscles of the larynx	Laryngeal cartilages	

TABLE 10-8. Pharyngeal Pouch Derivatives

Pouch Number	Structure	Comment
First	Mucosa of eardrum, tympanic cavity, mastoid antrum, auditory tube	
Second	Tonsillar fossa, surface epithelium of palatine tonsil	
Third	Thymus, inferior parathyroid glands	Thymus and inferior parathyroid glands migrate together inferiorly; if the parathyroid glands do not detach they can be carried into the mediastinum with the thymus
Fourth	Ultimobranchial body Superior parathyroid glands	Ultimobranchial body forms the C cells of the thyroid gland

(sternomastoid)—associated with the outer layer of deep fascia. These muscles can be used as anatomic landmarks to subdivide the neck into smaller triangles.

The sternocleidomastoid muscle passes superiorly and laterally from its two origins to its insertion (Table 10-9). The interval between the two heads is triangular and is closed by the outer investing layer of deep fascia and scant muscle fibers. It is a potential site for injection into or canalization of the subclavian vein located posteriorly to the sternoclavicular joint.

Spasm of the sternocleidomastoid produces both rotation and flexion of the head. Under this condition, the chin is rotated to the uninvolved side and then the head is flexed so that the mastoid process on the same side is pulled toward the shoulder. The chin now faces *away from* the involved side (torticollis, or wry neck).

The sternocleidomastoid muscle is innervated by the spinal portion of the accessory nerve with SVE fibers and by the cervical plexus (C2 and C3) with GSA fibers for proprioception.

The sternocleidomastoid muscle (Fig. 10-22) divides the neck into two large triangles, anterior and posterior.

Visceral Column

The three cylinders of fascia are held together by loose areolar connective tissue. The visceral column contains most of the major organs of the neck, namely, trachea, esophagus, larynx, pharynx, thyroid, and parathyroids (Fig. 10-23). It is surrounded by a loose visceral (pretracheal layer of cervical) fascia. The key landmarks in the visceral column are the inferior margin of the mandible, hyoid bone, thyroid, and cricoid cartilages.

The inferior margin of the mandible is the boundary between the neck and face.

The hyoid bone is a U-shaped bone found just inferior to the mandible (Fig. 10-23B). The hyoid bone has no direct bony articulations but instead is held in place by muscles, ligaments, and fascia. The hyoid bone has a small midline

TABLE 10-9. Attachment Sites of Sternomastoid and Trapezius Muscles

Muscle	Origin	Insertion	Action
Sternocleidomastoid	Tubular-like origin from manubrium, flat origin from medial third of the clavicle	Mastoid process of temporal bone	Rotates the head so that the chin moves to the contralateral side; two muscles acting together flex the head on the neck
Cervical portion of trapezius	Superior nuchal line, external occipital protuberance, nuchal ligament	Inserts on the lateral third of the clavicle; acromion, scapular spine	Cervical portion elevates scapula and clavicle; retracts scapula; draws head to one side or backward

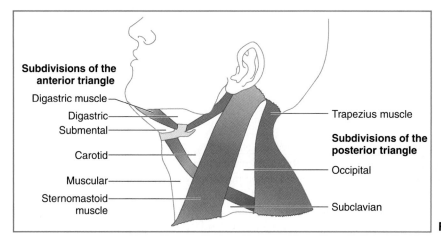

Figure 10-22. Triangles of the neck.

body anteriorly and two pairs of horn-like processes, or cornua. The greater cornu is the large process projecting posterosuperiorly from the body. The lesser cornu is the small process projecting superiorly from the articulation of the body and the greater cornu. The hyoid bone is at the level of the third cervical vertebra.

The thyroid cartilage (see Fig. 10-23A) is the major cartilage of the larynx and an important landmark in the neck. It is composed of two laminae, or plates, that meet anteriorly in the midline but are open posteriorly. The thyroid cartilage's laryngeal prominence (Adam's apple) is located anterosuperiorly and is more prominent in the male. Above the laryngeal prominence, a deep notch, the thyroid notch, separates the laminae. This notch is easily palpated, is found at the level of the fourth cervical vertebra, and easily identifies the midline. The oblique line of the thyroid cartilage is found on the body of each plate. It runs from approximately the base of the superior cornu to the inferior tubercle. The oblique line on the lateral aspect of the thyroid cartilage serves as the attachment site of the sternothyroid and thyrohyoid muscles.

The cricoid cartilage is found at the level of the transverse process of cervical vertebra C6.

Vertebral Column

The cervical vertebral column consists of seven cervical vertebrae and their intervertebral disks. Associated with it are the eight cervical spinal nerves and the muscles that are attached to the cervical vertebrae. The posterior, middle, and anterior scalene muscles are located on the lateral aspect of the vertebral column, and the longus coli and longus capitis muscles are located anteriorly on the vertebral column. The prevertebral fascia encloses these muscles plus the intrinsic back muscles in the cervical region and the cervical vertebral column. This layer of fascia forms the medial (deep) boundary of the posterior triangle of the neck.

Fascia of the Neck

Superficial Fascia

The superficial fascia of the neck contains the platysma muscle (Table 10-10). The platysma gives the anterior triangle of the neck its fullness. Loss of the platysma due to surgery produces a flat, flaccid, and expressionless neck.

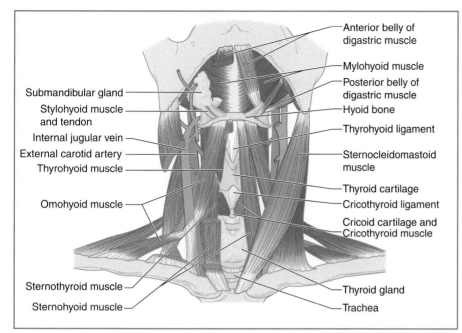

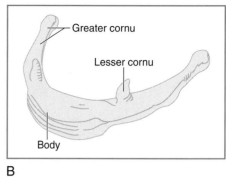

B

Figure 10-23. A, Visceral column of the neck. **B,** Hyoid bone.

Deep Fascia

The cervical fasciae enable structures to move over one another without difficulty during movements such as swallowing and twisting the neck. These fascial sheaths also define several fascial planes that will act as barriers to the spread of deep neck infection into adjacent regions. At the same time, they may serve to funnel the spread of infection along given planes to predictable locations.

Outer Investing (Superficial) Layer

The outermost cylinder of fascia is the outer investing layer of deep cervical fascia (Fig. 10-24). It is attached posteriorly to the cervical vertebrae (see Table 10-9). As it encircles the neck, it divides into two layers to enclose the trapezius on both its internal and external surfaces. At the anterior aspect of the trapezius, the two layers of this outer investing layer of deep fascia rejoin and form the tough external wall of the posterior triangle. At the anterior border of the posterior triangle, the outer investing layer of deep fascia again divides to encompass the sternocleidomastoid muscle. This fascia then rejoins to form one layer, which is continuous over the midline of the neck. Here, it forms the lateral and anterior walls of the anterior triangle.

Superiorly, the outer investing layer of deep cervical fascia splits over the submandibular gland to hold the gland in place and joins with the fascia over the parotid gland. This fascia forms the stylomandibular ligament found between the styloid process of the temporal bone and the posterior surface of the mandible. Inferiorly, the suprasternal space (of Burns) contains the jugular arch that connects the anterior jugular veins, and it may contain the sternal head of the sternocleidomastoid.

TABLE 10-10. Attachment Points of Outer Investing Layer of Deep Cervical Fascia

Direction	Point of Attachment
Anteriorly	Continuous across midline
Posteriorly	External occipital protuberance, spinous processes of cervical vertebrae, ligamentum nuchae, mastoid process of temporal bone
Superiorly	Hyoid bone and mandible, zygomatic arches, superior nuchal line of occipital bone
Inferiorly	Splits into two layers that attach to manubrium to form suprasternal space (of Burns), clavicle, acromion, spine of scapula

In summary, the outer investing layer of deep fascia forms the external (lateral) surface of both the anterior and posterior triangles and encloses the other two major fascial cylinders in the neck: the pretracheal layer of deep cervical fascia (enclosing the visceral column) and the prevertebral layer of deep cervical fascia (enclosing the vertebral column).

Pretracheal Layer

The pretracheal layer of deep cervical fascia (middle layer of deep fascia) is a thin layer that surrounds the visceral column (see Fig. 10-24). This visceral layer of deep cervical fascia is continuous anterosuperiorly to the cricoid cartilage and often

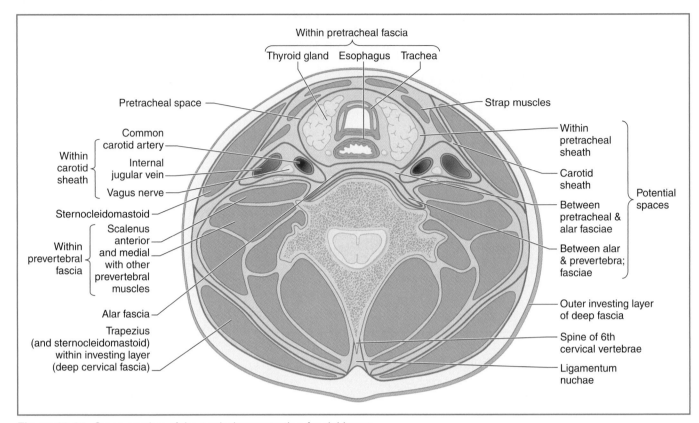

Figure 10-24. Cross-section of the neck demonstrating fascial layers.

to the hyoid bone. Posterosuperiorly it is called the bucco-pharyngeal fascia on the posterior lateral aspect of the pharynx to the base of the skull. The pretracheal fascia is the anterior portion of the visceral fascia below the hyoid bone, and it surrounds the thyroid gland, trachea, and esophagus. The pretracheal fascia also forms the false capsule of the thyroid gland.

The infrahyoid (strap) muscles, which insert into the hyoid bone and thyroid cartilage, are found anterior to the visceral column. Inferiorly two of the four strap muscles arise from the manubrium while the pretracheal layer of deep cervical fascia continues into the superior mediastinum to become continuous with the fibrous pericardium. The pretracheal layer of deep cervical fascia is described as covering the posterior surface of the infrahyoid muscles and the visceral column. The pretracheal space lies between the infrahyoid muscles and the pretracheal fascia associated with the trachea. The pretracheal space is anterior to the trachea and posterior to the strap muscles (Fig. 10-25). *Thus, infection in the visceral compartment can reach the superior mediastinum.* Infection in the pretracheal space typically results from an endoscopic instrument perforating the anterior esophageal wall or by a foreign body or trauma.

Prevertebral Fascia

The prevertebral fascia (see Figs. 10-24 and 10-25) invests the vertebral column. It also encloses muscles associated with the vertebral column including the scalene muscles, levator

scapulae, and the deep muscles of the neck, along with the phrenic nerve, cervical spinal nerves, and sympathetic trunk. This fascia is attached to the base of the skull and to the transverse processes of the cervical vertebrae. The prevertebral fascia covers the floor of the posterior triangle. It is reflected along the structures that lie anterior to the middle scalene muscle and posterior to the anterior scalene muscle to form the axillary sheath at the interscalene triangle. It surrounds the brachial plexus and subclavian artery. Therefore, infection deep to the prevertebral fascia can follow the axillary artery into the arm.

Alar Layer

An additional layer of prevertebral fascia is found between the pretracheal and the prevertebral fascial layers in front of the cervical vertebrae. This is the alar layer of fascia, which is a duplication of the prevertebral fascia that reinforces the vertebral column (see Figs. 10-24 and 10-25). It stretches between the transverse processes of the cervical vertebrae. *Thus, prevertebral fascia has two anterior layers that stretch between the transverse processes:* the anterior-most *alar layer* and the deeper *prevertebral layer.* The alar fascia is attached to the base of the skull, as is the rest of the prevertebral fascia. However, *inferiorly*, it passes forward to blend with the pretracheal fascia. The exact vertebral level where the alar fascia passes forward to fuse with the pretracheal fascia has been described as anywhere from C7 to T2.

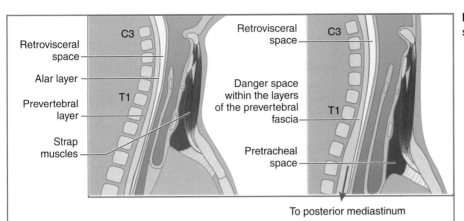

Figure 10-25. Subdivisions of the fascial spaces.

Labels in figure:
Retrovisceral space
Alar layer
Prevertebral layer
Strap muscles
C3
T1
Retrovisceral space
C3
Danger space within the layers of the prevertebral fascia
T1
Pretracheal space
To posterior mediastinum

CLINICAL MEDICINE

Spread of neck infection

The retrovisceral or retropharyngeal space is an important pathway for the spread of infection from the neck into the thorax. This space lies behind the visceral fascia and in front of the alar layer of prevertebral fascia. Posterior to the retrovisceral space is a potential space found between the *anterior layers* of prevertebral fascia, that is, the alar fascia and the prevertebral fascia proper.

The retrovisceral space is a potential space behind the visceral fascia and anterior to the alar layer of prevertebral fascia. This space is *confined to the neck,* since the alar fascia attaches anteriorly to the previsceral fascia.

The danger space is an important space found posterior to the alar layer of prevertebral fascia and anterior to the deeper layer of prevertebral fascia associated with the bodies of the vertebrae. Thus, the danger space lies between the alar layer and the deeper anterior layer of prevertebral fascia.

Both the retrovisceral and danger spaces reach the base of the skull. The retrovisceral space ends anywhere from C7 to T2, where the alar layer of fascia fuses with the posterior layer of the esophageal visceral fascia. However, the danger space extends through the posterior mediastinum to the diaphragm and contains only a loose connective tissue. Therefore, there is no inferior fascial barrier in the danger zone until the diaphragm. An infection that gains access to the danger zone has the potential to spread inferiorly to the diaphragm. This may lead to mediastinitis that has a very poor prognosis.

Pus or exudate from an infection deep to the prevertebral fascia associated with the anterior vertebral column can also migrate along the axillary sheath and subclavian artery or brachial plexus into the axilla.

Carotid Sheath

The carotid sheath (see Fig. 10-24) is a fascial specialization on the anterolateral surface of the neck enclosing three important structures of the neck. The fascial layers contributing to this sheath are the outer investing layer of deep cervical fascia on the deep (medial) surface of the sternocleido-mastoid muscle, the pretracheal layer of deep cervical fascia, and the prevertebral fascia.

The three structures enclosed in the carotid fascial sheath are the common and (superiorly) the internal carotid arteries located medially, internal jugular vein located laterally, and the vagus nerve located posteriorly and between the first two.

The carotid sheath extends from the base of the skull, encircling the carotid canal and jugular foramen, to the thorax. It is always well formed around the arteries but is thinner over the internal jugular vein, permitting the arteries to expand. A well-formed carotid sheath may exist only in the lower neck in relationship to the common carotid artery, whereas the upper portion may be poorly developed. The sympathetic trunk is described as either in the prevertebral fascia or posterior to the carotid sheath. The ansa cervicalis can be found embedded within the anterolateral surface of the carotid sheath in the carotid triangle.

●●● TRIANGLES OF THE NECK

The triangles of the neck are anatomic subdivisions of the neck that freely communicate with each other. They are a series of anatomic relationships that allow for the detailed description of smaller regions of the neck.

Posterior and Anterior Triangles

A lateral view of the neck presents a roughly quadrilateral cylinder. The neck is divided into posterior and anterior triangles by the sternocleidomastoid muscle (Fig. 10-26 and Table 10-11; see also Fig. 10-22).

Several structures pass from one triangle to another by passing medially (deep) to the sternocleidomastoid muscle. However, a few structures pass superficially to the sterno-cleidomastoid muscle. This is evidenced by the omohyoid muscle, which passes from the posterior triangle into the anterior triangle by passing deep to the sternocleidomastoid muscle while branches of the cervical plexus pass superficial to this muscle. The right and left anterior triangles freely communicate with each other across the midline. Indeed,

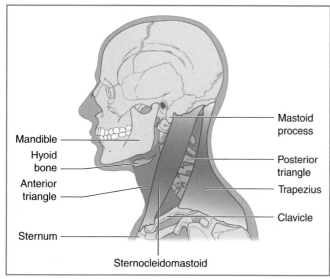

A

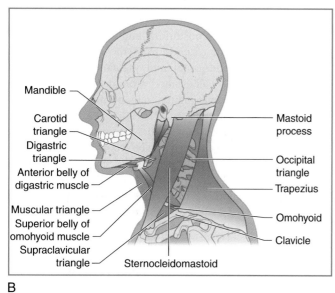

B

Figure 10-26. A, Division of the neck into triangles. **B,** Subdivisions of the triangles of the neck.

clinically a single anterior triangle is described between both sternocleidomastoid muscles.

Subdivisions of the Posterior Triangle

The posterior belly of the omohyoid muscle subdivides the posterior triangle into two smaller triangles (Fig. 10-27). This muscle has an unusual morphology. It has two muscular bellies attached to bones that are connected by means of a shared central or intermediate tendon (Table 10-12).

The omohyoid muscle has an inferior belly that arises from the scapula medial to the scapular (suprascapular) notch and the superior transverse scapular ligament to insert into the central tendon. The superior belly arises from the central tendon and inserts into the hyoid bone. The central tendon is found medial (deep) to the sternocleidomastoid muscle at the level of the sixth cervical vertebra. It is held in place by a loop of fascia that connects it to the clavicle. The omohyoid muscle is innervated by the ansa cervicalis.

The inferior belly of the omohyoid muscle divides the posterior triangle into the occipital and subclavian triangles. The occipital (neural) triangle is superior to the omohyoid muscle, and the subclavian (vascular) triangle is inferior to the omohyoid muscle.

The subclavian vein is not visible in this triangle because the first rib slopes inferiorly as it passes anteriorly. Thus, it is posterior to the clavicle at this point. Indeed, one clinical approach to the subclavian vein is along the medial inferior surface of the clavicle.

Scalene Muscles

The anterior scalene muscle (see Fig. 10-27) is a key landmark in the inferior aspect of the neck. It arises from the anterior tubercles of the transverse processes of C3–C6. The anterior scalene muscle inserts into the scalene tubercle of the first rib. This insertion separates the grooves found on the first rib for the subclavian vein and artery. Thus, the subclavian vein is always located *anterior* to the anterior scalene muscle, while the subclavian artery is always located *posterior* to the anterior scalene muscle. Because of the anteroinferior slope of the first rib, the subclavian vein does

---

TABLE 10-11. Boundaries of the Anterior and Posterior Triangles of the Neck

| | | Boundary | | |
Anterior	Posterior	Superior	Inferior	Deep
Posterior Triangle Sternocleidomastoid	Trapezius muscle	Apex of triangle	Middle third of clavicle	Small portion of semispinalis capitis, splenius capitis, levator scapulae, small portion of scalene muscles
Anterior Triangle Midline of the neck	Sternocleidomastoid muscle	Mandible	Apex of triangle	Strap muscles, cricothyroid, mylohyoid, middle and inferior pharyngeal constrictor muscles

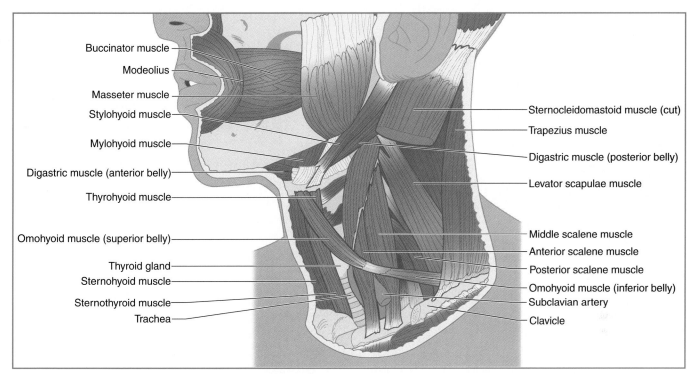

Figure 10-27. Muscles and vascular structures of the neck.

CLINICAL MEDICINE

Scalene Muscle Spasms

Spasm of the anterior scalene muscle may compress the structures found in relation to it. It may occlude the normal flow of blood to the upper limb by compressing the subclavian artery. It may compress the lower roots of the brachial plexus, affecting the neural supply to the arm, especially the root of the plexus that arises from spinal nerves C8 and T1 that supply the hand. Spasm could also compromise venous return from the upper limb by elevating the first rib. The subclavian vein crosses the first rib just in front of the anterior scalene muscle. The vein can be compressed when the rib is elevated.

TABLE 10-12. Subdivisions of the Posterior Triangle

Triangle	Boundaries	Content
Subclavian	Trapezius, sternocleidomastoid, and inferior belly of omohyoid muscles	Trunks of the brachial plexus, subclavian artery and many of its branches, long thoracic nerve
Occipital	Trapezius, sternocleidomastoid, and inferior belly of omohyoid muscles	Accessory nerve, cervical plexus branches, brachial plexus (dorsal scapular and suprascapular nerves), transverse cervical and suprascapular arteries

not rise above the plane of the clavicle. However, the subclavian artery rises slightly higher.

The middle scalene muscle is the largest of the scalene muscles and arises from the posterior tubercles of the transverse processes of C2–C6(C7). It inserts on the first rib, posterior to the insertion of the anterior scalene muscle and the groove for the subclavian artery. The middle scalene muscle is posterior to the subclavian artery and the roots of the brachial plexus.

The posterior scalene muscle is almost indistinguishable from the middle scalene muscle. It has the same origins as the middle scalene muscle, but it inserts on the second rib.

The scalene muscles flex the neck to the same (ipsilateral) side. With both sides working together, the scalene muscles can flex the neck forward on the chest. The scalene muscles can also act as accessory respiratory (inspiratory) muscles by

elevating the first and second ribs. The scalene muscles are innervated by the lower cervical (C4–C8) spinal nerves, with the anterior scalene innervated by C4–C6, the middle scalene innervated by (C3)C4–C8, and the posterior scalene innervated by C6–C8.

The anterior and the middle scalene muscles and the first rib form the boundaries of the interscalene (scalene) triangle (see Fig. 10-27). The roots of the brachial plexus and the subclavian artery pass through the interscalene triangle, which is in the occipital triangle. The subclavian vein passes anteriorly to the anterior scalene muscle and is not in the occipital triangle.

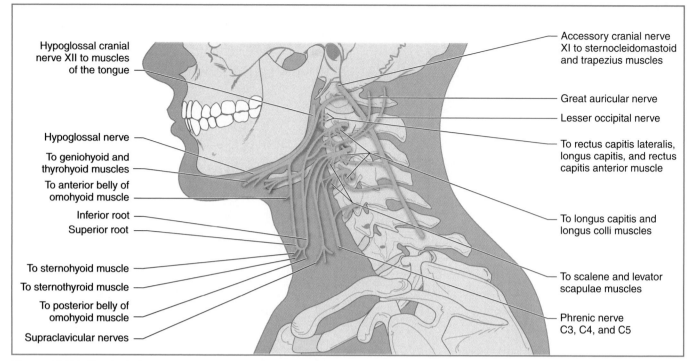

Hypoglossal cranial nerve XII to muscles of the tongue

Hypoglossal nerve

To geniohyoid and thyrohyoid muscles

To anterior belly of omohyoid muscle

Inferior root

Superior root

To sternohyoid muscle

To sternothyroid muscle

To posterior belly of omohyoid muscle

Supraclavicular nerves

Accessory cranial nerve XI to sternocleidomastoid and trapezius muscles

Great auricular nerve

Lesser occipital nerve

To rectus capitis lateralis, longus capitis, and rectus capitis anterior muscle

To longus capitis and longus colli muscles

To scalene and levator scapulae muscles

Phrenic nerve C3, C4, and C5

Figure 10-28. Cervical plexus.

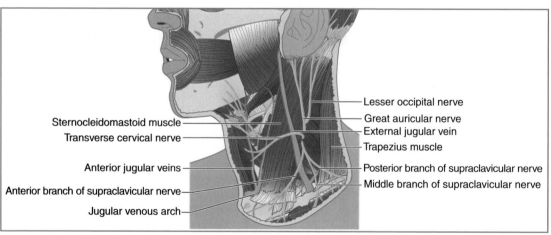

Sternocleidomastoid muscle

Transverse cervical nerve

Anterior jugular veins

Anterior branch of supraclavicular nerve

Jugular venous arch

Lesser occipital nerve

Great auricular nerve

External jugular vein

Trapezius muscle

Posterior branch of supraclavicular nerve

Middle branch of supraclavicular nerve

Figure 10-29. Sensory branches of the cervical plexus.

Cervical Plexus

The cervical plexus (see Fig. 10-28) is a looping plexus derived from the *ventral rami* of cervical spinal nerves (C1–C4). As such, it contains GSA and GSE fibers. Postganglionic sympathetic fibers from the superior sympathetic ganglion join it through gray rami communicantes. The cervical plexus is found deep (medial) to the sternocleidomastoid muscle, on the surface of or just lateral to the levator scapulae and middle scalene muscles. Its branches pass into both posterior and anterior triangles. The cervical plexus consists of the redistribution of the first four cervical spinal nerves in the form of three loops, along with the gray rami communicantes that are postganglionic sympathetic fibers from the superior cervical (sympathetic) ganglion. The first loop is derived from the ventral rami of cervical spinal nerves 1 and 2 (C1 and C2), the second loop is derived from C2 and C3, and the third loop is derived from C3 and C4. The cervical ventral rami and neural loops lie deep to the prevertebral fascia. However, many branches penetrate this fascia, such as the cutaneous branches and roots of the ansa cervicalis. The first cervical spinal nerve is most unusual in that it has *no* dorsal root ganglion and no cutaneous distribution.

Morphology of the Superficial (Cutaneous) Branches

All the sensory branches of the cervical plexus appear along the posterior margin of the sternocleidomastoid muscle, where the upper third and middle third of this muscle meet (Figs. 10-28 and 10-29 and Table 10-13).

TABLE 10-13. Cervical Plexus Branches

Loop of Cervical Plexus	Branches and Function
First loop, C1, C2	C1 has only motor branches and supplies muscles
Second loop, C2, C3	Lesser occipital (C2), great auricular, and transverse cervical nerves are cutaneous branches (C2, C3) and contain GSA and postganglionic sympathetic fibers Muscular nerves to longus capitis and cervicalis contain GSA, GSE, and postganglionic sympathetic fibers Branches join accessory nerve to provide GSA fibers for proprioception to sternocleidomastoid muscle
Third loop, C3, C4	Supraclavicular nerves (with cutaneous fibers) Sensory branches join accessory nerve to provide proprioception fibers to trapezius

The lesser occipital nerve (C2) follows the sternocleidomastoid's posterior margin to the mastoid process and penetrates the investing fascia (see Fig. 10-29). It is sensory to the region of the mastoid process and part of the occipital region posterior to the ear as well as the medial portion of the upper ear.

The great auricular nerve (C2 and C3) passes superiorly toward the ear, parallel with and posterior to the external jugular vein (see Fig. 10-29). It passes over (laterally to) the sternocleidomastoid muscle and is sensory to the skin over the angle of the mandible, the inferior aspects of the ear (lobe), and the adjacent mastoid process.

The transverse cervical nerve (C2 and C3) crosses the sternocleidomastoid muscle deep to the platysma and external jugular vein to supply the skin of the anterior triangle.

The supraclavicular nerves (C3 and C4) penetrate the investing layer of deep fascia, which is deep to the platysma. The supraclavicular nerves have medial, intermediate, and lateral branches, which supply cutaneous innervation to the lower neck, upper thoracic wall to the sternal angle and second rib as well as the shoulder tip, the acromion, and part of the upper scapula.

A meningeal branch communicates (runs piggyback) with the hypoglossal nerve into the posterior cranial fossa to help supply the meninges of this fossa.

Morphology of the Muscular Branches

The first three cervical nerves form the ansa cervicalis, which is a looping neural structure found on the carotid sheath (see Fig. 10-28). An ansa is any structure in the form of a loop or arc. The ansa cervicalis is a U-shaped structure composed of two branches. The superior root of the ansa cervicalis appears to be derived from the hypoglossal nerve; however, it actually carries fibers that are derived from the ventral ramus of the

cervical spinal nerve 1 (and possibly 2). The superior branch of the ansa cervicalis communicates (travels) only with the hypoglossal nerve. The other branch of the ansa cervicalis is derived from cervical spinal nerves C2 and C3 and is called the inferior root of the ansa cervicalis. The ansa cervicalis innervates three of the strap muscles: sternohyoid, sternothyroid, and omohyoid muscles.

The thyrohyoid and geniohyoid muscles are innervated by small branches of cervical spinal nerves 1 and 2 that initially run with the hypoglossal nerve in the same manner as the superior root of the ansa cervicalis. The cervical branches separate from CN XII to innervate the geniohyoid and thyrohyoid muscle as the nerve to the thyrohyoid muscle and a less obvious nerve to the geniohyoid muscle. All of these nerves are typical spinal nerves in that they carry general somatic motor, general somatic sensory, and postganglionic sympathetic fibers. *The postganglionic sympathetic fibers to the branches of the cervical plexus arise as gray rami communicantes from the superior cervical sympathetic ganglion.*

The phrenic nerve arises mainly from the ventral ramus of the cervical spinal nerve 4 with some fibers from C3 and C5. The roots of the phrenic nerve join at the lateral border of the anterior scalene muscle. This nerve runs inferiorly across the front of the anterior scalene muscle, deep to the prevertebral fascia. The phrenic nerve then enters the thorax by passing anteriorly to the subclavian artery, crossing the internal thoracic artery, and then passing posteriorly to the beginning of the brachiocephalic vein and through the superior thoracic aperture.

The dorsal rami of cervical spinal nerves 1 to 3 also provide sensory and motor fibers to the scalp and neck. The dorsal ramus of the second cervical nerve is the greater occipital nerve. It perforates the trapezius to provide cutaneous innervation to the superior dorsal scalp and posterior occipital region. The dorsal ramus of the third cervical nerve forms the third occipital nerve (occipitalis tertius), which provides cutaneous innervation to the dorsal aspect of the medial and inferior scalp and neck.

Circulation
Subclavian Artery

The subclavian arteries have different origins on the right and left sides. The right subclavian artery arises from the brachiocephalic trunk, dorsal to the sternoclavicular articulation. It arches laterally and slightly upward just above the level of the clavicle and leaves the neck by crossing the first rib externally to become the axillary artery. The left subclavian artery arises from the arch of the aorta and has to pass through the superior mediastinum to reach the root of the neck. The subclavian artery (Figs. 10-30 and 10-31) is subdivided into three parts by the anterior scalene muscle, which also separates it anteriorly from the subclavian vein. The first part of the subclavian artery lies medial to the anterior scalene muscle, the second part is found posterior to the anterior scalene muscle, and the third part is found lateral to the anterior scalene muscle.

The first part of the subclavian artery is crossed anteriorly by the following structures: the internal jugular and vertebral

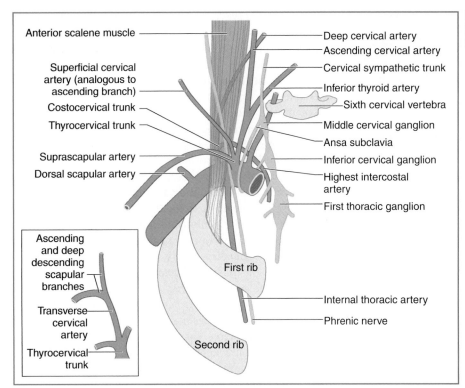

Anterior scalene muscle

Superficial cervical artery (analogous to ascending branch)

Costocervical trunk

Thyrocervical trunk

Suprascapular artery

Dorsal scapular artery

Deep cervical artery

Ascending cervical artery

Cervical sympathetic trunk

Inferior thyroid artery

Sixth cervical vertebra

Middle cervical ganglion

Ansa subclavia

Inferior cervical ganglion

Highest intercostal artery

First thoracic ganglion

Ascending and deep descending scapular branches

Transverse cervical artery

Thyrocervical trunk

First rib

Second rib

Internal thoracic artery

Phrenic nerve

A

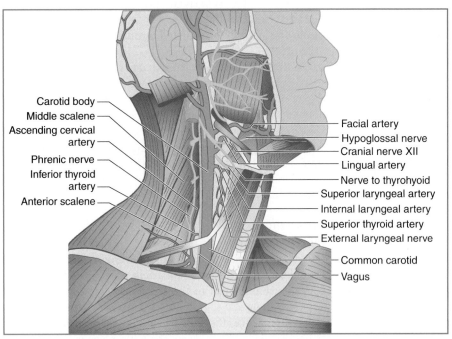

Carotid body

Middle scalene

Ascending cervical artery

Phrenic nerve

Inferior thyroid artery

Anterior scalene

Facial artery

Hypoglossal nerve

Cranial nerve XII

Lingual artery

Nerve to thyrohyoid

Superior laryngeal artery

Internal laryngeal artery

Superior thyroid artery

External laryngeal nerve

Common carotid

Vagus

B

Figure 10-30. A, Subclavian artery and its branches. **B,** External carotid artery, its branches, and related nerves.

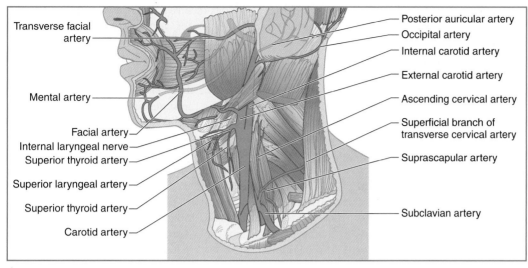

A

Transverse facial artery
Mental artery
Facial artery
Internal laryngeal nerve
Superior thyroid artery
Superior laryngeal artery
Superior thyroid artery
Carotid artery

Posterior auricular artery
Occipital artery
Internal carotid artery
External carotid artery
Ascending cervical artery
Superficial branch of transverse cervical artery
Suprascapular artery
Subclavian artery

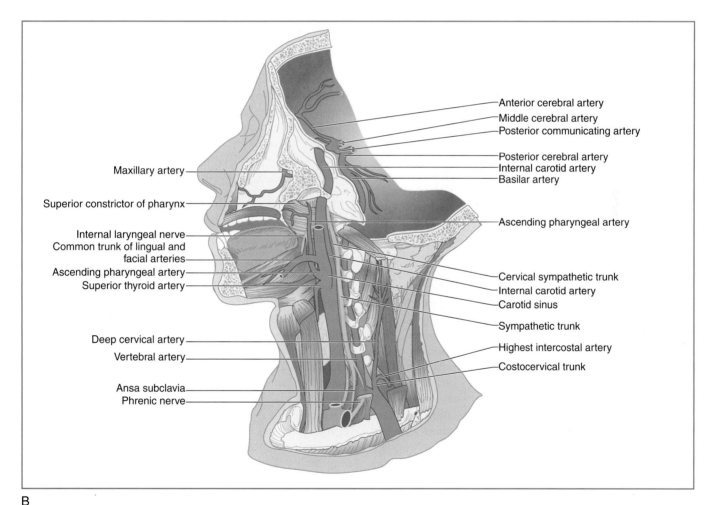

B

Maxillary artery
Superior constrictor of pharynx
Internal laryngeal nerve
Common trunk of lingual and facial arteries
Ascending pharyngeal artery
Superior thyroid artery
Deep cervical artery
Vertebral artery
Ansa subclavia
Phrenic nerve

Anterior cerebral artery
Middle cerebral artery
Posterior communicating artery
Posterior cerebral artery
Internal carotid artery
Basilar artery
Ascending pharyngeal artery
Cervical sympathetic trunk
Internal carotid artery
Carotid sinus
Sympathetic trunk
Highest intercostal artery
Costocervical trunk

Figure 10-31. A, Superficial branches of the carotid and subclavian arteries. **B,** Deep branches of the subclavian artery and branches of the carotid artery.

veins, the vagus and phrenic nerves, the ansa subclavia, vagal cardiac nerves, and sympathetic cardiac nerves. The ansa subclavia is a cord of the sympathetic trunk that forms a loop around the subclavian artery and connects the middle and inferior cervical sympathetic ganglia. The right recurrent nerve of the vagus also recurs around the right subclavian artery. The left subclavian artery rests upon the pleura of the apex of the lung. However, because of the differences in the origin of the subclavian arteries in the thorax, the lung's apex and pleura are inferior to the right subclavian artery.

Branches of the first part of the subclavian artery (see Figs. 10-30 and 10-31B) are the vertebral artery, thyrocervical trunk, and internal thoracic artery.

Vertebral Artery. The vertebral artery is the first branch of the subclavian artery. It arises from the subclavian artery's posterosuperior surface and runs upward between the anterior scalene muscle and the longus coli muscle (vertebral triangle) to enter the foramen transversarium in the transverse process of the sixth cervical vertebra (see Fig. 10-30). It ascends in the transverse foramina of the remaining cervical vertebrae. As it ascends, the vertebral artery gives rise to anterior spinal medullary branches that anastomose with the anterior spinal artery and the contralateral vertebral artery. This allows the right and left vertebral arteries to anastomose with each other.

The vertebral artery continues by bending around the lateral mass of the first cervical vertebra (atlas) to enter the vertebral canal between the posterior arch of the atlas and the occipital bone. The dorsal ramus of the first cervical spinal nerve is just inferior to the vertebral artery as it winds across the posterior arch. The vertebral artery then pierces the dura and arachnoid to lie in the subarachnoid space, where it gives rise to the anterior spinal and posteroinferior cerebellar arteries (see Fig. 10-31B). The latter artery typically gives rise to the posterior vertebral artery. However, the posterior spinal artery sometimes arises from the vertebral artery. The vertebral arteries continue into the posterior cranial fossa and unite to form the basilar artery that runs along the clivus in the subarachnoid space. The basilar artery has many branches including the anteroinferior cerebellar, labyrinthine, and superior cerebellar and terminates as the two posterior cerebral arteries. The posterior cerebral arteries participate with the internal carotid arteries in a collateral circulation called the circle of Willis.

A sympathetic plexus of postganglionic fibers that have their cell bodies in the inferior cervical sympathetic ganglion surrounds the vertebral artery.

The vertebral vein follows the artery but does *not* enter the vertebral canal. It originates as a plexus of veins in the suboccipital region. This plexus continues around the vertebral artery until the lower cervical vertebrae, where a single vein is formed that typically emerges through the transverse foramina of the sixth cervical vertebra to drain into the brachiocephalic vein. It usually receives a *small tributary* that passes through the foramen transversarium of the seventh cervical vertebrae when the vein passes through the sixth foramen transversarium. The vertebral vein does not appear in the cranial cavity or in the superior aspect of the vertebral canal. However, it does receive tributaries that do arise in the posterior cranial fossa or the vertebral canal. These include emissary veins that communicate with sigmoid sinus as well as tributaries from the internal vertebral plexus, which reach the vertebral vein by means of the intervertebral foramina.

Thyrocervical Trunk. The thyrocervical trunk (see Figs. 10-30 and 10-31A) arises from the superior surface of the first part of the subclavian artery. It splits into the inferior thyroid, the suprascapular, and the transverse cervical arteries.

Inferior Thyroid Artery. The inferior thyroid artery runs upward, anteriorly to the vertebral artery and longus colli muscle to pass along the medial border of the anterior scalene muscle. It turns medially at the level of the sixth cervical vertebra, behind the carotid sheath, to penetrate the fascia (false capsule of the thyroid gland) and reach the posterior aspect of the thyroid gland.

As the inferior thyroid artery passes posteriorly to the carotid sheath, it crosses behind, but sometimes in front of, the cervical sympathetic trunk and the middle cervical ganglion. The inferior thyroid artery comes into close but variable relationship to the recurrent laryngeal nerve (a branch of the vagus nerve), which is associated with the tracheoesophageal groove. The recurrent laryngeal nerve may pass posteriorly to the artery, anteriorly to the artery, or more often through its branches. This relationship is important during a thyroidectomy. At this point, the inferior thyroid artery gives off an inferior laryngeal branch that runs with the recurrent laryngeal nerve into the larynx. The inferior thyroid artery also helps supply the trachea, esophagus, parathyroid glands, and pharynx.

The *ascending cervical* branch of the inferior thyroid artery runs upward on the anterior surface of the anterior scalene muscle. It is just medial to the phrenic nerve, and it helps supply the muscles of the neck. The ascending cervical artery anastomoses with branches of the occipital and muscular branches of the vertebral arteries (see Fig. 10-31A).

Suprascapular Artery. The suprascapular artery is a branch of the thyrocervical trunk. It crosses the anterior surface of the *anterior scalene muscle*, the inferior trunk of the brachial plexus, and the third part of the subclavian artery. The suprascapular artery runs deep to the inferior belly of the omohyoid muscle to reach the suprascapular notch and then enters the supraspinous fossa of the scapula by passing superiorly to the superior transverse scapular (suprascapular) ligament. The suprascapular nerve, which also follows the inferior belly of the omohyoid, passes through the suprascapular notch inferiorly to the superior transverse scapular ligament (see Fig. 10-31A).

Transverse Cervical Artery. The transverse cervical artery is variable in its distribution. It arises from the thyrocervical trunk above the suprascapular artery and crosses anteriorly to the anterior scalene muscle and brachial plexus. In approximately 30% of cases, the artery divides into a superficial or ascending branch and a deep or descending branch (see Fig. 10-30A). The superficial branch runs on the deep surface of the trapezius while the deep branch descends on the deep surface of the levator scapulae to become the dorsal scapular artery.

However, in a large number of cases *only* the superficial branch arises from the thyrocervical trunk, which may be referred to as the *superficial cervical artery*. More commonly (70% of the time), the deep branch arises from the third part of the subclavian artery and is called the dorsal scapular artery. This artery descends on the anterior surface of the rhomboids to reach the inferior angle of the scapula. Here, the dorsal scapular artery anastomoses with the transverse cervical artery beneath the trapezius.

Internal Thoracic Artery. The internal thoracic artery (clinically referred to as the internal mammary artery) arises from the *inferior* surface of the first part of the subclavian artery opposite the origin of the thyrocervical trunk. It descends dorsally to the subclavian vein, the internal jugular vein, and the first costal cartilage to enter the thorax. The phrenic nerve crosses the internal thoracic artery. In the thorax, the artery is superficial to the endothoracic fascia.

Costocervical Trunk. The second part of the subclavian artery (see Fig. 10-31B) is found posterior to the anterior scalene muscle. The costocervical trunk is the only branch arising from the second part of the subclavian artery. It arises from the dorsal surface of the artery and passes posteriorly to divide into the highest intercostal artery and the deep cervical artery.

The highest intercostal artery is found dorsal to the pleura in the neck and ventral to the necks of the first and second ribs. It lies just *lateral* to the first thoracic sympathetic ganglion on the neck of the first rib. Here, it gives rise to the first and second posterior intercostal arteries, which enter the first and second posterior intercostal spaces to be distributed in a manner similar to that of the other intercostal arteries.

The deep cervical artery passes backward behind the seventh and eighth cervical nerves. It then runs upward between the semispinalis capitis and semispinalis cervicis muscles to supply the deep muscles of the neck. The deep cervical artery anastomoses with the occipital artery's descending branch and branches of the vertebral artery.

The subclavian vein is a continuation of the axillary vein at the lateral border of the first rib. It runs in the groove anterior to the anterior scalene muscle and does not rise above the plane of the clavicle, whereas the subclavian artery is slightly higher. The subclavian vein receives the external jugular vein and is then joined by the internal jugular vein posterior to the sternoclavicular joint to form the brachiocephalic vein. The subclavian vein is one of the veins catheterized for ongoing chemotherapy, parenteral hyperalimentation (supply of nutrients by means of a central venous line when the patient can not receive nutrition via the gastrointestinal tract), and cardiac catheterization.

C6 is an important landmark in the neck (analogous to the sternal angle in the thorax). The following relationships are found at this vertebral level:

1. The vertebral artery enters the transverse foramen.
2. The tendon of the omohyoid muscle crosses the carotid sheath.
3. The inferior thyroid artery passes behind the carotid sheath. This artery may pass in front of or behind the sympathetic

trunk and the middle cervical ganglion, and then it runs in close relationship to the recurrent laryngeal nerve.
4. The recurrent laryngeal nerve and inferior laryngeal artery (a branch of the inferior thyroid artery) enter the larynx at the junction of the inferior pharyngeal muscle and the esophagus.
5. The junctions between the pharynx and esophagus (pharyngoesophageal junction) and between the larynx and trachea are found at this vertebral level.

Anterior Triangle

The anterior triangle of the neck (see Fig. 10-22) is bounded superiorly by the mandible, posteriorly by the anterior border of the sternocleidomastoid muscle, and anteriorly by the midline (Table 10-14). The anterior triangles on both sides communicate freely with each other across the midline.

Digastric (Submandibular) Triangle

The digastric muscle (Table 10-15 and Fig. 10-32) has two bellies with a central tendon. The posterior belly is larger. This tendon is found just above the hyoid bone and is held to the hyoid bone by a loop of the outer investing layer of deep fascia as well as the insertion of the stylohyoid muscle.

Its dual innervation is representative of the dual embryologic origin of this muscle from both the first and the second pharyngeal arches.

The outer investing layer of deep cervical fascia forms the lateral boundary of the digastric triangle. Portions of the mylohyoid, hyoglossus, and superior pharyngeal constrictor muscles form the muscular paralingual or sublingual space (floor of this triangle).

The mylohyoid raphe is the midline connective tissue band that runs from the mandible to the hyoid bone. It joins the right and left mylohyoid muscles into a single functional unit that separates the neck from the floor of the mouth. *The mylohyoid muscle also forms an important transitional zone between the neck and the sublingual space.* The lateral (external) surface of the mylohyoid muscle is part of the medial boundary of the digastric triangle, while its medial (internal) surface serves as the inferolateral boundary of the paralingual (sublingual) space.

Many structures pass from the digastric triangle into the paralingual (sublingual) space by passing around the posterior margin of the mylohyoid muscle. This cleft, which can be referred to as the mylohyoid cleft (Fig. 10-33; see also Fig. 10-32), is found between the mylohyoid muscle and the hyoglossus muscle, and the structures that utilize this cleft include the hypoglossal nerve, the deep lobe of the submandibular gland, the submandibular duct, and the vena comitans of hypoglossal nerve. The hyoglossus muscle (see Fig. 10-33 and Table 10-15) ascends deep to the mylohyoid muscle to insert into the base of the tongue. It is thicker than the mylohyoid muscle. The *lingual artery and vein pass along the hyoglossus muscle's medial (internal) surface to reach the paralingual space and tongue* (see Fig. 10-33).

TABLE 10-14. Subdivisions of the Anterior Triangle

Triangle	Boundaries	Content
Digastric (submandibular)	Inferior margin of the mandible, anterior belly of the digastric, posterior belly of the digastric and stylohyoid muscles	Hypoglossal nerve (CN XII), mylohyoid branch of the inferior alveolar nerve of V₃, facial artery and vein, submandibular gland
Carotid	Posterior belly of the digastric, superior belly of the omohyoid, anterior border of the sternocleidomastoid	Common carotid; internal and external carotid arteries; external carotid artery branches: superior thyroid artery, lingual artery, facial artery, ascending and occipital pharyngeal arteries; vagus and its superior laryngeal, internal, and external laryngeal branches; sympathetic trunk; hypoglossal and ansa cervicalis nerves; nerve to thyrohyoid; internal jugular vein and associated deep cervical lymph nodes
Muscular	Midline of the neck, superior belly of the omohyoid and the sternocleidomastoid muscle	Remaining strap muscles, internal jugular vein
Submental	Hyoid bone, anterior belly of the digastric muscle and the midline	Submental lymph nodes that drain the floor of the oral cavity, tip of the tongue, lower lip

TABLE 10-15. Muscles of the Digastric Triangle

Muscle	Origin	Insertion	Action	Innervation
Digastric	Two bellies; posterior belly arises from mastoid notch of temporal bone	Inserts into anterior belly by means of intermediate tendon tethered to the hyoid bone by means of a fascial loop; anterior belly inserts into the internal surface of the mandible's body	With the mandible fixed, it assists in elevating hyoid bone, as in swallowing With hyoid bone fixed, it assists in depressing jaw	Posterior belly innervated by main trunk of facial nerve Anterior belly innervated by mylohyoid branch of mandibular nerve
Mylohyoid	Mylohyoid line of mandible	Mylohyoid raphe, body of hyoid bone	Elevates hyoid bone and tongue, depresses mandible when hyoid is fixed	Mylohyoid branch of inferior alveolar branch of V₃
Hyoglossus	Greater cornu of hyoid bone	Base of the tongue	Depresses and retracts tongue	Hypoglossal nerve (CN XII)
Superior pharyngeal constrictor	To be described with pharynx			
Stylohyoid	Styloid process of temporal bone	Hyoid bone	Elevates and retracts hyoid bone	Facial nerve

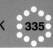

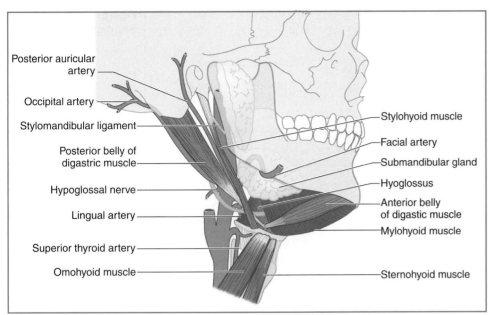

Figure 10-32. Digastric triangle.

Posterior auricular artery

Occipital artery

Stylomandibular ligament

Posterior belly of digastric muscle

Hypoglossal nerve

Lingual artery

Superior thyroid artery

Omohyoid muscle

Stylohyoid muscle

Facial artery

Submandibular gland

Hyoglossus

Anterior belly of digastic muscle

Mylohyoid muscle

Sternohyoid muscle

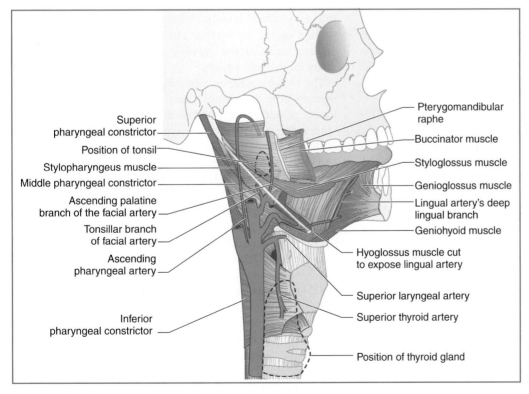

Superior pharyngeal constrictor

Position of tonsil

Stylopharyngeus muscle

Middle pharyngeal constrictor

Ascending palatine branch of the facial artery

Tonsillar branch of facial artery

Ascending pharyngeal artery

Inferior pharyngeal constrictor

Pterygomandibular raphe

Buccinator muscle

Styloglossus muscle

Genioglossus muscle

Lingual artery's deep lingual branch

Geniohyoid muscle

Hyoglossus muscle cut to expose lingual artery

Superior laryngeal artery

Superior thyroid artery

Position of thyroid gland

Figure 10-33. Lingual artery deep to the hyoglossus muscle.

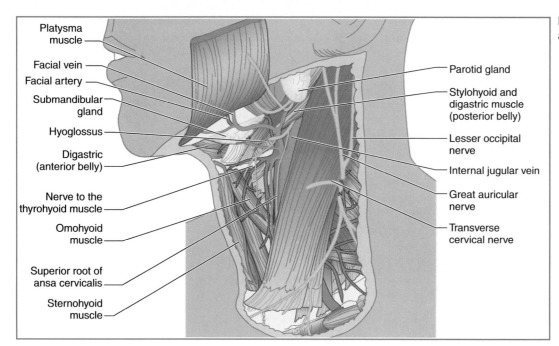

Platysma muscle

Facial vein

Facial artery

Submandibular gland

Hyoglossus

Digastric (anterior belly)

Nerve to the thyrohyoid muscle

Omohyoid muscle

Superior root of ansa cervicalis

Sternohyoid muscle

Parotid gland

Stylohyoid and digastric muscle (posterior belly)

Lesser occipital nerve

Internal jugular vein

Great auricular nerve

Transverse cervical nerve

Figure 10-34. Carotid and digastric triangles.

Only the most inferior fibers of the superior pharyngeal constrictor muscle are found in the digastric triangle.

The stylohyoid muscle (see Fig. 10-32 and Table 10-15) is found just anterior to the posterior belly of the digastric muscle. Close to its insertion into the hyoid bone, the stylohyoid muscle divides to encompass the central tendon of the digastric muscle.

Structures

The submandibular gland (Fig. 10-34; see also Fig. 10-32) is the largest structure in the digastric triangle (see Table 10-14). The investing layer of deep fascia divides into two layers that hold the gland in place. The external layer of this deep fascia attaches to the inferior borders of the mandible, while a deeper or internal layer of this deep fascia passes medially to the gland to attach to the mylohyoid ridge of the mandible. This arrangement of the fascia creates a submandibular space that holds the submandibular gland in the submandibular fossa of the mandible.

The submandibular gland has two parts: a large superficial lobe located in the digastric triangle and a smaller deep lobe that passes through the mylohyoid cleft into the paralingual (sublingual) space. The submandibular (Wharton's) duct runs with the deep lobe of the submandibular gland. The submandibular gland receives a glandular branch from the facial artery in the digastric triangle, postganglionic sympathetic fibers from the superior cervical sympathetic ganglion, and postganglionic parasympathetic fibers from the submandibular ganglion. This ganglion receives preganglionic fibers from the chorda tympani of the facial nerve, which runs with the lingual nerve. There are several lymph nodes on the external surface of the submandibular gland and a few within the gland's capsule.

The mylohyoid nerve is a branch of the inferior alveolar nerve (of V_3) and travels from the infratemporal region to the digastric triangle in the mylohyoid groove. This groove is found on the internal surface of the mandible just posterior to the mylohyoid muscle. This nerve then runs on the external surface of the mylohyoid muscle to innervate it and the anterior belly of the digastric muscle with SVE and GSA fibers for proprioception.

The hypoglossal nerve (see Fig. 10-32) enters the digastric triangle from the carotid triangle by passing medially (deep) to the posterior belly of the digastric muscle or its central tendon. The hypoglossal nerve passes along the deep surface of the submandibular gland. It then exits the digastric triangle and enters the mylohyoid cleft to reach the tongue.

The facial artery (see Fig. 10-31A) also passes deep to the posterior belly of the digastric muscle to reach the posterior surface of the submandibular gland. It runs posterior to, then deep (medially) to the gland. The facial artery then passes between the mandible and the submandibular gland onto the face. Here, it is found in a groove on the mandible just antero-inferior to the masseter muscle. In the digastric triangle, the facial artery has glandular, submental, and tonsillar branches.

The facial vein *passes superficially* to the submandibular gland. Thus, in the digastric triangle, the submandibular gland separates the deeply placed facial artery from the more superficially located facial vein.

The marginal mandibular and cervical branches of the facial nerve also pass *superficially* to the submandibular gland.

The submandibular lymph (Fig. 10-35) nodes lie either lateral to or in the superficial lobe of the submandibular gland. These nodes receive afferents from the cheek, floor and angle of the mouth, adjacent lips, and side of the tongue, and parotid and submental nodes. Efferents drain into the superior deep cervical nodes. The submandibular nodes usually are not palpable from the oral cavity.

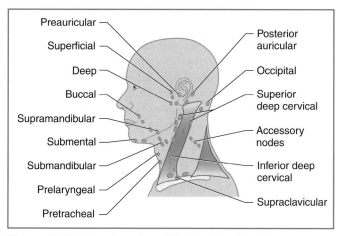

Figure 10-35. Lymph nodes of the head and neck.

Carotid Triangle

Structures

The middle pharyngeal constrictor muscle overlaps the superior pharyngeal constrictor muscle while the inferior pharyngeal constrictor muscle overlaps the middle pharyngeal constrictor. These muscles will be described with the pharynx.

The thyrohyoid muscle is a small muscle originating on the oblique line of the thyroid cartilage and inserting onto the hyoid bone. This strap muscle is innervated by branches from the first and second cervical spinal nerves that run with the hypoglossal nerve and branches as the nerve to the thyrohyoid (see Cervical Plexus, above).

The common boundary between the carotid and digastric triangles is the *posterior belly of the digastric muscle*. The following structures pass medially (deep) to the digastric muscle (see Figs. 10-32 and 10-33 and Table 10-15): sympathetic trunk, hypoglossal nerve, structures in the carotid sheath, and the external carotid artery. The important structures found superficial to the posterior belly of the digastric muscle are branches forming the external jugular vein, the cervical branch of the facial nerve that innervates the platysma muscle, and the lower pole of the parotid gland. *Thus, the posterior belly of the digastric muscle is an important landmark in locating the numerous structures associated with it.*

Carotid Arteries

The left common carotid artery has a thoracic origin while the right common carotid artery (see Fig. 10-31B) is a terminal branch of the brachiocephalic trunk. Both common carotid arteries run posteriorly to the sternoclavicular articulation and then upward in the neck deep to the sternocleidomastoid muscle.

The common carotid artery is found anterior to the lower cervical transverse processes until it reaches the lower apex of the carotid triangle (vertebral level C6). At the level of the cricoid cartilage, the common carotid artery can be compressed against the anterior (carotid) tubercle of the transverse process of the sixth cervical vertebra in order to stop or impede a hemorrhage of the common carotid artery or one of its branches.

The common carotid artery continues until the superior aspect of the thyroid cartilage (C4), where it splits into its two terminal branches: the external and internal carotid arteries (see Fig. 10-31A). There is significant variability in the position that the two arteries have to each other. This is of some importance, since arteriosclerotic plaque usually is found at the origin of the internal carotid artery or at the junction of the common and internal carotid arteries. The external carotid artery may also be involved. The external carotid artery is typically, but not always, anteromedial to the internal carotid artery. As they ascend, the internal carotid artery takes a more medial position and the external carotid artery a lateral position. The internal carotid artery continues superiorly within the carotid sheath until it reaches the carotid canal in the petrous portion of the temporal bone. The internal carotid artery does not give off any branches in the neck.

The carotid body and the carotid sinus (see Fig. 10-31A) are two specialized sensory organs associated with the bifurcation of the common carotid artery and its internal branch. The carotid sinus is a dilatation of the arterial wall of the junction of the common and internal carotid arteries. It functions as a baroreceptor, which is stimulated by elevated blood pressure. The carotid sinus is innervated by the carotid sinus nerve (nerve of Herring), a branch of CN IX, with a possible contribution from the vagus. The GVA fibers from the carotid sinus reach the CNS and stimulate control centers, which eventually affect the heart rate by slowing the heart. Carotid sinus syndrome results from hypersensitivity of the carotid sinus. In severe cases, it may result in unconsciousness (syncope). Denervation of the carotid sinus is a treatment for severe cases of carotid sinus syndrome.

The carotid body is a reddish-brown organ that functions as a chemoreceptor stimulated primarily by hypoxia (a low level of oxygen in the blood) or an excess of CO_2. It is located at the posteromedial surface of the common and internal carotid arteries and rises into the bifurcation of the internal and external carotid arteries. It consists of highly vascularized epithelial cells held in place by connective tissue and a fibrous capsule. The GVA fibers innervating the carotid body are from the carotid branch of the glossopharyngeal nerve. It is also stimulated by hypercapnia (an elevated level of carbon dioxide). When stimulated, it signals respiratory centers located in the brainstem to increase the rate and depth of breathing.

The external carotid nerve plexus is located on the external surface (adventitia) of the external carotid artery. This neural plexus consists of postganglionic sympathetic fibers mostly from the superior cervical sympathetic ganglia with some possible contribution from the middle cervical sympathetic ganglia.

External Carotid Artery

The external carotid artery has many branches that supply the upper part of the neck, the face, and the infratemporal, temporal, and occipital regions.

The three anterior branches of the external carotid artery (see Fig. 10-31A) are described below.

1. The superior thyroid artery arises just lateral to the thyroid cartilage and passes medially (deep) to the omohyoid

muscle. At or near its origin, it gives off a major branch, the superior laryngeal artery, which passes between the hyoid bone and the thyroid cartilage, penetrating the thyrohyoid membrane to enter the larynx. The internal branch of the superior laryngeal nerve (of the vagus) accompanies the superior laryngeal artery into the larynx. The external laryngeal branch of the superior laryngeal nerve accompanies the superior thyroid artery, which continues to the superior pole of the thyroid gland. The superior thyroid artery is often ligated close to the thyroid gland's superior pole to preserve the external laryngeal nerve, which supplies the cricothyroid muscle.

The superior thyroid artery descends just laterally to the thyroid cartilage to reach the superior pole of the thyroid gland. Along the way, it supplies the infrahyoid muscles (strap muscles). It then divides into the anterior medial and posterior lateral branches that supply the thyroid gland and adjacent structures. The anterior branch has an isthmus branch that anastomoses with the contralateral isthmus branch while the posterior branch anastomoses with the inferior thyroid artery. These anastomoses create an excellent collateral circulation.

2. The lingual artery arises just above the cornu of the hyoid bone and supplies the tongue. About 50% of the time, it arises as a common trunk with the facial artery. At its origin just above the posterior tip of the hyoid's greater cornu, the lingual artery curves superiorly and then inferiorly, forming a loop just before this artery passes forward, *medially (deep) to the hyoglossus muscle,* lying on the middle pharyngeal constrictor muscle (see Fig. 10-30B). This loop of the lingual artery is usually crossed laterally by the hypoglossal nerve, which completes a circle.

The lingual artery and vein are separated from the hypoglossal nerve by the hyoglossus muscle. However, the vena comitans nervi hypoglossi runs with the hypoglossal nerve in the mylohyoid cleft. The lingual artery has tonsillar and dorsal lingual branches before ending as the deep lingual and sublingual arteries.

3. The facial artery originates either as a common branch with the lingual artery or as a separate artery. In the digastric triangle, the facial artery gives rise to ascending palatine, submental, glandular, and two tonsillar branches.

The two posterior branches of the external carotid artery (see Fig. 10-31B) are the occipital and posterior auricular arteries.

1. The occipital artery arises from the external carotid artery inferiorly to the posterior belly of the digastric muscle. At this point, the hypoglossal nerve hooks laterally around both the external and the internal carotid arteries. As the hypoglossal nerve hooks around the occipital artery, the artery gives off a small sternocleidomastoid branch that supplies the sternocleidomastoid muscle. The occipital artery follows the inferior surface of the digastric muscle's posterior belly. This artery continues in the mastoid groove just medial to the mastoid notch. It passes between the attachments of the sternocleidomastoid and the trapezius muscles to be distributed with the greater occipital nerve on the back of the head. The occipital artery has meningeal branches that enter the posterior cranial fossa through the jugular foramen or hypoglossal canal and a descending branch that anastomoses with the deep cervical branch of the costocervical trunk of the subclavian artery.

2. The posterior auricular artery follows the superior margin of the posterior belly of the digastric muscle. This small artery travels inferiorly and then posteriorly to the ear with the posterior auricular branch of VII. The posterior auricular artery supplies the external ear, part of the parotid gland, and the skin behind the ear. This artery also has a stylomastoid branch that enters the stylomastoid foramen to help supply the middle ear.

The three ascending branches of the external carotid artery are as follows:

1. The maxillary artery is one of the two terminal branches of the external carotid artery. The maxillary artery branches from the external carotid artery after the external carotid artery has entered the parotid gland. The maxillary artery passes medially to the neck of the mandible to enter the infratemporal region. Its numerous branches are described with the infratemporal region.

2. The ascending pharyngeal artery (see Fig. 10-27) arises on the posteromedial (deep) surface of the external carotid artery near its origin. It passes medially (deep) to travel up between the internal carotid artery and the pharynx. The ascending pharyngeal artery passes over the superior border of the superior pharyngeal constrictor muscle to enter the pharynx. The ascending pharyngeal artery has tonsillar, palatine, and meningeal branches.

3. The superficial temporal artery is the other terminal branch of the external carotid artery in the parotid gland. It arises posteriorly to the neck of the mandible, passes over the zygomatic arch anteriorly to the auricle, and runs superiorly with the auriculotemporal branch of the mandibular nerve. The superficial temporal artery penetrates the deep fascia and passes over the zygomatic arch into the plane of the superficial temporal fascia, an unusual location for a major artery. The superficial temporal artery has a transverse facial branch that helps supply the face. This artery passes between the zygomatic arch and the parotid duct. The superficial temporal artery also has a zygomatico-orbital branch that runs above the zygomatic arch to anastomose with the arteries around the orbit. The superficial temporal artery divides into frontal and parietal branches and supplies the skin over the frontal and temporal regions and scalp. These branches of the superficial temporal artery anastomose with branches of the contralateral superficial temporal artery, and the superficial temporal artery's frontal division also anastomoses with the supraorbital and supratrochlear branches of the ophthalmic artery. The superficial temporal artery's parietal division anastomoses with the occipital artery.

Collateral Circulation of the Head and Neck

If necessary, the common carotid artery can be ligated at the level of the sixth cervical vertebra because of the excellent collateral circulation found in the head and neck. The extracranial collateral circulation (Table 10-16) includes anastomoses between the ipsilateral branches of the external carotid artery and subclavian artery, ipsilateral branches of the external carotid artery, and branches of both external carotid arteries.

The intracranial anastomoses consist of the two vertebral arteries that form the basilar artery that anastomose with the internal carotid arteries by means of the right and left posterior communicating branches. The cranial arterial circle (circle of Willis) is completed by the anastomoses of the right and left anterior cerebral arteries by means of the anterior communicating artery (Fig. 10-36).

Veins of the Carotid Triangle

The internal jugular vein begins at the jugular foramen as a continuation of the sigmoid and inferior petrosal sinuses. It receives branches from the common facial, lingual, pharyngeal, superior thyroid, and middle thyroid veins. The internal jugular vein's superior bulb is located in the jugular foramen, while its inferior bulb marks its caudal end just before it joins the subclavian vein to form the brachiocephalic vein. The internal jugular vein has valves only at its superior and inferior bulbs.

Innervation

The vagus nerve exits the skull through the jugular foramen. It has two sensory ganglia, the superior (jugular) ganglion and the inferior (nodose) ganglion, which are located in or inferior to the jugular foramen. The vagus nerve passes vertically down the neck in the carotid sheath, posteriorly and between the internal jugular vein and the internal carotid artery. Below the thyroid cartilage, the vagus nerve lies between the internal jugular vein and the common carotid artery. The nerve enters the thorax with the common carotid artery by passing anteriorly to the first part of the subclavian artery.

Branches of the Vagus Nerve in the Neck

The pharyngeal branch passes forward between the internal and external carotid arteries to reach the wall of the pharynx. It communicates with branches of CN IX and the sympathetic trunk to form the pharyngeal plexus. The pharyngeal fibers of the vagus supply all the muscles of the pharynx except the stylopharyngeus muscle, which is innervated by CN IX, and all the muscles of the soft palate except the tensor veli palatini, which is innervated by the mandibular nerve. The SVE fibers of the vagus that supply the muscles of the pharynx and larynx have their cell bodies in the nucleus ambiguus. This nucleus gives rise to SVE fibers that are distributed through both CN X and CN XI. Thus, this innervation is referred to as the "X–XI complex."

The superior laryngeal nerve arises just below the inferior ganglion of the vagus. It enters the carotid triangle medially to the carotid sheath. The superior laryngeal nerve passes medially (deep) to both the internal and external carotid arteries and divides into internal and external laryngeal branches. The internal laryngeal nerve follows the superior laryngeal artery while the external laryngeal nerve follows the superior thyroid artery.

Cardiac branches of the vagus join cardiac branches from the sympathetic trunk to form the *cardiac plexus*, which is

---

TABLE 10-16. Collateral Circulation of the Neck and Head

Anastomoses of Ipsilateral Arteries

Superior thyroid artery with inferior thyroid artery

Deep cervical branch of costocervical trunk with descending branch of occipital artery

Superficial temporal artery with occipital artery

Inferior labial artery of facial artery with mental artery of inferior alveolar artery

Infraorbital branch of maxillary artery with palpebral branches of ophthalmic artery

Transverse facial branch of superficial temporal with infraorbital branches of maxillary and branches of facial arteries

Anastomoses of Right and Left External Carotid Arteries

Right and left superior thyroid arteries

Right and left vertebral arteries via radicular branches to anterior spinal artery

Both superior and inferior labial branches of right and left facial arteries

Right and left superficial temporal arteries across scalp

Right and left nasal branches of facial arteries

Anastomoses of Internal and External Carotid Arteries

Dorsal nasal branch of ophthalmic artery with angular branch of facial artery

Anterior division of superficial temporal artery with supraorbital and supratrochlear branches of ophthalmic artery

Middle meningeal branch of maxillary artery with lacrimal branch of ophthalmic artery

Vertebral arteries via their basilar artery with the internal carotid arteries via the posterior communicating branches which help to form the cerebral arterial circle (of Willis)

---

found inferior to the aortic arch and anterior to the bifurcation of the trachea. The cardiac branches of the vagus have preganglionic parasympathetic fibers and GVA fibers.

The right and left recurrent laryngeal nerves supply sensory fibers to the larynx below the vocal cords and motor fibers to all the muscles of the larynx except the cricothyroid muscle. The right recurrent laryngeal nerve recurs around the right subclavian artery (Fig. 10-37). The left recurs around the arch of the aorta posteriorly to the ligamentum arteriosum. The recurrent laryngeal nerves run with the inferior laryngeal arteries (branches of the inferior thyroid arteries) to enter the larynx inferior to the cricopharyngeal portion of the inferior pharyngeal constrictor muscle, posterior to the cricothyroid joint, and anterior to the esophagus. Occasionally there is a nonrecurrent laryngeal nerve, which is found only on the right side, when there is a retroesophageal right subclavian artery. This is the result of the right subclavian artery arising from the distal portion of the left aortic arch. The fourth arch is lost with an aberrant right subclavian artery, and the right recurrent nerve arises higher in the neck and runs directly to the larynx or occasionally winds around the inferior thyroid artery.

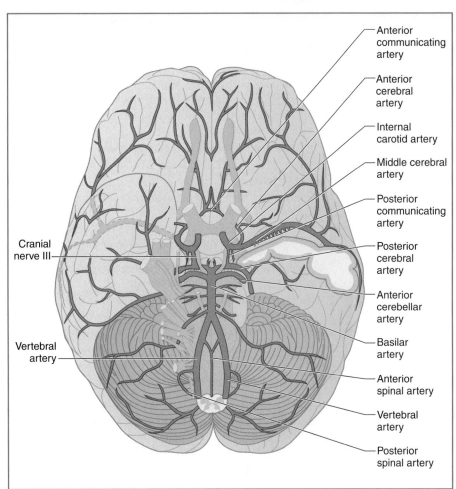

Figure 10-36. Cerebral arterial circle of Willis.

Anterior communicating artery

Anterior cerebral artery

Internal carotid artery

Middle cerebral artery

Posterior communicating artery

Posterior cerebral artery

Anterior cerebellar artery

Basilar artery

Anterior spinal artery

Vertebral artery

Posterior spinal artery

Cranial nerve III

Vertebral artery

As previously described, the hypoglossal nerve enters the superior aspect of the carotid triangle by winding around the external carotid artery, usually at the level of the occipital artery. It passes deep to the posterior belly of the digastric muscle to enter the digastric triangle. As the hypoglossal nerve crosses the carotid sheath, it *appears* to give rise to the superior root of the ansa cervicalis (see Cervical Plexus, above).

Cervical Sympathetic Trunk

The cervical sympathetic trunk (see Fig. 10-37) passes superiorly into the neck from the thorax embedded in the deep fascia posterior to the carotid sheath. It is directly behind the common or internal carotid arteries and medial to the vagus nerve. The cervical portion of the sympathetic trunk is found at the root of the neck, medial to the highest intercostal branch of the costocervical artery.

The cervical sympathetic ganglia give rise only to gray rami communicantes. The preganglionic fibers arise in the thorax from the lateral horn nuclei of T1–T4. These fibers then pass in the ventral roots of thoracic spinal nerves 1–4, ventral rami, and white rami communicantes of thoracic spinal nerves 1–4 to enter the sympathetic trunk and ascend into the neck.

Inferior, Middle, and Superior Cervical Sympathetic Ganglia

The inferior cervical ganglion (Fig. 10-38) usually fuses with the first thoracic ganglion, forming the cervicothoracic or stellate (star-shaped) ganglion. It is found anywhere from the level of the transverse process of C7 (vertebra prominens) to the level of the neck of the first rib. The stellate ganglion is posterior or posteromedial to the vertebral artery, while the highest intercostal artery is lateral to the ganglion. The inferior cervical ganglion has the following branches that contain postganglionic sympathetic fibers: inferior cardiac branches, vertebral branches that follow the vertebral artery, and gray rami communicantes to cervical spinal nerves 7 and 8.

The middle cervical ganglion is located at the level of the sixth cervical vertebra. The inferior thyroid artery passes either anteriorly to or posteriorly to this ganglion. Both the middle cervical ganglion and the inferior thyroid artery are posterior to the carotid sheath.

Often a loop (ansa subclavia) passes around the subclavian artery between the middle and inferior ganglia.

Branches of the middle cervical ganglion that contain postganglionic fibers are the gray rami communicantes to the fifth and sixth cervical spinal nerves, and the middle cardiac and thyroid branches.

The superior cervical ganglion is the largest of the three ganglia and is found posterior to the internal carotid artery and the carotid sheath. This ganglion stretches from the lower border of the first cervical vertebra to the third cervical vertebra.

The following are branches of the superior cervical sympathetic ganglion that contain postganglionic sympathetic fibers:

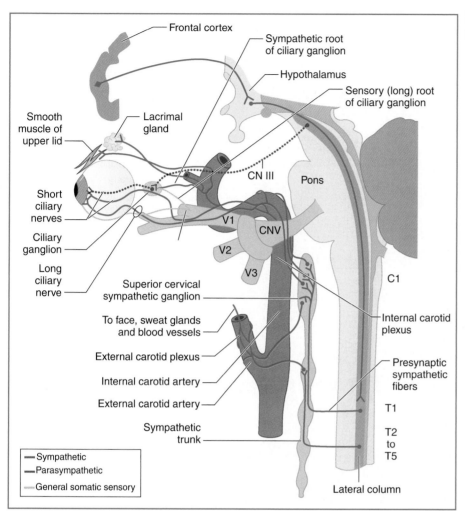

Figure 10-37. Cervical sympathetic pathway to the orbit, face, and cerebrum.

Labels within figure:
- Frontal cortex
- Sympathetic root of ciliary ganglion
- Hypothalamus
- Sensory (long) root of ciliary ganglion
- Smooth muscle of upper lid
- Lacrimal gland
- CN III
- Pons
- Short ciliary nerves
- V1
- CNV
- Ciliary ganglion
- V2
- C1
- Long ciliary nerve
- V3
- Superior cervical sympathetic ganglion
- Internal carotid plexus
- To face, sweat glands and blood vessels
- External carotid plexus
- Presynaptic sympathetic fibers
- Internal carotid artery
- External carotid artery
- T1
- Sympathetic trunk
- T2 to T5
- Sympathetic
- Parasympathetic
- General somatic sensory
- Lateral column

gray rami communicantes, which join the first four cervical nerves; superior cardiac branches; pharyngeal branches; *post-ganglionic branches that contribute to the external carotid nerve plexus*, which follows the external carotid artery and its branches to supply the face and head; and postganglionic fibers, which follow the internal carotid artery as the *internal carotid nerve or nervous plexus* to enter the skull and inner-vate the central arteries and orbit.

Muscular Triangle

The muscular triangle's superficial boundary is formed by the investing layer of deep cervical fascia, and the medial or deep boundary is formed by the pretracheal fascia (Table 10-17).

The contents of the muscular triangle (see Figs. 10-30B and 10-34 and Table 10-17) are the strap muscles and their neurovascular bundles. However, deep to the muscular triangle's strap muscles is the *visceral column*, which includes the *thyroid gland, pharynx, larynx, trachea, and esophagus* (Fig. 10-38).

The sternohyoid muscle arises from the posterior surface of the manubrium, the sternoclavicular joint, and the adjoining portion of the clavicle. The muscle runs superiorly and medially to insert on the body of the hyoid bone.

The sternothyroid muscle arises from the posterior surface of the manubrium and first costal cartilage. It runs superiorly, deep to the sternohyoid muscle, to insert on the oblique line of the thyroid cartilage. It draws the thyroid cartilage inferiorly. The sternothyroid muscle covers the lateral lobe of the thyroid gland.

The thyrohyoid muscle arises from the oblique line of the thyroid cartilage and passes superiorly over the thyrohyoid membrane. It inserts into the lower border of the body of the hyoid bone.

The superior belly of the omohyoid muscle is found in the muscular triangle. This muscle has already been described. The thyrohyoid and sternothyroid muscles lie deep to the anterior belly of the omohyoid and sternohyoid muscles.

During deglutition (swallowing), the strap muscles depress the hyoid bone and the thyroid cartilage.

The strap muscles are innervated by branches of the cervical plexus. The sternohyoid, sternothyroid, and both bellies of the omohyoid muscles are innervated by branches of the ansa cervicalis (cervical spinal nerves 1–3). The thyrohyoid muscle is innervated by a branch of the first and second cervical spinal nerves that communicate (travel) with the hypoglossal nerve. These muscles receive their innervation

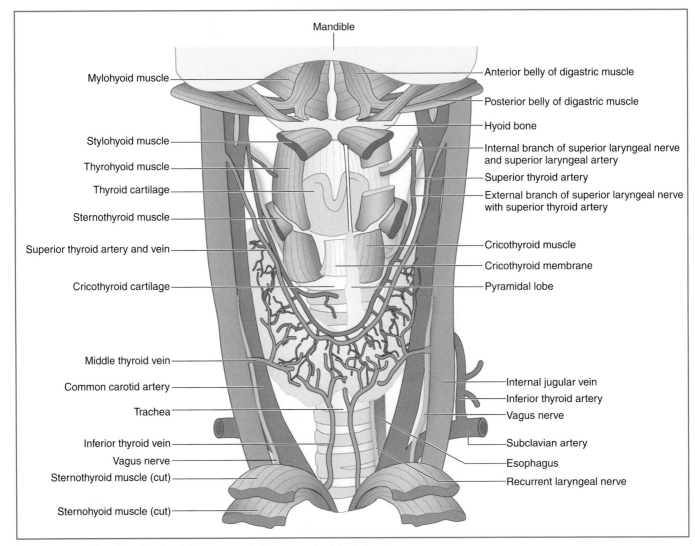

Figure 10-38. The thyroid gland, its venous drainage, and related structures.

relatively low in the muscular belly. Thus, the nerve supply can be spared if the muscle bellies are sectioned high. The strap muscles are sometimes bisected to expose the thyroid gland or visceral column.

Thyroid Gland

The thyroid gland is a brownish-red gland found deep to the long strap muscles (see Figs. 10-27 and 10-38). This gland enlarges during puberty in both sexes but is larger in females. It physiologically enlarges during menstruation and pregnancy.

The thyroid gland, like all glands, has its own true connective capsule. It is also wrapped in a variable fascia, derived from the pretracheal fascia, which forms the false capsule of the thyroid gland. The false capsule helps anchor the gland to the thyroid cartilage, the arch of the cricoid cartilage, and the rings of the trachea. The suspensory ligament of the thyroid gland (suspensory ligament of Berry) helps the thyroid gland adhere to the cricoid cartilage and trachea. The thyroid gland moves with the thyroid cartilage during swallowing. This is a

TABLE 10–17. Content of the Muscular Triangle		
Triangle	**Boundaries**	**Content**
Muscular	Anteriorly, midline of the neck; superiorly, hyoid bone; posteriorly, anterior border of the superior belly of the omohyoid and anterior border of the sternocleidomastoid	Strap muscles

maneuver that aids in the identification of a thyroid nodule during a physical examination.

The gland has two pear-shaped lateral lobes connected by a narrow midline isthmus. The superior aspect of each lobe extends as far as the oblique line of the thyroid cartilage. The inferior aspect of each lobe lies at the level of the fourth to sixth tracheal rings. The isthmus extends across the midline in front of the upper two or three tracheal rings lying superficially between right and left sternohyoids. There is often a pyramidal lobe present that extends superiorly from the isthmus, usually at the point where the isthmus joins the left lateral lobe. Occasionally, a fibromuscular structure, the levator glandulae thyroideae muscle, connects the isthmus to the body of the hyoid bone.

The thyroid gland develops from a down-growth of the foramen cecum of the tongue known as the thyroglossal duct. A remnant of this duct may connect the isthmus and the tongue. It may contain thyroid tissue or may be the site of cyst formation in the neck. The pyramidal lobe, if present, is the remnant of the inferior end of the thyroglossal duct.

Posterolateral to each lateral lobe is the common carotid artery in the posterior aspect of the carotid sheath, whereas the parathyroid glands are usually in the posterior aspect of the false capsule. The following structures are found posteromedial to the lateral lobes: the trachea, larynx (including part of the thyroid and cricoid cartilages, and cricothyroid membrane), lower pharynx, and esophagus. The esophagus is intimately associated with the left lateral lobe because the *esophagus lies somewhat to the left of the midline*. The tracheoesophageal groove containing the recurrent laryngeal nerve is more prominent on the right.

The thyroid gland has a rich blood supply, as is typical of endocrine glands.

The superior thyroid artery is a branch of the external carotid artery.

The inferior thyroid artery (a branch of the thyrocervical trunk) helps supply the thyroid gland (at cervical vertebral level 6), trachea, and esophagus, and it has an inferior laryngeal branch. The recurrent laryngeal nerve crosses either anteriorly or posteriorly to or between the branches of the inferior thyroid artery as it passes upward to the larynx. The inferior thyroid artery anastomoses with the superior thyroid artery on the posterior aspect of the lateral lobe of the thyroid gland. It also has branches to the parathyroid glands.

The thyroidea ima is a single artery found in a small percentage of the population. This artery has a variable origin. It may arise from the brachiocephalic trunk, the common carotid artery, or the arch of the aorta. It may be a source of bleeding during a tracheotomy.

The veins draining the thyroid gland are the superior, middle, and inferior thyroid veins. The superior thyroid vein drains the superior part of the thyroid gland into the internal jugular vein (see Fig. 10-38). The middle thyroid vein also drains into the internal jugular vein or may be absent. The inferior thyroid veins either join together anterior to or between the branches of the trachea and drain into the left brachiocephalic vein, or drain separately into the two brachiocephalic veins. The arteries and veins that supply the thyroid gland form a plexus between the false and true capsules of the thyroid gland.

The four parathyroid glands are small, ovoid masses usually located in the false capsule of the thyroid gland. The parathyroids have a very variable location because of their migration during development. The superior parathyroid glands are derived from the fourth pharyngeal pouch and usually are found above the inferior parathyroids derived from the third pouch. The superior parathyroids are often located at the level of the cricoid cartilage while the two inferior glands are often found posterior to the inferior poles of the thyroid gland.

Since the inferior parathyroids are derived from the third pharyngeal pouch, as is the thymus, their migration may be highly variable. The inferior parathyroids are typically carried inferiorly to the fourth pouch derivatives, the superior parathyroids, by the descent of the thymus. However, they can separate very early and remain in the neck as high as the hyoid bone, or fail to separate from this primordium and descend into the superior and even the anterior mediastinum.

The inferior thyroid artery usually supplies both parathyroid glands and part of the thyroid gland. Sometimes, the superior thyroid artery supplies the superior parathyroid glands. The presence of a defined hilum, which receives the arteries, aids in the identification of the parathyroid glands.

Submental Triangle

The submental triangle is bounded anteriorly by the midline of the neck, laterally by the anterior belly of the digastric muscle, and inferiorly by the body of the hyoid bone. The floor of the triangle is formed by the mylohyoid muscle. The contents of the submental triangle are the beginning of the anterior jugular vein and the submental lymph nodes. These nodes drain the chin, medial portion of the lower lip, adjacent gums, and floor of the mouth (sometimes from both sides). Efferents drain into the submandibular and jugulo-omohyoid nodes.

●●● VENOUS DRAINAGE OF THE NECK

The veins of the neck lie superficial or deep to the deep fascia. They vary considerably in size, and one system of veins can drain into the other.

Superficial Veins

The external jugular vein is formed by the posterior division of the retromandibular vein and the posterior auricular vein on the lateral surface of the sternocleidomastoid muscle just inferior to the parotid gland. The external jugular vein pierces the deep cervical fascia and runs in the superficial fascia across the sternocleidomastoid muscle. In the posterior triangle, the external jugular vein again pierces the deep cervical fascia to empty into the subclavian vein. At this point, the deep cervical fascia can hold a lacerated external jugular open, allowing air to enter the vein and produce an air embolus.

The paired *anterior jugular veins* begin in the suprahyoid region. They descend near the midline to drain laterally into the subclavian vein or external jugular vein. The two anterior jugular veins are connected above the jugular notch by the jugular venous arch in the suprasternal space.

Deep Veins

The internal jugular vein begins at the superior jugular bulb located at the jugular foramen. The sigmoid sinus and the inferior petrosal sinus pass through the jugular foramen to drain into the superior bulb of the internal jugular vein.

As the internal jugular vein passes inferiorly, it receives the following veins:

- The facial vein unites with the anterior division of the retromandibular vein to form a common facial vein.
- The lingual vein and the venae comitantes nervi hypoglossi drain the dorsal and lateral parts of the tongue.
- The pharyngeal veins drain the pharyngeal plexus on the outer surface of the pharynx.
- The superior, middle, and inferior thyroid veins have been described.

As described in the Vertebral Artery section, the vertebral vein begins in the suboccipital venous plexus. It communicates with emissary veins and the internal vertebral venous plexus, and it receives the occipital vein.

●●● LYMPHATIC DRAINAGE OF THE NECK

The lymph nodes (see Fig. 10-35) drain the external head and neck and eventually empty into the thoracic duct or right main lymphatic (jugular) duct. The nodes are arranged as a horizontal chain and several vertical chains that eventually reach the venous circulation.

The horizontal chain is a collar-like chain of nodes located high in the neck and lower portion of the head (see Fig. 10-35). It consists of the submental nodes (under the chin), the submandibular nodes (associated with the submandibular gland under the mandible), the pre- and postauricular nodes (located either anteriorly or posteriorly to the ear), and the occipital nodes (see Fig. 10-35). Understanding how the nodes drain is important for understanding how disease spreads from a primary site to the involved nodes. Enlarged lymph nodes are an important diagnostic sign indicating the primary site of a lesion.

Horizontal Chain of Cervical Lymph Nodes

The submental nodes receive afferent lymphatics from the skin of the chin, tip of the tongue, middle portion of the lower lip, and mucous membranes of the mouth. These nodes have efferent lymphatics that travel to the submandibular nodes or the deep cervical chain of lymph nodes (jugulo-omohyoid node).

The submandibular nodes receive afferents from the submental nodes, the preauricular nodes and buccal (along the facial artery) nodes, the lower portion of the nasal cavity, the nose, cheeks, gums of the upper and lower jaws, tongue, and lateral part of the lower lip. The efferent lymphatics from these nodes drain into the superior deep cervical nodes (i.e., the jugulodigastric node, which is associated with the digastric muscle and is the principal node that drains the tongue).

The preauricular nodes include the anterior auricular and parotid nodes. The anterior auricular nodes are always located anterior to the tragus. They drain the superficial ear, temporal region, and lateral conjunctiva and are often enlarged as a result of conjunctivitis.

The parotid nodes include superficial and deep nodes. The superficial nodes are located external to the parotid capsule. These nodes drain the eyelids, scalp, anterior external auditory meatus, and tympanic membrane. The deep nodes are located in the parotid gland and drain the most of the external auditory meatus, nose, and superficial parotid nodes.

The posterior auricular nodes lie on the mastoid process and drain the adjacent scalp, external auditory meatus, and ear.

The occipital nodes lie along the occipital artery and drain the occipital region.

The vertical chains are the superficial cervical nodes that lie along the external jugular vein, the deep cervical nodes that are intimately associated with the internal jugular vein, and the accessory nodes, which are associated with the accessory nerve in the posterior triangle and drain the posterior scalp and occipital region (see Fig. 10-35).

The superficial cervical nodes receive afferents from the cutaneous nodes of the face and the parotid, occipital, and auricular regions. The efferents drain into the deep cervical nodes. These nodes lie along the external jugular vein, superficial to the sternocleidomastoid muscle.

Deep Cervical Nodes: Superior and Inferior Components

The numerous deep cervical nodes form a chain that is associated with the carotid sheath. They lie close to the internal jugular vein and extend from the base of the skull to the root of the neck. The deep cervical nodes are divided into superior and inferior groups approximately at the level where the omohyoid muscle's central tendon crosses the common carotid artery and the internal jugular vein.

The superior deep cervical nodes receive afferents from the upper portion of the neck (i.e., the buccal, parotid, submental, and submandibular nodes). They also drain the superficial and deep structures of the neck. The jugulodigastric node is located where the digastric muscle crosses the carotid sheath usually just posterior to the angle of the mandible. This node receives afferents from the pharynx and preauricular and parotid nodes and is the main node of the palatine tonsil. The retropharyngeal nodes are located posterior to the pharynx in the retropharyngeal space. They drain into the nasal cavities and pharynx. The retropharyngeal nodes drain into the adjacent superior deep cervical nodes. Finally, the juguloomohyoid node receives efferents from the above nodes, including the tip of the tongue, and is located at the point where the central tendon of the omohyoid muscle crosses the carotid sheath.

The midline prelaryngeal (Delphian) node is usually a single node located over the cricothyroid membrane. The afferent lymphatics to these nodes are from the lower larynx, upper trachea, and thyroid gland. The efferents drain into the inferior deep cervical nodes (usually the jugulo-omohyoid nodes). The location of the prelaryngeal node is variable; it may lie alongside or in front of the larynx and trachea.

The inferior deep (supraclavicular) cervical nodes drain the entire head and neck and are lateral and posterior to the internal jugular vein. These nodes receive afferents from the back of the neck and scalp, most of the superior deep cervical nodes, some of the lower tracheal nodes, and often some of the arm (axilla).

●●● ORBIT

The orbit is a four-sided pyramidal space with its apex located posteriorly at the optic foramen. Each cavity is essentially a socket for the eyeball and its associated structures. The seven bones that form the orbit are the frontal, zygomatic, sphenoid, palatine, ethmoid, lacrimal, and maxilla. There are no sharp divisions between most of the four walls. The medial walls of the two orbits are parallel to the midsagittal plane. However, the lateral walls make a 45-degree angle with the midsagittal plane and medial wall at the orbital apex. The apex of the orbit is at the optic foramen, which transmits the optic nerve and ophthalmic artery with postganglionic sympathetics.

The orbital margin, or aditus, is the external aperture of the orbit (Fig. 10-39). It is really quadrilateral in shape with rounded angles and has also been described as a "square circle." The zygomatic, maxillary, and frontal bones form the margin of the orbit (see Fig. 10-39A).

The margin is the strongest aspect of the orbit. The superior orbital margin is formed by the frontal bone. The lateral margin is the strongest border and is formed by the zygomatic bone and some of the frontal bone's zygomatic process. The inferior margin is formed by the zygomatic and maxillary bones, which articulate near the middle of this margin. The medial margin is formed mostly by the maxilla's frontal process with a contribution from the maxillary process of the frontal bone.

The orbital margin is not the greatest diameter of the orbit. The greatest orbital diameter is located just inside the orbital margin. The following openings are associated with the margin: the supraorbital notch or foramen, the zygomaticofacial foramina on the facial surface of the zygomatic bone, and the infraorbital foramen below the margin in the maxilla. These openings allow several neurovascular bundles to reach the face. The supraorbital notch often has a foramen leading to the frontal paranasal sinus. However, several other neurovascular bundles leave the orbit to reach the face by passing across the orbital margin.

The superior boarders, or roof, of the orbit is slightly concave and separates the orbit from the anterior cranial fossa (see Fig. 10-39B and Table 10-18). The orbital plate of the frontal bone and the lesser wing of sphenoid bone form the orbital roof. The anteromedial aspect of the orbital plate contains part of the frontal sinus.

The roof has two important landmarks: the fossa for the lacrimal gland located anterolaterally and the trochlear spine for the trochlea (pulley) of the superior oblique muscle located anteromedially. The trochlea is located medial to the supraorbital notch, slightly posterior to the margin (see Fig. 10-39A).

The optic foramen is located between the lesser wing and body of the sphenoid bone. The lesser wing is connected to the body by means of two roots or spicules of bone. The inferior spicule (orbital strut) is more prominent and separates the optic foramen from the superior orbital fissure.

The floor of the orbit is smaller than the roof (see Fig. 10-39). It comprises the orbital surface of the maxilla, the orbital surface of the zygomatic bone, and the orbital process of the palatine bone. Landmarks include the infraorbital groove, which leads to the infraorbital canal for the infraorbital neurovascular bundle, which passes anteriorly through the infraorbital canal and foramen onto the face. The floor separates the orbit from the maxillary sinus. It is one of the thinnest of the orbital walls. It is prone to blow-out fractures produced by a rapid elevation in pressure caused by a blow to the anterior orbit.

The lateral wall of the orbit consists of the greater wing of the sphenoid bone, the orbital surface of the zygomatic bone, and to a varying degree the zygomatic process of the frontal bone (see Fig. 10-39B). It is the strongest (thickest) wall of the orbit and separates the orbit from both the temporal region and middle cranial fossa. Important landmarks include the orbital tubercle of the zygomatic bone and the spine of the greater wing.

The orbital tubercle of the zygomatic bone (Whitnall's tubercle) is just internal to the orbital margin on the zygomatic bone and inferior to the zygomaticofrontal suture (see Fig. 10-39A). It is an important anatomic anchor for many connective tissue structures.

Posteriorly, the spine for the lateral rectus muscle is located on the greater wing approximately halfway along the border of the superior orbital fissure (see Fig. 10-39B). This spine serves as the lateral attachment point for the common tendinous ring (anulus of Zinn) and the lateral rectus muscle.

Posteriorly, the superior orbital fissure is found between the lateral wall and the roof of the orbit. This gap is between the lesser and greater wings of the sphenoid bone, and is widest at its medial side (see Fig. 10-39A). The superior orbital fissure communicates with the middle cranial fossa and transmits CN III, IV, the ophthalmic division of V and VI, and the superior ophthalmic vein. This vein drains into the cavernous sinus. Filaments from the cavernous plexus, consisting of the postganglionic sympathetic fibers of the internal carotid plexus as well as the ophthalmic branch of the middle meningeal artery, also pass through the superior orbital fissure.

Anteriorly, the zygomatico-orbital foramen is found in the orbital surface of the zygomatic bone (see Fig. 10-39B). This foramen leads to the zygomaticofacial foramina on the anterior surface of the zygomatic bone. The zygomaticotemporal foramen is located on the posterior (temporal) surface of the zygomatic bone. These openings transmit neurovascular bundles.

The inferior orbital fissure is located between the greater wing of the sphenoid bone (above), the orbital process of the palatine bone, plus the orbital surface of the maxilla (below) (see Fig. 10-39A). This fissure allows the orbit to

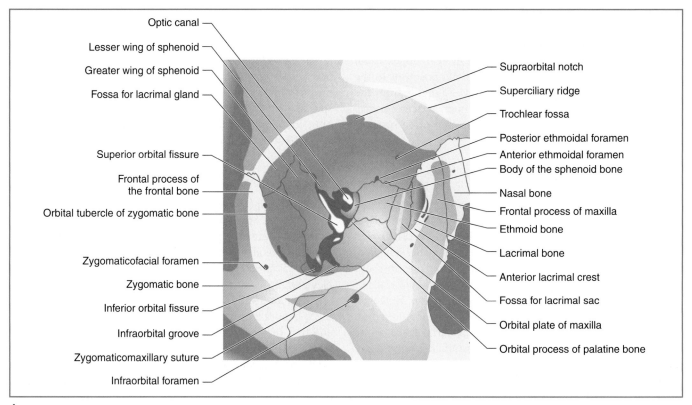

A

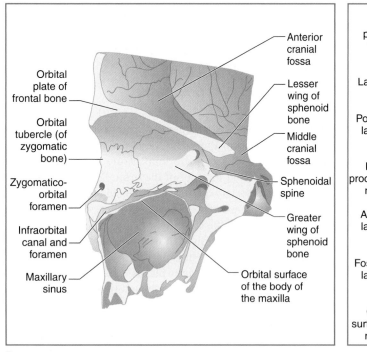

B

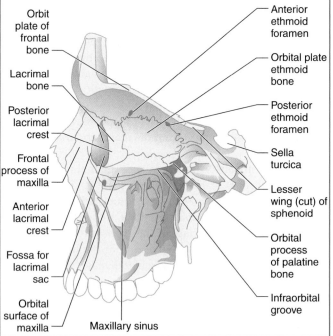

C

Figure 10-39. A, Bony orbit. **B,** Lateral orbital wall. **C,** Medial wall of the orbit.

TABLE 10-18. Important Landmarks Associated with the Bony Orbit

Orbital Wall	Structure
Superior (roof)	Trochlear spine, fossa for lacrimal gland
Lateral	Lateral spine of great wing, orbital tubercle of zygomatic bone, zygomatico-orbital foramen
Inferior (floor)	Infraorbital groove and canal, nasolacrimal canal
Medial	Anterior and posterior ethmoidal foramina, anterior and posterior lacrimal crests, fossa for lacrimal sac

communicate with both the pterygopalatine fossa and the infratemporal fossa. It transmits neurovascular bundles, which are branches of the maxillary artery and nerve (i.e., the infraorbital neurovascular bundle and the zygomatic nerve). It also transmits communicating branches of the pterygoid plexus of veins, which communicate with the inferior ophthalmic vein and infraorbital vein. It also transmits the postganglionic parasympathetic fibers from the pterygopalatine ganglion, which run with the zygomatic nerve.

The orbit's medial wall consists of the frontal process of the maxilla, the lacrimal bone, the orbital plate (lamina papyracea) of the ethmoid bone, and the body of the sphenoid bone (see Fig. 10-39C). It is vertical and separates the orbit from the nasal cavity and some of the paranasal sinuses. The anterior and posterior ethmoidal foramina are located in the suture between ethmoid and frontal bones. They transmit the anterior and posterior ethmoidal vessels and nerves through the ethmoidal canals into the anterior cranial fossa. The orbital plate of the ethmoid bone is very thin. It separates the orbit from the ethmoidal cells.

These neurovascular bundles supply the ethmoidal cells and frontal and sphenoid paranasal sinuses as well as having meningeal branches in the anterior cranial fossa. The anterior ethmoidal neurovascular bundle also supplies the anterior third of the nasal cavity by means of the internal nasal nerves and most of the dorsal surface of the nose by means of the external nasal nerve.

Two important landmarks on the medial wall are the anterior lacrimal crest on the frontal process of the maxillary bone and the posterior lacrimal crest of the lacrimal bone. These crests of bone help define the fossa for the lacrimal sac and also serve as important attachment points for connective tissue structures.

The medial palpebral ligament inserts on the anterior lacrimal crest. The following structures are attached to the posterior lacrimal crest: a small part of the medial palpebral ligament, the medial check ligament, the medial end of the suspensory ligament, the medial cornu of the levator palpebrae muscle, and the lacrimal portion of the orbicularis oculi (Fig. 10-40).

The fossa for the lacrimal sac is a depression between the lacrimal bone's posterior lacrimal crest and the frontal process of the maxilla (i.e., between anterior and posterior lacrimal crests) (see Fig. 10-39C). This fossa communicates with the inferior meatus of the nose by means of the nasolacrimal canal, which is formed by the articulation of the lacrimal bone, the frontal process of the maxilla, and the inferior conchae.

Orbital Fascia

The orbital fascia helps organize the orbit and support the eye.

The periorbita consists of the periosteum that is loosely associated with the bones of the orbit. It is continuous with the periosteum of the face anteriorly across the margin of the orbit. Posteriorly the periorbita is continuous with the endosteal layer of the cranial dura mater at the optic foramen (see Fig. 10-40).

The dura of the neurocranium enters the orbit through the optic foramen with the optic nerve and separates into its two components: an inner meningeal dural layer and an external endosteal (periosteal) layer. The inner layer of meningeal dura continues over the optic nerve as the external sheath of optic nerve and is attached to the outer two-thirds of the sclera. The internal sheath of the optic nerve consists of arachnoid and pia and continues around the optic nerve to the eyeball. Thus, the subarachnoid space filled with CSF is extended out in the orbit to the eyeball's optic disc. Changes in the CSF pressure in the region of the chiasmatic subarachnoid cistern will be transmitted to the optic disc and can produce a swelling of the disc called papilledema.

The additional derivatives of the periorbita are the orbital septum; a tendinous pulley; the trochlea, for the superior oblique muscle; and the common tendinous ring of extraocular muscles (anulus of Zinni).

The orbital septum is found on the posterior surface of the orbicularis oculi muscle in the eyelid (Fig. 10-41). It is attached to the orbital margin, where it is continuous with the periorbita. The orbital septum also attaches to the adjacent margins of the tarsal plates and acts as a facial barrier to the spread of infection. *Orbital fat will not invade the lids unless hernias develop in the septum.* Numerous structures normally penetrate this septum including branches of the ophthalmic nerve, artery, and veins.

The fascial sheath of the eyeball (Tenon's capsule) is the delicate fascia that surrounds the eyeball except for the cornea (Fig. 10-42). It firmly attaches to the sclera *just posterior to the true limbus.* The fascia of the eyeball forms a socket-like structure that helps suspend the eyeball. It is not continuous with the optic sheath but is a continuation of the muscular fascia. Anteriorly, the fascia of the eyeball blends with the bulbar conjunctiva and is firmly attached to the sclera posterior to the sclerocorneal junction. Tenon's capsule is not a socket for a true ball-and-socket joint. The eye moves slightly in Tenon's capsule, and then the capsule and the

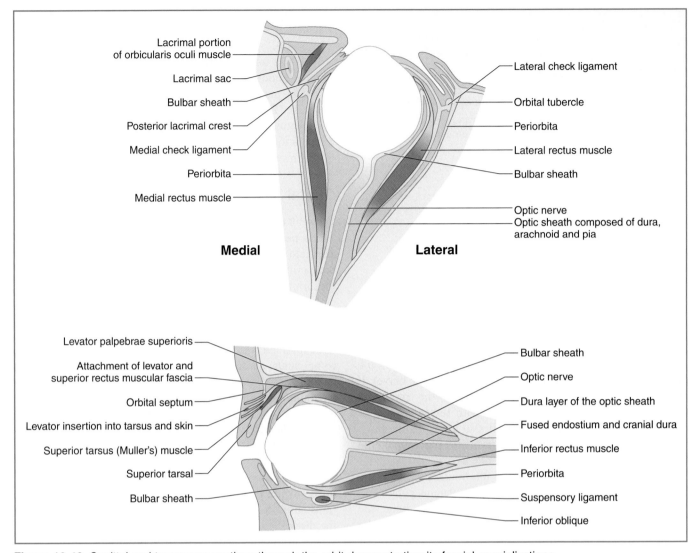

Figure 10-40. Sagittal and transverse sections through the orbit demonstrating its fascial specializations.

eye move together. This latter situation is due to the movement of both the muscular fascial connections to Tenon's capsule as well as the muscular insertions into the sclera.

Muscular fascia, or epimysium, surrounds each extraocular muscle. Muscular fascia is thickened near the eyeball. It has a tubular-like arrangement that expands to become continuous with the fascia of the eyeball.

In addition, there are strong extensions or expansions from the muscular fascia of the medial and lateral rectus muscles (see Fig. 10-40). These extensions are the medial and lateral check ligaments, which attach to the posterior lacrimal crest and the orbital tubercle, respectively. They help stabilize the position of Tenon's capsule and the eye, which is essential for normal binocular vision.

The fascia of the inferior rectus and inferior oblique muscles blends together to form the suspensory ligament (of Lockwood) (see Fig. 10-40), which is a continuous hammock below the eye that supports the eye. This has also been described as an

expansion of the fascia of the eyeball. The suspensory ligament narrows as it attaches medially to the posterior lacrimal crest and laterally to the orbital tubercle of the zygomatic bone. The following structures attach to the orbital tubercle: the lateral check ligament, suspensory ligament, lateral palpebral ligament, and lateral cornu of the levator palpebral muscle.

A well-developed fibromuscular system is found in the orbit. It consists of the extraocular muscles and the connective tissue attachments that pass from muscle to muscle or from muscle to bone. This arrangement produces a muscular cone with a central intraconal space occupied by the optic nerve and other important neurovascular structures. The fibromuscular system is well developed around the eye and close to the apex of the orbit. However, the fibromuscular system is incomplete posterior to the eye, allowing neurovascular bundles to either enter or leave the muscular cone. The vertical stability of the eye is dependent on the suspensory

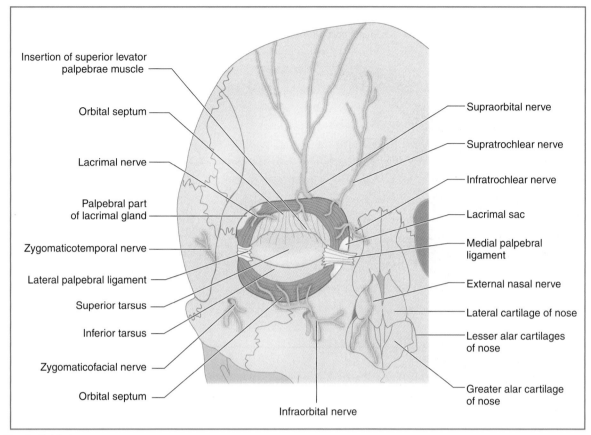

Insertion of superior levator palpebrae muscle

Orbital septum

Lacrimal nerve

Palpebral part of lacrimal gland

Zygomaticotemporal nerve

Lateral palpebral ligament

Superior tarsus

Inferior tarsus

Zygomaticofacial nerve

Orbital septum

Supraorbital nerve

Supratrochlear nerve

Infratrochlear nerve

Lacrimal sac

Medial palpebral ligament

External nasal nerve

Lateral cartilage of nose

Lesser alar cartilages of nose

Greater alar cartilage of nose

Infraorbital nerve

Figure 10-41. Orbital septum.

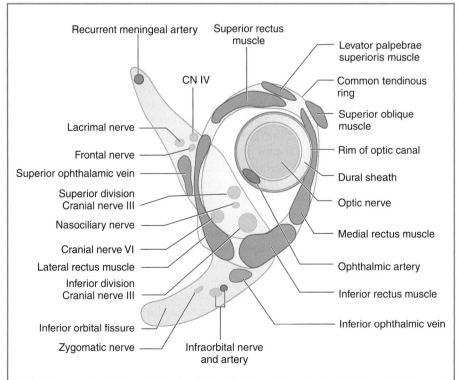

Recurrent meningeal artery

Superior rectus muscle

Levator palpebrae superioris muscle

Common tendinous ring

CN IV

Lacrimal nerve

Frontal nerve

Superior ophthalamic vein

Superior division Cranial nerve III

Nasociliary nerve

Cranial nerve VI

Lateral rectus muscle

Inferior division Cranial nerve III

Inferior orbital fissure

Zygomatic nerve

Infraorbital nerve and artery

Superior oblique muscle

Rim of optic canal

Dural sheath

Optic nerve

Medial rectus muscle

Ophthalmic artery

Inferior rectus muscle

Inferior ophthalmic vein

Figure 10-42. Passage of neurovascular structures into the orbit in relationship to the common tendinous ring.

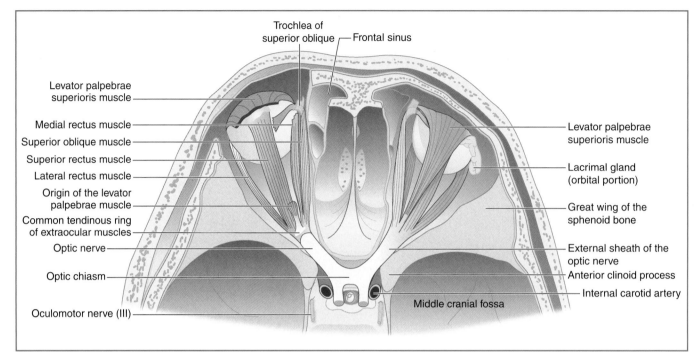

Figure 10-43. Levator palpebrae superioris.

ligament, while the anteroposterior stability of the eye is dependent on the check ligaments, the periorbital fat, and the pull of the oblique and rectus muscles.

The most likely wall to fracture is the inferior wall. Restriction of upward gaze is often a sequela of a blow-out fracture of the orbital floor. The inferior oblique or inferior rectus muscle is rarely trapped at the fracture. Restriction is usually due to capture of the orbital fibroadipose tissue herniating in the maxillary sinus or captured by the fracture.

Extraocular Muscles

There are seven voluntary muscles in the orbit. Six are attached to and move the eyeball while the seventh elevates the upper eyelid (Fig. 10-43). There are also smooth muscle fibers that cross the inferior orbital fissure and smooth muscle fibers in the eyelids.

The six skeletal muscles that attach to the eyeball are the four rectus ("straight") muscles and the two oblique muscles. The six muscles are arranged in pairs. Each muscle has a fascial sheath that contributes to the bulbar fascia (Tenon's capsule; see Fig. 10-40). Each muscle inserts into the sclera behind the cornea.

The four rectus muscles arise from a common origin that takes the form of the anulus that surrounds the optic foramen and the middle portion of the superior orbital fissure. It is derived from the periorbita and is the common tendinous ring of extraocular muscles, or anulus of Zinn (see Fig. 10-42). The four rectus muscles arising from the fibrous ring form a cone of muscles. The fibrous ring is actually oval in shape and is completed by tendinous bridges over the inferior and medial parts of the superior orbital fissure and attaches to the spine of the lateral rectus muscle and is on the greater wings of the sphenoid bone.

The common tendinous ring is composed of two tendons derived from the periorbita. The anulus surrounds the optic foramen and the middle part of superior orbital fissure. The two divisions of the oculomotor nerve—the nasociliary and the abducent nerves—enter the orbit through the interval of the superior orbital fissure enclosed by the anulus (see Fig. 10-42). The ophthalmic artery enters with the optic nerve through the optic foramen, also within the anulus. The lacrimal and frontal branches of the ophthalmic nerve and the trochlear nerve enter above the anulus while branches of the maxillary nerve enter the orbit through the inferior orbital fissure below the anulus.

The levator palpebrae superioris muscle arises from the inferior surface of the lesser wing of the sphenoid bone, above the superior rectus muscle. It has "multiple" insertions, none of which are *into the eye* (see Fig. 10-40). These insertions include the following:

- Fibers that run over the superior tarsus attach to the anterior aspect of the tarsal plate. Some of these fibers continue through the orbital septum and the palpebral portion of the orbicularis oculi to insert into the superficial fascia of the upper eyelid.
- The middle portion inserts into the superior surface of the superior tarsus. *This portion contains smooth muscle fibers, the superior tarsal or Müller's muscle.* The smooth muscle is responsible for the tone of the eyelid and is innervated by postganglionic sympathetic fibers.

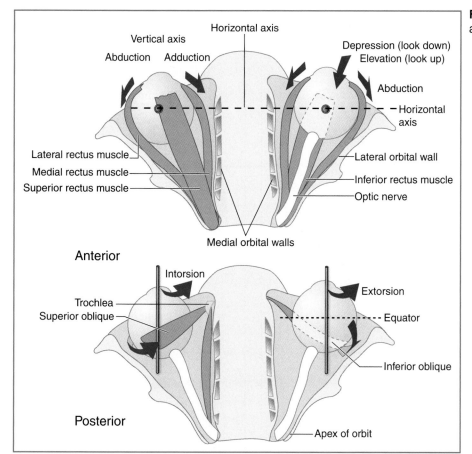

Figure 10-44. Rectus muscles and the axes of movement.

- Fibers that insert into the superior conjunctival fornix help elevate the conjunctiva during elevation of the upper lid.
- Fibers that expand medially and laterally form the cornua that insert into the anterior and posterior lacrimal crests medially and the orbital tubercle of Whitnall laterally.

The levator palpebrae superioris muscle elevates the upper lid and pulls the superior conjunctival fornix out of the way when the lid is retracted. The levator palpebrae superioris muscle is the antagonist to the palpebral portion of the orbicularis oculi muscle during blinking.

The functions of six of the extraocular muscles that act upon the eye are quite complex. Only the major functions will be considered here. Duction is rotational movement of the eye. The eye rotates in three planes: vertical, horizontal, and anteroposterior or sagittal (Fig. 10-44). When the cornea is directed medially (nasally), the eye rotates in its vertical axis and is adducted, and when the cornea is directed laterally (temporally), the eye is abducted (Fig. 10-45). When the cornea is directed upward it is elevated, and when the cornea is directed downward, it is depressed. The eye rotates in its horizontal axis to achieve elevation or depression (see Fig. 10-44). The eye can also rotate inward or outward upon its sagittal axis to achieve intorsion or extorsion (see Fig. 10-44).

The four rectus muscles arise from the anulus and insert on the sclera anterior to the equator of the eyeball close to the limbus of the cornea (see Figs. 10-44 and 10-45AB). The medial rectus muscle inserts closest to the limbus on the nasal (medial) side of the globe. It has the greatest mechanical advantage of all the rectus muscles to adduct the eye. The lateral rectus muscle abducts (laterally deviates) the eye. The insertion of the medial and lateral rectus muscles allows for horizontal motion, specifically, abduction or adduction about a vertical axis (see Fig. 10-45A).

The superior and inferior rectus muscles elevate and depress the eye when they rotate the eye in the horizontal axis. They adduct the eye in the vertical axis. In addition, they produce a rotation of the eye inward toward the nose or outward toward the temporal region. These actions are intorsion (superior rectus) or extorsion (inferior rectus), and this rotation revolves around an anteroposterior (sagittal) axis (see Fig. 10-45B).

Superior and Inferior Oblique Muscles

The oblique muscles insert into the sclera posterior to the equator; thus, they will elevate or depress the posterior aspect of the eye producing the opposite position for the cornea. Hence, the superior oblique will elevate the posterior aspect of the eye and therefore depress the cornea (see Figs. 10-44 and 10-45C).

The superior oblique muscle is the longest and most slender muscle. It is found at the superior and medial side of the orbit. It arises from the body of the sphenoid bone. It runs

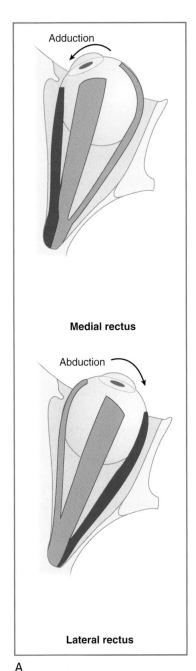

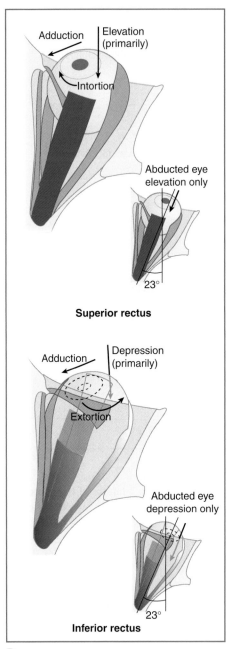

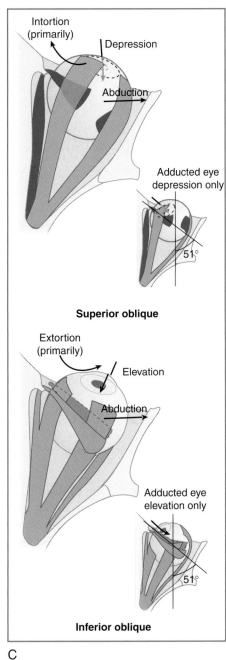

Figure 10-45. A, Movements of the medial and lateral rectus muscles. **B,** Movements of the superior and inferior rectus muscles. The superior rectus elevates the abducted eye. **C,** Movements of the eye produced by the oblique muscles. From the adducted position, the superior oblique depresses the eye and the inferior oblique elevates the eye.

forward just above the medial rectus muscle to form a rounded tendon that is surrounded by a synovial sheath as it passes through a fibrocartilaginous pulley (trochlea). This tendon then passes laterally and posteriorly, running beneath the superior rectus muscle to insert into *the superior lateral quadrant of the eye posterior to the equator.* This muscle depresses, intorts, and abducts the eye (see Fig. 10-45C).

The inferior oblique muscle is the shortest of the extraocular muscles. It arises anteriorly from the floor of the orbital surface of the maxilla just laterally to the fossa for the lacrimal sac and nasolacrimal canal. The muscle runs laterally between the inferior rectus tendon and the orbital floor and then between the eyeball and the lateral rectus muscle. It inserts into the lateral inferior quadrant of the sclera, posterior to

TABLE 10-19. Actions of Recti and Obliques Acting in Concert with Other Extraocular Muscles

Muscle	Action When Eye Is Abducted	Action in Primary Gaze	Action When Eye Is Adducted
Superior rectus	Elevation	Elevation Adduction Intorsion	Intorsion
Inferior rectus	Depression	Depression Adduction Extorsion	Extorsion
Superior oblique	Intorsion	Depression Abduction Intorsion	Depression
Inferior oblique	Extorsion	Elevation Abduction Extorsion	Elevation

the equator, between the superior and lateral rectus muscles. The inferior oblique muscle elevates, abducts, and extorts the eye (see Fig. 10-45C).

Muscle Action

Both the superior rectus and inferior oblique muscles elevate the eye, and the inferior rectus and superior oblique muscles depress the eye. The superior rectus and superior oblique muscles also intort the eye, whereas the inferior rectus and inferior oblique muscles extort the eye. The superior rectus elevates the eye, while the inferior rectus depresses the eye. The superior and inferior rectus muscles insert somewhat medial to the visual axis of the eye. Thus, the superior rectus muscle can also intort and adduct the eye, while the inferior rectus muscle can extort and adduct the eye (Table 10-19).

Innervation of the Orbit

The optic nerve (CN II) consists of the axons of the retina's ganglion cells. These cells receive impulses from the bipolar cells, which in turn receive impulses from the receptor cells, the rods and cones. The optic nerve takes a sinuous course that allows for unrestricted movements of the eye without damage to the nerve.

The oculomotor nerve contains GSE and GVE fibers. The oculomotor nerve passes between the superior cerebellar and posterior cerebral arteries, running anteriorly on the lateral side of the posterior communicating artery. This nerve enters the dura that forms the roof and then the lateral wall of the cavernous sinus. The oculomotor nerve is initially above the trochlear nerve. However, as they run anteriorly in the lateral wall of the cavernous sinus, the oculomotor nerve crosses the trochlear nerve medially (see Fig. 10-19B) so that the trochlear nerve is now superior to the oculomotor nerve. CN

III then passes through the superior orbital fissure in the annular ring and into the muscular cone. It separates into its two divisions prior to entering the orbit (Fig. 10-46). In the cavernous sinus, the oculomotor nerve has communications with the ophthalmic nerve, which receives GSA fibers for proprioception, and with the internal carotid plexus to receive postganglionic sympathetic fibers. In the orbit, the abducent nerve lies inferolateral to the divisions while the nasociliary lies between the divisions of CN III.

The divisions of the oculomotor nerve are as follows:
- The smaller superior division crosses the lateral aspect of the optic nerve to reach the superior rectus and levator palpebrae muscles (see Fig. 10-46). These are GSE fibers. However, postganglionic sympathetic fibers from the cavernous sinus plexus may run with this part of the oculomotor nerve to reach the superior tarsal (Müller's) muscle.
- The inferior division of CN III passes inferiorly and laterally to the optic nerve to supply the medial and inferior rectus muscles as well as the inferior oblique muscle. This division first lies on and then runs on the lateral side of the inferior rectus muscle to reach the posterior surface of the inferior oblique muscle (see Fig. 10-46).

A short, thick branch, the "motor root of the ciliary ganglion," arises from the inferior division of the oculomotor nerve. It reaches the posteroinferior aspect of the ciliary ganglion and synapses in the ciliary ganglion. This ganglion is located between the optic nerve and the lateral rectus muscle, approximately 1 cm from the apex of the orbit. The motor root of the ciliary ganglion contains preganglionic parasympathetic fibers that synapse in the ciliary ganglion (Fig. 10-47). The postganglionic parasympathetic fibers that leave the ciliary ganglion make up most of the short ciliary nerves and innervate the ciliaris and sphincter pupillae muscles.

The location of the preganglionic parasympathetic fibers in the oculomotor nerve is thought to change as CN III passes through the posterior and middle cranial fossae. Before the cavernous sinus, the parasympathetic fibers are superficially located at the periphery of the nerve. Here, they are the first fibers affected by compression. However, in the cavernous sinus and anterior to the sinus, the parasympathetic fibers are deeply placed as the GSE motor fibers are separated into superior and inferior divisions.

Other nerves enter but do not synapse in the ciliary ganglion. They *run through* this ganglion. These latter nerves include the sensory root of the ciliary ganglion from the nasociliary branch of ophthalmic nerve (see Fig. 10-47). The sensory root of the ciliary ganglion consists of sensory fibers (GSA) from the cornea, sclera, iris, and ciliary body. These sensory fibers also travel in the long ciliary branches of the nasociliary nerve, which do not traverse the ciliary ganglion but travel medial to the optic nerve to reach the eye.

The internal carotid nerve consists of postganglionic sympathetic fibers (see Fig. 10-37). The sympathetic fibers in the cavernous sinus are referred to as the cavernous plexus. Some of these fibers form a sympathetic root that *passes through*

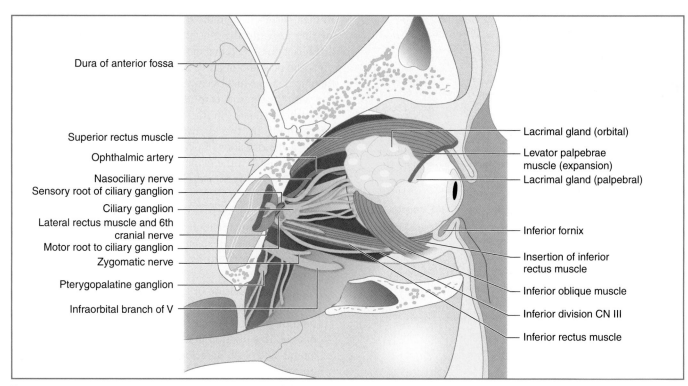

Figure 10-46. Distribution of the oculomotor nerve (CN III).

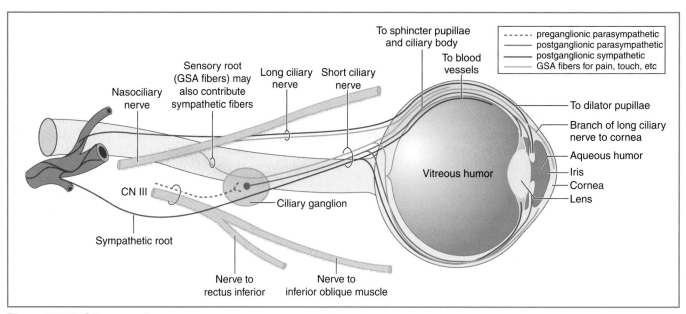

Figure 10-47. Ciliary ganglion.

the ciliary ganglion and the short ciliary nerves to reach the dilator pupillae muscle of the eye. Cavernous plexus postganglionic sympathetic fibers could also join the ophthalmic nerve and its nasociliary branch to travel with the long ciliary nerves to reach the eye (see Fig. 10-47).

The trochlear nerve (GSE fibers) supplies the superior oblique muscle. It runs inferior to the free margin of the tentorium cerebelli to pierce the dura and enter the lateral wall of the cavernous sinus. The trochlear nerve passes laterally to the oculomotor nerve as it runs superiorly to change positions

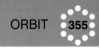

Horner Syndrome

Horner syndrome is due to the loss of sympathetic innervation to the head. This loss can be from a lesion in either the central or the peripheral nervous system (PNS). This discussion focuses on the loss of sympathetics in the PNS resulting from the loss of either preganglionic or postganglionic sympathetic fibers.

Symptoms due to the loss of the preganglionic sympathetic fibers that synapse in the superior cervical sympathetic ganglion are produced by loss of CNS control of this ganglion. The result is loss of function of all the effectors innervated by the postganglionic fibers from the superior cervical sympathetic ganglion.

The resulting symptoms include droopy eyelid (ptosis), constriction of the pupil (miosis), absence of sweating (anhydrosis), and flushing of the face (face feels hot).

These symptoms are due to a loss of the sympathetic innervation to several structures in the head. The loss of function of the superior tarsal muscle, which helps produce the tone in the eyelid, results in a slight ptosis. The loss of function of the dilator pupillae muscle, which dilates the pupil, allows the antagonist constrictor pupillae muscle, innervated by parasympathetic fibers, to constrict the pupil. The loss of function of the sympathetics, which regulate the sweat glands and blood vessels of the face, allow the face to become hot and dry. These symptoms result from loss of ability to constrict the facial blood vessels and loss of innervation to the sweat glands.

Partial Horner syndrome can be produced by disruption of the postganglionic sympathetic fibers that run with the internal carotid artery (the internal carotid nerve plexus). The patient would not have anhydrosis and flushing of the face, since the external carotid plexus is not involved.

with the CN III (see Fig. 10-19B). The trochlear nerve enters the orbit through the superior orbital fissure above the anulus and the other motor nerves. The trochlear nerve passes superiorly to the origin of the levator palpebrae muscle to enter the orbital surface of the superior oblique muscle (see Fig. 10-37).

The abducent nerve (GSE fibers) enters the dura after a long run in the subarachnoid space. Here, it is vulnerable to pressure changes in the CSF or to stretching due to brain displacement. In the cavernous sinus, the abducent nerve passes laterally to the internal carotid artery. Here, it is vulnerable to increased pressure resulting from an aneurysm of the internal carotid artery or a thrombosis lodged in the sinus. The abducent nerve innervates the lateral rectus muscle (Fig. 10-48).

The ophthalmic division of the trigeminal nerve (ophthalmia nerve) is the sensory nerve to the orbit and many surrounding regions. It carries only GSA fibers whose neuronal cell bodies are located in the trigeminal ganglion. The ophthalmic nerve divides into lacrimal, frontal, and nasociliary branches before passing through the superior orbital fissure (see Fig. 10-19B).

The lacrimal nerve enters the orbit through the narrowest part of the superior orbital fissure. It runs along the superior border of the lateral rectus muscle, close to the periorbita, to reach the lacrimal gland, the adjacent conjunctiva and the lateral aspect of the upper eyelid. It is sensory to the region near this gland and to the adjacent conjunctiva and the upper eyelid. The lacrimal branch communicates with the zygomaticotemporal branch of the maxillary nerve. Postganglionic parasympathetic fibers from the pterygopalatine ganglion to the lacrimal gland first communicate with the zygomatic nerve and then with the zygomaticotemporal nerve before forming a separate independent communicating nerve that joins the lacrimal nerve (of V_1). The lacrimal branch of the ophthalmic nerve carries only GSA fibers for cutaneous sensation from the lateral portion of the upper eyelid until it is joined by the communicating branch (see Fig. 10-48).

The frontal nerve enters the superior orbital fissure and then runs anteriorly between the levator palpebrae superioris muscle and the periorbita. The frontal nerve divides into the supratrochlear and supraorbital branches (see Fig. 10-48). The supratrochlear nerve turns medially above the pulley (trochlea) of superior oblique muscle. It pierces the orbital septum to supply the conjunctiva, skin of the superior eyelid (medial part), and lower and most medial part of the forehead with sensory fibers. The supraorbital nerve runs anteriorly on the superior surface of the levator palpebrae superioris muscle and then through the supraorbital foramen onto the forehead. It supplies the eyelid and skin of the forehead to the vertex. The supraorbital nerve also supplies the frontal sinus as it passes through the supraorbital foramen.

The nasociliary nerve is deeply placed in the orbit (Fig. 10-49; see also Fig. 10-48). It is the only branch of the ophthalmic nerve that enters the superior orbital fissure inside the anulus and muscular cone. The nasociliary nerve passes between the two divisions of the oculomotor nerve, laterally to the optic nerve. It crosses the optic nerve with the ophthalmic artery by passing between the optic nerve and the superior rectus muscle. Upon reaching the medial wall of the orbit, the nasociliary nerve runs anteriorly between the superior oblique and medial rectus muscles. It has long ciliary branches, a posterior ethmoidal branch, an infratrochlear branch, and ends as the anterior ethmoidal nerve (see Fig. 10-49).

The anterior ethmoid nerve passes through anterior ethmoidal foramen and canal to enter the anterior cranial fossa above the cribriform plate but below the meningeal dura. The anterior ethmoidal nerve supplies the dura with its anterior meningeal branches (GSA fibers). Its internal nasal branches pass through the nasal slit, found close to the cribriform plate at the base of the crista galli, to enter the nasal cavity as lateral and medial internal nasal nerves (see Fig. 10-49). The lateral internal nasal nerve has a branch that emerges between the nasal bone and lateral nasal cartilage as the external nasal branch to be sensory to the dorsal aspect of the nose. The anterior ethmoidal nerve supplies the ethmoidal air cells and part of the frontal air sinus. It also supplies the meninges and finally the mucous membranes of the anterior third of the nasal cavity as well as the nose.

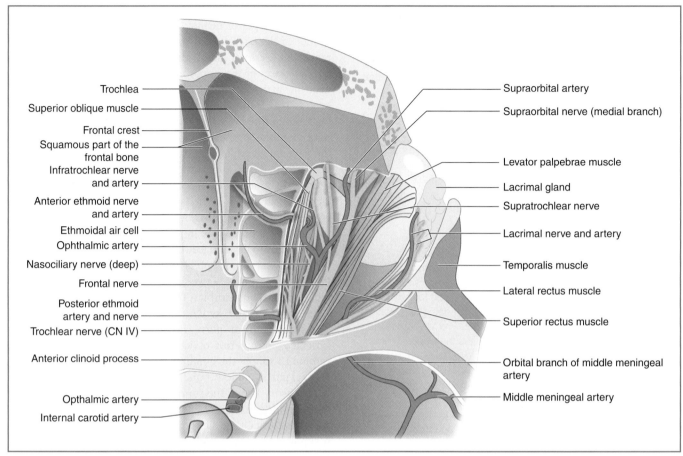

Figure 10-48. The orbit as seen from above.

The infratrochlear branch continues anteriorly to pass through the orbital septum. It supplies the medial aspect of both eyelids and base of the nose as well as the conjunctiva, lacrimal sac, and lacrimal caruncle.

The two or three long ciliary nerves are sensory branches of the nasociliary nerve that supply the iris, ciliary body, cornea, and sclera with GSA fibers. They pass medial to the optic nerve and ciliary ganglion to reach the eye and have no direct relationship to the ganglion (see Figs. 10-47 and 10-49). The sensory root of the ciliary ganglion has been described with the ciliary ganglion (see Fig. 10-47).

The posterior ethmoidal nerve runs through the posterior ethmoidal canal to supply the mucous membrane and periosteum of posterior ethmoidal air cells, the sphenoid sinus, and the meninges in the posterior part of the anterior cranial fossa.

The ophthalmic nerve receives GSA proprioceptive fibers from the oculomotor, trochlear, and abducent nerves in the cavernous sinus. Proprioception fibers from the extraocular muscle spindles and Golgi tendon apparatus are general somatic sensory fibers that initially ran with the motor nerves to these muscles. These GSA fibers join the ophthalmic nerve. Finally, the oculomotor and ophthalmic nerves receive postganglionic sympathetic fibers from the internal carotid plexus in the cavernous sinus.

Circulation

The ophthalmic artery arises from the internal carotid artery (Fig. 10-50). It enters the orbit inferior and lateral to the optic nerve as they both pass though the optic foramen. The ophthalmic artery then passes over the optic nerve, running from lateral to medial to reach the medial wall of the orbit. It takes the same course as the nasociliary nerve. The ophthalmic artery then runs forward, sandwiched between the medial rectus and superior oblique muscles. The artery runs along the inferior border of the superior oblique muscle to divide into its two terminal branches, the supratrochlear and dorsal nasal arteries. Although its course is similar to that of the nasociliary nerve, it is never referred to as the nasociliary artery.

The lacrimal artery arises close to the optic foramen. It leaves the muscular cone to travel with the lacrimal nerve along the superior border of the lateral rectus muscle to the lacrimal gland, conjunctiva, and eyelid. It gives rise to its terminal branches, the upper and lower lateral palpebral arteries. The lateral palpebral arteries cross the eyelid to anastomose with the medial palpebral arteries. These latter arteries are direct terminal branches of ophthalmic artery. The two superior arterial arches thus formed are found in the eyelid, one

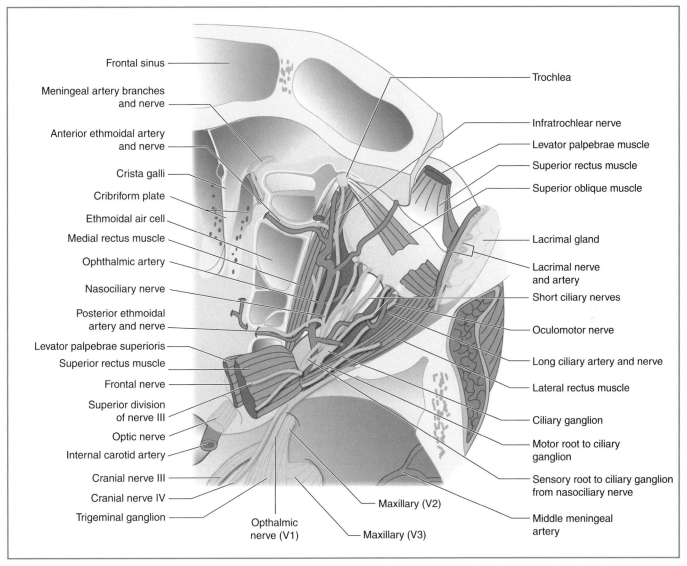

Figure 10-49. Deeper view of the nasociliary nerve and its many branches.

between the tarsal plate and orbicularis oculi muscle (the marginal arcade) and the other in the pretarsal space between the insertions of the levator palpebrae superioris muscle (peripheral arcade). There is only one inferior arcade for the inferior eyelid. Zygomatico-orbital, transverse facial, supraorbital, infraorbital, and angular arteries anastomose with branches of these arches. The lacrimal artery also gives rise to a zygomatic artery, which has zygomaticofacial and zygomaticotemporal branches. Finally, a recurrent branch of the lacrimal artery passes through the superior orbital fissure to anastomose with an orbital branch of the middle meningeal artery. In rare cases, it can replace the lacrimal artery, and it is one of the two embryonic possibilities for the development of the ophthalmic artery.

The supraorbital artery passes over the optic nerve, leaves the muscular cone usually on the medial side of the superior rectus muscle, and runs forward over the levator palpebrae superioris muscle with the frontal nerve. Both structures pass

through the supraorbital foramen to supply the skin, muscles, and pericranium of the forehead. It also supplies muscular branches to the superior rectus and levator palpebrae superioris muscle.

The posterior ethmoidal artery passes through the posterior ethmoidal foramen to supply the posterior ethmoidal air cells, posterior portion of the anterior cranial fossa (anterior meningeal branches), and the sphenoid air sinus.

The anterior ethmoidal artery passes through the anterior ethmoidal foramen and canal with the anterior ethmoidal branch of the nasociliary nerve. This artery supplies the anterior and middle ethmoidal air cells and a small portion of the frontal sinus. After entering the anterior cranial fossa, the anterior ethmoidal artery gives off anterior meningeal branches and then descends into the cribiform plate or its nasal cavity by passing through the cribiform plate or its nasal slit on the side of the crista galli. These nasal branches help supply the anterior third of the nasal cavity and external nose.

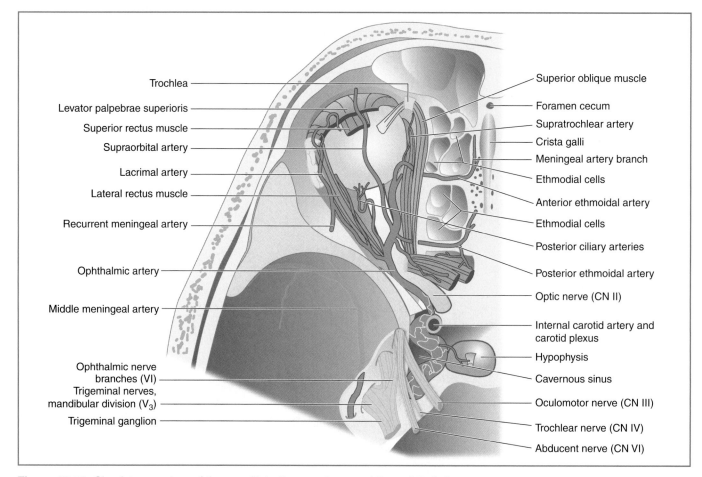

Figure 10-50. Circulatory system of the eye. Note the prominence of the ophthalmic artery.

The medial palpebral arteries help form the vascular arches of the eyelids. They anastomose with the lateral palpebral arteries, which are branches of the lacrimal artery.

The supratrochlear and the dorsal nasal arteries are the two terminal branches of the ophthalmic artery that leave the orbit at its medial angle. The supratrochlear artery leaves the orbit below the trochlea but then runs superiorly to join the supratrochlear nerve.

The dorsal nasal artery is the other terminal branch. It emerges above the medial palpebral ligament and anastomoses with the angular artery.

Branches of Ophthalmic Artery

The central artery of the retina is the first and one of the smallest branches of the ophthalmic artery. It runs for a short distance inferiorly to the sheath of the optic nerve. It then pierces the nerve to run forward in the center of the optic nerve and enters the retina at the optic disc. The central artery has small branches that supply the pia of the internal sheath and the optic nerve itself. The central artery of the retina bifurcates and terminates as the superior and inferior

nasal and temporal arteries. These latter arteries run between the hyaloid membrane and the neuroretina and soon enter the nervous layer deep to its internal limiting membrane. Terminal capillary plexus extends until the inner nuclear layer. Thus, branches of the central artery do not reach the outer layers of the retina; namely, rods, cones, and pigmented epithelium.

Ciliary arteries include two to three long and many short posterior ciliary arteries, whereas the anterior ciliary arteries arise from muscular arteries.

Short posterior ciliary arteries are 6 to 12 in number. They surround the optic nerve to pierce the sclera just peripherally to the lamina cribrosa of the eye. The short posterior ciliary arteries supply the choroid and the external portion of the retina (i.e., pigmented epithelium, rods, and cones). In addition, the short posterior ciliary arteries form a possible arterial anastomosis around the optic nerve disc called the circle of Zinn or Zinn-Haller. This arterial circle consists of branches of the short posterior ciliary arteries that supply the dura of the external sheath and adjacent sclera. These branches anastomose with each other. They are located in the sclera and help nourish the lamina cribrosa, sclera, and optic nerve disc. The circle of Zinn is the only potential anastomosis between branches of the central artery of the retina and the short ciliary arteries. This cilioretinal anastomosis is found in about 10% to 20% of the population. It can be important in occlusion of the central artery, since it can actually preserve some of or all of a patient's vision.

The long posterior ciliary arteries are usually two in number. They pierce the sclera medially and laterally to the short ciliary arteries and nerves. The long posterior ciliary arteries run anteriorly in the perichordal space to reach the ciliary body, where they help form the major arterial circle of the iris. Branches of the major arterial circle of the iris enter the iris and anastomose to produce a minor arterial circle close to the pupil. The long posterior ciliary arteries help supply the anterior aspect of the choroid, ciliary body, and iris.

The anterior ciliary arteries are branches of the muscular arteries that supply the four rectus muscles. Usually two anterior ciliary arteries branch from each muscular artery except for the artery to the lateral rectus muscle, which has only one anterior ciliary branch. The anterior ciliary arteries penetrate the sclera just posteriorly to the muscle insertion to help form the major arterial circle of the iris by anastomosing with the long posterior ciliary arteries.

Ophthalmic Veins

For the most part, the veins of the orbit follow the branches of the ophthalmic artery. The superior ophthalmic vein is joined by the anastomosis of the supraorbital vein with a branch of the facial vein (nasofrontal vein). This large vein passes posteriorly in the orbit and receives its tributaries including the central vein of the retina and the superior vorticose veins. It passes through the superior orbital fissure above the anulus to empty into the cavernous sinus. The central vein may also send a branch that directly empties into the cavernous sinus.

The inferior ophthalmic vein is smaller than the superior. It is formed by a plexus that lies anteriorly on the orbital floor. As it passes posteriorly, it receives tributaries from the eyelid, lacrimal sac, and vorticose veins. The inferior ophthalmic vein sends a communicating branch through the inferior orbital fissure to anastomose with the pterygoid plexus of veins and the infraorbital vein that drains into the pterygoid plexus of veins. The inferior ophthalmic vein then usually joins the superior ophthalmic vein but can pass independently through the superior orbital fissure to empty into the cavernous sinus.

●●● TEMPORAL, INFRATEMPORAL, AND PAROTID REGIONS

Temporal Fossa

The temporal fossa is located on the lateral side of the head (see Fig. 10-1C). The superior temporal line is its anterior, superior, and posterior boundaries (see Fig. 10-1C). It marks the attachment site of the deep temporal fascia. The medial wall of the temporal region consists of the squamous portion of the frontal bone, the temporal surface of the greater wing of the sphenoid bone, the parietal bone, and the squamous portion of the temporal bone. The inferior temporal line follows the superior temporal line and denotes the peripheral origin of the temporalis muscle.

The infratemporal crest found on the greater wing of the sphenoid bone is the anatomic marker that separates the temporal from the infratemporal region (Fig. 10-51). The zygomatic arch is found just lateral to the infratemporal crest and approximates this separation. The zygomatic arch (see Fig. 10-51) is formed by the zygomatic process of the temporal bone, the zygomatic bone, and the zygomatic process of the maxilla. The space between the infratemporal crest and the zygomatic

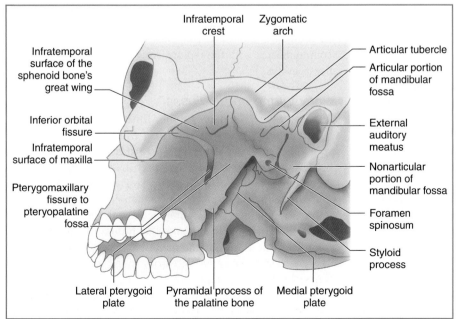

Labels on figure:
- Infratemporal crest
- Zygomatic arch
- Infratemporal surface of the sphenoid bone's great wing
- Inferior orbital fissure
- Infratemporal surface of maxilla
- Pterygomaxillary fissure to pteryopalatine fossa
- Articular tubercle
- Articular portion of mandibular fossa
- External auditory meatus
- Nonarticular portion of mandibular fossa
- Foramen spinosum
- Styloid process
- Lateral pterygoid plate
- Pyramidal process of the palatine bone
- Medial pterygoid plate

Figure 10-51. Lateral inferior view of temporal and infratemporal fossae with disarticulated mandible.

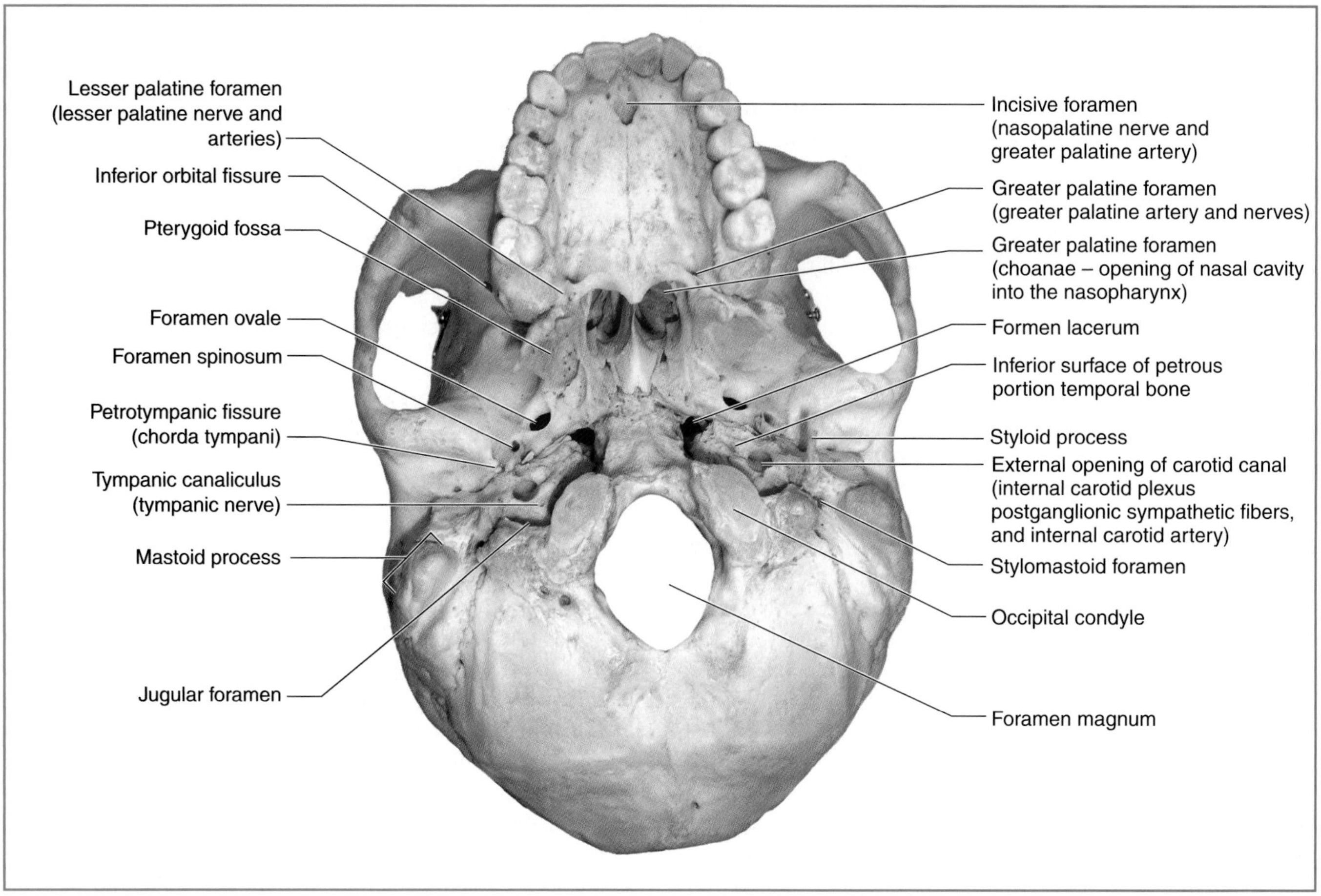

Lesser palatine foramen (lesser palatine nerve and arteries)
Inferior orbital fissure
Pterygoid fossa
Foramen ovale
Foramen spinosum
Petrotympanic fissure (chorda tympani)
Tympanic canaliculus (tympanic nerve)
Mastoid process
Jugular foramen
Incisive foramen (nasopalatine nerve and greater palatine artery)
Greater palatine foramen (greater palatine artery and nerves)
Greater palatine foramen (choanae – opening of nasal cavity into the nasopharynx)
Formen lacerum
Inferior surface of petrous portion temporal bone
Styloid process
External opening of carotid canal (internal carotid plexus postganglionic sympathetic fibers, and internal carotid artery)
Stylomastoid foramen
Occipital condyle
Foramen magnum

Figure 10-52. Base of the skull.

arch allows the temporalis muscle to pass into the infratemporal regions (see Fig. 10-51).

The temporalis muscle occupies the temporal fossa. It is covered by the deep temporal fascia, which attaches to the superior temporal line and becomes continuous with the pericranium. This fascia is a very strong outer investing layer of deep fascia that divides to attach to both internal and external surfaces of the zygomatic arch. The zygomatico-orbital branch of the superficial temporal artery often passes to the orbital region by running above the zygomatic arch.

The major neurovascular structures found in the temporal region are the superficial temporal artery and vein and the auriculotemporal branch of V_3. This artery is a terminal branch of the external carotid artery, which arises in the retromandibular region. The superficial temporal artery penetrates the outer investing layer of deep fascia inferior to the zygomatic arch to lie in the plane of the superficial fascia. This very unusual location for a major artery allows a physician to take an arterial pulse just superior to the zygomatic arch.

Infratemporal Fossa

The infratemporal fossa is located on the lateral aspect of the skull (see Fig. 10-51). Its superior boundary is the inferior surface of the greater wing of the sphenoid bone and squamous portion of the temporal bone, its medial boundary is the lateral plate of the pterygoid plate, its lateral boundary is the posterior margin of the neck and ramus of the mandible, and its inferior margin is closed by the insertion of the medial pterygoid muscle (Fig. 10-52). The infratemporal fossa contains several of the masticatory (chewing) muscles, the maxillary artery, pterygoid plexus of veins, mandibular nerve (V_3) and its branches, and small branches of CNs V_2, VII, and IX. It communicates with the regions surrounding it through many passageways.

Bony Infratemporal Fossa

The superior boundary of this fossa is composed of the *infratemporal (inferior) surface of the greater wing of the sphenoid bone*, while the *inferior surface of the squamous portion of the temporal bone* contributes to the temporomandibular joint (Fig. 10-53; see also Figs. 10-51 and 10-52). The infratemporal surface of the sphenoid bone contains two important openings that communicate with the middle cranial fossa: the foramen ovale and the foramen spinosum. The foramen ovale transmits the mandibular nerve (V_3), an emissary vein, sometimes an accessory meningeal artery, sometimes the lesser petrosal branch of IX. The lesser petrosal branch of IX typically enters the infratemporal fossa through the suture between the greater wing of the sphenoid bone

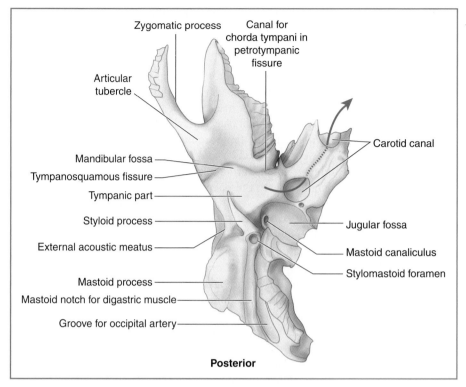

Figure 10-53. Inferior view of right temporal bone for chorda tympani.

and the petrous portion of the temporal bone. The foramen spinosum transmits the middle meningeal artery and the recurrent meningeal branch of V_3 (see Figs. 10-52 and 10-53). The spine of the sphenoid bone is located just posterior to the foramen spinosum and is the superior attachment of the sphenomandibular ligament (see Fig. 10-52).

The mandibular fossa of the temporal bone and articular tubercle of the temporal bone are the superior aspect of the temporomandibular joint (Figs. 10-54 and 10-55). The tympanosquamous fissure, which separates the mandibular fossa into a smooth articular portion and a rough nonarticular portion, extends medially to meet the petrotympanic fissure (see Fig. 10-53). As indicated by its name, this latter fissure is located between the tympanic and petrous portions of the temporal bone. The petrotympanic fissure has a small opening for the communication between the middle ear and infratemporal region, which transmits the *chorda tympani* of the facial nerve.

The lateral pterygoid plate of the sphenoid bone and the pyramidal process of the palatine bone mark the medial wall of the infratemporal fossa. The sphenoid bone's pterygoid process consists of *lateral and medial plates*. The lateral and medial plates are fused anteriorly but separated posteriorly (see Fig. 10-52). The pterygoid process projects inferiorly from the junction of the sphenoid bone's greater wing and its body.

The anterior wall of the infratemporal fossa is formed by the *posterior (infratemporal) surface of the maxilla* (see Figs. 10-51 and 10-52). The pterygomaxillary fissure is formed by the angle between the maxilla and the lateral pterygoid process. It transmits structures between the infratemporal fossa and the deeper-lying pterygopalatine fossa, including the maxillary artery, for further distribution to the posterior

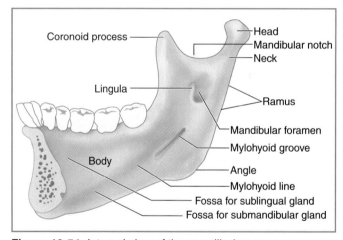

Figure 10-54. Internal view of the mandibular ramus.

nasal cavity and palate. The pterygomaxillary fissure also transmits the lateral division of the maxillary nerve (infraorbital and zygomatic nerves) into the infratemporal fossa from the pterygopalatine fossa.

The inferior orbital fissure is found anterosuperiorly between the infratemporal surface of the maxilla and the orbital process of the palatine bone located inferiorly and the greater wing of the sphenoid bone located superiorly (see Figs. 10-51 and 10-52). It transmits the infraorbital neurovascular bundle and the zygomatic nerve, along with a communicating branch from the pterygoid plexus of veins from the infratemporal region into the orbit.

The ramus of the mandible is the lateral boundary of the infratemporal fossa. Significant landmarks on the medial surface of the mandibular ramus are the mandibular foramen; the

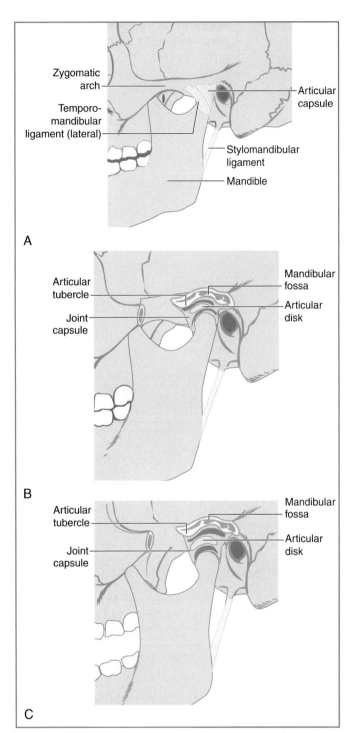

Figure 10-55. Lateral view of temporomandibular joint. **A,** Temporomandibular ligaments and joint at rest. **B,** An elevated jaw. **C,** A depressed jaw after both gliding and hinging.

adjacent lingula, which serves as the inferior attachment of the sphenomandibular ligament; and the mylohyoid groove (see Fig. 10-54). The mandibular foramen is the entrance to the mandibular canal, which extends to the mental symphysis. The mandibular canal opens onto the chin by means of the mental foramen, which is a passageway for the mental neurovascular branches of the inferior alveolar neurovascular bundle.

The mylohyoid groove on the internal surface of the mandible carries the mylohyoid neurovascular bundle to the digastric triangle, and the mylohyoid line marks the origin of the mylohyoid muscle.

Projecting superiorly from the ramus of the mandible are two bony structures (see Fig. 10-54). Anteriorly, the coronoid process marks the insertion for the temporalis muscle; posteriorly, the mandibular condyle, or head, forms the inferior portion of the temporomandibular joint (see Fig. 10-51). Between the condyle and the coronoid process lies the mandibular notch, through which the masseteric neurovascular bundle runs to the deep face and masseter muscle.

Temporomandibular Joint

The temporomandibular (TM) joint is formed by the superiorly located mandibular fossa and articular tubercle of the temporal bone and the inferiorly located mandibular condyle. The mandibular condyle is ellipsoid in shape. It is separated from the mandibular fossa and articular tubercle of the temporal bone by an articular disk.

The TM joint is stabilized in part by a connective tissue articular capsule that is reinforced anterolaterally by the lateral (TM) ligament (see Fig. 10-55). Other important ligaments influencing function are the sphenomandibular ligament from the sphenoid spine to the mandibular lingula and the stylomandibular ligament.

The articular capsule is rather loosely attached superiorly to the tympanosquamous fissure and the margins of the mandibular fossa and the articular tubercle. However, it is firmly attached inferiorly to the neck of the mandible. The upper fibers of the lateral pterygoid muscle insert into the articular capsule and articular disk.

The articular disk is primarily dense fibrous connective tissue with some fibrocartilage that divides the TM joint into two cavities: superior and inferior (see Fig. 10-55). The disk is thicker between the condyle and mandibular fossa, but it thins as it contacts the posterior slope of the articular tubercle. The superior surface of the articular disk conforms to the morphology of the mandibular fossa and articular tubercle. Thus, its superior surface is convex posteriorly and concave anteriorly. Inferiorly, the articular disk has a concave surface to conform to the condyle. The articular disk follows the mandibular condyle during gliding movements because it is loosely attached to the superior portion of the capsule but firmly attached to the condyle.

Actions of the Temporomandibular Joint

The TM joint makes both hinge and gliding movements (see Fig. 10-55). Movement of the jaw, such as for chewing and speech, is due to a gliding motion that occurs in the superior TM joint cavity. The axis of the gliding motion passes transversely through both mandibular lingulae and their attached sphenomandibular ligaments. This transverse axis allows for considerable movement without applying tension to the inferior alveolar neurovascular bundle that enters the mandibular foramen. The *hinging movement is maximized after gliding has occurred.*

CLINICAL MEDICINE

Spontaneous Dislocation of the TM Joint

Laxity of the articular capsule and lateral ligament along with any activity that results in maximal opening of the mouth may allow the condyle to dislocate anteriorly to the articular tubercle. Reduction of the jaw requires depressing the mandible sufficiently to allow the mandibular head to pass under the articular tubercle. Owing to the strength of the masticatory muscles, spasm of the muscles usually requires the use of muscle relaxants.

Protrusion is a forward gliding movement, which is produced by the mandibular head and articular disk sliding motion. The mandibular head and disk move as a unit out of the fossa down onto the articular tubercle. This action occurs between the superior surface of the articular disk and the temporal bone. The condyle and disk are pulled forward together by the lateral pterygoid with the aid of the medial pterygoid and masseter muscles, producing protrusion of the jaw.

Retraction is the return of the condyle from the articular tubercle to the mandibular fossa. Elevation is the movement of the mandible in closing of the mouth, and depression of the mandible is opening of the mouth. A side-to-side movement produces grinding of the articular surfaces of the teeth.

Musculature

The four major masticatory muscles are all derived from the first pharyngeal arch. The infratemporal fossa contains most of the medial and the lateral pterygoid muscles. The temporalis arises superiorly in the temporal region and inserts into the coronoid process in the infratemporal region. The masseter is located *laterally* to the mandibular ramus and is therefore completely outside the infratemporal fossa, being located in the deep face. Other muscles involved in opening of the mouth are the digastric, mylohyoid, and geniohyoid muscles.

The roughly rectangular masseter aids in elevating and protruding the jaw and making a small, side-to-side movement (Fig. 10-56 and Tables 10-19 to 10-21). The masseter is supplied by the masseter's branch of V_3 and a branch of the maxillary artery. This neurovascular bundle passes from the infratemporal fossa to the deep surface of the masseter through the mandibular notch.

The fan-shaped, broad origin of the temporalis leads to a progressively narrower anteroinferior tendon that passes deep to the zygomatic arch, enters the infratemporal fossa, and inserts on the coronoid process and anterior border of the ramus of the mandible. The temporalis closes (elevates) and retracts the jaw and maintains the position of rest. The deep temporal branches of both mandibular nerve and maxillary artery pass over the infratemporal crest deep to the temporal muscle.

The two heads of the lateral pterygoid muscle pull the mandibular condyle and articular disk down and forward. It

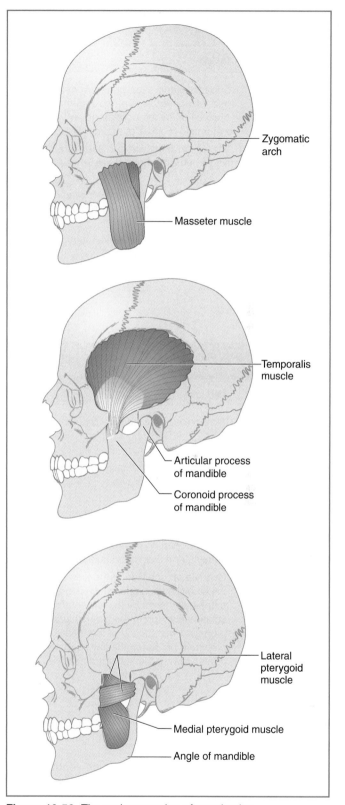

Figure 10-56. The major muscles of mastication.

is the only one of these four major chewing muscles that acts to depress (open) the jaw (Fig. 10-57). The lateral pterygoid can help produce lateral deviation (side-to-side movement) aided by the medial pterygoid and the contralateral temporalis

TABLE 10-20. Major Muscles of Mastication

Muscle	Origin	Insertion	Action
Masseter	Superficial and deep origins from lateral and inferior surfaces of the zygomatic process of the temporal bone and zygomatic process of the maxilla	Lateral surface of the ramus and angle of the mandible	Elevation and protrusion of the jaw and a small side-to-side (grinding) movement
Temporalis	Inferior temporal line and deep temporal fascia of the temporal fossa	Coronoid process and anterior border of the ramus of the mandible	Elevation and retraction of the jaw and maintenance of the position of rest
Lateral pterygoid	Infratemporal surface greater wing of the sphenoid and lateral surface of the lateral pterygoid plate	Neck of the mandible and the articular disk and capsule of the temporomandibular joint	Depression and protrusion of the jaw and lateral deviation (side-to-side movement)
Medial pterygoid	Medial surface of the lateral pterygoid plate, tuberosity of maxilla	Medial surface of the mandibular ramus and angle	Elevation, protrusion, and grinding movements of the jaw

TABLE 10-21. Masticatory Actions of the Mandible

Action	Muscles
Elevation (closing the mouth)	Temporalis, masseter, medial pterygoid
Depression (opening the mouth)	Lateral pterygoid, digastric, mylohyoid, and geniohyoid (and gravity)
Protrusion	Lateral pterygoid, medial pterygoid, masseter
Retraction	Posterior portion of temporalis (pulling condyle and disk into mandibular fossa)
Lateral deviation (grinding motion due mostly to gliding with little hinging)	Condyle on one side of the jaw deviates to the stabilized condyle, which is held in the mandibular fossa by the temporalis with considerable force; the contralateral lateral pterygoid with the aid of the medial pterygoid protrudes the jaw so that the jaw rotates toward the stabilized condyle

Innervation

The mandibular nerve (V_3) is the only trigeminal division containing both general somatic afferent (GSA) and special visceral efferent (SVE) fibers (Fig. 10-58). The mandibular nerve's main trunk enters the infratemporal region through the foramen ovale deep to the lateral pterygoid muscle (Fig. 10-59; see also Fig. 10-57). Before it divides into anterior and posterior divisions, the mandibular nerve's *main trunk* supplies the medial pterygoid, tensor tympani, and tensor veli palatini muscles. The recurrent meningeal branch is a small branch of the main trunk that reenters the middle cranial fossa through the foramen spinosum with the middle meningeal artery to help supply the dura mater of the middle cranial fossa with GSA fibers.

The smaller anterior division supplies the lateral pterygoid, masseter, and temporalis muscles (see Figs. 10-57 and 10-58) with innervation containing SVE and proprioceptive GSA fibers. The anterior division also has a buccal nerve (long buccal nerve) that runs between the two heads of the lateral pterygoid muscle and then anteriorly between the mandibular ramus and buccinator muscle onto the face. This buccal nerve carries cutaneous sensation from the cheek. It also has numerous branches that pierce the buccinator to supply sensation from the lateral (buccal) surface of the oral cavity. *The buccinator muscle is supplied with SVE fibers by the buccal branches of the facial nerve, since it is derived from the second pharyngeal arch.*

The larger posterior division of V_3 is mainly sensory, but it also has motor fibers. The lingual nerve runs anteroinferiorly on the surface of the medial pterygoid muscle and passes inferiorly to the superior pharyngeal constrictor muscle, to the floor of the mouth (Fig. 10-59; see also Fig. 10-58). This nerve carries GSA fibers from the anterior two thirds of the tongue and adjacent gums (Fig. 10-60).

The inferior alveolar nerve also passes along the lateral surface of the medial pterygoid muscle just posterior to the

muscles, which act as a stabilizer. Alternating contraction of these muscles produces a grinding motion (see Fig. 10-56). The strong grinding movements, which are necessary to macerate food, can be accomplished only when one condyle is stable so that the mandible can rotate about it as the contralateral condyle is protruded and retracted.

The medial pterygoid muscle inserts on the medial surface of the mandibular ramus and angle (see Fig. 10-56). The medial pterygoid can affect closure, protrusion, and grinding movements of the jaw.

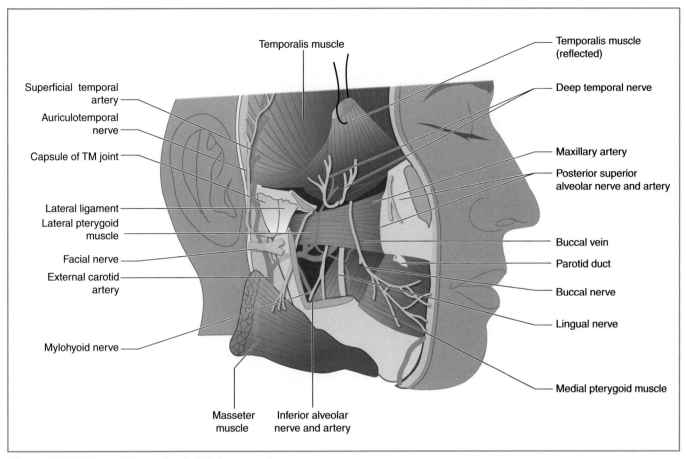

Figure 10-57. Pterygoid muscles in infratemporal fossa.

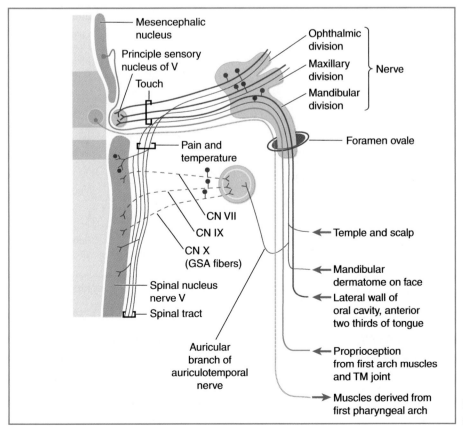

Figure 10-58. Mandibular nerve, sensory, and motor pathways.

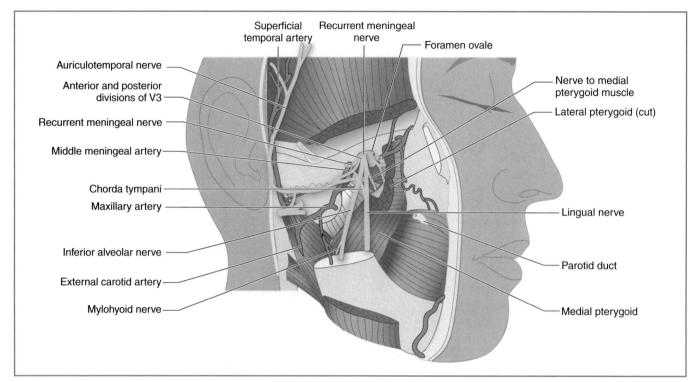

Figure 10-59. Deep infratemporal structures.

lingual nerve (see Fig. 10-59). At this point, the inferior alveolar nerve carries both motor and sensory fibers. The mylohyoid nerve arises from the posterior surface of the inferior alveolar nerve just before it enters the mandibular foramen and canal (see Figs. 10-58 and 10-59). The mylohyoid nerve runs in the mylohyoid groove on the internal surface of the mandible to reach the anterior aspect of the digastric triangle and supply the mylohyoid muscle and the anterior belly of the digastric muscle (see Fig. 10-56).

The inferior alveolar nerve enters the mandibular foramen and canal (see Figs. 10-59 and 10-60). It carries GSA fibers from the lower teeth and gums (see Fig. 10-58). The inferior alveolar nerve's mental branch passes through the mental foramen and supplies the skin of the chin and the lower lip with GSA fibers.

The auriculotemporal nerve arises as two roots from the posterior division of V_3. The two roots encircle the middle meningeal artery, unite, and then pass medially to the neck of the mandible to reach the retromandibular region (Fig. 10-60; see also Fig. 10-57). Here, the auriculotemporal nerve passes medially, then posteriorly, and finally laterally to the superficial temporal artery to become cutaneous, carrying general sensation from the auricular tragus, anterior part of external auditory meatus, anterior part of tympanic membrane, upper ear, and adjacent temporal region.

A nerve block of the lower jaw is usually accomplished by an injection via the intraoral route into the infratemporal region, close to the mandibular foramen (see Fig. 10-60). The goal is to anesthetize the teeth of the lower jaw by anesthetizing the inferior alveolar nerve. However, the chin and lower lip are also anesthetized. The lingual nerve runs

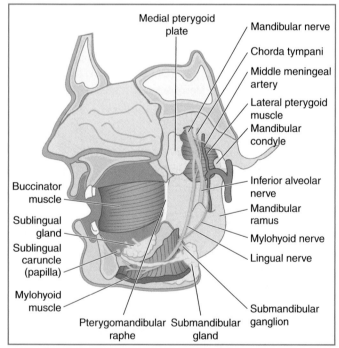

Figure 10-60. Medial view of infratemporal region and floor of the mouth.

just anteriorly to the inferior alveolar nerve on the medial pterygoid muscle. The bolus of anesthesia is always injected close to the inferior alveolar nerve, never into it. As such, the bolus may also involve the lingual nerve, anesthetizing the anterior two thirds of the tongue (to the midline) and adjacent gums.

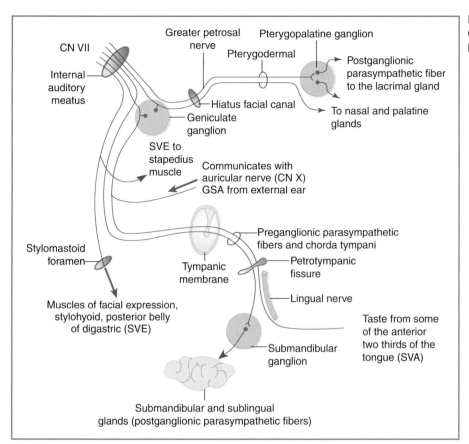

Figure 10-61. Chorda tympani branch of CN VII communicates with the lingual branch of the mandibular nerve.

Branches of CN VII and CN IX That Communicate with V₃

Branches that communicate with V_3 are destined to reach the floor of the mouth or the retromandibular region.

The chorda tympani branch of the facial nerve carries special visceral afferent fibers for taste and preganglionic parasympathetic fibers (Fig. 10-61; see also Fig. 10-60). It enters the infratemporal region through the petrotympanic fissure (see Figs. 10-50 and 10-53) and joins the lingual nerve in the infratemporal region and travels with the lingual nerve to reach the paralingual (sublingual) space (see Fig. 10-60). The taste fibers arise from taste buds on the anterior two thirds of the tongue and have their cell bodies in the geniculate ganglion located in the facial canal (see Fig. 10-61). The preganglionic parasympathetic fibers synapse in the submandibular ganglion, which is attached to the lingual nerve by two nerve roots. The postganglionic fibers pass directly to the adjacent submandibular gland or return to the lingual nerve to supply the sublingual gland (see Fig. 10-61). Preganglionic parasympathetic fibers from CN IX enter the middle ear via the tympanic canaliculus to provide GSA fibers to the mucoperiosteum. The accompanying preganglionic parasympathetic fibers continue through the roof of the middle ear (tegmen tympani) as the lesser petrosal nerve (Fig. 10-62).

The lesser petrosal branch of the glossopharyngeal nerve carries preganglionic parasympathetic fibers through the suture between the temporal and sphenoid bone's greater wing to synapse in the otic ganglion, which is located just medial to the main trunk of V_3 (see Fig. 10-62). Postganglionic parasympathetic fibers run with the auriculotemporal branch of V_3 to innervate the parotid gland.

Circulation

The maxillary artery is the larger of the two terminal branches of the external carotid artery (Fig. 10-63). It arises in the retromandibular region and passes medially to the mandibular neck and laterally to the sphenomandibular ligament. The artery then runs either superficially or deep to the lateral pterygoid muscle to ultimately exit the infratemporal fossa through the pterygomaxillary fissure. The external carotid plexus supplies postganglionic sympathetic fibers that run with the maxillary artery and its various branches. These postganglionic sympathetic fibers supply the parotid gland and travel with the middle meningeal artery (see Fig. 10-62).

The first part of the maxillary artery, which is medial to the neck of the mandible, gives off the following branches. The deep auricular artery runs through the parotid gland to supply the external auditory canal and external tympanic membrane surface. The anterior tympanic artery passes through the petrotympanic fissure to form a vascular circle around the tympanic membrane with the stylomastoid branch of the posterior auricular artery. The inferior alveolar artery and nerve enter the mandibular foramen to supply the teeth and periodontal ligaments of the lower jaw and the mental artery to the chin. The middle meningeal artery passes between the two roots of the auriculotemporal nerve, through the foramen spinosum, into the middle cranial fossa to supply the meninges of the

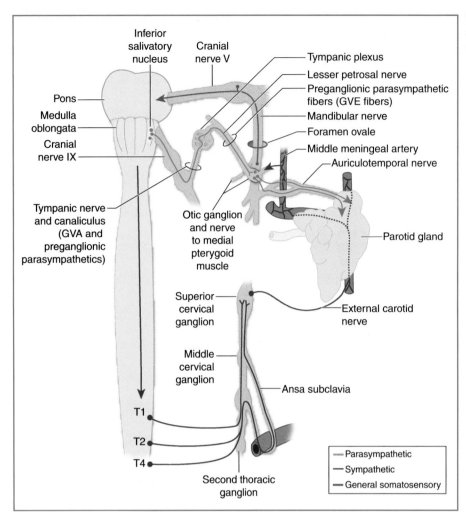

Figure 10-62. Parasympathetic and sympathetic pathways to the parotid gland.

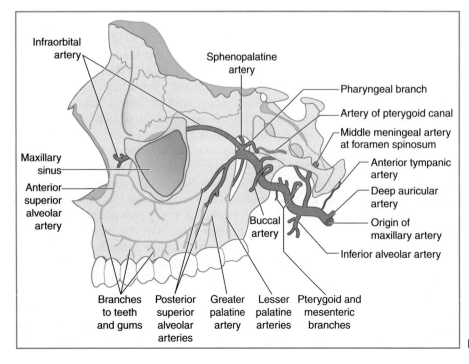

Figure 10-63. Maxillary artery.

middle and most of the anterior cranial fossa and the adjacent bone.

The second part of the maxillary artery provides muscular branches such as the deep temporal, pterygoid, masseteric, and buccal branches. Branches of the third part of the maxillary artery arise in the pterygopalatine fossa.

Veins

These veins are in the form of a venous plexus closely associated with the lateral pterygoid muscle. The pterygoid plexus of veins communicates with the face, orbit, and dural sinuses including the cavernous sinus. These communications allow the pterygoid plexus of veins to be a route for the spread of infection from the face to the deep face, orbit, or dural sinuses. It can also serve as a pathway for a thrombus due to extraction of an upper molar to travel from the infra-orbital vein to the pterygoid plexus, orbit, or cavernous sinus. The pterygoid plexus of veins drains into a short maxillary vein, which joins the superficial temporal vein to form the retromandibular vein.

Parotid Space (Parotid Bed)

The parotid is the largest of the three major salivary glands and occupies the parotid space (see Tables 10-15, 10-17, and 10-22) along with several neurovascular structures. This gland extends anteriorly over the masseter muscle in a variable manner. Occasionally, an accessory portion of the gland becomes detached along the parotid duct. The parotid gland can also extend anteromedially to the margin of the medial pterygoid muscle. Thus, the superficial and deep parts of this gland can be connected by a narrow portion. The facial nerve branches emerge from the larger lateral portion of the parotid gland.

The parotid gland is encapsulated in a strong fascia derived from the outer investing layer of deep fascia. The deep fascia

TABLE 10-22. Boundaries of the Parotid Region (Parotid Bed)

Boundary	Structures
Anterior	Posterior margin of mandibular ramus, masseter muscle anterolaterally, medial pterygoid anteromedially
Medial	Styloid process and attached muscles, internal jugular vein, internal carotid artery, pharyngeal wall
Posterior	Mastoid process, sternocleidomastoid muscle
Lateral	Outer investing layer of deep fascia
Superior	External auditory meatus, temporomandibular joint
Inferior	Sternocleidomastoid muscle, stylohyoid and posterior belly of the digastric muscle

CLINICAL MEDICINE

Parotid Tumors

The parotid gland is involved in approximately 70% of all salivary gland tumors, and approximately 70% of these are benign. The malignant tumors are usually slow growing. The use of fine-needle biopsy allows for most decisions to be made prior to surgery. The major concern with all parotid surgery is the preservation of facial nerve branches. However, after nerve sparing resections of the lateral portion of the parotid gland, a large percentage of patients develop gustatory sweating (Frey's syndrome). This syndrome is characterized by sweating on one side of the face upon eating or other gustatory stimuli. This is due to damage to the skin capsule and branches of the auriculotemporal nerve that carry postganglionic parasympathetic fibers to the parotid gland. It is suspected that the damaged autonomic fibers regenerate and erroneously innervate the adjacent sweat glands. In the past, surgical procedures required sectioning the tympanic plexus on the promontory of the middle ear, which was not always successful. However, the recent use of botulinum toxin injected into the affected skin field often results in improvement in this condition within 1 week.

produces a strong superficial layer that extends superiorly to the zygomatic bone.

Several neurovascular structures pass through the parotid gland. The external carotid artery divides into its two terminal branches—maxillary and superficial temporal—in the parotid gland, while the maxillary vein and superficial temporal vein form the retromandibular vein within the parotid gland. The vein is typically superficial to the artery. The transverse facial branch of the superficial temporal artery may emerge from the anterior surface of the gland, while the external carotid's posterior auricular branch may emerge from the posterior surface.

The facial nerve exits the stylomastoid foramen and passes laterally to the styloid process to enter the parotid gland. Here, it divides into a superior (temporofacial) and an inferior (cervicofacial) division, which in turn split into five major divisions: temporal, zygomatic, buccal marginal, mandibular, and cervical. These five divisions typically have numerous branches.

The neurovascular structures that lie medial to the gland are the internal carotid artery, internal jugular vein, and the auriculotemporal nerve associated with its medial fascial border. The auriculotemporal and temporal nerves both emerge from the superior margin of the parotid gland. They can be easily identified by the fact that the auriculotemporal nerve emerges posterior to the superficial temporal artery and then crosses the artery anterior to ascend into the temporal region (see Figs. 10-57 and 10-59).

The parotid duct extends from the anterior border of the gland approximately the breadth of a finger below the zygomatic arch. However, there is some variability in the course of the duct including a duct that arises low and runs obliquely upward. The duct crosses the masseter muscle and penetrates the buccinator muscle to open into the vestibule of the mouth

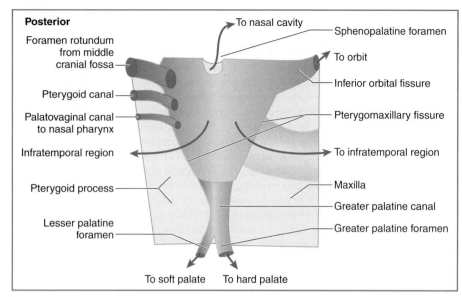

Posterior

Foramen rotundum from middle cranial fossa

Pterygoid canal

Palatovaginal canal to nasal pharynx

Infratemporal region

Pterygoid process

Lesser palatine foramen

To nasal cavity

Sphenopalatine foramen

To orbit

Inferior orbital fissure

Pterygomaxillary fissure

To infratemporal region

Maxilla

Greater palatine canal

Greater palatine foramen

To soft palate   To hard palate

A

Figure 10-64. A, Passageways of the pterygopalatine fossa. **B,** Arrangement of the sphenoid, palatine, and maxilla to form the pterygopalatine fossa.

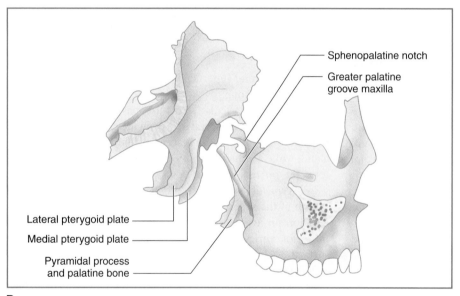

Sphenopalatine notch

Greater palatine groove maxilla

Lateral pterygoid plate

Medial pterygoid plate

Pyramidal process and palatine bone

B

by means of a small papilla located opposite the second upper molar.

The parotid gland is supplied by branches of the external carotid artery and is innervated by postganglionic sympathetic fibers from the external carotid nerve and postganglionic parasympathetic fibers from the otic ganglion (see Fig. 10-62).

PTERYGOPALATINE FOSSA

The pterygopalatine fossa is a small pyramid-shaped region found posterior to the maxilla and posteroinferior to the orbit. This fossa is different from most anatomic regions in that it does not contain muscles, glands, or special sense organs. It is a redistribution center for numerous neurovascular structures. Therefore, the pterygopalatine fossa region is characterized by passageways. Indeed eight major passageways allow it to communicate with the surrounding regions.

The pterygopalatine fossa communicates with the middle cranial fossa, nasopharynx, nasal cavity, hard and soft palate, orbit, and infratemporal region (Fig. 10-64).

Bony Architecture

The pterygopalatine fossa is bounded by the maxilla, palatine, and sphenoid bones (Fig. 10-64B). It is located posterior to the maxilla, lateral to the perpendicular plate of the palatine bone, and anterior to the pterygoid process of the sphenoid bone. It is a small, pyramidal region whose apex faces caudally.

Posterior Wall

The posterior wall of the pterygopalatine fossa is formed by the sphenoid bone's pterygoid process along with a small portion of the greater wing (Fig. 10-65). There are three passageways in the posterior wall (see Figs. 10-64A and 10-65).

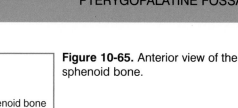

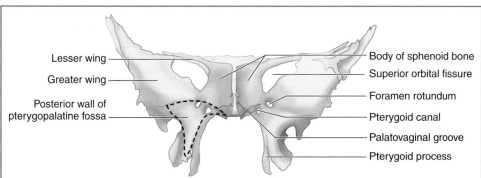

Figure 10-65. Anterior view of the sphenoid bone.

Two communicate with the middle cranial fossa, and the third communicates with the nasopharynx (see Fig. 10-64A).

The foramen rotundum leads from the middle cranial fossa into the superolateral aspect of the pterygopalatine fossa.

The pterygoid canal (see Figs. 10-64A and 10-65) starts in the anterior wall of the foramen lacerum in the middle cranial fossa. It passes through the floor of the sphenoidal air sinus into the pterygopalatine fossa. The pterygoid canal's anterior opening is found slightly inferior and medial to the opening of the foramen rotundum. The anterior end of the pterygoid canal is larger than the posterior opening because the pterygopalatine ganglion is located approximately at the anterior opening.

The pharyngeal (palatovaginal) canal is formed by the articulation of the palatovaginal groove on the inferior surface of the body of the sphenoid bone with the palatine bone. It is a very narrow passageway that starts just medially and slightly inferiorly to the pterygoid canal and ends in the nasopharynx posteriorly to the pharyngotympanic (auditory) tube (see Fig. 10-65).

Medial Wall

The palatine bone is L-shaped and forms the medial boundary of the pterygopalatine fossa (Fig. 10-66). The long (vertical) arm of the L is the perpendicular plate that separates the pterygopalatine fossa from the nasal cavity. The short arm of the L is the horizontal process of the palatine bone. It extends medially from the inferior end of the perpendicular plate and forms the posterior fourth of the hard palate. It does not directly participate in the formation of the pterygopalatine fossa.

The pyramidal process (see Fig. 10-66) of the palatine bone extends posteriorly and laterally to insert into the sphenoid bone's pterygoid notch to complete the pterygoid fossa.

The sphenopalatine notch is found on the superior aspect of the perpendicular plate between the anteriorly located orbital process and a posteriorly located sphenoidal process (see Fig. 10-66). The sphenopalatine notch is converted into the sphenopalatine foramen when the palatine bone articulates with the body of the sphenoid bone. The sphenopalatine foramen is the passageway that allows this fossa to communicate with the posterior aspect of the nasal cavity. The palatine

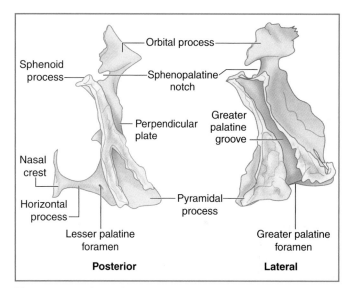

Figure 10-66. Lateral and posterior views of the palatine bone.

bone's sphenoidal process articulates with the body of the sphenoid bone to form the pharyngeal canal, which ends in the nasopharynx.

Anterior Wall

The posterior surface of the maxilla forms the anterior wall of the pterygopalatine fossa (see Fig. 10-64B). It also forms the anterior wall of the adjacent infratemporal region. This fossa can communicate with the orbit through the medial end of the inferior orbital fissure.

The pterygopalatine fossa communicates with the hard and soft palates by means of the greater and lesser palatine canals and foramina. The palatine bone has a deep groove, the greater palatine groove, on the lateral surface of the perpendicular plate. Upon articulation of the palatine bone with the maxilla, this groove becomes the greater palatine canal (Fig. 10-67). This canal ends as the greater palatine foramen, which allows the pterygopalatine fossa to communicate with the hard palate. However, the lesser palatine canal runs from the greater palatine canal to the lesser palatine foramina and soft palate through the pyramidal process of the palatine bone.

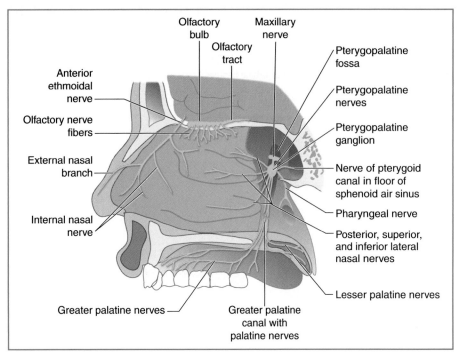

Figure 10-67. Lateral side of the nasal cavity and palate with dissected perpendicular plate of palatine bone to visualize pterygopalatine fossa demonstrates V$_2$, pterygopalatine nerves, pterygopalatine ganglion, palatine nerves, and other branches of V$_2$.

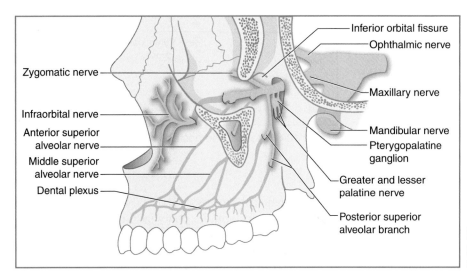

Figure 10-68. Lateral division and pterygopalatine branches of the maxillary nerve.

Lateral Wall

The pterygomaxillary fissure is the lateral wall of the pterygopalatine fossa. It is located between the maxilla and the lateral plate of the pterygoid process (see Figs. 10-51 and 10-52). The maxilla is also inferior to the boundary of the inferior orbital fissure allowing the infratemporal region to communicate with the orbit. While the maxilla is a shared boundary for both the pterygomaxillary and the inferior orbital fissures, these two fissures are at right angles to each other (Fig. 10-68).

Neurovascular Bundles

The pterygopalatine fossa contains the maxillary nerve, branches of CN VII (including its pterygopalatine ganglion) sympathetic fibers, and the third portion of the maxillary artery and vein (see Fig. 10-68).

Maxillary Nerve

The maxillary nerve has only GSA fibers (see Fig. 10-68). In the middle cranial fossa, the maxillary nerve gives rise to meningeal branches that cross the floor of the fossa to reach and then be distributed with the middle meningeal artery. The maxillary nerve passes through the foramen rotundum into the superolateral aspect of the pterygopalatine fossa. Here, the maxillary nerve divides into lateral and medial branches. The medial branches are the two pterygopalatine (also called ganglionic) branches. The larger lateral branches include zygomatic, posterosuperior alveolar, and infraorbital branches (see Figs. 10-67 and 10-68).

Lateral Branches of the Maxillary Nerve

The infraorbital nerve is the largest of the lateral branches. This nerve passes through the inferior orbital fissure onto the orbital floor. Here, it supplies small branches to the periorbita and passes through the infraorbital groove into the infraorbital canal and foramen onto the face (see Fig. 10-68).

In the infraorbital canal, the infraorbital nerve gives off anterosuperior alveolar nerves and middle superior alveolar nerves. These nerves supply the mucoperiosteum of the maxillary air sinus. They then continue through the lateral and anterior walls of the maxillary sinus to reach the alveolar processes, where they form most of the dental (alveolar) plexus that supplies branches to the dentition and gums of the upper jaw (see Fig. 10-68).

Posterosuperior alveolar nerves pass through the pterygopalatine fissure onto the infratemporal surface of the maxilla. Here, they enter the small posterosuperior alveolar foramina to supply the posterior aspect of the maxillary sinus and the molars. Thus, *the posterosuperior alveolar nerves enter the maxilla from the infratemporal region.* The middle and anterosuperior alveolar nerves reach the dentition through the internal surfaces of the walls of the maxillary sinus.

The zygomatic nerve enters the orbit through the inferior orbital fissure with the infraorbital nerve. Here, it divides into zygomaticofacial and zygomaticotemporal branches, which enter small foramina including the zygomatico-orbital found in the orbital surface of the zygomatic bone. The zygomaticofacial nerves reach the face by means of the zygomaticofacial foramina on the anterior surface of the zygomatic bone. The zygomaticotemporal branches reach the temporal region by means of the zygomaticotemporal foramen on the posterior (temporal) surface of the zygomatic bone. The zygomaticotemporal nerve passes between the temporalis muscle and zygomatic bone and pierces the deep temporal fascia to reach the skin of the temporal region lateral to the orbit. Before leaving the orbit, the zygomaticotemporal nerve gives a communicating branch, carrying postganglionic parasympathetic fibers, to the lacrimal nerve.

Medial Branches of the Maxillary Nerve

The medial branches of the maxillary nerve are the pterygopalatine (ganglionic) branches that pass through the pterygopalatine ganglion *without synapsing* (Fig. 10-69). The pterygopalatine nerves enter the ganglion and emerge as the pharyngeal, posterosuperior lateral nasal, nasopalatine, greater palatine, and lesser palatine nerves. These branches of the maxillary nerve supply part of the nasopharynx, posterior

two thirds of the nasal cavity, hard palate, and some of the soft palate with general somatic sensory fibers. However, they receive postganglionic parasympathetic fibers from the facial nerve's pterygopalatine ganglion and in some cases possibly postganglionic sympathetic fibers as well.

Facial Nerve Branches

The facial nerve branches in the pterygopalatine fossa are the nerve of the pterygoid canal, the pterygopalatine ganglion, and the postganglionic branches that arise in this ganglion (see Fig. 10-69).

The hiatus of the canal for the greater petrosal nerve is a small opening found at the first turn of the facial canal. This hiatus allows the greater petrosal branch of CN VII to exit onto the anterior surface of the petrous temporal bone in the middle cranial fossa. The greater petrosal nerve continues under the trigeminal ganglion to reach the foramen lacerum. It then passes anteriorly beneath the internal carotid artery, which is also passing horizontally across the top of this foramen. At the anterior end of the foramen lacerum, the deep petrosal nerve, which is a branch of the internal carotid plexus, joins the greater petrosal nerve. The *greater and deep petrosal nerves* now enter the pterygoid canal to reach the pterygopalatine fossa as the nerve of the pterygoid canal (vidian nerve).

The greater petrosal nerve has three types of functional fibers: preganglionic parasympathetic, general visceral afferent, and special visceral afferent fibers. The deep petrosal nerve contains postganglionic sympathetic fibers. Thus, the nerve of the pterygoid canal contains preganglionic parasympathetic fibers as well as general and special visceral sensory fibers from the greater petrosal nerve and the postganglionic sympathetic fibers from the deep petrosal nerve. The postganglionic sympathetic fibers have their cell bodies in the superior cervical ganglion.

The nerve of the pterygoid canal enters the pterygopalatine fossa to find the pterygopalatine ganglion at the canal's anterior opening. Only the preganglionic parasympathetic fibers synapse in this ganglion. All other fibers merely pass through this ganglion. The postganglionic parasympathetic fibers that arise in the pterygopalatine ganglion reach their final destination by running with branches of the maxillary nerve. Thus, the glands of the nasal cavity will receive postganglionic parasympathetic fibers from the pterygopalatine ganglion that run with the posterior lateral nasal and nasopalatine branches of the maxillary nerve to the lateral and septal walls of the nasal cavity. The postganglionic parasympathetic fibers to the glands of the hard palate run with the greater palatine nerve.

A more complicated route is used by the postganglionic parasympathetic fibers that innervate the lacrimal gland (see Fig. 10-69). These fibers arise in the pterygopalatine ganglion and run laterally in the pterygopalatine nerves to reach the zygomatic nerve. The postganglionic parasympathetic fibers enter the orbit with the zygomatic nerve through the inferior orbital fissure. They follow the zygomaticotemporal branch to reach the lateral wall of the orbit. Just before the zygomaticotemporal nerve leaves the orbit, the postganglionic parasympathetic fibers that ran "piggyback" with it separate from

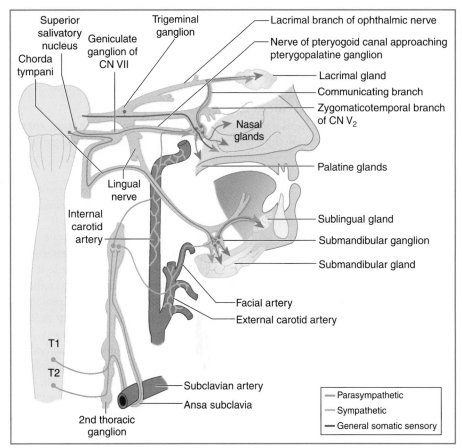

A

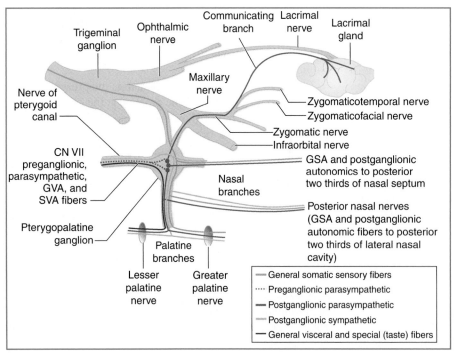

B

Figure 10-69. A, Distribution of fibers from the pterygopalatine ganglion. **B,** Facial nerve branches associated with the pterygopalatine fossa.

the zygomaticotemporal nerve as a communicating branch. These postganglionic parasympathetic fibers pass superiorly along the lateral wall of the orbit to communicate with the ophthalmic nerve's lacrimal branch to reach and innervate the lacrimal gland. It is thought that the postganglionic sympathetic fibers of the deep petrosal nerve follow the same course to innervate the lacrimal gland.

The cell bodies located in the geniculate ganglion of the facial nerve give rise to sensory fibers in the greater petrosal nerve and then in the nerve of the pterygoid canal. These general visceral sensory and special visceral sensory fibers pass through the pterygopalatine ganglion and then run with the lesser palatine nerve to reach the soft palate. Most of the fibers in the lesser palatine nerve are supplied by the facial nerve with only a minority of fibers from the maxillary nerve. The special visceral sensory fibers innervate the taste buds that are located on the anterior portion of the soft palate, just anterior to the sulcus terminalis of the tongue. Note that *not all taste buds are confined to the tongue.*

Circulation

The infraorbital artery (see Fig. 10-63) arises in the infra-temporal region and follows the infraorbital nerve through the inferior orbital fissure. The branches of the infraorbital artery follow the branches of the nerve including anterior and middle superior alveolar branches that pass through the maxillary air sinus. Posterosuperior alveolar arteries follow the posterosuperior alveolar nerves and enter the maxilla through the infratemporal surface.

The third portion of the maxillary artery passes through the pterygomaxillary fissure from the infratemporal region into the pterygopalatine fossa. The branches of this artery then pass through the eight passageways that allow this fossa to communicate with the surrounding regions. The branches of the third portion of the maxillary artery are, for the most part, named for the passageways that they use, for example, the artery of the pterygoid canal (see Fig. 10-63).

The artery of the pterygoid canal passes through the ptery-goid canal to supply the nerve of this canal as well as the sphenoid air sinus and adjacent nasal pharynx. Other arteries include the pharyngeal branch, sphenopalatine artery, and descending palatine artery.

The veins follow the arteries.

●●● ORAL CAVITY (MOUTH)

The oral cavity (mouth) is the entrance to the digestive system.

The boundaries of the oral cavity are different from those of the floor of the mouth, since the oral cavity is defined by mucous membranes, including those covering the floor of the mouth (Tables 10-23 and 10-24).

The lips are multifunctional structures as described in the chapter on the face that can act as a sphincter at the entrance of the mouth. The lips have two epithelial surfaces: an external layer of thin skin and an internal layer of mucous membrane of the vestibule.

The skin of the lips is very thin, revealing a highly vascular region, the vermilion zone. This accounts for the color of the lips. The skin of the face meets the vermilion zone at the vermilion border. The skin of the lips has sparse glands and requires continual moistening by the tongue. This accounts for the drying of the lips (chapped lips) in dry weather.

The facial nerve provides motor innervation to the orbicularis oris (see Fig. 10-12). However, the sensory inner-vation for the upper lip is the infraorbital branches of the maxillary nerve, and the lower lip is innervated by the mental branch of the mandibular nerve. A common symptom of facial nerve palsy is drooling from the corner of the mouth owing to weakness of the orbicularis oris.

Vestibule

The dental arches (complete structure associated with the dentition) divide the oral cavity into two parts: the vestibule and the oral cavity proper. The vestibule of the oral cavity is the U-shaped region found between the mucous membranes covering the lips and cheeks and the dental arches, gums, and teeth. The vestibule communicates with the external environment by means of the rima oris, the elongated opening or fissure between the lips. The vestibule communicates with the oral cavity proper by means of the spaces between the occlusal

TABLE 10-23. Boundaries of the Oral Cavity

Boundary	Structures
Anterior	Lips
Posterior	Oropharyngeal isthmus, formed by the palatoglossal arches, palate, and sulcus terminalis of the tongue
Lateral	Oral mucosa covering the buccinator muscle
Superior	Hard palate
Inferior	Mucous membranes of the tongue and extending to the dental arches

TABLE 10-24. Boundaries of the Oral Cavity Proper

Boundary	Structures
Anterior	Alveolar arches covered by mucosa and gingiva
Posterior	Palatoglossal arches
Lateral	Alveolar arches covered by mucosa and gingiva
Superior	Hard palate
Inferior	Mostly tongue and some mucous membranes between inferior tongue and alveolar arch of the mandible

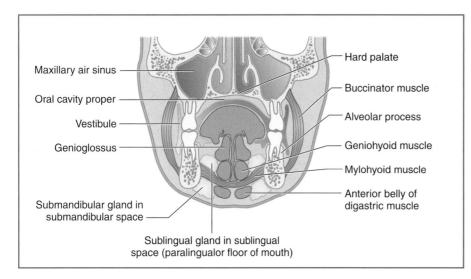

Figure 10-70. Coronal section through the oral cavity.

Labels: Maxillary air sinus, Oral cavity proper, Vestibule, Genioglossus, Submandibular gland in submandibular space, Sublingual gland in sublingual space (paralingualor floor of mouth), Hard palate, Buccinator muscle, Alveolar process, Geniohyoid muscle, Mylohyoid muscle, Anterior belly of digastric muscle

surfaces of the teeth as well as the space between the last molar and the pterygomandibular fold.

Both superiorly and inferiorly, the mucosa of the labial and buccal walls becomes continuous with the mucosa on the alveolar arches, producing vault-like arches or fornices (Fig. 10-70). The alveolar processes (hollow sac-like bony cavities) of the maxilla and mandible dental arches contain the sockets for the roots of the teeth.

Extra or enlarged folds of the mucous membrane, referred to as the superior and inferior labial frenula, extend from the lips across the fornix to become continuous with the mucosa of the alveolar processes (Fig. 10-71).

The gingiva (gum) is the dense connective tissue covering the apical portion of the alveolar processes and the necks of the teeth.

The posterior boundary of the oral cavity communicates with the oropharynx by means of the oropharyngeal isthmus (isthmus of fauces). The fauces is the space between the oral cavity of the mouth and the pharynx. It is bounded by the soft palate, the palatoglossal arch, and the sulcus terminalis of the tongue (see Fig. 10-71). The palatoglossal arch is formed by the mucous membrane overlying the palatoglossus muscle (see Fig. 10-71).

Palate

The palate is subdivided into a hard palate, consisting of the anterior two thirds of the palate, and the soft palate, consisting of the posterior one third (Fig. 10-72). The hard palate separates the oral cavity from the nasal cavity. The palatine processes of the two maxillary bones and the horizontal processes of the palatine bones form the hard palate. Just posterior to the incisors is the incisive fossa, which is a depression that contains the incisive foramen (see Fig. 10-72A). This opening is the palatine end of the incisive canals (see Fig. 10-52), which start in the floor of the right and left nasal passageways. The incisive canals have a Y-shaped configuration with the base of the canal being the incisive foramen and fossa on the hard palate.

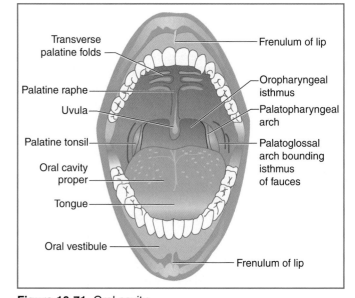

Labels: Transverse palatine folds, Palatine raphe, Uvula, Palatine tonsil, Oral cavity proper, Tongue, Oral vestibule, Frenulum of lip, Oropharyngeal isthmus, Palatopharyngeal arch, Palatoglossal arch bounding isthmus of fauces, Frenulum of lip

Figure 10-71. Oral cavity.

Posteriorly, the horizontal process of the palatine bones has a greater palatine foramen. The lesser palatine foramina are in the pyramidal process of the palatine bone (see Fig. 10-52). These openings communicate with the pterygopalatine fossa by means of the greater palatine canal (see Figs. 10-64B and 10-66). The two horizontal processes of the palatine bones produce a posterior nasal spine (see Fig. 10-72A), which is a bony attachment point for some of the soft palate structures.

Hard Palate
Mucoperiosteum

The incisive papilla is an oval elevation that marks the presence of the incisive foramen. This papilla is located posterior to the incisors. This landmark allows for the identification of the passageway for the nasopalatine branch of V_2 that innervates

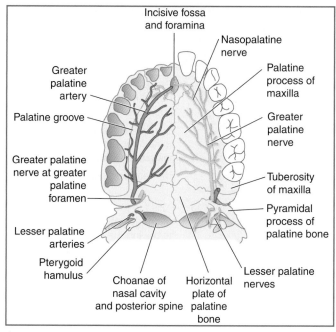

A

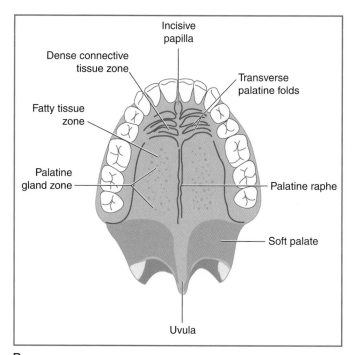

B

Figure 10-72. A, Innervation and blood supply to the hard palate. **B,** Mucoperiosteum of the hard and soft palates.

papilla, posterior to this region is a fatty (adipose) region of the mucoperiosteum, and then starting at the level of the molars and extending into the soft palate is the glandular region.

The mucoperiosteum of the hard palate receives GSA fibers from the greater palatine branches of the maxillary nerve. The greater palatine nerves descend in the greater palatine canal and emerge onto the hard palate through the greater palatine foramen (see Fig. 10-67). These nerves, accompanied by the greater palatine artery, run anteriorly to supply most of the hard palate. The incisive region is supplied by the nasopalatine branches of the maxillary nerve that descend on the nasal septum and pass through the incisive canal and foramen onto the hard palate.

The palatine glands receive postganglionic parasympathetic fibers from the pterygopalatine ganglion (see Fig. 10-67). These fibers run with the greater and lesser palatine branches of the maxillary nerve. The greater palatine nerve provides GSA fibers to the hard palates. The lesser palatine nerves communicate with the nerve of the pterygoid canal and carry GVA fibers from CN VII along with some SVA fibers for taste from the soft palate (see Figs. 10-67 and 10-69A) and some GSA fibers from V_2. The lesser palatine nerves help innervate the soft palate and tonsillar region. The tonsillar branch of the glossopharyngeal nerve also provides most of the GVA fibers to the tonsillar region and the soft palate.

Circulation

The maxillary artery ends by passing through the pterygomaxillary fissure as the third part of the maxillary artery, which then gives rise to several branches. Its descending palatine branch gives rise to the greater and lesser palatine arteries in the greater palatine canal (see Fig. 10-72A). The greater palatine artery emerges through the greater palatine foramen, passes forward on the hard palate, and sends a branch through the incisive foramen and canal onto the nasal septum. Thus, the incisive canal is a two-way street for the nasopalatine nerve and greater palatine artery. The lesser palatine arteries pass through the lesser palatine foramina into the soft palate.

Soft Palate

The soft palate (Table 10-25; see also Fig. 10-72A) is part of the oral pharynx. It is a fibromuscular structure that can separate the oropharynx from the nasopharynx during swallowing, mastication, coughing, sneezing, etc. The soft palate is a flexible structure that has epithelium on both the nasopharynx and the oropharynx surfaces. The anterior aspect of the soft palate is attached to the posterior margin of the palatine bones. The posterior free surface has a prominent midline process, the uvula.

Muscles

The muscles of the soft palate are arranged as elevators, tensors, and depressors (see Table 10-25).

The tensor veli palatini muscle (Figs. 10-73 and 10-74) arises from the lateral wall of the cartilaginous portion of the

this portion of the hard palate and upper incisors. A midline palatine raphe starts at the incisive papilla. It is more obvious in children than in the aged. Transverse palatine rugae radiate laterally from the palatine raphe and incisive papillae.

The mucosa of the hard palate (see Fig. 10-72B) is firmly bound to the underlying periosteum. However, the mucoperiosteum is subdivided into three regions; anteriorly is the dense connective tissue region associated with the incisive

TABLE 10-25. Muscles of the Soft Palate

Muscle	Origin	Insertion	Action
Tensor veli palatini	Scaphoid fossa of sphenoid bone, lateral surface of auditory tube cartilage	Palatine aponeurosis	Tenses soft palate, preventing the palate from being inverted Opens the auditory tube
Levator veli palatini	Petrous temporal bone and auditory tube cartilage	Palatine aponeurosis	Elevates and pulls the palate posteriorly, helps segregate the nasopharynx and oropharynx
Musculus uvulae	Posterior palatine spine	Posterior mucosa of the soft palate	Shortens and raises the uvula
Palatoglossus	Inferior surface of the palatine aponeurosis	Side and dorsum of the tongue	Pulls the palatoglossal arch anteriorly and medially, narrowing the isthmus of the fauces and separating the oral cavity from the pharynx
Palatopharyngeus	Anterior larger portion from the inferior aspect of the palatine aponeurosis, and smaller portion from the superoposterior aspect of the palate	Thyroid cartilage, muscles of the pharynx Pharyngobasilar fascia	Elevates the larynx and pharynx and depresses the soft palate, aids in swallowing

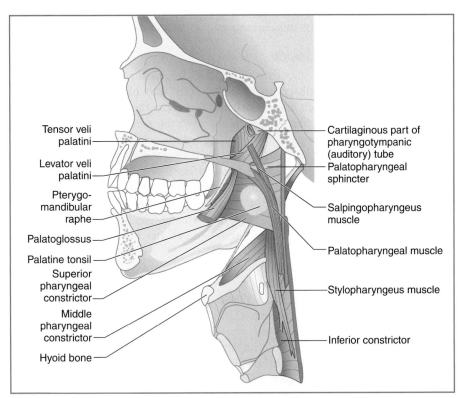

Figure 10-73. Lateral view of the pharynx.

auditory tube and the scaphoid fossa of the sphenoid bone, which is located on the superior aspect of the medial pterygoid plate just below the pterygoid canal's opening. The tensor muscle passes inferiorly and then its tendon hooks around the pterygoid hamulus and inserts medially into the palatine aponeurosis (see Fig. 10-74). This aponeurosis is formed by both tensor veli palatini muscles and is also attached to the horizontal palatine processes. The palatine aponeurosis serves as the backbone of the soft palate. The mandibular nerve innervates the tensor veli palatini. Although the tensor helps tense the soft palate, its primary action is to open the auditory tube by pulling down on the cartilage of its lateral wall.

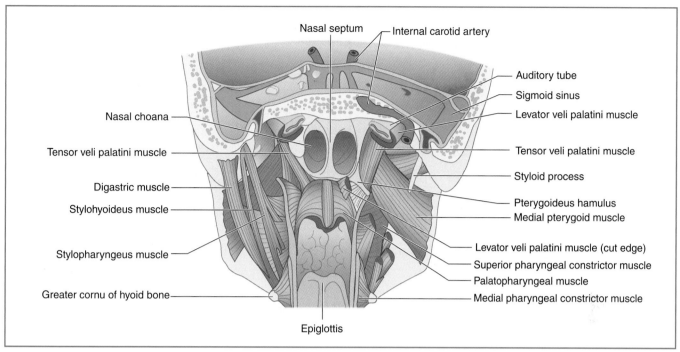

Figure 10-74. Muscles of the soft palate and pharynx.

The levator veli palatini muscle passes medially in the interval between the base of the skull and the superior pharyngeal constrictor muscle to insert into the palatine aponeurosis (see Fig. 10-73).

During swallowing, the superomedial fibers of the superior pharyngeal constrictor muscle, along with a thinner posterior portion of the palatopharyngeus, contract to produce the palatopharyngeal sphincter, or Passavant's ridge (see Fig. 10-73). This lip-like ridge on the posterolateral wall of the nasopharynx meets the elevated soft palate to separate the nasopharynx from the oropharynx.

The more prominent anterior fibers of the palatopharyngeus muscle unite and pass in the palatopharyngeal fold to be joined by some of the fibers of the salpingopharyngeus muscle to elevate the larynx and pharynx.

Innervation

The tensor veli palatini is derived from the first pharyngeal arch and thus is innervated by the mandibular nerve. It is uncertain whether the other muscles are derived from pharyngeal arch 4 or 6. These soft palate muscles receive SVE fibers from the nucleus ambiguus. Therefore the innervation includes fibers from the cranial portion of the accessory nerve (X–XI). It is distributed by the vagus nerve and its contribution to the pharyngeal plexus.

The few GSA fibers from the soft palate are found in the lesser palatine branches of V_2. These nerves also carry postganglionic parasympathetic fibers from the pterygopalatine ganglion to the palatine glands. They may also transmit some postganglionic sympathetic fibers. GVA fibers for visceral sensation and reflexes such as the gag reflex and SVA fibers

for taste are supplied by the lesser palatine nerves and are from CN VII.

Palatine Tonsil

The palatine tonsil is found in the tonsillar fossa between the palatoglossal and palatopharyngeal arches (called the isthmus of the fauces). It is oval shaped in the superior-inferior axis and has a medial and lateral surface. The lateral surface is embedded in the wall of the pharynx. The palatine tonsil receives its primary supply from the tonsillar branches of the facial artery. The other arteries that also help supply it are the lingual artery's tonsillar branch, the maxillary artery's lesser palatine branch, the facial artery's ascending palatine branch, and the ascending pharyngeal artery's descending branch (see Fig. 10-33).

The innervation of the fauces consists of GVA fibers, which are primarily carried by the tonsillar branch of the glossopharyngeal nerve, but some are also in the lesser palatine nerve. These latter fibers are from CN VII and its greater petrosal nerve.

Tongue

The tongue (Figs. 10-75 and 10-76) is a muscular organ that plays an important part in swallowing, sucking, and speech. It has a root and body. The covering of the tongue and the adjacent mucosa form the inferior boundary of the oral cavity but not the floor of the mouth. This latter region is bounded by the mylohyoid muscle that separates the mouth from the digastric triangle. It is also referred to as the sublingual space, since this gland is its major occupant (see Fig. 10-70).

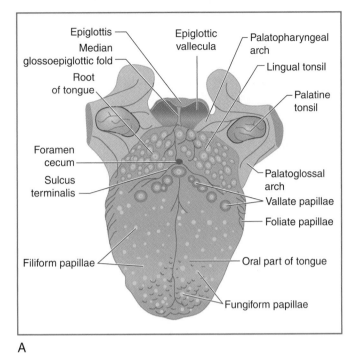

A

B

Figure 10-75. Dorsal (**A**) and inferior (**B**) surfaces of the tongue.

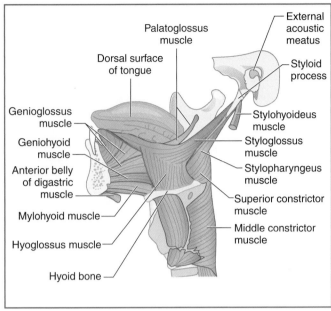

A

B

Figure 10-76. A, Extrinsic muscles of the tongue. **B,** Coronal section of the tongue.

The root of the tongue is attached to the mandible, hyoid bone, palate, and styloid process by means of the tongue's extrinsic muscles (see Fig. 10-76).

The body of the tongue is the more mobile portion found in the oral cavity, formed by intrinsic muscles, small salivary glands, taste buds, and connective tissue.

The surfaces of the tongue are the dorsal and inferior surfaces. These surfaces meet at the lateral margin of the tongue. The dorsal surface faces the palate when the mouth is closed and is visible upon protrusion of the tongue. The inferior surface is covered with a thinner mucous membrane that is continuous with the mucous membrane of the oral cavity. The anterior tip, or apex, of the tongue is the most mobile portion of the tongue.

The dorsum of the tongue is marked by a median longitudinal sulcus that denotes the underlying median septum (see Fig. 10-75A). The median septum divides the tongue into two halves and is attached to the hyoid bone. The median sulcus and septum reflect the development of the tongue in part from the bilateral lingual swellings. If these swellings fail to fuse, the tongue could be either bifid or cleft-shaped.

A V-shaped depression, the sulcus terminalis, is found on the dorsum of the tongue (see Fig. 10-75A). The apex of the sulcus terminalis faces posteriorly toward the depression, known as the foramen cecum. The sulcus terminalis separates the anterior two thirds (body) of the tongue from the posterior one third (root). The root of the tongue faces the oropharynx while the body is in the oral cavity. Thus, the sulcus terminalis marks the separation of the oral cavity from the oropharynx (see Fig. 10-71).

The dorsal surface of the tongue has many projections of its mucous membrane, called lingual papillae, which contain

TABLE 10-26. Extrinsic Muscles of the Tongue

Muscle	Origin	Insertion	Action
Styloglossus	Anterior aspect of styloid process	Side of the tongue and hyoglossus muscle	Retracts and elevates the tongue
Palatoglossus	Inferior surface of soft palate	Insertion of the styloglossus	Raises the tongue, narrows oropharyngeal isthmus
Hyoglossus	Greater cornu and body of hyoid bone, adjacent stylohyoid ligament	Side of the tongue along with inferior longitudinal intrinsic and styloglossus muscles	Retracts the tongue and, working with the genioglossus, depresses the tongue
Genioglossus	Superior mental spine	Hyoid bone, mostly into the tongue from tip to epiglottis	Anterior fibers retract the tip of the tongue Posterior fibers protrude the tongue

specialized receptors, or taste buds. However, not all papillae have taste buds.

The vallate (circumvallate) papillae are the largest of the specializations that contain taste buds (see Fig. 10-75A). The vallate papillae lie just anterior to the sulcus terminalis and thus are in the anterior two thirds of the tongue. The anterior two thirds of the tongue also has foliate papillae found posteriorly near the margin. Filiform papillae are the most numerous and are found on the dorsum of the tongue. They do not have taste buds, but their coarse structure increases friction and may aid in the movement of material by the tongue. Fungiform papillae are not easily found upon gross inspection. They appear near the lateral margins and dorsal surface of the anterior two thirds of the tongue.

Taste buds are also located on the posterior third of the tongue, epiglottis, soft palate, and anterior palatine arches in infants. The taste buds on the soft palate and epiglottis involute during postnatal development.

Other distinguishing structures on the dorsum of the tongue are the foramen cecum and the lingual tonsil. The foramen cecum is the remnant of the thyroglossal duct that gives rise to the thyroid gland. The lingual tonsil covers the surface of the posterior third of the tongue (see Fig. 10-75A). The lingual tonsils, palatine tonsils, and pharyngeal tonsils form a ring of protective lymphatic tissue called Waldeyer's lymphatic ring.

The mucous membranes on the dorsum of the root continue toward the epiglottis in the form of three folds. The central fold is the median glossoepiglottic fold, while the peripheral folds are the two lateral glossoepiglottic folds (see Fig. 10-75A). The folds produce two depressions, the valleculae epiglotticae (epiglottic valleys), which are sites for the flow of food and liquid during swallowing.

Muscles

The muscles of the tongue are intrinsic and extrinsic. The extrinsic muscles arise outside the tongue and insert into the tongue, namely, styloglossus, hyoglossus, genioglossus, and palatoglossus. The extrinsic muscles of the tongue all insert into the tongue; thus, they have "-glossus" as their suffix (see Fig. 10-76A and Table 10-26).

The styloglossus muscle passes from the styloid process anteriorly, inferiorly, and medially along the inferior border of the superior pharyngeal constrictor muscle into the side of the tongue and hyoglossus muscle. The styloglossus muscle can help the vertical intrinsic muscle elevate the sides of the tongue, while the center remains depressed, for example, during drinking.

The hyoglossus muscle passes superiorly to insert into the side of the tongue along with the inferior longitudinal intrinsic and the styloglossus muscles. Its relationships in the digastric triangle have already been discussed.

The genioglossus muscle expands into a fan-shaped muscle that inserts into the tongue. The genioglossus is the only muscle that can protrude the tongue. If weak or paralyzed, the tongue will deviate to the weak side. The genioglossus muscle is attached to the mandible, along with the geniohyoid muscle, and helps keep the tongue from falling backward and obstructing the airway. If a patient lapses into unconsciousness, the mandible can be pulled forward at the mandibular angle to keep the airway clear.

Intrinsic Muscles

The intrinsic muscles of the tongue can be identified by the location and direction of muscle fibers. Starting at the dorsum of the tongue, the intrinsic muscles are listed below (Fig. 10-76B).

- The superior longitudinal muscle is located just deep to the mucosa of the dorsal surface of the tongue. It arises in part from the septum and extends from the tip almost to the root of the tongue. It helps retract and shorten the tongue. This muscle also turns the lateral margins upward, producing a medial trough.
- The transverse muscle arises from the median septum and extends to the dorsum and sides of the tongue. It helps lengthen and vertically thicken the tongue.

- The vertical muscle arises from the mucosa and extends inferiorly and laterally to the sides of the tongue. It flattens (broadens) and thereby lengthens the tongue.
- The inferior longitudinal muscle is found in the inferior lateral border of the tongue between the genioglossus and hyoglossus. It blends with the styloglossus muscle. The inferior longitudinal muscle helps retract and thereby shorten the tongue.

Inferior Surface of the Tongue

The epithelium on the inferior surface of the tongue is thinner and not as rough as on the dorsal surface. A lingual frenulum extends in the median plane from the inferior surface almost to the tip of the tongue (see Fig. 10-75B). On either side of the lingual frenulum is a swelling called the sublingual caruncle, which contains the orifices of the submandibular ducts. A fold of tissue called the plica fimbriata (fold running from the lingual frenulum) passes just laterally to the frenulum toward the apex (see Fig. 10-75B). The deep lingual vein and to a lesser extent the deep lingual artery can be observed between the inferior surface of the tongue and the plica fimbriata. The vein is usually visible through the thin epithelium of the inferior surface of the tongue.

Innervation

All intrinsic muscles and extrinsic muscles are derived from the occipital somites and are innervated by the hypoglossal nerve except for the palatoglossus muscle. The X-XI complex by means of the pharyngeal plexus innervates the palatoglossus, which is derived from the branchial arches.

The epithelium of the tongue is derived from different arches. The sensory innervation of the surface of the tongue is complex and represents the extensive embryologic contributions of the branchial arches. The epithelium of the anterior two thirds of the tongue is derived from the ectoderm of the first arch and is innervated by GSA fibers carried by the lingual branch of the mandibular nerve. Some of the taste fibers for the anterior two thirds of the tongue are from the chorda tympani of the facial nerve. However, the vallate and foliate papillae are innervated by the glossopharyngeal nerve.

The epithelium of the posterior third of the tongue is derived from the endoderm of the third and a little of the fourth pharyngeal arches and is innervated by GVA fibers from the glossopharyngeal nerve. This cranial nerve also provides the taste fibers for most of the posterior one third of the tongue. However, the vagus nerve provides some taste fibers for the root of the tongue, vallecula, and adjacent epiglottis.

Blood Supply to the Oral Cavity

The lingual artery passes medially (deep) to the hyoglossus muscle just above the tip of the greater cornu of the hyoid bone (see Fig. 10-33). The lingual artery gives rise to a tonsillar branch to the palatine tonsil and dorsal lingual artery to the dorsum and root of the tongue. The lingual artery has a sublingual branch to the sublingual gland and then continues as the deep lingual artery (arteria profunda

linguae). This artery continues anteriorly on the inferior surface of the tongue to the tip of the tongue.

The deep lingual vein starts close to the tip of the tongue. It is very prominent under the mucous membrane on the tongue's inferior surface. The deep lingual vein is joined by the sublingual vein and follows the hypoglossal nerve laterally to the hyoglossus muscle. It is often referred to as the accompanying vein of the hypoglossal nerve (vena comitans nervi hypoglossi) or the ranine vein.

The lingual vein starts as dorsal lingual veins that drain the dorsum and side of the tongue. The lingual vein follows the lingual artery medial to the hyoglossus muscle, where it is often joined by the deep lingual vein to drain into the internal jugular vein. The deep lingual vein can also drain into the facial vein.

Paralingual or Sublingual Space

Floor of the mouth is not a term recognized by *Nomina Anatomica*. Other terms used are paralingual or sublingual fascial space. This space is located between the oral cavity's mucous membrane, which stretches from the inferior aspect of the tongue to the dental arch's gingiva as its superior boundary, and the mylohyoid muscle laterally and the genioglossal muscle medially as its inferior boundary. It is also referred to as the sublingual portion of the submandibular space (see Fig. 10-70). The submandibular space also includes the space surrounding the submandibular gland in the digastric triangle. This portion of the submandibular space is referred to as the submaxillary space. The different parts of the submandibular space communicate with each other by means of the mylohyoid cleft and with the peripharyngeal space. As such, it can serve as a pathway for infection from the mouth into the sublingual space, to the submaxillary space, to the parapharyngeal space, and even to the retropharyngeal space.

The important structures to be considered are the submandibular gland and its duct, the sublingual gland, the hypoglossal and lingual nerves, and the lingual vessels (Fig. 10-77A; see also Fig. 10-76B). Most of these structures have been discussed above or in other sections. Here, we will concentrate on several interesting relationships.

The mylohyoid cleft (see Fig. 10-32) is found between the mylohyoid and hyoglossus muscles. Each mylohyoid muscle arises from the mylohyoid line and inserts into the hyoid bone and the mylohyoid raphe. The two mylohyoid muscles together are referred to as the diaphragma oris (see Fig. 10-70).

The submandibular gland's deep lobe and duct (Wharton's duct) enter the floor of the mouth from the digastric triangle by passing through the mylohyoid cleft. The duct continues between the mylohyoid and genioglossus muscles, and then between the sublingual gland and the genioglossus muscle, until it opens onto the sublingual caruncle.

The submandibular gland is innervated by means of preganglionic parasympathetic fibers in the chorda tympani (facial nerve) that synapse in the submandibular ganglion. Postganglionic fibers run from the ganglion, which is situated

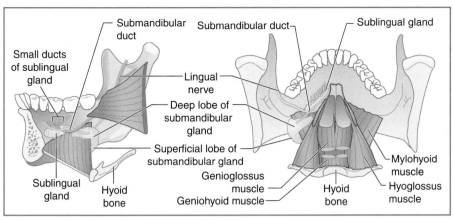

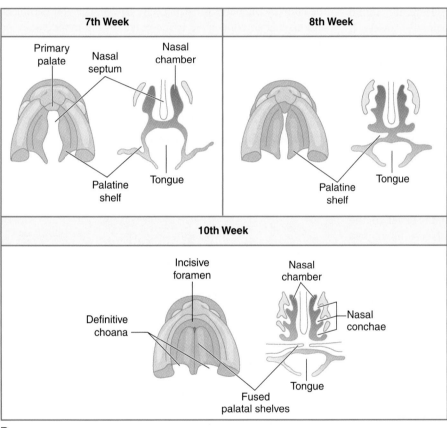

Figure 10-77. A, Floor of the mouth. **B,** Development of the palate.

below the lingual nerve, directly to the gland. Postganglionic sympathetic fibers from the superior cervical sympathetic ganglion run with the facial artery and its glandular branch and also supply the gland. Most of the blood supply is from the facial artery's glandular branch and the sublingual branch of the lingual artery.

The sublingual gland is found in the floor of the mouth. It is located between the inferior mucous membranes of the mouth and mylohyoid muscle, lateral to the genioglossus, and medial to the sublingual fossa of the body of the mandible (see Fig. 10-77A).

The superior surface of the sublingual gland raises a sublingual plica (fold) in the mucous membranes of the oral cavity alongside the inferior aspect of the tongue (see Fig. 10-75B). The sublingual plica receives the numerous small ducts (of Rivinus) from the sublingual gland. Several of the anterior ducts unite to form the sublingual duct (of Bartholin) that empties into the submandibular duct. The sublingual gland receives its autonomic innervation from the same nerves as the submandibular gland. However, the sublingual gland blood supply is from the sublingual branches of the lingual and submental arteries.

CLINICAL MEDICINE

Cleft Palate

If the palatine shelves do not fuse properly with each other, the resulting condition is called cleft palate. If the shelves do not fuse with the primary palate, cleft lip results. Cleft palate is more prevalent in females because the fusion process takes place a week later in gestation, which allows extra time for the process to be disrupted by teratogens. Retin A and the anticonvulsant phenytoin cause an increase in facial abnormalities, including cleft lip and palate.

The hypoglossal nerve enters the mylohyoid cleft inferior to the submandibular gland (see Fig. 10-32). Here, it is found between the submandibular gland and hyoglossus muscle. It continues with the deep lingual vein, inferior to the submandibular duct, on the hyoglossus muscle. Anteriorly, the nerve lies on the genioglossus muscle and communicates with the lingual nerve.

The lingual nerve enters the floor of the mouth from the infratemporal region, where it receives the chorda tympani nerve (see Fig. 10-77A). The lingual nerve emerges inferior to the superior pharyngeal constrictor muscle on the lateral side of the styloglossus muscle. Here, the lingual nerve comes into contact with the mandibular body about 1 cm below and 1 cm posterior to the last molar. The submandibular ganglion is located just inferior to the nerve at about the level of the posterior margin of the mylohyoid muscle. Nerve fibers pass between the lingual nerve and submandibular ganglion and then from the ganglion to the submandibular gland.

The lingual nerve has an interesting course as it continues in the floor of the mouth. It continues on the lateral side of the submandibular duct, then passes below the duct, and finally is found on the medial side of the duct as it passes around the submandibular duct. The lingual nerve is now medial to both the submandibular duct and sublingual gland lateral to the genioglossus muscle. The submandibular duct continues forward to end as one to three openings in the sublingual caruncle (papillae).

Development of the Palate

At the end of the second month, a partition develops between the developing nasal cavity and oral cavity. The intermaxillary process extends posteriorly into the oral cavity, forming the anterior aspect of the partition, the primary palate (see Fig. 10-77B). The posterior portion of the partition comes from the two shelf-like processes called the palatine shelves. These processes are formed from neural crest cells, which migrate into the maxillary processes. The palatine shelves initially grow inferiorly along the lateral side of the developing tongue; however, by the ninth week they rotate into a horizontal position superior to the tongue and fuse in the midline to form the secondary palate. Mesenchyme in the ventral portion of the secondary palate undergoes endochondral ossification to

form the definitive hard palate. Mesenchyme in the dorsal aspect of the secondary palate condenses to form the soft palate.

●●● NASAL CAVITY AND PHARYNX

The nose, which includes the external nose and nasal cavity, is the beginning of the respiratory tract superior to the hard palate. The external nose leads to the nasal cavity, which is continuous with the nasopharynx. The nose and nasal cavity are divided into two right and left passageways by a midline septum. The nose is the site of olfaction and is responsible for warming, filtering, and moistening the inspired air.

The external nose has an apex, dorsal surface (dorsum), and root of the nose. The nose is penetrated anteriorly beneath the apex by the nares (nostrils) (Fig. 10-78). The alar cartilages and associated connective tissue make up the mobile alae, or wings, of the nostrils.

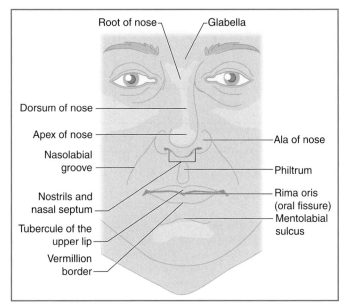

A

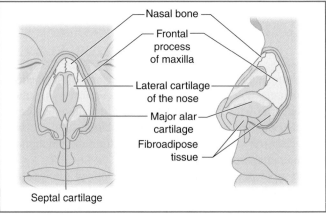

B

Figure 10-78. A, External nose. **B,** Cartilages of the nose.

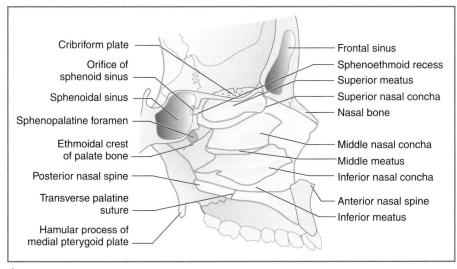

Cribriform plate
Orifice of sphenoid sinus
Sphenoidal sinus
Sphenopalatine foramen
Ethmoidal crest of palate bone
Posterior nasal spine
Transverse palatine suture
Hamular process of medial pterygoid plate

Frontal sinus
Sphenoethmoid recess
Superior meatus
Superior nasal concha
Nasal bone
Middle nasal concha
Middle meatus
Inferior nasal concha
Anterior nasal spine
Inferior meatus

A

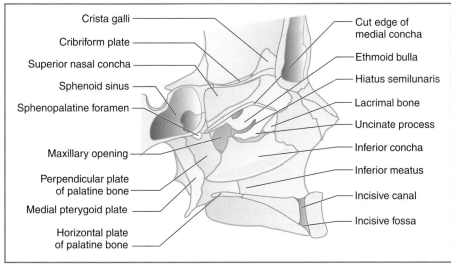

Crista galli
Cribriform plate
Superior nasal concha
Sphenoid sinus
Sphenopalatine foramen
Maxillary opening
Perpendicular plate of palatine bone
Medial pterygoid plate
Horizontal plate of palatine bone

Cut edge of medial concha
Ethmoid bulla
Hiatus semilunaris
Lacrimal bone
Uncinate process
Inferior concha
Inferior meatus
Incisive canal
Incisive fossa

B

Figure 10-79. A, Lateral wall of bony nasal cavity and adjacent regions. **B,** Bony lateral wall of the nasal cavity with superior and middle conchae cut away.

The skeleton of the nose consists of cartilage, nasal bones, frontal process of maxilla, and nasal process of frontal bones. The cartilage extends anteriorly from the nasal and frontal process of maxilla and consists of septal, paired lateral and alar nasal cartilages along with small accessory cartilages (see Fig. 10-78B).

The nose expands from the nares (nostrils) to the nasal cavity, which has a vestibule, meatuses, and choanae (posterior openings) into the nasopharynx. A meatus is a passageway, and a concha is a structure shaped like a shell. In the nasal cavity, these are parts of the ethmoid bone or, in the case of the inferior concha, a separate bone.

The bony nasal cavity consists of parts of the nasal bone; the nasal portion of the frontal, ethmoid, palatine, maxillae and sphenoid bones. The two nasal cavities are separated by a septum.

The curved roof of the bony nasal cavity consists of nasal bone, frontal bone, the cribriform plate of the ethmoid bone, and the body of the sphenoid bone, which is occupied by a

sphenoidal sinus (Fig. 10-79). Its inferior boundary is the hard palate consisting of the maxilla's palatine process and the palatine bone's horizontal process.

The medial wall consists of the nasal septum, which is formed by cartilage and bone. The bony structures are the perpendicular plate of the ethmoid, and the vomer. Smaller contributions arise from adjacent bones such as the nasal and frontal bones superiorly and the crest of the maxilla and palatine bones inferiorly. The vomer has a groove on both surfaces for the right and left nasopalatine nerves and the accompanying septal branches of the sphenopalatine arteries.

The lateral wall is irregular. It consists of parts of the nasal, lacrimal, frontal, maxilla, and ethmoid bones as well as the perpendicular plate of the palatine bone (see Fig. 10-79). Extending medially from the ethmoid are two curved processes: the superior and middle conchae. The inferior concha articulates with the maxilla and palatine bones (see Fig. 10-79).

All of the paranasal sinuses open onto the meatuses of the lateral nasal wall or into the sphenoethmoid recess. Some of these openings are small, such as the ethmoidal foramina. Others are easily observed in a bony skull or cadaver (Fig. 10-80B; see also Fig. 10-79).

The nasal surface of the maxilla is characterized by a gaping opening that becomes narrowed by the articulation of the maxilla with the palatine bone's perpendicular plate, the inferior concha, and the overlapping articulation with the ethmoid bone's hook-like uncinate process (see Fig. 10-79B). The addition of mucous membrane and periosteum changes the morphology of the lateral wall. These structures greatly narrow the original opening into the maxillary opening (see Fig. 10-79A).

With the mucoperiosteum in place, the three conchae and the meatuses become more apparent (see Fig. 10-80). However, the conchae hide most of the openings to the sinuses (Table 10-27). Just internal to the nares is the vestibule of the nose, which is marked by the presence of coarse hairs to help prevent the passage of particulate material into the nose. This leads to the antrum of the middle concha (see Fig. 10-80A). Directly inferior to each concha is a meatus, termed the superior, middle, and inferior meatuses. These passageways are associated with the entrance of the paranasal sinuses whose functions in humankind are not clear. They may play a role in the enlargement of the skull while adding proportionally less to the weight of the skull.

The sphenoethmoidal recess, which receives the opening of the sphenoid sinus, is superior to the superior concha and anterior to the sphenoid sinus. Below the superior concha is the superior meatus, which receives the opening of the posterior ethmoidal cells. Below the middle concha lies the ethmoidal bulla and hiatus semilunaris (see Figs. 10-79B and 10-80B). The ethmoidal bulla is a bulge on the ethmoid bone, while the hiatus semilunaris is found between the ethmoid bulla and uncinate process of the ethmoid bone.

The ethmoid bulla receives the openings of the anterior ethmoidal air cells, while the hiatus semilunaris may receive the opening to the frontonasal duct and the maxillary sinus. Whereas the frontonasal duct typically drains into the ethmoidal infundibulum and then into the hiatus semilunaris, the infundibulum sometimes has a blind end and the frontal sinus then empties directly into the middle meatus. The maxillary sinus often has an accessory ostium located inferior to the hiatus semilunaris.

Inferior to the inferior concha lies the exit of the nasolacrimal canal. This canal is formed by the frontal process of the maxilla, lacrimal bone, and inferior concha. It transmits the nasolacrimal duct, which is part of the lacrimal apparatus. The nasolacrimal duct drains tears from the conjunctival sac into the inferior meatus.

The sphenopalatine foramen communicates with the pterygopalatine fossa. This opening allows neurovascular bundles to enter the nasal cavity and supply the mucoperiosteum and bones of the posterior two thirds of the lateral wall and septum of the nasal cavity. The sphenopalatine foramen is found slightly superior to the posterior margin of the middle concha.

The two choanae are the posterior openings of the nasal cavities into the nasopharynx.

Innervation of the Nasal Cavity

The anterior ethmoid nerve is a branch of the nasociliary nerve. Its internal (lateral) nasal branches supply the anterosuperior third of the nasal cavity. The nasal cavity's posteroinferior two thirds is supplied by posterior lateral nasal branches of the maxillary nerve. The sense of smell is supplied by the olfactory nerve, composed of numerous neuroepithelial cells whose processes pass through the olfactory foramina of the cribriform plate to synapse in the olfactory bulb. Parasympathetic fibers reach the nasal cavity from the pterygopalatine ganglion with the maxillary nerve branches.

The internal nasal branches of the anterior ethmoidal nerve enter the nasal cavity through or adjacent to the nasal slits of the cribriform plate as lateral internal nasal and septal branches. They supply GSA fibers to the anterior third of the lateral wall and give rise to the external nasal nerve that passes between the nasal bone and lateral cartilage to reach the external nose. The septal internal nasal branches supply the anterior third of the septum (see Fig. 10-80C).

The posterosuperior lateral nasal and nasopalatine nerves pass through the sphenopalatine foramen from the pterygopalatine fossa into the nasal cavity to supply most of the sensory innervation to the posterior two thirds of the nasal cavity. The posteroinferior lateral nasal nerves, from the greater palatine nerve, supply the inferior portion of the posterior two thirds of lateral wall.

The nasopalatine branch passes across the roof of the nasal cavity close to the opening of the sphenoid air sinus and down the nasal septum to supply the posterior two-thirds of the nasal septum (see Fig. 10-80B). It then enters the incisive canal and foramen to reach the hard palate just posterior to the incisor teeth.

Facial nerve branches in the pterygopalatine fossa have already been discussed.

Blood Supply to the Nasal Cavity

The maxillary artery's sphenopalatine branch passes through the sphenopalatine foramen from the pterygopalatine fossa into the nasal cavity (see Fig. 10-80C). In life, this foramen is covered by mucoperiosteum, and the artery is in this layer of tissue along with the accompanying nerves. The sphenopalatine artery has lateral and septal branches that supply the posterior two thirds of the nasal cavity.

The septal branches of the sphenopalatine artery follow the nasopalatine nerve but do not pass through the incisive foramen with the nasopalatine nerve to reach the hard palate. Instead, branches of the greater palatine artery pass from the hard palate through the incisive canal onto the septum of the nasal cavity. Thus, the anterior portion of the nasal septum is supplied by both the septal branch of the sphenopalatine artery and the greater palatine artery. In addition, the facial artery's superior labial branch and the anterior ethmoidal artery's septal branch also anastomose with these arteries at a point on the septum located just superior to the internal end of the nasal vestibule that is referred to as Kiesselbach's

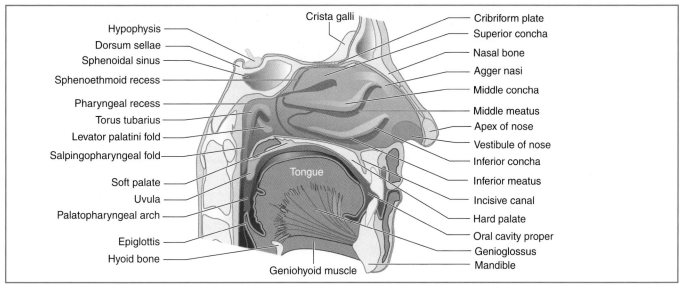

A

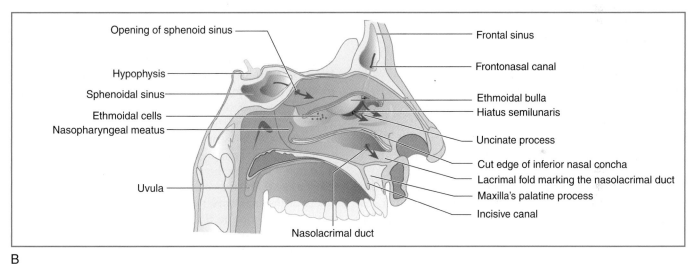

B

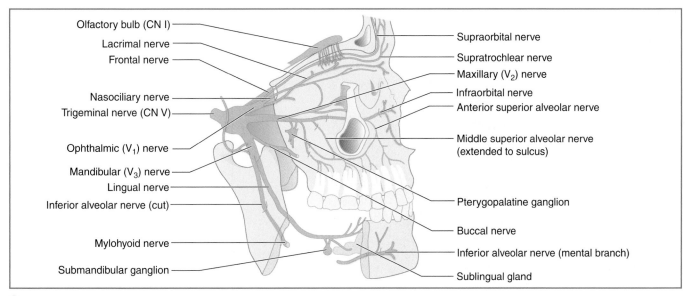

C

Figure 10-80. A, Lateral wall of the nasal cavity. **B,** Entrance of paranasal sinuses in the wall of the nasal cavity. **C,** Lateral nasal wall with branches of V_3, V_1, and CN I.

TABLE 10-27. Location of the Openings of the Sinuses and Innervation of the Mucoperiosteum

Sinus	Location of Opening	Innervation
Sphenoid	Sphenoethmoid recess	Posterior ethmoid branches of nasociliary nerve
Anterior ethmoid	Ethmoidal infundibulum, which typically ends in hiatus semilunaris	Anterior ethmoid nerves
Middle ethmoid	Ethmoid bulla	Anterior and posterior ethmoid nerves
Posterior ethmoid	Superior meatus	Posterior ethmoidal nerves
Frontonasal duct of frontal sinus	Ethmoid infundibulum or anterior to hiatus semilunaris	Supraorbital branches of CN V_1
Maxillary	Hiatus semilunaris, accessory ostium in middle meatus bellow hiatus semilunaris	Superior alveolar branches of maxillary nerve

TABLE 10-28. Boundaries of the Pharynx

Boundary	Structures
Superior	Body of sphenoid and basilar portion of occipital bones
Posterior	Buccopharyngeal and prevertebral fascia, pharyngeal constrictor muscles, and C1 to C6
Lateral	Styloid process, stylopharyngeus muscle, medial pterygoid muscle, carotid sheath and its content, and thyroid gland
Anterior	Continuous with nasal and oral cavities and larynx
Inferior	Esophagus

area. Kisselbach's area is a common site of epistaxis (nosebleed). Epistaxis often results from prolonged breathing of cold, dry air; use of anticoagulants such as aspirin or warfarin; nonsteroidal anti-inflammatory drugs; trauma to the nose; and even nose picking.

Pharynx

The pharynx is a fibromuscular tube whose anterior surface is open and continuous with the nasal cavity, oral cavity, and larynx (Fig. 10-81 and Table 10-28). The pharynx is therefore divided into a nasopharynx, oropharynx, and laryngopharynx. The pharynx is specialized to serve both deglutition and respiration, two functions that are incompatible with each other, so mechanisms are present that normally prevent these functions from occurring simultaneously.

In many respects the anterior portion of the nasopharynx can be considered a continuation of the nasal cavity. GSA fibers in the maxillary nerve's pharyngeal branch innervate the anterosuperior portion of the nasopharynx. However, the nasopharynx distal to the ostium (opening) of the pharyngotympanic (auditory) tube and the rest of the pharynx is

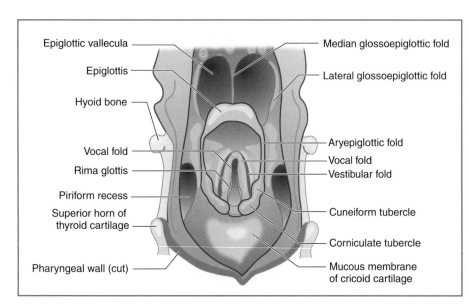

Epiglottic vallecula
Epiglottis
Hyoid bone
Vocal fold
Rima glottis
Piriform recess
Superior horn of thyroid cartilage
Pharyngeal wall (cut)

Median glossoepiglottic fold
Lateral glossoepiglottic fold
Aryepiglottic fold
Vocal fold
Vestibular fold
Cuneiform tubercle
Corniculate tubercle
Mucous membrane of cricoid cartilage

Figure 10-81. Anterolateral walls of the laryngopharynx viewed from posterior aspect.

CLINICAL MEDICINE

Transsphenoidal Pituitary Hypophysectomy

One method of gaining access to a pituitary adenoma is through the nasal cavity and nasopharynx. The superior boundary of the nasopharynx consists of the body of the sphenoid and occipital bones. The hypophyseal fossa that contains the pituitary gland is in the superior surface of the sphenoid sinus. The surgeon makes an incision in one nostril to reach the nasal cavity and then the anterior wall or roof of the nasopharynx (body of sphenoid) bone, sphenoid air sinus, and its common boundary with the sella turcica. Using minimally invasive techniques, the surgeon excises the tumor and part or all of the pituitary gland. A graft may be necessary to stop the leakage of CSF and/or blood. After surgery, the patient is assessed to determine the need for hormone replacement therapy.

CLINICAL MEDICINE

Infected Adenoids

Enlarged or infected adenoids are common in children and typically involute between the ages of 8 and 10 years. However, they may also produce nasal obstruction, mouth breathing, frequent ear or sinus infections, difficulty swallowing, and sleep apnea. The first line of treatment of infected adenoids is antibiotics. Children's adenoids may eventually shrink on their own. However, greatly enlarged or continuously infected adenoids may require surgical removal.

innervated by GVA fibers of the glossopharyngeal and vagus nerves.

The pharyngotympanic tube is marked by the torus tubarius, which is the circular terminal end of the auditory tube's cartilage. This cartilage is an upside-down C-shaped structure. The anterior end of the C-shaped cartilage has an anterior connective tissue fold running to the palate, while the posterior end of the C-shaped cartilage has the salpingopharyngeal muscular fold running to the pharynx. The salpingopharyngeal fold is produced by the salpingopharyngeus muscle (see Fig. 10-80A). The levator veli palatini muscle also makes a fold, which appears to descend inferiorly from the opening of the torus tubarius (see Fig. 10-80A). Posterior to the torus tubarius is the pharyngeal recess.

The pharyngotympanic tube connects the nasopharynx to the middle ear (tympanic cavity). When open, it equilibrates the pressure within the middle ear with that in the pharynx and therefore the environment. It is composed of cartilaginous and bony components. As they meet at a slight angle, the canal narrows. The pharyngotympanic tube is a potential path for the spread of infection from the pharynx to the middle ear. Otitis media or middle ear infection is more prevalent in very young children because their auditory tubes do not open as readily as those of adults. The inability to adequately open and ventilate the middle ear with fresh air leads to an anaerobic environment where infections may thrive. The cartilaginous portion of the tube is typically closed and opened only upon swallowing or yawning, mostly owing to the contraction of the tensor veli palatini muscle.

The pharyngeal tonsils are a group of unencapsulated lymphoid tissue associated with the mucous membrane of the posterior and superior nasopharynx. Enlargement of this lymphoid tissue especially in children is referred to as adenoids; however, this term is often used interchangeably with pharyngeal tonsil.

The oral pharynx stretches from the soft palate superiorly to the top of the epiglottis inferiorly. Most of the oropharynx has been described with the oral cavity. The oral pharynx's lateral wall was described with the oral cavity. The posterior wall is found anterior to the prevertebral fascia pharyngeal constrictor muscles, and C2 and C3 vertebrae. The oral pharynx can be isolated from the nasal cavity by the soft palate interfacing with palatopharyngeal sphincter (see Fig. 10-73).

The laryngopharynx extends from the superior border of the epiglottis to the esophagus, which begins at the cricoid cartilage's inferior border. Anterior is the laryngeal inlet (see Fig. 10-81), while posterior is the musculofascial wall and C4–C6 vertebrae. Lateral to the laryngeal inlet are the piriform recesses, which are found between the thyrohyoid membrane and thyroid lamina laterally, and the aryepiglottic fold with attached cartilages medially (see Fig. 10-81). The piriform recesses can be the site of a lodged foreign body or even swallowed pills in the aged.

The laryngopharynx narrows inferiorly to conform to the entrance to the esophagus, the cricopharyngeal sphincter. This slit-like opening at rest can enlarge to accommodate the passage of food.

The laryngeal wall consists of four layers: mucous membrane, pharyngobasilar fascia, muscles, and buccopharyngeal fascia.

The muscle layer can be described as an outer circular layer and an inner longitudinal layer. The three pharyngeal constrictors, which make up the outer layer, are arranged so that the inferior one overlaps the middle constrictor, which in turn overlaps the superior. This arrangement has been likened to three funnels or flowerpots, one inserted unto the other. Thus, the inferior pharyngeal is the most evident and the middle and superior pharyngeal constrictors less so (Fig. 10-82 and Table 10-29).

The pharyngeal constrictors are not completely circular. They arise from fixed lateral cartilaginous, ligamentous, and bony points, so they are not present anteriorly and leave spaces between them or between the superior constrictor and the skull laterally (see Fig. 10-82B). However, they are complete posteriorly to insert into the pharyngeal raphe, which extends from the pharyngeal tubercle of the occipital bone to the cricopharyngeus muscle (see Fig. 10-82B and Table 10-29).

These intervals are completed by the fascia of the pharynx, but they still allow muscles, nerves, and arteries to enter the pharyngeal wall (see Fig. 10-82A and Table 10-29). The stylo-glossus muscle accompanied by the glossopharyngeal nerve and lingual nerve pass inferiorly to the superior pharyngeal

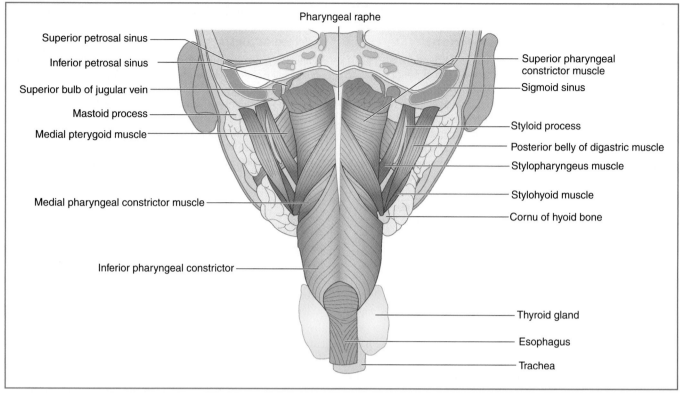

Pharyngeal raphe

Superior petrosal sinus

Inferior petrosal sinus

Superior bulb of jugular vein

Mastoid process

Medial pterygoid muscle

Medial pharyngeal constrictor muscle

Inferior pharyngeal constrictor

Superior pharyngeal constrictor muscle

Sigmoid sinus

Styloid process

Posterior belly of digastric muscle

Stylopharyngeus muscle

Stylohyoid muscle

Cornu of hyoid bone

Thyroid gland

Esophagus

Trachea

A

Continued on page 391

Figure 10-82. A, Posterior view of the pharynx.

TABLE 10-29. Muscles of the Pharynx

Muscle	Origin	Insertion	Action
Pharyngeal Constrictor Circular Muscles			
Superior pharyngeal constrictor	Side of tongue, mylohyoid line, pterygoid hamulus, pterygomandibular raphe (if present)	Pharyngeal raphe and pharyngeal tubercle	Constricts pharynx; tone aids in maintaining pharyngeal wall
Middle pharyngeal constrictor	Greater and lesser horns of hyoid bone and the stylohyoid ligament that attaches to the lesser horn	Pharyngeal raphe	
Inferior pharyngeal constrictor	Two parts (1) thyropharyngeus: the oblique line of the thyroid cartilage and a small slip from it to the inferior cornu, and; (2) cricopharyngeus: cricoid cartilage and a tendon from the thyroid cartilage to the cricoid cartilage over the cricothyroid muscle	Becomes continuous with esophageal fibers	Sphincter function at the laryngopharyngeal and esophageal junction
Longitudinally Oriented Muscles			
Palatopharyngeus	See oral cavity and pharynx		
Stylopharyngeus	Medial side of styloid process	Fibers spread out into pharyngeal wall and with palatopharyngeus into posterior border of thyroid cartilage	Elevate pharynx and larynx

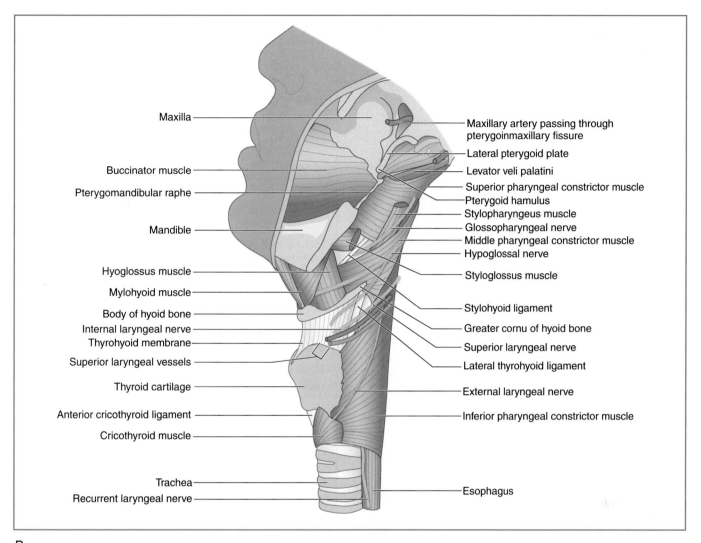

Maxilla

Maxillary artery passing through pterygoinmaxillary fissure

Lateral pterygoid plate

Levator veli palatini

Buccinator muscle

Superior pharyngeal constrictor muscle

Pterygomandibular raphe

Pterygoid hamulus

Stylopharyngeus muscle

Glossopharyngeal nerve

Mandible

Middle pharyngeal constrictor muscle

Hypoglossal nerve

Styloglossus muscle

Hyoglossus muscle

Mylohyoid muscle

Body of hyoid bone

Stylohyoid ligament

Internal laryngeal nerve

Greater cornu of hyoid bone

Thyrohyoid membrane

Superior laryngeal nerve

Superior laryngeal vessels

Lateral thyrohyoid ligament

Thyroid cartilage

External laryngeal nerve

Anterior cricothyroid ligament

Inferior pharyngeal constrictor muscle

Cricothyroid muscle

Trachea

Recurrent laryngeal nerve

Esophagus

B

Figure 10-82 cont'd. B, Lateral intervals between the pharyngeal constrictor muscles.

constrictor. The styloglossus muscle, which arises medially from the infratemporal region (Table 10-30), enters the floor of the mouth by passing through the interval between the superior and middle pharyngeal constrictors and is joined by the glossopharyngeal nerve on its external surface.

The fascia of the pharynx is thought to be derived from the epimysium of the muscle. These fascial layers are located both internally and externally to the muscle layer. The internal layer is the pharyngobasilar fascia. It is substantially thicker where it completes the spaces left on either side of the superior pharyngeal constrictor and the skull. It is attached to the base of the skull, petrous temporal bone, and laterally located structures, such as the posterior margin of the medial pterygoid plates, pterygomandibular raphe, mylohyoid line, stylohyoid ligament, hyoid bone, thyroid cartilage, and cricoid cartilage. As such, it provides a firm layer that, with the help of the muscle layer, prevents distortion and collapse of the pharyngeal wall, thereby maintaining an open airway.

The external layer of fascia is the buccopharyngeal fascia, which is continuous with the pretracheal fascia. It extends superiorly to the skull base and laterally to cover the buccinator muscle.

Innervation of the Pharynx

The muscles of the pharynx, except the stylopharyngeus and tensor veli palatini muscles, receive SVE (branchiomotor) fibers from the pharyngeal plexus, which arises from the vagus nerve but carries fibers from the cranial portion of the accessory nerve. Sympathetic fibers arise from the superior cervical sympathetic ganglion and run with the branches of the external carotid plexus and the external carotid artery's branches to the pharynx.

The sensory innervation of the nasopharynx superior and posterior to the torus tobarius is GSA fibers from the palatine branch of the maxillary nerve and the posterior nasal branches. The rest of the nasopharynx, oropharynx, and superior portion

TABLE 10-30. Lateral Intervals Between the Pharyngeal Constrictor Muscles

Description of Space	Structures Passing Through Space
Between skull and superior pharyngeal constrictor	Levator veli palatini, pharyngotympanic tube, ascending pharyngeal artery
Between superior and middle pharyngeal constrictors	Stylopharyngeus muscle and associated glossopharyngeal nerve
Between middle and inferior pharyngeal constrictors	Through thyrohyoid membrane and superior laryngeal nerve and artery
Between inferior pharyngeal constrictor and esophagus	Recurrent laryngeal nerve and inferior laryngeal artery

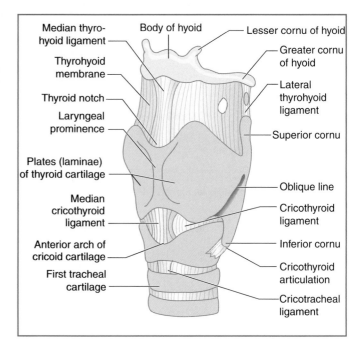

A

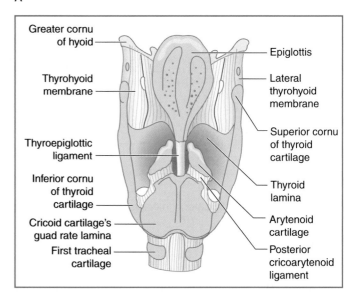

B

Figure 10-83. Anterolateral view (**A**) and posterior view (**B**) of the larynx.

of the laryngopharynx is supplied with GVA fibers from the glossopharyngeal nerve. The remainder of the laryngopharynx is supplied with GVA fibers from the internal laryngeal and recurrent laryngeal nerves.

The major blood supply to the pharynx is the ascending pharyngeal arteries and superior and inferior thyroid arteries.

●●● LARYNX

The larynx is a multifunctional organ, responsible for vocalization, speech, and singing, and it is a sphincter of the respiratory system, especially during swallowing. The larynx is anterior to the laryngopharynx, prevertebral fascia, and C3–C6 vertebrae. It is superficially placed anteriorly in the midline, just internally to the skin and fascia. Lateral to the midline, the larynx is also covered by the strap muscles and in part by the upper poles of the thyroid gland's lateral lobes. Directly lateral to the larynx are the carotid sheaths, their contents, and the sternomastoid muscles. The laryngeal inlet extends from the laryngopharynx to the laryngeal cavity, which starts at the aryepiglottic folds (see Fig. 10-81).

The larynx is made up of a cartilaginous skeleton system held together by ligaments, membranes, and muscles. This framework consists of individual cartilages (thyroid, cricoid, epiglottis) and paired cartilages (arytenoid, corniculate, and cuneiform) (Fig. 10-83).

The thyroid cartilage (see Figs. 10-38 and 10-83A) is the major cartilage of the larynx. It is composed of two laminae that meet anteriorly at an approximately 90-degree angle in the midline and are open posteriorly (see Fig. 10-83B). Many structures are attached close to this angle. The thyroid cartilage's laryngeal prominence ("Adam's apple") and thyroid notch are found at the level of the fourth cervical vertebrae. The oblique line of the thyroid cartilage is found on the body of each plate and serves as the attachment of the sternothyroid and thyrohyoid muscles.

The thyroid cartilage (see Fig. 10-83) has two pairs of hornlike projections (cornua) extending from the posterior surface of the thyroid cartilage. The superior projections (superior cornua) of the thyroid cartilage are attached to the hyoid bone by the lateral aspects of the thyrohyoid membrane (lateral thyrohyoid ligaments). The inferior projections (inferior cornua) of the thyroid cartilage articulate with the junction of the lamina and arch of the cricoid cartilage.

The cricoid cartilage (Fig. 10-84) is found at the level of the transverse process of vertebra C6. Its posterior surface (lamina) is wider than its narrow anterior arch and projects

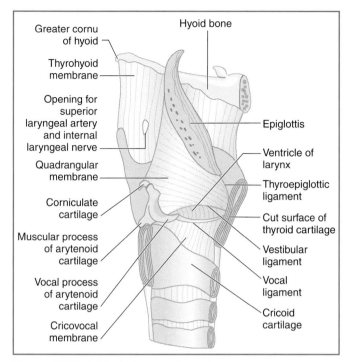

Greater cornu of hyoid

Thyrohyoid membrane

Opening for superior laryngeal artery and internal laryngeal nerve

Quadrangular membrane

Corniculate cartilage

Muscular process of arytenoid cartilage

Vocal process of arytenoid cartilage

Cricovocal membrane

Hyoid bone

Epiglottis

Ventricle of larynx

Thyroepiglottic ligament

Cut surface of thyroid cartilage

Vestibular ligament

Vocal ligament

Cricoid cartilage

Figure 10-84. Intrinsic laryngeal membranes.

superiorly inside the thyroid cartilage of the larynx. The cricoid cartilage is the only complete ring-like cartilage of the larynx and trachea, making it a likely site of obstruction of the respiratory tract by a foreign body; the rings of the trachea are found just inferior to the cricoid cartilage. The cricoid cartilage's posterior surface (quadrate lamina) is wider than its narrow anterior arch. The cricoid cartilage is relatively stable.

The epiglottis is a thin plate of elastic fibrocartilage that expands superiorly and narrows inferiorly, giving it a tear-drop shape (see Fig. 10-83). Its free end extends above the hyoid bone and tongue and forms the anterior aspect of the laryngeal inlet and posterior aspect of the epiglottic valleculae (Fig. 10-85). The stem of the epiglottis is held to the laryngeal prominence by the thyroepiglottic ligament. Laterally, the epiglottis is attached to the arytenoid cartilages by the aryepiglottic folds. These ligaments stabilize the inferior stem. They also allow the free surface a degree of flexibility, which allows it to bend posteriorly during swallowing. The bolus moves over the bent epiglottis, which covers the laryngeal inlet, and is channeled into the piriform recesses of the laryngopharynx.

The arytenoid cartilages are paired (see Fig. 10-83B). The arytenoid cartilage articulates with the posterolateral surfaces of the cricoid cartilage's quadrate lamina (see Figs. 10-83A and 10-84). Each pyramid-shaped arytenoid cartilage has an anterior vocal process and a lateral muscular process. The vocal ligament attaches to the vocal process (see Fig. 10-85A). The arytenoid cartilage swivels on the cricoid cartilage at the cricoarytenoid joint, which allows for adduction and abduction of the vocal process and therefore the vocal cord.

The intrinsic ligaments and membranes of the larynx include the quadrangular membrane and the two parts of the cricothyroid ligament, which are the anterior cricothyroid ligament and the cricovocal (conus elasticus) ligament (see Figs. 10-84 and 10-85B).

The quadrangular membrane attaches to the epiglottis and arytenoid cartilage (see Fig. 10-85B). It forms the aryepiglottic ligament, which in turn forms the core of the aryepiglottic fold (see Fig. 10-85A). Inferiorly, the quadrangular membrane has a free margin that stretches from the arytenoid cartilage to the epiglottis. It forms the vestibular ligament in the vestibular fold (see Figs. 10-84 and 10-85). The two vestibular folds are referred to as the false vocal cords. Each vestibular ligament is the lower boundary of the laryngeal vestibule (see Figs. 10-84 and 10-85). The space between the right and left vestibular folds is the rima vestibuli. A rima is a narrow opening between two symmetric parts.

The cricothyroid membrane extends from the arch of the cricoid cartilage to the inferior border of the thyroid cartilage. The cricovocal membrane (see Figs. 10-84 and 10-85) is the anterior portion of the cricothyroid membrane. It slopes superomedially to attach to the arytenoid's vocal process posteriorly and to the thyroid plate angle located anteriorly (see Fig. 10-85B). This free superior margin is thickened between these two points as the vocal ligament, which is covered by the vocal fold. The two vocal folds are the true vocal cords, and the space between them is the rima glottidis.

The laryngeal vestibule extends from the laryngeal inlet to the vestibular folds (see Fig. 10-85). The ventricles are located between the vestibular folds and the vocal folds (see Fig. 10-85).

The muscles of the larynx can be divided into extrinsic and intrinsic groups. The extrinsic muscles are muscles of the neck that elevate or depress the larynx. These include the sternohyoid, sternothyroid, and thyrohyoid, as well as the inferior pharyngeal constrictor muscle. The palatopharyngeus and stylopharyngeus elevate the thyroid cartilage while the geniohyoid muscle elevates and moves the hyoid and therefore the larynx anteriorly during swallowing.

The intrinsic muscles consist of three functional groups: muscles that act on the inlet, muscles that regulate the size of the rima glottis, and muscles that act on the vocal cords (Table 10-31; see also Fig. 10-85C). Only the posterior cricoarytenoid muscle abducts (opens) the rima glottis. All of the remaining muscles that attach to the arytenoid cartilage adduct (close) the rima glottis. The cricothyroid muscles can tense the vocal cords while the vocalis muscle fine-tunes the vocal cords by relaxing specific portions of the cords (see Fig. 10-85C).

Innervation and Blood Supply of the Larynx

The vagus nerve's superior and recurrent laryngeal branches innervate the larynx (Fig. 10-86). The superior laryngeal nerve divides into an internal and external branch. The internal laryngeal nerve (internal branch of superior laryngeal) enters the larynx by passing through the thyrohyoid membrane with the superior laryngeal artery, which is a branch of the superior

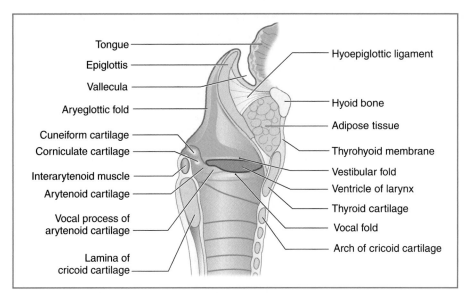

Tongue
Epiglottis
Vallecula
Aryeglottic fold
Cuneiform cartilage
Corniculate cartilage
Interarytenoid muscle
Arytenoid cartilage
Vocal process of arytenoid cartilage
Lamina of cricoid cartilage

Hyoepiglottic ligament
Hyoid bone
Adipose tissue
Thyrohyoid membrane
Vestibular fold
Ventricle of larynx
Thyroid cartilage
Vocal fold
Arch of cricoid cartilage

A

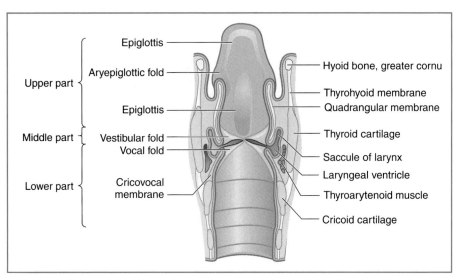

Upper part
Epiglottis
Aryepiglottic fold
Epiglottis

Middle part
Vestibular fold
Vocal fold

Lower part
Cricovocal membrane

Hyoid bone, greater cornu
Thyrohyoid membrane
Quadrangular membrane
Thyroid cartilage
Saccule of larynx
Laryngeal ventricle
Thyroarytenoid muscle
Cricoid cartilage

B

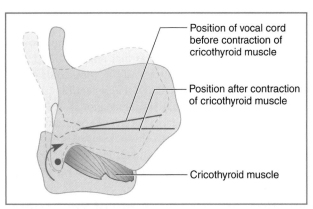

Position of vocal cord before contraction of cricothyroid muscle

Position after contraction of cricothyroid muscle

Cricothyroid muscle

C

Figure 10-85. A, Interior of the larynx. **B,** Coronal section of the larynx demonstrating the cricothyroid and cricovocal. **C,** Cricothyroid muscle tilting downward and forward to relax vocal cords.

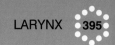

TABLE 10-31. Intrinsic Muscles of the Larynx

Muscle	Origin	Insertion	Action
Muscles That Act on the Laryngeal Inlet			
Thyroepiglottic	Fibers from posterior surface of thyroid cartilage	Epiglottis	Depresses base of epiglottis
Aryepiglottic	Located in aryepiglottic fold, from apex of the arytenoid cartilage	Epiglottis	Pulls the epiglottis posteriorly and tenses the aryepiglottic folds to act as a weak sphincter
Muscles That Act on the Rima Glottidis			
Lateral cricoarytenoid	Arch of the cricoid cartilage	Muscular process of ipsilateral arytenoid cartilage	Pulls muscular process of arytenoid cartilage anteriorly, so that process pivots medially, adducting the vocal folds
Posterior cricoarytenoid	Posterior surface of the lamina of the cricoid cartilage quadrilateral plate	Muscular process of arytenoid cartilage	Pulls muscular process of arytenoid cartilage so that it pivots laterally, abducting the vocal folds
Transverse (inter) arytenoid	Unpaired muscle, arises from posterior surface and lateral border of the arytenoid cartilage	Posterior surface and lateral border of contralateral arytenoid cartilage	Pulls arytenoid cartilages together, adducting the vocal folds
Oblique arytenoid	Muscular process of arytenoids	Crosses posterior surface obliquely to apex of contralateral arytenoid cartilage	Pulls arytenoid cartilages together, adducting the vocal folds narrowing inlet
Muscles That Act on the Vocal Cords			
Thyroarytenoid	Posterior surface of thyroid cartilage and adjacent cricothyroid ligament	Anterolateral surface of arytenoid cartilage	Pulls arytenoid cartilage to thyroid cartilage, relaxing and adducting vocal cords
Vocalis	Medial fibers of thyroarytenoid, stretches from thyroid cartilage	Vocal ligament and vocal process of arytenoid cartilage	Shortens and relaxes parts of vocal cord
Cricothyroid	Cricoid cartilage and its arch	Inferior cornu of thyroid cartilage and its posteroinferior lamina	Tilts thyroid cartilage anteriorly and inferiorly, stretching the vocal cords and increasing pitch

thyroid artery. The internal laryngeal nerve carries sensory (GVA) fibers to the larynx above the vocal cords for the sensory arm of the cough reflex that clears the larynx and some autonomic fibers to the glands of the larynx. The internal laryngeal nerve also contains taste (SVA) fibers to the epiglottis and adjacent root of the tongue.

The external laryngeal nerve (external branch of superior laryngeal) runs with the superior thyroid artery (see Fig. 10-82B). As the two approach the superior pole of the thyroid gland, they diverge. The external laryngeal nerve passes anteroinferior with the superior thyroid artery to innervate the cricothyroid muscle (tensing the vocal cords) and a small portion of the inferior pharyngeal constrictor muscle, the cricopharyngeus muscle (see Fig. 10-82B).

The recurrent laryngeal nerve supplies all of the other intrinsic muscles of the larynx. It enters the larynx with the inferior laryngeal artery, which is a branch of the inferior thyroid artery (see Fig. 10-86). The recurrent laryngeal nerve provides branchiomotor (SVE) and sensory fibers to all the intrinsic muscles of the larynx except the cricothyroid muscle. The GSA fibers provide proprioception from these muscles, and general visceral sensory (GVA) fibers provide general sensation below the vocal cords.

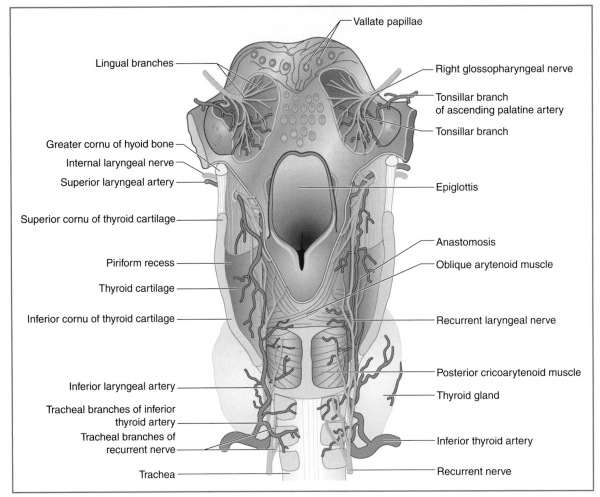

Figure 10-86. Laryngeal neurovascular bundles.

CLINICAL MEDICINE

Injury to the Superior Laryngeal Nerve

When one of the recurrent laryngeal nerves is injured, the denervated vocal cord is found in a paramedian plane but not totally adducted to the midline. The transverse arytenoid receives its innervation from both recurrent laryngeal muscles. When one recurrent nerve is involved, the voice becomes breathy because phonation requires adduction of both vocal cords. In most cases of involvement of one recurrent nerve, the voice eventually gets better because of compensation of the contralateral vocal cord. However, if both vagus nerves are involved, then the vocal cords may lie in the midline, thereby completely blocking respiration.

Loss of the external laryngeal nerve produces a qualitative change in the voice. Normally, the cricothyroid muscle lengthens the vocal cord and causes the cord to tense, which increases the voice's pitch. Loss of the cricothyroid muscle causes a reduction in the ability to tense the vocal cord, leaving it somewhat shortened and flaccid. The voice is weak and easily fatigued, the pitch is lower, and the singing voice is diminished or lost.

Concurrent loss of the internal laryngeal branch of the superior laryngeal nerve results in a sensory deficit on the involved side affecting the afferent arm of the cough reflex. The patient coughs more to clear the aditus (laryngeal inlet).

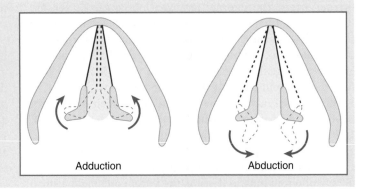

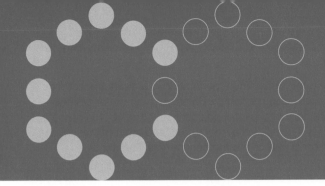

Case Studies

CASE STUDY 1: Shingles

A 76-year-old man saw his physician because of a sharp pain in his left chest. Since he has hypertension, he is worried about a heart attack. In discussing his symptoms, the patient indicates that the pain started about 2 days ago as a vague tingling, itchy feeling and progressed to a sharp, stabbing pain on the skin. The pain is localized to a strip or band of skin at the level of his left nipple and slightly above. The man was able to take a deep breath but with considerable discomfort. He did not appear to have any muscle weakness.

Upon physical examination followed by an ECG, there was no sign of heart disease. The physician decides that the patient most likely has shingles and prescribes acyclovir to try to reduce the intensity of this viral disease. About 3 days later, the patient developed a painful rash that was distributed to a strip or band of skin on the left side of his thoracic wall. This is an important sign that the patient has shingles, produced by the varicella-zoster virus, which also causes chickenpox (see Chapter 2).

1. What type of pain did the patient have?

2. How did the location of the rash verify the physician's diagnosis?

3. Which one of the following categories of neuronal cell bodies is infected by the varicella-zoster virus (choose one): somatic motor, somatic sensory, preganglionic parasympathetic, postganglionic parasympathetic, preganglionic sympathetic, postganglionic sympathetic?

4. For each of the following symptoms list (1) the appropriate category of involved neuron and (2) the location of its cell bodies.

   a. Paralysis and atrophy of skeletal muscles

   b. Hot and dry skin with no pain or cutaneous loss of sensation

   c. Loss of sensation

CASE STUDY 2: Bacterial Meningitis

A 3-year-old child returned home from preschool with fever, headache, lethargy, a stiff neck, nausea, and vomiting. Her parents, being worried about her health, immediately sought medical help at a nearby emergency room. The child was isolated and examined. The concern was that the child had meningitis. Viral meningitis is usually self-limiting, but bacterial meningitis is life threatening. The sequelae (symptoms that evolve over time) include fever, headache, altered mental status (confusion and lethargy), photophobia, rash, stiff neck, nausea, and vomiting, especially in children. Many of these symptoms may be due to increased intracranial pressure and inflamed sensory nerves (see Chapter 3).

The patient often but not always has some or all of the above symptoms. Neck stiffness occurs in the great majority of bacterial meningitis cases.

1. Why are Brudzinski's and Kernig's signs painful and therefore significant signs of bacterial meningitis?

2. Where is the bacterial infection, and how does it cause pain?

3. How would you obtain a sample for culture and white cell count?

4. Where would you perform this procedure?

5. Which landmarks would you use to determine the correct location to obtain your sample?

6. What are the risks if you do not choose the correct location?

CASE STUDY 3: Coronary Heart Disease

A 58-year-old man who is overweight and has a sedentary lifestyle complains of pressure-like, retrosternal pain that tends to move down the inside of his left arm. The pain appears when the man walks up stairs or exercises but subsides upon rest.

The patient seeks medical help. His physician diagnoses angina pectoris. During a subsequent attack, the pain increases in severity and duration and does not ease with rest. The patient goes to the emergency room, where he complains that the pain has become unbearable. He also has cold sweats, nausea, vomiting, and shortness of breath. Sublingual nitroglycerin relieves the symptoms, but the patient is admitted to the coronary care unit for observation.

Blood chemistries are performed. Levels of creatine phosphokinase, lactose dehydrogenase, troponin I, and troponin T are measured and are found to be normal.

The diagnosis is atherosclerotic coronary artery disease. Coronary angiography reveals incomplete obstruction of three major coronary vessels (see Chapter 4).

1. **Considering your knowledge of the circulation of the heart, which three vessels probably are involved?**

2. **If only the patient's right coronary artery was occluded, which parts of the heart would not be receiving proper blood supply?**

3. **If the posterior interventricular artery was occluded, which valve most likely would be affected?**

4. **What are creatine phosphokinase, lactate dehydrogenase, troponin I, and troponin T, and where are they found?**

5. **Why does the patient feel pain down the inside of his left arm?**

6. **Why does nitroglycerin relieve his symptoms?**

CASE STUDY 4: Peptic Ulcer Disease (PUD)

Peptic ulcers occur in both the first and second parts of the duodenum (duodenal ulcers) and stomach (gastric ulcers). However, they are more commonly found in the duodenum. The single most common symptom is dyspepsia (upset stomach), which is characterized by epigastric pain, often with a burning, gnawing sensation and nausea. These symptoms can be aggravated by fasting and relieved by eating or by antacids in some but not all individuals. Thus, these symptoms are not specific or sensitive enough to be critical diagnostic criteria for PUD.

Asymptomatic ulcers have been found in people who were taking nonsteroidal anti-inflammatory drugs (NSAIDs). Indeed, NSAIDs are a contributing factor along with *Helicobacter pylori*. Since most patients with PUD are infected with *H. pylori*, endoscopy with biopsy for this microorganism is diagnostic for most patients.

Although uncommon, perforation is a distinct possibility. An ulcer located in the first part of the duodenum or stomach may perforate to involve adjacent structures or regions. Most ulcers are found in the duodenum, and most of these are in the anterior wall of the duodenum (see Chapter 5).

1. **Name the structure(s) and region(s) that could be involved by an anterior perforation of the duodenum bulb.**

2. **Name the structure(s) and region(s) that could be involved by a posterior perforation of the duodenal bulb.**

3. **Name the structure(s) and region(s) that could be involved by a posterior perforation of the of the stomach's wall.**

4. **Name the structures that could be involved by an anterior perforation of the stomach.**

5. **If the gastric ulcer occurs at the gastric incisure (notch). What structures could be involved?**

6. **Hemorrhage is the most common cause of death in PUD patients. Which type of perforation is most likely to produce this hemorrhage?**

7. **A perforation can produce a direct communication between the stomach and the peritoneal cavity, allowing contents of the GI tract to enter the peritoneal cavity. What are the potential accompanying complications and symptoms?**

CASE STUDY 5: Renal Calculus

A 44-year-old woman enters the emergency room with the help of her husband at 5 AM. When the ER physician was taking her history, she indicated that she was nauseated, and she vomited. After vomiting, her pain was reduced but not eliminated. The patient went to bed, thinking that she had a bad flu. The pain persisted with chills, fever, and the need to urinate but with dysuria (difficulty in urinating).

When asked to locate the pain, the patient points to the right flank (side of the back from the 12th rib to the third lumbar vertebra). She indicates that the pain started in her back but got worse and also began to shoot down her side into her groin.

She has had no other recent illness. Although she has a fever of 101°F, her vital signs are normal. Physical examination of the abdomen revealed distention with considerable costovertebral tenderness.

The patient's urine was dark with the color indicating blood in her urine (hematuria). The ER physician ordered a CT scan that demonstrated a kidney stone (renal calculus) in the ureter at the brim of the pelvis (see Chapter 6).

1. Where can kidney stones typically obstruct the flow of urine?

2. Why is the costovertebral region tender to palpation?

3. Which dermatomes are involved in pain from the loin or the groin pain?

4. Which nerves are involved in referred pain from the kidney or from the ureter?

5. A patient would perceive the pain as coming from which structures in the female groin or in the male groin?

6. Where is the obstruction? What is your reasoning?

CASE STUDY 6: Testicular Cancer

A 28-year-old male goes to his physician because he noticed a small lump in his right testicle 3 weeks ago. It is not painful, but he is concerned. The physician immediately orders blood tests and an ultrasound of the scrotum. Ultrasound confirms the presence of an intratesticular mass. Examination reveals elevated levels of three proteins: β-human chorionic gonadotropin (β-hCG), lactate dehydrogenase, and α-fetoprotein.

A diagnosis of testicular cancer is made, and the patient is sent for a radiograph of the chest and CT scan of the abdomen (see Chapter 7).

1. What is the purpose of the radiograph of the chest and CT scan of the abdomen?

2. What is the embryologic explanation for the lymphatic drainage?

3. During surgical removal of the affected testicle, which arteries must be ligated?

4. If in the process of surgical removal of the right testicle, cancerous cells are seeded to the scrotum, where would these cells metastasize to?

5. Some patients also have sensitivity of the breasts. How can this be explained?

6. What is the largest risk factor for testicular cancer?

CASE STUDY 7: Compartment Syndrome

A 43-year-old construction worker was brought to the emergency room after falling from a scaffold. He has a compound fracture of the right leg. Radiographs reveal that both the right tibia and fibula are broken in the mid-shaft region. He is prepared for surgery, and the orthopedist repairs the leg by inserting a rod into the tibia.

The next day some alarming symptoms develop. The patient has difficulty dorsiflexing the toes on his right foot against resistance, and he has decreased sensation in the first dorsal web space.

These symptoms are characteristic for a serious complication known as compartment syndrome. Compartment syndrome is defined as increased pressure within a small confined space that compromises the circulation and function of tissues within that space. If the pressure becomes too high, the muscle tissue becomes ischemic, and any neural tissue present can be affected (see Chapter 8).

1. On the basis of the symptoms described, which compartment is involved?

2. How could the circulation to the compartment be assessed?

3. What symptoms would you anticipate if one of the other two compartments was involved?

4. Why is the leg particularly susceptible to compartment syndrome?

CASE STUDY 8: Separation of the Shoulder

A 45-year-old woman fell down a flight of stairs and in addition to extensive bruising noticed impairment of her left upper extremity. Radiographs revealed no fractures. However, the examining physician noted the following signs: her arm was extended at the elbow, adducted, and internally rotated. The physician also noted sensory loss to the lateral aspect of the arm, forearm, and hand (see Chapter 9).

1. Paralysis or weakness of what muscles might explain the extended elbow?

2. Which nerve(s) provide innervation to these muscles?

3. Paralysis or weakness of what muscles might explain the adducted arm?

4. Which nerve(s) provide innervation to these muscles?

5. Paralysis or weakness of what muscles might explain the internally rotated arm?

6. Which nerve(s) provide innervation to these muscles?

7. Which nerves are responsible for the sensory loss noted by the physician?

8. What do all these nerves have in common?

9. How might you discriminate between an injury that simply stretches the upper portion of the brachial plexus and one that involves the actual avulsion (pulling out) of the upper roots of the brachial plexus?

Case Study 9: Facial Nerve Palsy

A 19-year-old male goes to his college health clinic with symptoms of a runny nose, an earache, and a cold (see Chapter 10).

1. What would you examine, and why?

2. If there were signs of inflammation in the pharynx, how would infection travel from the nasopharynx to the middle ear?

3. Upon further questioning, the patient revealed that he seemed to have some dryness of his right eye. After finding no signs of infection, the physician asked the patient to blink several times. What is this procedure testing? What other muscles would you test and what are your expected results? Why was there some dryness of the right eye?

4. However, the facial muscle deficits were not accompanied by any signs of ear infection or loss of facial sensation. Vision, as tested with a Swellen chart, was normal when the patient wore his glasses. Which parts of the face are tested for cutaneous sensation? How would you test for motor function of the mandibular nerve?

5. What test would you use to determine if cranial nerves III, IV, and VI were involved?

6. After considering the results of the history and physical examination, especially considering the pain in the ear without any signs of inflammation, the physician suspected facial nerve palsy and prescribed a regimen of prednisone and acyclonic treatment. A blood sample was drawn, and the patient was asked to return for a follow-up visit. What was the purpose of the blood test, and what was the possible etiology of the facial nerve palsy that suggested this regimen?

7. What other symptoms could accompany facial nerve palsy?

8. How would the finding that the defect involved only muscles of the face below the orbit without any of the other symptoms be explained?

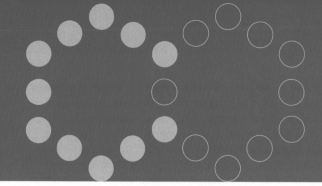

Case Study Answers

CASE STUDY 1: Shingles

1. Because the pain was highly localized to the chest wall and not diffuse or found somewhere else on the body wall, it was most likely somatic pain. Visceral pain from the heart was not suggested by the location of the pain and was subsequently ruled out by the physical examination and ECG. Although cardiac pain can be sharp, it is typically diffuse and may radiate to other parts of the body wall.

2. The rash was confined to one or two bands, or strips, of skin on the left side only. The rash stopped at the midline. These strips of skin correspond to dermatomes. A cutaneous infection would not be restricted to one side or to one or two dermatomes. The varicella-zoster virus can lie dormant in the cell body of a neuron; once activated, it migrates along the axon of the sensory neuron, producing the sensory disorders until it reaches the skin and produces the eruptions.

3. Somatic sensory.

4a. GSE; ventral horn of the spinal cord.

4b. GVE; postganglionic sympathetic chain ganglia.

4c. GSA; dorsal root ganglia.

CASE STUDY 2: Bacterial Meningitis

1. Brudzinski's sign: Involuntary flexion at the knee and hip produces a net reduction of stretch on the sciatic nerve (whose roots are L4, L5, S1–S3), which in turn reduces tension on the lumbosacral spinal meninges. Kernig's sign: The test is considered positive if it elicits pain in neck, head, or back that can be relieved by hip and knee flexion. Hip and knee extension stretches the lumbosacral meninges. The patient cannot fully extend the knee because of pain.

2. The microorganisms are in the cerebrospinal fluid in the subarachnoid space. They produce an inflammation of the meninges that also affects the spinal nerve root and some of the cranial nerves.

3. The gold standard for bacterial meningitis diagnosis is lumbar puncture and culture of the cerebrospinal fluid.

4. Since the spinal cord ends at vertebral level L1–L2 and the dural and arachnoid end at the level of S2, the subarachnoid space is enlarged between L2 and S2 as the lumbar cistern.

5. Lumbar puncture is typically done at spinal levels L4–L5 or L3–L4. The key is to locate the L3–L4 interspace by using an imaginary line from the one iliac crest to the contralateral iliac crest. This line passes through the spine of L4 vertebrae.

6. In a child of this age, there could be an increased risk of damage to the spinal cord at the level of L2.

CASE STUDY 3: Coronary Heart Disease

1. Right coronary, left anterior descending, and circumflex arteries.

2. Typically SA node, AV node, wall of right atrium, wall of right ventricle, and posterior third of the interventricular septum.

3. Mitral valve.

4. These enzymes all are found in various organs including muscle. However, the isozymes tested to diagnose a heart attack are specific for myocardium. Their levels would be elevated following a myocardial infarction. However, the levels of some of the isoenzymes appear early and others later; troponin I and T and CK-MB are elevated within hours and LDH within 2–3 days. This allows for the determination of the time and severity of the infarct. Since this patient's isozyme levels are in the normal range, he has not suffered a myocardial infarction.

5. This region (dermatomes) of the upper arm has its neuronal cell bodies located in the same dorsal root ganglion (T1–T2) and synapsing in the same spinal cord segments (T1–T2) as the general visceral sensory fibers from the heart. These axons converge on the same second-order neurons in the involved spinal cord segments. The CNS cannot clearly discern whether the

pain is from the body wall or the viscera (heart). The heart also receives sensory fibers from spinal cord segments T3 and T4. General visceral sensory fibers for pain usually follow the sympathetic innervation of the thoracic and abdominal organs.

6. Nitroglycerin is a vasodilator and can be absorbed through the mucous membranes of the inferior surface of the tongue and adjacent tissues. This allows for immediate delivery of this vasodilator to the circular system and coronary arteries.

CASE STUDY 4: Peptic Ulcer Disease (PUD)

1. The right lobe of the liver and the adjacent biliary tree, and the peritoneal cavity.

2. The bile duct and the gastroduodenal artery and its branches, such as the right gastroepiploic artery, posterior superior pancreaticoduodenal artery, and head of the pancreas.

3. Pancreas and lesser peritoneal sac.

4. Liver, adjacent biliary tree, and greater peritoneal sac. Rarely a fistula can form between the duodenum and common bile duct, or between the stomach and transverse colon.

5. Right and or left gastric vessels and possibly the adjacent anterior vagal branches to the pylorus.

6. Posterior perforation of the duodenal bulb involves the gastroduodenal artery or one of its branches. The perforation at the incisure also could involve the gastric vessels.

7. The patient would have sudden, severe epigastric pain that could spread to the rest of the abdomen owing to acute peritonitis. If it spread via the right paracolic gutter, then the pain would also be localized in the right lower quadrant.

CASE STUDY 5: Renal Calculus

1. Obstructing kidney stones can be found at the ureteropelvic junction (junction of the renal pelvis and ureter), at the brim of the pelvis, and in the intramural portion of the ureter (the portion in the wall of the bladder).

2. The patient had chills and fever, indicating the presence of a secondary infection. Pyelonephritis is an infection of the kidney and renal pelvis that often produces flank and costovertebral angle tenderness. The pain is elicited by pressing on the costovertebral angle. The pain is most likely due to the location of the subcostal nerve posterior to the swollen kidney.

3. The involved dermatomes are T11 and T12 for the loin and L1 for the groin. Pain does *not* appear in the tenth thoracic dermatome, which includes the umbilicus.

4. General visceral afferent fibers from the kidney and ureter travel with the sympathetic nerves back to the spinal cord. The sympathetics to the kidney and superior portion of the ureter arise in spinal cord segments T10–T12, while the lower portion of the ureter is supplied by sympathetics arising in spinal cord segment L1. Therefore, the pain is referred to the dermatomes corresponding to these spinal cord segments.

5. Structures that are supplied by lumbar spinal nerve L1. In the female groin, the involved structures would be the labium majus and adjacent thigh. In the male groin, the involved structures would be the scrotum, sometimes the base of penis, and adjacent thigh. These structures receive their sensory innervation from L1.

6. Initially with flank pain the obstruction is in the calices or the ureteropelvic junction. With groin pain, the renal calculus is typically in the lower ureter, where the ureter crosses the pelvic brim or in the intramural portion of the ureter.

CASE STUDY 6: Testicular Cancer

1. Testicular cancer can spread very quickly. Tumor cells of the testes typically metastasize to the lumbar lymph nodes near the renal vessels. The radiograph of the chest and CT scan can show evidence of metastases to the lymph nodes and other organs in the region.

2. The testes begin development in the lower thoracic region and then descend to their final location in the scrotum. Thus, their lymphatic drainage and blood supply reflect their more superior location earlier in life.

3. The testes are supplied by the testicular artery, the artery of the vas deferens, and the cremasteric artery, so branches of all three must be ligated.

4. The lymphatic drainage of the scrotum is to the superficial inguinal lymph nodes, not to the lumbar lymph nodes.

5. Normal males have no circulating β-hCG. Some testicular cancers, nonseminomas, are correlated with elevated levels of hCG, which causes enlargement and tenderness of breast tissue.

6. Cryptorchidism is the largest risk factor. Even after undescended testes are surgically moved into the scrotum, it remains the largest risk factor.

CASE STUDY 7: Compartment Syndrome

1. The dorsiflexors of the toes are located in the anterior compartment of the leg. They receive their motor innervation from the deep peroneal nerve. The deep peroneal nerve also provides sensory innervation to the first dorsal web space; therefore, loss of sensation to that region also points to the anterior compartment.

2. The anterior tibial artery supplies the anterior compartment. It becomes superficial in the area of the dorsum of the foot, where it changes its name to dorsalis pedis. Therefore, the physician can check for a pulse in this region.

3. If the lateral compartment were involved, the symptoms would be weakness of eversion of the ankle and loss of sensation over the dorsum and lateral side of the foot with the exception of the first dorsal web space. If the posterior compartment were involved, there would be weakness in plantar-flexion.

4. The deep fascia of the leg is particularly dense and unyielding. Under normal circumstances, this facilitates venous return because muscle contraction pushes against the veins, since the compartments cannot expand. However, under abnormal conditions, it can quickly compromise the proper functioning of the neurovascular structures within the compartment.

CASE STUDY 8: Separation of the Shoulder

1. Active flexion of the elbow requires the action of the biceps brachii, brachialis, and brachioradialis.

2. The musculocutaneous nerve provides innervation to the biceps brachii, brachialis, and brachioradialis. The radial nerve provides innervation to brachioradialis and a small part of the brachialis muscle.

3. Active abduction of the arm requires the action of the deltoid, supraspinatus, and serratus anterior.

4. The axillary nerve provides innervation to the deltoid muscle. The suprascapular nerve provides innervation to the supraspinatus muscle, and the long thoracic nerve innervates the serratus anterior.

5. The teres minor and the infraspinatus muscles are responsible for lateral rotation of the arm.

6. The axillary nerve innervates the teres minor muscle, and the suprascapular nerve innervates the infraspinatus muscle.

7. The lateral arm is supplied by the axillary nerve; the lateral forearm by the lateral antebrachial cutaneous nerve, which is the terminal portion of the musculocutaneous nerve; and the lateral portion of the hand by branches of the median and radial nerves.

8. They are all derived from spinal cord levels C5 and C6, which indicate that this is an injury to the upper portion of the brachial plexus. This can happen when there is a forceful separation of the shoulder from the laterally deviated head, as might happen in a tumble down a flight of stairs or from being thrown from a motorcycle.

9. Since the long thoracic nerve (nerve to the serratus anterior) arises from the roots of the brachial plexus, the physician should test the serratus anterior by itself by asking the patient to push against the wall and looking for winging of the scapula.

CASE STUDY 9: Facial Nerve Palsy

1. The external and middle ear, oral and nasal pharynx, and horizontal chain of lymph nodes, looking for signs of bacterial or viral infection. In this case, all appeared to be normal.

2. Via the pharyngotympanic (auditory) tube.

3. The physician is testing the muscles of facial expression starting with the orbicularis oculi and the other muscles of facial expression. Weakness of the orbicularis oris was noted (some inability to smile on this right side), and upon further examination there was weakness of the orbicularis oculi (weakness in closing the eye) and frontalis (wrinkling the forehead) muscles. There was some dryness of the eye because the orbicularis oculi spreads the tear film.

4. Ophthalmic nerve (forehead), maxillary nerve (cheek under lower eyelid, sensory component of mandibular nerve (chin), and C2–C3 spinal nerves, which provide cutaneous sensation over the angle of the mandible. The cornea can be tested with a wisp of cotton. To test the muscle of mastication, the patient is asked to protrude the chin and move it to the right and left against resistance.

5. Have the patient follow your fingers in the cardinal fields of gaze. In this case, this procedure indicated that cranial nerves VI, V, and VI were not involved.

6. To test for varicella-zoster virus, which can cause facial nerve palsy.

7. There could be a change in hearing (hyperacusis, or an increase in hearing, most obvious when using a telephone, is due to loss of innervation to the stapedius muscle), diminished submandibular and sublingual gland salivation and taste on the anterior two-thirds of the tongue due to loss of chorda tympani to the submandibular ganglion, and loss of lacrimation and drying of the nasal cavity on the affected side due to loss of innervation of the lacrimal gland and nasal glands innervated by branches of the pterygopalatine ganglion, which is supplied by the greater petrosal nerve.

8. An upper motor neuron lesion would result in only a partial facial nerve lesion because the frontalis and orbicularis oculi muscles receive bilateral upper motor neurons to both facial motor nuclei. This could be due to a cerebrovascular accident or an infarct.

Index

Page numbers followed by f indicate figures; those followed by t indicate tables; and those followed by b indicate boxed material.

A

Abdomen, 77–126
 blood supply to, 134f
 cross-section of, 121f, 132f
 inguinal region of, 85–90
 innervation of, 98–99, 98b
 pain in, 98–99, 98b
 versus pelvis, 141–142
 peritoneum in. *See* Peritoneum.
 structures of, 134f. *See also specific organs, eg,* Esophagus; Pancreas; Stomach.
  congenital abnormalities of, 125–126, 125f
  development of, 99–102, 123–236
 wall of. *See* Abdominal wall.
Abdominal wall
 anterior, 78–85
  bony components of, 79–80, 81f
  fascia of, 79, 80f–82f, 82, 83t, 86f
  inguinal region of, 85, 86f
  innervation of, 83–85, 84f
  layers of, 79–80, 80f, 81f
  ligaments of, 83, 83f, 83t
  muscles of, 80–85, 80f–84f
  quadrants of, 78, 78f, 79t
  regional divisions of, 78, 78f, 79t
  skin of, 79
  vasculature of, 84f, 85
 versus pelvic wall, 142
 posterior, 127–140. *See also* Kidney.
  blood supply to, 134f, 137–139, 138t, 139f, 139t
  bones of, 127, 128f
  lymphatic system of, 139–140, 140t
  muscles of, 127, 128f, 129t. *See also* Diaphragm.
  nervous system of, 128f, 136–137, 137t
  structures in, 127, 128f
  suprarenal gland in, 128f, 131, 131f, 134f, 135–136, 136t
  ureter in, 130f, 134f, 135, 153f
Abdominopelvic cavity, 141–142
Abducent nerve (VI), 313f, 315, 315f, 316, 349f, 350, 358f
Abduction
 of eye, 351–353, 351f, 352f, 353t
 of hand, 281, 282f
 of shoulder, 246, 246f
Abductor digiti minimi muscle
 of lower limb, 227f, 233, 233f, 234t, 235f, 239f
 of upper limb, 283, 284f, 285f, 285t
Abductor hallucis muscle, 213t, 233, 233f, 234t, 235f, 239f
Abductor pollicis brevis muscle, 282–283, 284f, 284t
Abductor pollicis longus muscle, 274, 275t, 276f, 278f, 281, 282f, 283
Abductor pollicis longus tendon, 279f
Abductor pollicis muscle, 284f
Abscess, ischioanal, 189b
Accessory duct (of Santorini), 121
Accessory hemiazygos vein, 73, 74f

Accessory nodes, 344
Accessory renal arteries, 133
Acetabular fossa, 197, 198f
Acetabular labrum, 197
Acetabular notch, 197, 198f
Acetabulum, 142–144, 143f, 197
Achilles tendon, 213t, 225
Acoustic (auditory) meatus, 293f, 297f, 299, 299t
Acromial end, of clavicle, 246, 246f
Acromioclavicular joint, 248–249, 249f
Acromion, 247, 247f, 249f, 254f
Action potential, in nodes of Ranvier, 12b
Adam's apple (thyroid cartilage), 322, 323f, 343, 391f, 392–393, 392f, 394f, 396f
Adduction
 of eye, 351–353, 351f, 352f, 353t
 of hand, 281, 282f
 of shoulder, 246, 246f
Adductor brevis muscle, 211f, 212f, 213t, 219f
Adductor canal, 212f, 216–217, 218f
Adductor (medial) compartment, of thigh, 209, 210f, 211, 212f, 213t
Adductor hallucis muscle, 234t, 236, 236f, 239f
Adductor hiatus, 210, 212f, 214f, 216–217, 219f
Adductor longus muscle, 209, 210f–212f, 213t, 219f
Adductor magnus muscle, 203f, 209, 211f, 213t, 214f, 218f, 219f
Adductor pollicis brevis muscle, 284f
Adductor pollicis fascia, 282
Adductor pollicis muscle, 283, 285f, 288f
Adductor tubercle, 206
Adenoids, 389, 389b
Aditus (orbital margin), 345
Adrenal (suprarenal) gland, 128f, 131, 131f, 134f, 135–136, 136t
Afferent (sensory) neurons, 11f, 12
 morphology of, 17b
 visceral, 16
Agger nasi, 387f
Air, in pleural cavity (pneumothorax), 47b
Alar layer, of prevertebral fascia, 324, 324f, 325f
Alar part, of nasalis muscle, 304
Alcock's (pudendal) canal, 189f, 191
Allantois, 165, 165f
Alveolar arteries, 375
Alveolar canal, 293f
Alveolar cells, 48b
Alveolar foramina, 373
Alveolar nerves, 372f, 373, 387f
Alveolar processes, 376, 376f
Amniotic cavity, 6, 6f
Amphiarthrodial joints, 6
Ampulla of Vater, 122
Anal canal, 157f, 158–160, 158t
 lymphatic system of, 160–161, 160f
 relationships of, 161, 161t
Anal columns, 157f, 158
Anal sinuses, 157f, 158
Anal sphincters, 157f, 159, 180f, 190–191, 190f
Anal triangle, 178–179, 179f, 189–191, 189f, 190f

Anal valves, 157f, 158
Anal verge (anocutaneous line), 157f, 158
Anastomosis, 3
 cilioretinal, 358–359
 of colon arteries, 112
 cruciate, in lower limb circulation, 204–205, 206f
 of duodenal arteries, 105
 of facial arteries, 307–308
 of facial veins, 308
 of head and neck arteries, 338–339, 339t, 340f
 of scalp arteries, 301–302
 of shoulder arteries, 260f, 261
 of vertebral arteries, 332
Anatomic position, 1–4, 2f, 2t, 3b, 3f
Anatomic snuffbox, 281, 281f
Anconeus muscle, 263, 266t, 267f, 268f, 276f, 278f
Androgen insensitivity syndrome, 170b
Angina pectoris, 61
Angiotensin II, 135b
Angle of inclination, of femur, 198
Angle of the acromion, 247, 247f
Angular artery, 300f
Ankle joint
 blood supply to, 228f, 231
 bones of, 220, 221f, 222f, 223
 fascia of, 221f, 224
 gout in, 223b
 innervation of, 228f, 230–231
 ligaments of, 229–230, 230f
 lymphatic system of, 231
 movement of, 220, 221f, 229
 muscles of, 224–226, 224f, 225f, 226t, 227f, 227t, 228f
Annular ligament, of ulna, 262, 262f
Annulus fibrosus, 58
Anococcygeal ligament, 152f, 190, 190f
Anococcygeal nerves, 205f
Anococcygeal raphe, 149, 180f, 190f, 191
Anocutaneous line (anal verge), 157f, 158
Anorectal hiatus, 147f
Anorectal junction, 158
Anoxia, 49b
Ansa cervicalis, 328f, 329
Ansa subclavia, 330f, 331f, 332
Antebrachial cutaneous nerve, 245, 264f, 267f, 268f, 283f
Antebrachial fascia, 283f
Anterior auricular muscles, 304
Anterior axillary line, 43, 43f
Anterior cardiac veins, 54f, 57
Anterior cerebellar artery, 340f
Anterior cerebral artery, 331f, 340f
Anterior ciliary artery, 359
Anterior circumflex humeral artery, 269f
Anterior clinoid process, 296f, 350f
Anterior communicating artery, 340f
Anterior compartment
 of arm, 262–263, 264f, 266t
 of leg, 225–226, 227t, 228f
 of thigh, 207–209, 209t, 210f
Anterior cranial fossa, 293–296, 294f–296f, 295t, 296b
Anterior cricothyroid ligament, 391f
Anterior cruciate ligament, 215–216, 215b, 215f, 216f, 217f

Anterior cutaneous nerves of neck, 306f
Anterior ethmoid groove, 295f
Anterior ethmoidal artery, 356f, 357, 357f, 358f
Anterior ethmoidal foramen, 346f
Anterior ethmoidal nerve, 355–356, 356f, 357f, 372f, 386
Anterior femoral cutaneous nerve, 212f
Anterior fontanelle, 292, 294f
Anterior gluteal line, 198, 198f
Anterior intercostal artery, 41
Anterior intermuscular septum, of leg, 223f
Anterior interosseous artery, 277f, 279f
Anterior interosseous nerve, 277f, 288f
Anterior interventricular artery, 56, 56f
Anterior jugular vein, 328f, 343
Anterior lacrimal crest, 346f, 347
Anterior meningeal artery, 311
Anterior papillary muscle, 58, 58f, 59f
Anterior position, 1, 2f, 2t
Anterior recess of the ischioanal fossa, 189–190, 189f
Anterior scalene muscle, 244f, 326–327, 326f, 327f, 330f
Anterior spinal artery, 340f
Anterior superior alveolar nerve, 387f
Anterior tibial artery, 225f, 228f, 231, 240f
Anterior tibial recurrent artery, 228f
Anterior triangle, of neck
    boundaries of, 325–326, 326f, 326t, 333
    carotid, 322f, 326f, 334t, 337–341
    digastric (submandibular), 322f, 326f, 333, 334t, 335f, 336
    muscular, 322f, 334t, 335f, 341–343, 342f, 342t
    subdivisions of, 333, 334t
    submental, 322f, 334t, 343
Anterior trunk, of brachial plexus, 244
Anterolateral (sphenoidal) fontanelle, 292, 294f
Anteromedial intermuscular septum, of thigh, 211f
Anteversion, of uterus, 174, 174f
Anulus fibrosus, 28–29
Anulus of Zinn (common tendinous ring), 349f, 350, 350f
Anus, 159, 180f. See also subjects starting with Anal.
Aorta, 60, 60f, 68, 68f, 69f, 134f
    abdominal, 134f, 137–138, 138t
    branches of, 137–138, 138t
    development of, 66f, 68–69, 69f, 70t
    diaphragmatic hiatus for, 129
Aortic arches, 68–69, 69f, 70t
Aortic impression, 47f
Aortic sinuses (of Valsalva), 55, 59f, 60, 60f
Aortic valve, 59f, 60, 60f, 62, 63f
Aortic vestibule, 60
Aorticorenal ganglion, 98f, 108
Apex, of orbit, 345
Apical ectodermal ridge, 196
Aponeurosis, of abdominal wall, 79, 80f, 82–83, 82f
Appendicitis, psoas sign in, 209b
Appendicular artery, 110, 110f, 111f
Appendicular skeletal system, 5, 23
Appendix, 109–110, 109f, 110f
    congenital abnormalities of, 125–126, 125f
    development of, 122–126, 123f–125f
Arachnoid, 29, 29f–31f, 309f, 311
Arachnoid granulations, 309f, 311
Arachnoid trabeculae, 311
Arachnoid villi, 309f, 311
Arches
    of foot, 231–232, 232f
    pharyngeal, 319, 320f, 321t

Arcuate artery, of foot, 240f
Arcuate eminence, 298
Arcuate ligaments, 128f
Arcuate line, 80f, 81f, 83, 127, 128f, 142f, 143
Arcuate pubic ligament, 180f, 181
Arcus tendineus, 147f, 148f, 149, 153f, 181f, 189f
Arm. See also Forearm; Shoulder region.
    blood supply to, 266, 269, 269f
    bones of, 260–261, 261f–263f. See also individual bones.
    definition of, 242f, 261
    innervation of, 263, 264f, 266, 267f
    muscles of, 262–263, 264f, 266t
Arteriae rectae, 106, 106f
Arterioles, 3, 3f
Arteriosclerosis, 3b
Artery(ies), 3, 3f
    to abdominal wall
        anterior, 84f, 85
        posterior, 134f, 137–139, 138t, 139f, 139t
    to anal canal, 160
    to ankle joint, 228f, 231
    to back muscles, 32
    to bladder, 160f, 163
    to duodenum, 105, 106f
    to dura mater, 311
    to esophagus, 72, 72t
    to face, 301f, 307–308
    to foot, 239, 240f
    to forearm, 278–279, 279f
    to foregut, 99–100, 99f
    to gallbladder, 117f, 120
    to genital system
        female, 171f, 177t
        male, 168t
    to gluteal region, 204–205, 206f
    to hand, 289, 290f
    to hindgut, 99–100, 99f
    to hip joint, 204–205, 206f
    to ileum, 104f, 106, 108
    to jejunum, 104f, 106, 108
    to kidney, 131f, 133, 134f
    to knee joint, 206f, 212f, 219–220, 219f
    to larynx, 393, 395, 396f
    to leg, 225f, 228f, 231
    to liver, 114, 117f, 118
    to mediastinum, 68–69, 69f
    to midgut, 99–100, 99f
    to nasal cavity, 387f, 388
    to orbit, 356–359, 358f
    to palate, 377, 377f
    to pelvis, 154–156, 154t, 155f
    to prostate gland, 168, 168t
    to pterygopalatine fossa, 368f, 375
    to scalp, 301–302, 301f
    to shoulder region, 259, 260f, 261
    to spleen, 119f, 120–121
    to stomach, 99–100, 99f
    to suprarenal gland, 136, 136t
    to testis, 148f, 166
    to thigh, 206f, 212f, 219–220, 219f
    of thoracic wall, 40f, 41
    to thymus, 66
    to uterus, 171f, 175
    to vagina, 176, 177t
    to wrist, 278–279, 279f
Artery of the ductus, 154t, 167–168, 168t
Articular capsule, of elbow joint, 262, 263f
Articular cartilage, histology of, 198b
Articular muscle of knee, 208f
Articular nerve, 238f
Articular processes, vertebral, 25, 25f, 26f
Aryepiglottic folds, 393, 394f
Aryepiglottic ligament, 393

Aryepiglottic muscle, 395t
Arytenoid cartilage, 392f–394f, 393
Arytenoid muscle, 395t, 396f
Ascending cervical artery, 330f, 331f
Ascending palatine artery, 396f
Ascending pharyngeal artery, 331f, 335f, 338
Atelectasis, 49b
Atherosclerosis, 3b, 220b
Atlantoaxial joint, 26f, 27
Atlas, 26, 26f, 28
Atrial artery, 55
Atrial septum, 57–58, 57f, 64f, 65, 65f, 66f
Atrioventricular bundle, 60f, 62f
Atrioventricular canal, 64f, 66f
Atrioventricular groove (coronary sulcus), 53, 55
Atrioventricular node, 58, 62, 62f
Atrioventricular orifice, 58, 59, 59f
Atrioventricular septum, 62f
Atrium
    development of, 62–65, 63f–66f, 65t
    left, 59
    primitive, 63, 63f
    right, 54f, 57
Auditory (acoustic) meatus, 293f, 297f, 299, 299t
Auditory (pharyngotympanic) tube, 298, 378f, 379f
Auerbach's (myenteric) ganglion, 317
Auricle
    of ear, muscles of, 300f, 303t, 304
    of left atrium, 59
Auricular artery, 300f, 302, 331f, 335f, 338
Auricular muscles, 304
Auricular nerve, 303t, 306f, 317, 328f, 329, 336f
Auricular nodes, 344
Auricular vein, 308, 343
Auricularis anterior muscle, 300f
Auricularis superior muscle, 300f
Auriculotemporal nerve, 305f, 306f, 307
Auscultation
    of heart sounds, 62, 63f
    of lung, 48
Autonomic nervous system, 14–16. See also Parasympathetic nervous system; Sympathetic nervous system.
    parasympathetic division of, 16, 18f, 19t
    sympathetic division of, 14–15, 15f, 16t, 17t, 19t
    visceral afferent neurons with, 16
Avascular necrosis, 202b
Axial skeletal system, 5, 23. See also Vertebrae and vertebral column.
Axilla, 250, 250f
Axillary artery, 259, 260f, 261, 269f
Axillary fascia, 251f
Axillary lines, 43, 43f
Axillary nerve, 243f, 250f, 256t, 258f, 259, 265f, 268f, 269f
Axillary vein, 269, 270f
Axis, 26–27, 26f, 28
Axons, 11, 12f
Azygos system of veins, 41, 67–68, 68f, 70, 71f
    diaphragmatic hiatus for, 129
    impression of, 47f

B

Back, 23–33. See also Spinal cord; Vertebrae and vertebral column.
    development of, 27–28, 28f, 32
    joints of, 28–29
    ligaments of, 29
    muscles of, 31–32, 33t
    spinal meninges of, 29–30, 29f–31f

Bacterial meningitis, 397, 401
Bare area of the pericardium, 52
Baroreceptors, 61
Bartholin's glands, 186, 186f, 187f
Basal plates, 20f, 21
Basilar artery, 331f, 332, 340f
Basilar plexus, 312f, 313f, 314
Basilic vein, 269, 270f, 271f, 279f
Batson's plexus, 163, 168, 309
"Bed of the stomach," 95–96, 96f
Benign prostatic hyperplasia, 169b
Biceps brachii muscle, 262–263, 264f, 265f, 266t, 267f, 271f
Biceps brachii tendon, 257f, 271f
Biceps femoris muscle, 201f, 203f, 211, 214f, 214t, 224f, 227f
Biceps femoris tendon, 225f
Bicipital aponeurosis, 264f, 265f, 271f
Bicipital (intertubercular) groove, 248, 248f
Bicuspid valve, 60f
Bilaminar embryo, 6, 6f, 8f
Bile, 120
Bile ducts
    extrahepatic, 122–123, 123f
    innervation of, 107t
Biopsy, of liver, 113–114
Bladder, 155f, 160f, 161–163, 162f
Blood, in pleural cavity (hemothorax), 47b
Blood supply, 3–4, 3b, 3f
    to abdominal wall
        anterior, 84f, 85
        posterior, 134f, 137–139, 138t, 139f, 139t
    to anal canal, 159–160, 159f
    to ankle joint, 228f, 231
    to back muscles, 32
    to bladder, 160f, 163
    to diaphragm, 42
    to dura mater, 311
    to epididymis, 166
    to esophagus, 70, 72, 72t
    to face, 301f, 307–308
    to foot, 239, 240f
    to forearm, 278–279, 279f
    to gallbladder, 117f, 120
    to genital system
        female, 171f, 177t
        male, 168t
    of gluteal region, 204–205, 206f
    to hand, 289, 290f
    to hip joint, 204–205, 206f
    to ileum, 104f, 106, 106f, 108
    to jejunum, 104f, 105, 106, 106f, 108
    to kidney, 131f, 133, 134f
    to knee joint, 206f, 212f, 219–220, 219f
    to larynx, 393, 395, 396f
    to leg, 225f, 228f, 231
    to liver, 114, 117f, 118–119
    to lung, 49
    to nasal cavity, 387f, 388
    to oral cavity, 382
    to orbit, 356–359, 358f
    to ovary, 171, 171f, 177t
    to palate, 377, 377f
    to pancreas, 119f, 121
    to pelvis, 154–156, 154t, 155f
    to pericardium, 53
    to perineum, 191–193, 192f, 193f
    to pleura, 46
    to prostate gland, 168, 168t
    to pterygopalatine fossa, 368f, 375
    to scalp, 301–302, 301f
    to shoulder region, 259, 260f, 261
    to spleen, 119f, 120–121
    to stomach, 99–100, 99f
    to suprarenal gland, 136, 136t

Blood supply (cont'd)
    to testis, 148f, 166
    to thigh, 206f, 212f, 219–220, 219f
    to thoracic wall, 40f, 41
    to thymus, 66–67
    to trachea, 69
    to uterine tubes, 171f, 172–173, 177t
    to uterus, 171f, 175, 177t
    to vagina, 176, 177t
    to wrist, 278–279, 279f
Bone(s), 5. See also individual bones.
    of abdominal wall, 79–80, 81f, 127, 128f
    of ankle joint, 220, 221f, 222f, 223. See also individual bones.
    carpal, 270, 271f, 272
    classification of, 5
    of face, 292f–293f, 295f, 302
    of forearm, 270, 271f, 272
    formation of, 5b, 247b
    of gluteal region and hip joint, 197–198, 198f
    of hand, 270, 271f, 272
    histology of, 25b
    of leg, 220, 222f, 223. See also individual bones.
    of nose, 385–386, 385f
    of orbit, 345–347, 346f, 347t
    of pelvis, 142–145, 142f–145f, 197–198, 198f
    of pterygopalatine fossa, 360–362, 370f–372f
    shapes of, 5
    of shoulder region, 246–248, 246f–248f
    of thigh, 199f, 205–206, 208f. See also Femur.
    of thoracic wall, 35–38, 36f–38f. See also Rib(s).
    of wrist, 270, 271f, 272, 281, 282f
Brachial artery, 250f, 260f, 266, 267f–269f, 269, 271f, 274f, 279f
Brachial cutaneous nerve, 267f, 268f, 270f
Brachial fascia, 251f
Brachial plexus, 241–246
    cords of, 243f, 244–246, 265f
    functional fibers in, 241–242
    injury of, 245b
    roots of, 242, 243f, 245
    trunks of, 242, 243f, 244–245, 244f
Brachial vein, 269, 270f
Brachialis artery, 265f
Brachialis muscle, 264f, 265f, 266t, 267f, 268f, 271f, 272f, 277f
Brachiocephalic artery, 54f, 68
Brachiocephalic vein, 41, 54f, 67–68, 68f, 71f, 333
Brachiocephalic vein impression, 47f
Brachioradialis muscle, 264f, 271f, 272f, 273, 274f, 278f
Brachioradialis tendon, 277f
Brain, development of, 19–21, 20f
Breast, 39, 41
Broad ligament, of uterus, 170f, 173f, 174–175, 186f
Bronchi, 48–51, 48f, 49t, 50f
Bronchial arteries, 49
Bronchial veins, 49
Bronchiectasis, 49b
Bronchioles, 49
Bronchomediastinal nodes, 41, 50
Bronchopulmonary nodes, 50
Bronchopulmonary segments, 49
Brudzinski's sign, 31b, 397, 401
Brunner's glands, 106b
Buccal artery, 308
Buccal nerve, 303t, 305, 305f, 306f, 307, 387f
Buccal nodes, 308, 344
Buccinator muscle, 300f, 303t, 304–305, 327f, 335f, 376f, 391, 391f

Buccopharyngeal fascia, 324, 391
Buccopharyngeal membrane, 308f, 309
Buck's fascia of the penis, 183, 183f, 184f
Bulb
    olfactory, 372f, 387f
    of penis, 182, 182f
    sinovaginal, 178
    of vaginal vestibule, 185, 185f, 186f
Bulbar sheath, 348f
Bulbocavernosus muscle, 187f
Bulbospongiosus muscle, 181f, 182f, 183, 185, 185f, 186f, 190f
Bulbourethral (Cowper's) gland, 167f, 180f, 181
Bulbus cordis, 63, 63f
Bundle block, 62b
Bundle branches, 62, 62f

C
Calcaneal tendon, 213t, 224f
Calcaneocuboid ligament, 230f
Calcaneofibular ligament, 227f, 230f
Calcaneonavicular (spring) ligament, 230f, 232–233, 233f
Calcaneus, 213t, 220, 221f, 224f, 232f, 233f
Calculi, renal, 398–399, 402
Calvaria, 292, 293f
Calyces, renal, 130f, 133
Camper's fascia, 79, 87
Canal (of Dorello), 315
Canalicular phase, of lung development, 50
Cancer
    breast, 39, 41
    cervical, 176b
    testicular, 399, 402
Capillaries, 3, 3f
Capitate, 271f, 272, 282f
Capitis muscles, 33t
Capitulum, 263f
    of humerus, 261, 261f
    of ulna, 271f
Capsule
    of elbow joint, 262, 262f
    of knee, 215, 215f
    of thyroid gland, 342
Cardiac catheterization, 269b
Cardiac impression, 47f
Cardiac looping, 63, 63f
Cardiac muscle, 5–6
Cardiac nerve, 68f
Cardiac notch, 46f, 48
Cardiac plexus, 60, 71f, 339
Cardiac portion, of stomach, 94f, 95
Cardiac tamponade, 53b
Cardiac veins, 54f, 55f, 56–57
Cardinal (transverse cervical) ligament, 150f, 151, 156, 175, 175f
Carotid arteries, 68, 68f, 300f, 311, 313f, 323f, 330f, 331f, 337–339, 339t, 340f, 342f, 365f
    anastomosis of, 338–339, 339t, 340f
    development of, 68–69, 69f
Carotid body, 330f, 337
Carotid canal, 297t, 298, 298f
Carotid groove, 296f, 297f, 298
Carotid nerve, 353–354
Carotid nerve plexus, 337, 341, 341f
Carotid sheath, 324f, 325, 344
Carotid sinus, 331f, 337
Carotid sinus nerve (nerve of Herring), 337
Carotid sulcus, 297t
Carotid triangle, 322f, 326f, 334t, 337–341
Carotid tubercle, 26
Carpal articular surface, of radius, 270, 271f
Carpal bones, 270, 271f, 272
Carpal tunnel, 279, 280f, 281b

Cartilage
  histology of, 198b
  of larynx, 322, 323f, 343, 391f, 392–393, 393f, 394f
  of nose, 349f, 384–385, 384f
  of thoracic cage, 36f, 37, 38, 38f
Cartilaginous joints, 6, 6t
Case studies, 397–403
Catheterization, cardiac, 269b
Cauda equina, 31f
Caudal limb, in midgut development, 122–123
Caudal position, 1, 2f, 2t
Caudate lobe, of liver, 114, 116f
Cavernous nerves, 154
Cavernous plexus, 353–354
Cavernous sinus, 298f, 310, 310f, 312f, 313f, 314, 315f, 316b
Cecal diverticulum, 123
Cecum, 109, 110f
  development of, 122–126, 123f–125f
  innervation of, 107t
Celiac artery, 96, 96f, 97f, 99, 99f, 138t
Celiac ganglia, 97–98, 98f
Celiac plexus, 97
Celiac trunk, 134f
Central artery of retina, 358
Central canal, 20–21
Central nervous system
  development of, 19–21, 20f
  overview of, 11, 11f, 12f
Central tendon
  of perineum (perineal body), 152f
  of sternocleidomastoid muscle, 326
Central vein of retina, 359
Cephalic vein, 251f, 269, 270f, 271f, 279f
Cerebellar artery, 332, 340f
Cerebellar fossa, 310f
Cerebral artery, 311, 331f, 340f
Cerebral fossa, 310f
Cerebral vein, 310f, 312, 313f
Cerebrospinal fluid, 30b, 309f, 311
Cervical artery, 244f, 258f, 259, 260f, 330f, 332–333
Cervical ganglion, 330f
Cervical ligaments, 151
Cervical nerves, 303t, 305, 305f, 328f, 329, 336f
Cervical nodes, 344–345
Cervical pleura, 44
Cervical plexus, 253t, 327f, 328–329, 328f, 329t
Cervical spinal nerves, 244
Cervical sympathetic ganglion, 331f, 340–341, 341f
Cervical sympathetic trunk, 330f, 331f, 340, 341f
Cervical vertebrae, 24f, 25–27, 26f
Cervicalis muscle, 33t
Cervicoaxillary canal, 244
Cervicothoracic (stellate) ganglion, 241–242, 340–341, 341f
Cervix, 171f, 173–176, 173f, 176b
Check ligaments, 348, 348f
Cheek
  innervation of, 306f, 307
  muscles of, 300, 304–305
Chemoreceptors, 61
Chiasmatic sulcus, 296f
Chondrocranium, 292
Chordae tendinae, 58, 58f, 59f
Chyme, 94
Ciliary artery, 357f, 358–359, 358f
Ciliary ganglion, 316, 341f, 353–354, 354f, 357f
Ciliary nerve, 341f, 356, 357f
Circle of Willis, 332, 339, 340f

Circle of Zinn (Zinn-Haller), 358–359
Circulation
  collateral, 3
    at elbow, 279, 279f
    in gut, 99
    of head and neck, 338–339, 339t, 340f
  fetal, 62–65, 63f–66f, 65t
  in heart, 53
  lymphatic, 3–4
Circumflex artery, 54f, 55f, 56, 56f
Circumflex femoral artery, 210f
Circumflex humeral artery, 268f, 269f
Circumflex iliac artery, 206f, 207f, 211f
Circumflex iliac vein, 207f
Circumflex scapular artery, 260f, 261
Circumvallate (vallate) papillae, 380f, 381
Cisterna chyli, 73
Cisterns, of subarachnoid space, 29
Claudication, intermittent, 220b
Clavicle, 244f, 246, 246f
Clavicular notches, 38
Claw hand, 287b
Cleft palate, 384b
Clinoid process, 296, 296f, 350f
Clitoris, 185, 185f–187f
  deep dorsal vein of, 152f
  development of, 187–188, 188f
  dorsal nerve of, 180f, 186f, 191–192, 192f
Clivus, 299
Cloaca, 164–166
Cloacal membrane, 158, 165–166, 165f, 187
Cluneal nerve, 202f, 203f, 214f
Coccygeus muscle, 147f, 148t, 149, 153f, 155f
Coccyx, 143f, 145, 179f, 180f
Coelomic epithelium, 169f
Colic arteries, 111, 111f, 112f
Colic flexures, 109f, 110
Colic vein, 118f
Collateral circulation, 3
  at elbow, 279, 279f
  in gut, 99
  of head and neck, 338–339, 339t, 340f
Collateral ligaments
  of ankle, 230, 230f
  of elbow, 262
  of finger, 288f
  of knee, 208f, 215–216, 215f–217f, 227f
Colles fascia, 184, 184f
Colliculus seminalis (seminal hillock, verumontanum), 168
Colon, 108–113
  appendix in, 109–110, 109f, 110f
  ascending, 107t, 109f, 110
  blood supply to, 111–112, 111f
  cecum in, 109, 109f
  descending, 107t, 109f, 111
  development of, 122–126, 123f–125f
  diameter of, 108–109
  function of, 108
  innervation of, 107t, 112–113
  lymphatic system of, 112, 112f
  sigmoid, 107t, 109f, 111
  transverse, 109f, 110–111
Common carotid artery, 330f, 337, 342f, 343
Common digital nerves
  of lower limb, 235f, 239f
  of upper limb, 284f, 287
Common facial vein, 308
Common fibular (peroneal) nerve, 203, 204, 205f, 214f, 214t, 224f, 227f, 228, 228f, 231, 238f
Common hepatic artery, 97f
Common hepatic duct, 117f, 120, 122
Common iliac artery, 134f, 137–138, 155f, 211f

Common iliac vein, 104f, 134f, 138–139
Common interosseous artery, 269f, 277f, 278, 279f
Common palmar digital artery, 283f, 290f
Common fibular (peroneal) nerve, 203, 204, 205f, 214f, 214t, 224f, 227f, 228, 231, 238f
Common plantar digital nerves, 232f
Common tendinous ring, 349f, 350, 350f
Communicating artery, 340f
Compartment syndrome, 399, 402–403
Compressor urethrae muscle, 180f, 181
Conchae, 385, 385f, 386, 387f
Conduction system, of heart, 61–62, 62f
Condyles
  of femur, 199f
  of tibia, 208f, 222f
Condyloid canal, 299, 299t
Confluence of sinuses, 313f
Congenital defects
  of abdominal structures, 125–126, 125f
  of diaphragm, 42–43
  of heart, 64–65, 65f, 67f
  of midgut, 125–126, 125f
  of palate, 384b
Conjoined tendon (falx inguinalis), 83, 85, 86f, 87
Conjugate distances, of pelvis, 146f, 147
Conoid ligament, 249, 249f
Conoid tubercle, of clavicle, 246, 246f
Constrictor muscles, pharyngeal, 334t, 335f, 337, 378f–380f, 389, 390f, 390t, 391f, 392t
Conus arteriosus (infundibulum), 58, 58f, 66f
Conus elasticus (cricovocal ligament), 393
Conus medullaris, 29, 29f–31f, 31
Convergence theory, of referred pain, 18, 19f
Coracoacromial ligament, 249f, 250, 264f
Coracobrachialis muscle, 252f, 263, 266t
Coracoclavicular ligament, 249, 249f
Coracohumeral ligament, 249f, 250
Coracoid process, 247f, 248, 249f
Cords, of brachial plexus, 243f, 244–246
Corniculate cartilage, 393f, 394f
Coronal plane, 1, 2f, 2t
Coronal suture, 292f, 293f, 294f
Coronary artery(ies), 54f, 55–56, 56f
  disease of, 397–398, 401–402
Coronary ligament
  of abdomen, 93f, 100, 114, 116f
  of knee, 216f
Coronary sinus, 55f, 56, 57, 57f
Coronary sulcus, 53, 55
Coronary vein, 97
Coronoid fossa, of humerus, 261
Coronoid process, of ulna, 261, 261f
Corpus cavernosum penis, 182, 182f, 183f, 184f
Corpus spongiosum penis, 182, 182f, 184f
Corpus sterni, 38
Corrugator supercilii muscle, 300f, 303t, 304
Cortex
  of kidney, 130f, 133
  of suprarenal gland, 135, 136
Costal cartilages, 36f, 37, 38, 38f
Costal pleura, 44, 45f
Costal surface, of lung, 47
Costocervical trunk, 330f, 333
Costoclavicular ligament, 246, 246f
Costodiaphragmatic recess, 45, 46f, 133b
Costomediastinal recess, 45
Costotransverse joint, 36f, 37
Costovertebral joint, 36f, 37
Costoxiphoid ligament, 251f
Cowper's (bulbourethral) gland, 167f, 180f, 181

Cranial dura mater, 309–311
Cranial fossae
anterior, 293–296, 294f–296f, 295t, 296b
middle, 294f, 296, 296f–298f, 297t, 298, 299b
posterior, 294f, 297f, 298f, 299, 299t
Cranial limb, in midgut development, 122, 123f
Cranial nerves. *See also specific nerves.*
in cranial fossae
anterior, 296
middle, 298
posterior, 299
development of, 317, 319, 320f, 321t
dural venous sinuses and, 313f, 314–315, 315f
of face, 305, 305f, 307
Cranial position, 1, 2f, 2t
Craniosacral outflow (parasympathetic nervous system), 16, 18f, 19t
Cremaster fascia, 86f
Cremaster muscle, 80f, 81f, 86f, 88
Cremaster reflex, 88
Cremasteric artery, 166, 168t
Cribriform fascia, 205, 207f
Cribriform plate, of ethmoid bone, 293, 294f, 295–296, 295f, 295t, 297f, 385f, 387f
Cricoarytenoid joint, 393
Cricoarytenoid ligament, 392f, 396f
Cricoarytenoid muscle, 395t
Cricoid cartilage, 323f, 392–393, 392f–394f
Cricopharyngeus muscle, 389, 395
Cricothyroid cartilage, 342f
Cricothyroid ligament, 323f, 391f, 392f, 393
Cricothyroid membrane, 342f, 393
Cricothyroid muscle, 323f, 342f, 391f, 393, 394f, 395t
Cricotracheal ligament, 392f
Cricovocal ligament (conus elasticus), 393
Cricovocal membrane, 393, 393f, 394f
Crista galli, 294f–296f, 295–296, 357f, 385f, 387f
Crista terminalis, 57, 57f
Cross-section, 1, 2t
Cruciate anastomosis, in lower limb circulation, 204–205, 206f
Cruciate ligaments, 215–216, 215b, 215f–217f
Crura
of clitoris, 185, 185f
of diaphragm, 127
of heart, 55, 56f
of penis, 181–182, 182f
Crural fascia, 195, 223–224, 223f
Cryptorchidism, 90b
C-shaped cartilage, of pharynx, 389
Cubital fossa, 269–270, 271f
Cubital vein, 269, 270f, 271f
Cuboid bone, 220, 221f, 232f
Cul-de-sac (pouch of Douglas, rectouterine pouch), 151, 152f, 156, 157f, 158, 170f, 174
Cuneiform bones, 220, 221f, 232f
Cuneiform cartilage, 394f
Cuneonavicular ligament, 230f
Cupola, 44–45, 45f
Cutaneous nerve of forearm, 265f, 268f
Cutaneous nerve of thigh, 128f, 193f, 204f, 207f, 210f
Cyst(s), Gartner's, 178, 178f
Cysterna chyli, 160f
Cystic artery, 96f, 114, 117f, 119f, 120
Cystic duct, 119–120, 122
Cystohepatic triangle, 96f, 117f, 118

D
Dartos muliebris, 186
Dartos tunic, 184, 184f
Deep artery of clitoris/penis, 180f
Deep brachial artery, 266, 268f, 269f
Deep cardiac plexus, 60
Deep cervical artery, 330f, 331f, 333
Deep circumflex iliac artery, 85, 206f, 211f
Deep facial vein, 308
Deep fascia, 4f, 5
of abdominal wall, 79, 82
of neck, 323–324, 323t, 324f
Deep femoral artery, 206f, 219, 219f
Deep fibular (peroneal) nerve, 231, 237f, 238f
Deep infrapatellar bursa, 208f
Deep inguinal ring, 86f, 87, 91f
Deep palmar arch, 279f, 288f, 289, 290f
Deep perineal fascia, 183, 183f, 186f
Deep peroneal nerve, 228f, 240f
Deep petrosal nerve, 373, 375
Deep plantar artery, 240f
Deep position, 1, 2t
Deep transverse metacarpal ligament, 286f
Deep ulnar artery, 289, 290f
Delphian (midline prelaryngeal) node, 344
Deltoid ligament, 230, 230f
Deltoid muscle, 251f, 252f, 254–255, 254f, 256f–258f, 256t, 264f, 267f, 268f
Deltoid tuberosity, 248, 248f
Deltopectoral triangle, 251f, 255
Dendrites, 11, 12f
Denonvilliers' fascia (rectovesical septum), 151, 158, 162, 167, 168, 190f
Dens, 26–27, 26f
Dental arches, 375–376
Dental (alveolar) plexus, 372f, 373
Denticulate ligaments, 29f, 30
Depression, of eye, 351–353, 351f, 352f, 353t
Depressor anguli oris muscle, 300f, 303t, 305
Depressor labii inferioris muscle, 300f, 303t, 305
Depressor septi muscle, 303t, 304
Dermatome, 9, 9f, 21
Dermis, 4
Dermomyotome, 9, 9f
Detrusor urinae muscle, 163
Diaphragm
pelvic, 147f, 148f, 148t, 149–150, 176
respiratory, 41–43, 127–130
blood supply to, 42
development of, 42–43, 42f
fascia of, 129–130
function of, 41
innervation of, 41–42
insertions of, 127, 129t
openings in, 128–129, 128f, 129t
origins of, 127, 128, 129t
paralysis of, 42b
Diaphragma oris, 382
Diaphragma sellae, 310, 310f, 311
Diaphragmatic nodes, 41
Diaphragmatic pleura, 44–46, 45f
Diaphragmatic surface
of heart, 53, 55f
of lung, 47
of spleen, 120
Diarthrodial joints, 6, 6t
Digastric muscle, 322f, 323f, 327f, 333, 334t, 335f, 336f, 337, 342f, 376f, 379f, 380f
Digastric (submandibular) triangle, 322f, 326f, 333, 334t, 335f, 336
Digital arteries
of lower limb, 232f, 239f
of upper limb, 283f, 289b

Digital nerves
of lower limb, 232f, 235f, 237f, 239f
of upper limb, 287
Diploë bone, 292, 314
Diploic veins, 312, 314
Direct hernia, inguinal, 88b, 91f
Disks, intervertebral, 24, 25f, 26f, 28–29
Dorsal artery of clitoris/penis, 180f, 192f, 193
Dorsal carpal arch, 289, 290f
Dorsal cutaneous nerve, of foot, 237f
Dorsal horns, of spinal cord, 13, 13f
Dorsal interosseous artery, of hand, 278f
Dorsal interosseous muscles
of foot, 236–237, 236f, 240f
of hand, 286, 286f, 288f
Dorsal mesentery, liver development from, 99f, 100, 101f
Dorsal mesogastrium, 99f
liver development from, 100
peritoneal ligament development from, 101–102, 102f
stomach development from, 95
Dorsal metacarpal artery, 290f
Dorsal metatarsal artery, 240f
Dorsal motor nucleus, 317
Dorsal muscles, of foot, 233, 233f, 234t, 235f–237f, 236–237
Dorsal nasal artery, 300f, 307, 358
Dorsal nasal nerve, 306f
Dorsal pedis arteries, 239
Dorsal position, 1, 2f, 2t
Dorsal ramus, of spinal cord, 13f, 14
Dorsal root, 13–14, 13f, 20f, 21
Dorsal root ganglia, 13, 13f
Dorsal scapular artery, 244f, 260f, 330f, 332–333
Dorsal scapular nerve, 243f, 244f, 245, 250f, 253t, 258–259, 258f
Dorsalis pedis artery, 228t, 231, 239f, 240f
Dorsiflexion, of ankle joint, 221f, 229
Dorsum sellae, 296, 296f, 297f, 299, 313f
Duction, of eye, 351–353, 351f, 352f, 353t
Ducts of Rivinus, 383
Ductus, artery of, 154t, 167–168, 168t
Ductus arteriosus, 63, 66f
patent, 65
Ductus deferens, 89f, 155f, 162, 162f, 166–167, 167f, 168t
Duodenal papilla of Vater, 104, 105f
Duodenojejunal flexure, 103f, 104f, 105, 106b
Duodenojejunal junction, 109f
Duodenum, 102f, 103–105, 104f, 105f
bile duct in, 122
peptic ulcer disease of, 398, 402
Dura mater
cranial, 29–30, 29f–31f, 309–311, 309f
spinal, 29–30, 29f–31f
Dural venous sinuses, 311–315. *See also individual venous sinuses.*
cranial nerves and, 313f, 314–315, 315f
locations of, 311–312, 312f, 313f
midline unpaired, 310f, 312, 312f, 313f, 314
paired, 312f, 313f, 314, 315f
venous drainage into, 314

E
Ear, muscles of, 300f, 303t, 304
Echocardiography, transesophageal, 72b
Ectoderm, limb development from, 196
Ectomenix, 292
Ectopic pregnancy, 173b
Edema, 3b
pulmonary, 49b
Edinger-Westphal nucleus, 316

Efferent (motor) neurons, 12, 12f, 17b
Ejaculatory duct, 162f, 167, 167f, 168
Elbow joint
    collateral circulation around, 279, 279f
    cubital fossa of, 269–270, 271f
    movement of, 262, 263f
    muscles of, 262–263, 264f, 266t
Elevation, of eye, 351–353, 351f, 352f, 353t
Embolism, pulmonary, 49b
Embryology, 6–9, 6f–9f, 7b
    of anal canal, 158, 164–166, 165f
    of back, 32
    of back muscles, 32
    of bladder, 164–166, 165f
    of cranial nerves, 317
    of diaphragm, 42–43, 42f
    of face, 294f, 302, 308–309, 308f, 319,
        320f, 321t
    of gastrointestinal system, 122–126,
        123f–125f
    of genital system
        female, 169f, 177–178, 178f, 187–188,
            188f, 189t
        male, 169–170, 169f, 187–188, 188f, 189t
    of heart, 62–65, 63f–66f, 65t
    of inguinal canal, 88–90, 89f, 91f
    of kidney, 130, 134–135
    of liver, 100
    of lower limb, 195–197, 196b, 197f
    of lung, 44, 45f, 50–51, 50f
    of mediastinal vessels, 68–69, 69f, 70t
    of meninges, 31
    of midgut, 122–126, 123f–125f
    of nervous system, 8, 9f, 19–21, 20f
    of ovary, 169f, 171
    of palate, 383f, 384
    of pancreas, 100, 102–103, 103f
    of pericardium, 52
    of peritoneum, 90, 124
    of pleural cavity, 43–44, 44f
    of rectum, 164–166, 165f
    of skull, 292, 294f
    of spinal cord, 30–31
    of spleen, 120
    of stomach, 95, 99–101, 99f, 101f
    of suprarenal gland, 136
    of thoracic cavity, 43–44, 44f
    of upper limb, 195–197, 196b, 197f
    of vertebrae, 27–28, 28f
Emissary foramen (of Vesalius), 298
Emissary veins, 309f, 312, 313f, 314
Emphysema, 49b
Empyema, 47b
End artery, 3
Endoabdominal (transversalis) fascia, 5, 80f,
    81f, 82, 84f, 86f, 87, 90, 91f, 129–130,
    184f
Endocardial tubes, heart development from,
    63
Endochondral bone formation, 247b
Endoderm, 7, 7f, 8f
Endoneurium, 12b
Endopelvic fascia, 5, 150, 150f, 153f
Endosteal layer, of dura mater, 309, 309f
Endosteum, 301
Endothoracic fascia, 5
Epiarterial bronchus, 48
Epiblast, 6–8, 6f, 8f
Epicardium, 51, 52f, 54f
Epicondyles
    of femur, 199f, 206
    of humerus, 261, 261f
Epicranial aponeurosis, 300, 300f, 309f
Epicranius, 300
Epicranius (occipitofrontalis) muscle, 300,
    303t

Epidermis, 4
Epididymis, 162f, 166, 168t
Epidural space, 29, 30f, 309
Epigastric arteries, 41, 84f, 85, 206f, 207f,
    210f–212f
Epigastric region, 78, 78f
Epigastric vein, 85
Epiglottis, 387f, 389, 392f, 393, 393f
Epimere, back muscle development from, 32
Epimysium (muscular deep fascia), 5
Epineurium, 12b
Epiploic (omental) appendices, 109, 109f
Epiploic (omental) foramen, 91, 92f, 94f
Episiotomy, 187, 187f
Eponyms, 1
Erectile tissues, 181–182, 182f
Erector spinae muscles, 32, 33t
Esophageal artery, 97f
    diaphragmatic hiatus for, 128–129
Esophageal impression, 47f
Esophageal plexus, 72, 97, 98f
Esophageal veins, 118f
Esophagus, 70, 71–73, 71f, 94, 94f, 343
    blood supply to, 70, 72, 72t
    dorsal mesentery of, 42
    echocardiography probe in, 72b
    innervation of, 70, 107t
    reflux into, 94b
Ethmoid bone, 293, 295f, 296, 345, 346f,
    347, 385, 385f, 386
Ethmoid sinuses, 295f, 386t
Ethmoidal air cell, 357f
    of frontal bone, 295f
Ethmoidal artery, 311, 356f–358f, 357
Ethmoidal bulla, 385f, 386, 387f
Ethmoidal canals, 295t
Ethmoidal cells, 387f
Ethmoidal foramen, 346f, 347
Ethmoidal infundibulum, 386t
Ethmoidal nerve, 311, 355–356, 356f, 357f,
    372f, 386
Ethmoidal notch, of frontal bone, 295, 295f
Eversion, of ankle joint, 221f, 229–230
Expiration
    abdominal muscles in, 80–81
    respiratory muscles in, 47
Expression, facial, muscles of, 300f, 303t,
    304–305, 304f
Extension
    of ankle joint, 221f, 229
    of elbow joint, 262, 263f
    of hand, 281, 282f
    of wrist, 270
Extensor carpi radialis brevis muscle,
    273–274, 275t, 276f, 278f
Extensor carpi radialis brevis tendon, 279f
Extensor carpi radialis longus muscle,
    273–274, 275t, 276f, 278f
Extensor carpi radialis longus tendon, 279f
Extensor carpi ulnaris muscle, 274, 275t,
    276f, 278f
Extensor carpi ulnaris tendon, 279f
Extensor compartment, of forearm, 272f,
    273–274, 273t–275t
Extensor digiti minimi muscle, 274, 275t,
    276f, 278f
Extensor digiti minimi tendon, 279f
Extensor digitorum brevis muscle, 235t, 237,
    237f
Extensor digitorum muscle
    of lower limb, 223f, 226, 227f, 227t, 228f
    of upper limb, 274, 275t, 276f
Extensor digitorum tendons, 279f
Extensor hallucis brevis muscle, 235t, 237, 237f
Extensor hallucis longus muscle, 226, 227t,
    228f, 240f

Extensor hallucis longus tendon, 227f, 228t,
    237f
Extensor indicis muscle, 275t
Extensor indicis tendon, 279f
Extensor pollicis brevis muscle, 274, 275t,
    276f, 278f, 281, 281f
Extensor pollicis brevis tendon, 279f
Extensor pollicis longus muscle, 275t, 276f,
    278f, 281, 281f
Extensor pollicis longus tendon, 279f
Extensor retinaculum
    of ankle, 213t, 221f, 224
    of wrist, 276f, 278f
External acoustic meatus, 293f
External anal sphincter muscle, 190–191,
    190f
External auditory meatus, 293f
External carotid artery, 300f, 301–302, 301f,
    323f, 331f, 337–338, 365f
External carotid nerve plexus, 341, 341f
External esophageal venous plexus, 72
External genitalia
    female, 184–187, 185f–187f
    male, 181–184, 181f–184f
External iliac arteries, 139t, 155f, 206f, 210f,
    211f
External iliac nodes, 175
External iliac veins, 138–139, 210f
External intercostal muscle, 38–39, 39f, 40f,
    252f
External jugular vein, 312f, 339, 343
External laryngeal nerve, 330f, 391f, 395
External nasal nerve, 307, 349f
External oblique aponeurosis, 80f, 86f
External oblique muscle, of abdominal wall,
    80–81, 80f–82f, 254, 254f
External pudendal artery, 193, 210f, 212f
External rectal venous plexus, 159, 159f
Exteroceptors, 12
Extorsion, of eye, 351–353, 351f, 352f, 353t
Extrahepatic duct, 114, 118
Extraocular muscles, 348–353, 349f–352f,
    353t
Extraperitoneal (extraserous, subserous)
    fascia, 4f, 5, 82, 83, 86f, 87, 130,
    150–151
Eye. See Orbit.
Eyelid, muscles of, 304, 304f

F
Face, 302–309
    blood supply to, 301f, 307–308
    bones of, 292f–293f, 295f, 302
    definition of, 302
    development of, 294f, 302, 308–309, 308f
    innervation of, 295t, 303t, 305, 305f, 306f,
        307
    lymphatic system of, 308
    muscles of, 300f, 303t, 304–305, 304f
    veins of, 308
Facial artery, 300f, 307–308, 331f, 335f, 336,
    336f, 338
Facial canal, hiatus of, 297f, 297t, 298, 373
Facial nerve (VII), 300, 305f, 306f, 313f, 336
    branches of, 373, 374f, 375
    function of, 316–319
    palsy of, 400, 403
Facial nodes, 308
Facial vein, 308, 312f, 336, 336f, 344
Falciform ligament, 93f, 99f, 100, 101f, 102f,
    114, 115f, 116f
Fallopian tubes, 171f, 172–173, 172f, 173f
False capsule, of thyroid gland, 342
False (greater) pelvis, versus lesser pelvis,
    144f, 145–146
False ribs, 37

False vocal cords (vestibular folds), 393
Falx cerebelli, 309–310
Falx cerebri, 296, 309–310, 310f, 312, 312f, 313f
Falx inguinalis (conjoined tendon), 83, 85, 86f, 87
Fascia, 4–5, 4f
    of abdominal cavity, 93–94
    of abdominal wall, 79
    of ankle joint, 221f, 224
    of diaphragm, 129–130
    of gluteal region, 200–201, 201f
    of hand, 281–282, 283f
    of hip joint, 200–201
    of kidney, 130–131, 131b
    of leg, 221f, 223, 223f
    of lower limb, 195
    of neck, 322–324
        deep, 323–324, 323t, 324f
        superficial, 322
        in visceral column, 321, 323f, 323t
    of orbit, 347–348, 348f, 349f, 350
    of pelvis, 147f, 150f, 151, 152f
    of perineum, 181f
    of pharynx, 389
    of thigh, 205, 207f
    of urogenital triangle
        male, 183–184, 184f
        urogenital diaphragm, 179, 181
Fascia lata, 195, 205, 207f
Fat, in superficial fascia, 4–5, 4f
Fauces, isthmus of, 376
Feeding tubes, gastrostomy for, 96b
Female
    bladder development in, 164–166, 165f
    bladder of, 161–163
    pelvis of, 143f–146f, 146–147, 146t
    rectal examination of, 161t
    urethra of, 163, 164f
    urogenital triangle of
        superficial pouch in, 184–187, 185f–187f
        urogenital diaphragm in, 179, 180f, 181
Female genital system, 170–178. See also
        Ovary; Uterus.
    blood supply to, 177t
    development of, 177–178, 178f, 187–188, 188f, 189t
    innervation of, 177t
    uterine (fallopian) tubes in, 171f, 172–173, 172f, 173f
    vagina in, 176–177, 177t
Feminization, of males, 170b
Femoral artery, 138, 193, 205, 206f, 210f–212f, 216, 218f, 219, 219f, 220b
Femoral canal, 216, 218f
Femoral circumflex artery, 205, 206f, 211f, 219, 219f
Femoral cutaneous nerves, 136, 137, 137t, 186f, 191, 202, 203f, 205f, 207f
    anterior, 212f
    intermediate, 210f, 211f
    lateral, 136, 137, 137t, 210f, 211f
    posterior, 186f, 191, 203, 203f
Femoral nerve, 128f, 136, 137, 137t, 204f, 209t, 210f–212f, 217, 218f
Femoral ring, 216, 218f
Femoral sheath, 216, 218f
Femoral triangle, 212f, 216
Femoral vein, 210f, 212f, 216, 218f
Femur, 198, 199f
    avascular necrosis of, 202b
    distal, 205–206
    shaft of, 205–206
Fetus, circulation of, 62–65, 63f–66f, 65t
Fibroblast growth factor, in limb development, 196

Fibroids, uterine, 174b
Fibromuscular system, of orbit, 348
Fibrous capsule, of knee, 215, 215f
Fibrous joints, 6, 6t
Fibrous pericardium, 52, 52f
Fibrous trigone, 60f
Fibula, 206, 208f, 220, 222f
Fibular artery, 228f, 231
Fibular (lateral) collateral ligament, 208f, 215, 217f, 227f
Fibular nerve, 223f, 228t, 237f, 238f
Fibularis (peroneus) brevis muscle, 225, 226t, 227f, 228f
Fibularis (peroneus) brevis tendon, 237f
Fibularis (peroneus) longus muscle, 223f–225f, 225, 226t, 227f, 228f, 236, 236f
Fibularis (peroneus) longus tendon, 233f, 237f
Fibularis (peroneus) tertius muscle, 226, 227t
Filiform papillae, 380f, 381
Filum terminale, 30, 30f, 31f
Fimbriae ovarica, 172, 172f
Fingers. See Hand.
First atrial artery, 55
Fissures, of lung, 47–48, 47f
Fixation, in midgut development, 123f, 124, 124f
Flexion
    of ankle joint, 221f
    of elbow joint, 262, 263f
    of hand, 281, 282f
    of wrist joint, 270
Flexor carpi radialis muscle, 272, 273t, 275t, 288f
Flexor carpi radialis tendon, 277f, 280f
Flexor carpi ulnaris muscle, 272, 273t, 275t, 276f
Flexor carpi ulnaris tendon, 279f, 285f
Flexor compartment, of forearm, 266t, 272–273, 272f, 273t
Flexor digiti longus tendon, 239f
Flexor digiti minimi brevis muscle, 285f
Flexor digiti minimi muscle
    of lower limb, 234t, 235f, 236, 236f
    of upper limb, 283, 284f, 285t
Flexor digitorum brevis muscle, 234t
Flexor digitorum brevis tendon, 233f, 235f, 239f
Flexor digitorum longus muscle, 213t, 223f, 224f, 225, 226t, 233, 235f
Flexor digitorum longus tendon, 233f
Flexor digitorum profundus muscle, 273, 275t, 277f, 279f
Flexor digitorum profundus tendon, 279f, 285f, 286f
Flexor digitorum superficialis muscle, 272, 273, 273t, 274f, 275t
Flexor digitorum superficialis tendon, 279f, 285f
Flexor hallucis brevis muscle, 234t, 236, 236f, 239f
Flexor hallucis longus muscle, 213t, 224f, 225, 225f, 226t, 235f
Flexor hallucis longus tendon, 236f, 239f
Flexor hallucis tendon, 239f
Flexor pollicis brevis muscle, 283, 284f
Flexor pollicis longus muscle, 273, 275t, 277f
Flexor pollicis longus tendon, 280f, 285f, 286f
Flexor retinaculum
    of ankle, 224f, 239f
    of wrist, 274f, 278, 280f, 285f, 286f
Floating ribs, 37
Floor
    of mouth, 326, 376f, 382–384, 383f
    of orbit, 345
Fluid movement, across capillary walls, 3b

Foliate papillae, 380f, 381
Fontanelles, 292, 294f
Foot, 231–239
    arches of, 231–232, 232f
    blood supply to, 239, 240f
    definition of, 195, 196f
    function of, 231
    innervation of, 234t, 235f, 238–239, 238f, 239f
    ligaments of, 232–233, 233f
    muscles of, 233, 233f, 234t, 235f–237f, 235t, 236
Foramen cecum, 294f, 295b, 296, 358f, 380, 380f
Foramen lacerum, 294f, 296f, 297f, 297t, 298, 298f, 373
Foramen magnum, 294f, 297f, 299, 299t, 310f
Foramen ovale
    of heart, 64
    of skull, 294f, 296f, 297f, 297t, 298, 313f
Foramen rotundum, 296f, 297f, 297t, 298, 315f, 370f, 371, 371f
Foramen spinosum, 294f, 296f, 297f, 297t, 298
Forced expiration, 47
Forearm, 270–281. See also Elbow joint; Wrist.
    anatomic snuffbox in, 281, 281f
    blood supply to, 278–279, 279f
    bones of, 270, 271f, 272
    carpal tunnel in, 279, 280, 281b
    definition of, 242f
    extensor compartment of, 272f, 273–274, 273t, 274f, 275t
    flexor compartment of, 266t, 272–273, 272f, 273t
    innervation of, 275–278, 275t, 277f, 278f
    muscles of
        extensor, 272f, 273–274, 273t, 274f, 275t
        flexor, 266t, 272–273, 272f, 273t
Foregut, arterial supply of, 99–100, 99f
Foreskin (prepuce), 183f, 184
Fornix, of vagina, 173f, 174
Fossa navicularis, 183, 183f, 187f
Fossa ovalis, 57, 57f
Fourchette, 187f
Fovea capitis, 198
Fractures
    of anterior cranial fossa, 296b
    of middle cranial fossa, 299b
    of orbital wall, 350
Frontal bone, 292f–295f, 293, 297f, 302, 345, 346f, 347, 385, 385f
Frontal nerve, 315, 315f, 349f, 355, 356f, 357f, 387f
Frontal process, of maxilla, 293f, 302
Frontal sinus, 350f, 357f
    duct of, 386t
Frontal (metopic) suture, 292, 294f
Frontalis muscle, 300, 300f, 303t, 304f
Frontonasal canal, 387f
Frontonasal duct, 386t
Frontonasal process, face development from, 308, 308f
Fundiform ligament of penis, 182f
Fundus
    of gallbladder, 116f, 119
    of stomach, 94f, 95
    of uterus, 173, 173f, 175f
Fungiform papillae, 380f, 381

G

Galea aponeurotica, 300, 300f, 309f
Gallbladder, 104, 105f, 116f, 117f, 119–120
    duct system of, 122
    innervation of, 107t

Ganglia, 13–16, 13f, 15f, 16t, 21
  aorticorenal, 98f, 108
  Auerbach's (myenteric), 317
  cardiac, 60
  celiac, 97–98, 98f
  cervical, 330f, 331f, 340–341, 341f, 374f
  cervicothoracic (stellate), 241–242,
    340–341, 341f
  ciliary, 316, 341f, 353–354, 354f, 357f
  geniculate, 317, 319, 374f, 375
  inferior (nodose), 319, 339
  jugular (superior), 317, 339
  mesenteric, 98f, 113
  otic, 317
  pterygopalatine, 354f, 372f, 373, 374f, 375,
    379, 387f
  spiral, 319
  submandibular, 316–317, 374f, 384, 387f
  thoracic, 330f
  trigeminal, 313f, 314, 315f, 318, 357f, 358f
Gartner's cyst, 178, 178f
Gastric arteries, 96, 96f, 97f, 117f, 119f, 120,
  121
Gastric veins, 72, 97, 118f
Gastrocnemius muscle, 201f, 213f, 223f, 224,
  224f, 226t, 227f, 228t
Gastrocnemius tendon, 224f
Gastrocolic ligament, 95, 110
Gastroduodenal artery, 96, 96f, 97f, 105, 117f
Gastroesophageal reflux disease, 94b
Gastrointestinal tract. *See also specific
    structures, eg,* Colon; Esophagus;
    Stomach.
  nervous system of, 107t
Gastro-omental artery, 93f, 96, 97f, 117f, 119f
Gastro-omental vein, 97, 118f
Gastrophrenic ligament, 93f, 95
Gastrosplenic artery, 120
Gastrosplenic ligament, 92f, 93f, 95, 99f,
  101–102, 101f, 102f
Gastrostomy, 96b
Gastrulation, 6–8, 7f, 8f
Gemellus muscles, 200, 200t, 202f, 203f, 214f
General somatic efferent and afferent fibers
  in brachial plexus, 241
  in cranial nerves, 316–317, 318t
  of face, 305, 305f
General visceral efferent and afferent fibers,
  19, 19t
  in abdominal pain, 98
  in cranial nerves, 316–319, 318t
  to diaphragm, 41–42
  to heart, 60–61, 61f
  to ileum, 108
  to jejunum, 108
  to lung, 50
  to pelvis, 154
  to stomach, 98
  to visceral pleura, 46
Genicular artery, 218f
Geniculate ganglion, 317, 319, 374f, 375
Genioglossus muscle, 335f, 376f, 380f, 381,
  381t, 387f
Geniohyoid muscle, 329, 376f, 380f, 387f
Genital folds, 188f
Genital system. *See also* Female genital
    system; Male genital system.
  ambiguous, 170b
Genital tubercle, 165f, 187–188, 188f, 189t
Genitalia, external
  female, 184–187, 185f–187f
  male, 181–184, 181f–184f
Genitofemoral nerve, 88, 128f, 136, 137,
  137t, 191, 204f, 207f
Genitoinguinal ligament, 88, 90
Germ cells, 177

Germinal epithelium, 171
Gerota's (renal) fascia, 130–131, 131b
Glabella, 292f, 295f, 384f
Glans penis, 182, 182f
Glenohumeral joint, 249f
Glenohumeral ligaments, 249f, 250
Glenoid fossa, 247f, 248
Glenoid labrum, 247f, 248
Glomerular basement membrane, 135b
Glossoepiglottic fold, 380f, 381
Glossopharyngeal nerve (IX), 313f, 317–319,
  382, 391f, 396f
Gluteal arteries, 154t, 155, 155f, 202f, 203f,
  204, 206f, 211f
Gluteal lines, 198, 198f
Gluteal nerve, 151, 202f, 203, 204f, 205f
Gluteal region and hip joint, 197–205
  blood supply to, 204–205, 206f
  bones of, 197–198, 198f
  definition of, 195, 196f
  fascia of, 200–201, 201f
  innervation of, 200t
  movement at, 197, 198f
  muscles of, 198, 200, 200t, 202f, 203f
    injection into, 204b
  nerves of, 202–204, 205f
Gluteal tuberosity, 199f
Gluteus maximus muscle, 198, 200, 200t,
  201f, 202f, 203f, 214f
Gluteus medius muscle, 200, 200t, 201f, 202f,
  203f
Gluteus minimus muscle, 200, 200t, 202f
Gomphosis, 6t
Gonad(s). *See also* Ovary; Testis.
  development of
    female, 177–178, 178f
    male, 169–170, 169f, 170f
Gonadal arteries, 104f, 134f
Gonadal ridges, 169, 169f
Gonadal veins, 104f, 134f, 139, 139f
Goodell's sign, 174
Gout, 223b
Gracilis muscle, 210, 211f, 212f, 213t, 214f,
  218f, 224f
Gray matter, 11, 13, 13f
Gray ramus communicans, 14–15, 15f, 341
Great auricular nerve, 306f, 328f, 329, 336f
Great cardiac vein, 54f, 55f, 56
Great cerebral vein (of Galen), 310f, 312,
  312f
Great pancreatic artery, 119f
Great saphenous vein, 207f, 210f, 212f, 223f,
  228t
Great scapular (spinoglenoid) notch, 247,
  247f
Greater occipital nerve, 300, 306f
Greater omentum, 92f, 94f, 95, 101–102,
  101f, 124, 124f
Greater palatine artery, 377, 377f
Greater palatine canal, 370f, 371, 376
Greater palatine foramen, 370f, 371, 371f,
  376, 377
Greater palatine groove, 371, 371f
Greater palatine nerve, 372f, 373, 374f, 377,
  377f, 386
Greater pelvis, versus lesser pelvis, 144f,
  145–146
Greater petrosal nerve, 298, 373, 375
Greater sac, 102f
Greater sciatic foramen, 146, 146t
Greater splanchnic nerves, 74–75, 98
  of duodenum, 105–106, 107t
  of heart, 71f
  of stomach, 97
Greater trochanter, 198, 199f, 204f
Greater tuberosity, of humerus, 248

Greater tympanic artery, 298
Greater vestibular (Bartholin's) glands, 186,
  186f, 187f
Greater wing, of sphenoid bone, 296, 298,
  350f, 371, 371f
Gubernaculum, 88, 89f
Guyon's canal, 278

H
Hair, 4
Hamate, 271f, 272, 282f
Hamstring muscles, 210–211, 214f, 214t. *See
  also individual muscles.*
Hand, 281–290
  blood supply to, 289, 290f
  bones of, 270, 271f, 272
  claw deformity of, 287b
  definition of, 242f
  fascia of, 281–282, 283f
  innervation of, 286–289, 288f, 289f
  movements of, 281, 282f
  muscles of, 282–286, 284f–288f, 284t,
    285t
Hard palate, 376–377, 377f
Haustra, 109, 109f
Head
  of body. *See specific structures, eg,* Face;
    Oral cavity; Skull.
  of humerus, 248, 248f
  of ulna, 270, 271f
Headache, causes of, 316b
Heart, 53–65
  apex of, 53, 54f, 55
  auscultation of, 62, 63f
  base of, 53, 55f
  borders of, 53, 55f
  chambers of, 53
  circulation in, 53
  conduction system of, 61–62, 62f
  congenital defects of, 64–65, 65f, 67f
  coronary arteries of, 54f, 55–56, 56f
  development of, 62–65, 63f–66f, 65t
  innervation of, 60
  interior of, 57, 57f–60f
  location of, 53
  lymphatic system of, 62
  pericardium of. *See* Pericardium.
  referred pain from, 60–61, 61f
  sulci of, 54f, 55, 55f
  surfaces of, 53, 54f, 55, 55f
  tamponade of, 53b
  venous drainage of, 54f, 55f, 56–57
Hematoma, subdural, 312b
Hemiazygos vein, 73
  diaphragmatic hiatus for, 129
Hemorrhoidal plexus, 159–160
Hemorrhoids, 159–160
Hemothorax, 47b
Hepatic arteries, 93f, 96f, 97f, 114, 117f,
  118
Hepatic duct, 117f, 120, 122–123, 123f
Hepatic flexure, 103f, 110
Hepatic portal vein, 118–119, 118f
Hepatic veins, 118–120, 118f
Hepatoduodenal ligament, 92f, 94f, 99f, 100,
  101, 104, 114, 116f
Hepatogastric ligament, 92f, 94f, 99f, 100,
  114, 116f
Hepatopancreatic ampulla, 122
Hepatorenal pouch (of Morrison), 131
Hernia
  diaphragmatic, 42–43
  inguinal, 88b
  physiologic, in midgut development,
    122–123, 123f
Herpes zoster, 397, 401

Hesselbach's triangle, 87, 88b
Hiatus semilunaris, 385f, 386, 386t, 387f
Hilton's white line (intersphincteric line), 157f, 158
Hilum, 4
  of kidney, 133
  of lung, 47
  of spleen, 120, 120f
Hindgut, arterial supply of, 99–100, 99f
Hip bones, 79, 81f, 142–145, 142f–145f, 197–198, 198f. *See also individual bones.*
Hip joint. *See Gluteal region and hip joint.*
Horizontal chain, of lymph nodes, 344
Horizontal plane, 1, 2t
Horner syndrome, 355b
HOX genes, in limb development, 196b
Human papillomavirus, 176b
Humeral circumflex arteries, 258f, 260f, 261
Humerus
  distal, 261, 261f
  proximal, 248, 248f, 249f
Hymen, 178, 178f, 186f
Hyoepiglottic ligament, 394f
Hyoglossus muscle, 333, 334t, 335f, 336f, 380f, 381, 381t, 391f
Hyoid bone, 244f, 321–322, 323f, 342f, 343, 387f, 390f, 392f
Hyparterial bronchi, 48–49
Hypertension, portal, 159–160
Hypoblast, 6, 6f
Hypochondriac regions, 78, 78f
Hypodermis (superficial fascia), 4–5, 4f
Hypogastric nerves, 152, 152f, 153f, 153t, 175
Hypogastric plexus, 98f, 151–152, 152f, 153t, 154, 169, 175
Hypogastric (suprapubic) region, 78–79, 78f
Hypoglossal canal, 294f, 297f, 299, 299t
Hypoglossal nerve (XII), 311, 313f, 316, 328f, 329, 330f, 334t, 335f, 336, 340, 382, 384, 391f
Hypomere, back muscle development from, 32
Hypophysectomy, transsphenoidal approach to, 389b
Hypophysis (pituitary gland), 311, 313f, 389b
Hypothenar muscles, 283, 284f, 285t, 286
Hypoxia, 49b

I
Ileal artery, 111f
Ileocecal valve, 109, 110
Ileocolic artery, 110, 110f–112f, 111
Ileocolic vein, 118f
Ileum, 106, 106f, 107t, 108, 108b, 108t, 126
Iliac arcuate line, 127, 128f
Iliac arteries, 84f, 85, 104f, 134f, 137–138, 138t, 154–156, 155f, 204, 206f, 207f, 210f, 211f
Iliac crest, 144, 144f
Iliac fossa, 142f, 144, 144f
Iliac nodes, 160f, 172f, 175
Iliac spine, 142f, 144, 144f, 145f, 179f, 198f
Iliac veins, 84f, 104f, 134f, 138–139, 139f, 207f, 210f
Iliacus muscle, 128f, 129, 129t, 208, 209t, 210, 210f, 211f
Iliococcygeus muscle, 147f, 148f, 148t, 149, 153f
Iliocostalis muscle, 33t
Iliofemoral ligament (Y ligament of Bigelow), 201, 204f, 219f
Iliohypogastric nerve, 83–85, 128f, 136–137, 137t, 204f
Ilioinguinal nerve, 83–84, 87, 128f, 136–137, 137t, 191, 204f, 207f

Iliolumbar artery, 154t, 155, 155f
Iliopectineal (iliopubic) eminence, 142
Iliopsoas muscle, 127, 208, 209t, 212f, 218f
Iliopubic tract, 90
Iliotibial tract, 200–201, 201f, 214f, 216f, 218f, 227f
Ilium, 79, 81f, 127, 128f, 142f–145f, 144–145, 198, 198f
Impressions
  on esophagus, 71–72
  on femur, 199f
  on liver, 114, 115f, 116f
  on lung, 47–48, 47f
  on spleen, 120, 120f
Incisive canal, 377, 387f
Incisive foramen, 376, 377f
Incisive fossa, 376, 377f, 385f
Incisive papilla, 376–377, 377f
Indirect hernia, inguinal, 88b, 91f
Infection
  adenoidal, 389b
  cavernous sinus, 316b
  neck, spread of, 325b
  varicella-zoster virus, 397, 401
Inferior alveolar nerve, 387f
Inferior cervical ganglion, 330f, 340–341, 341f
Inferior cluneal nerve, 202f, 203f, 214f
Inferior concha, 385f, 386
Inferior epigastric artery, 85, 206f, 211f
Inferior extensor retinaculum, 237f
Inferior (nodose) ganglion, 319, 339
Inferior (petrous) ganglion, 319
Inferior gemellus muscle, 200, 200t, 202f, 203f, 214f
Inferior gluteal artery, 154t, 155f, 156, 203f, 204, 205, 206f, 211f
Inferior gluteal line, 198, 198f
Inferior gluteal nerve, 202f–205f, 203
Inferior hypogastric plexus, 152, 152f, 153f, 153t, 154, 169
Inferior labial artery, 300f, 307
Inferior laryngeal artery, 395f, 396f
Inferior longitudinal muscle, 380f, 382
Inferior meatus, 385f, 386
Inferior mesenteric artery, 99, 99f, 110–111, 111f, 112f, 134f, 138t
Inferior mesenteric vein, 112, 118f
Inferior oblique muscle, of orbit, 348f, 351–353, 351f, 352f, 352t, 354f
Inferior ophthalmic vein, 349f, 359
Inferior orbital fissure, 345, 346f, 347, 349f, 370f, 372
Inferior orbital margin, 345
Inferior palatine constrictor muscle, 378f
Inferior peroneal retinaculum, 227f, 237f
Inferior petrosal sinus, 312f, 313f, 314, 390f
Inferior petrosal sulcus, 296f
Inferior pharyngeal constrictor muscle, 335f, 389, 390f, 390t, 391f, 392t
Inferior phrenic artery, 42
Inferior position, 1, 2f, 2t
Inferior rectal artery, 192f, 193, 193f, 203f
Inferior rectal nerve, 193f, 203f
Inferior rectal vein, 118f, 159, 159f, 192f, 193
Inferior rectus muscle, 348f, 349f, 351, 351f, 352f, 352t, 353, 354f
Inferior sagittal sinus, 310f, 312, 312f
Inferior salivatory nucleus, 317
Inferior subscapular nerve, 243f
Inferior tarsus muscle, 349f
Inferior temporal line, 293f
Inferior thoracic aperture, 38
Inferior thyroid artery, 66, 330f, 332, 342f, 343, 396f
Inferior thyroid vein, 68f, 342f, 343

Inferior trunk, of brachial plexus, 242, 243f
Inferior ulnar collateral artery, 266, 267f, 269f, 279f
Inferior vena cava, 53, 55f, 57, 57f, 134f, 138–139, 139t
  diaphragmatic opening for, 128
  relationships of, 139t
Inferior vesical artery, 154t, 155f, 156, 168
Inferolateral surface, of bladder, 161, 162f
Infraglenoid tubercle, 247f, 248
Infrahyoid (strap) muscle, 324, 324f, 325f, 341–342
Infraorbital artery, 300f, 308, 349f, 368f, 375
Infraorbital canal, 346f
Infraorbital foramen, 292f, 300f, 302, 302t, 345, 346f
Infraorbital groove, 345, 346f
Infraorbital nerve, 306f, 307, 349f, 354f, 371, 372f, 375, 387f
Infrapatellar bursa, 208f, 215f, 227f
Infrapatellar fat pad, 215f
Infraspinatus muscle, 255, 256f–258f, 256t, 258
Infraspinous fossa, 247, 247f
Infratemporal fossa, 360–369
Infratrochlear artery, 356f
Infratrochlear nerve, 306f, 307, 349f, 356, 356f, 357f
Infundibulopelvic ligament, 170, 170f, 171f
Infundibulum
  of hypophysis, 311, 313f
  of ovary, 172, 172f
Infundibulum (conus arteriosus), 58, 58f, 66f
Inguinal canal, 85–90
  boundaries of, 85, 86f, 87
  contents of, 87–90, 88t, 89f, 91f
  hernia in, 88b
  openings of, 86f, 87
Inguinal ligament, 80f, 81f, 83, 83f, 85, 86f, 87, 128f, 144f
Inguinal nodes, 160f, 172f, 207f
Inguinal regions, 78f, 79
  versus inguinal canal, 85
Inguinal ring, 86f, 87, 88b, 91f
Injection, to gluteal region, 204b
Inner investing layer of deep fascia, 4f, 5, 150, 184f
Innermost intercostal muscle, 39, 39f, 40f
Inspiration, muscle activity in, 46–47
Interarytenoid muscle, 394f
Interatrial septum, 57–58, 57f, 64f, 65, 65f, 66f
Interatrial shunt, 63
Intercavernous sinus, 312f, 313f, 314
Interclavicular ligament, 249f
Intercondylar eminence, of tibia, 208f
Intercondylar fossa, of femur, 199f, 206
Intercondylar line, of femur, 199f
Intercostal arteries, 41, 49, 330f, 331f, 333
Intercostal muscles, 38–39, 39f, 40f, 46–47, 252f
Intercostal nerves, 40f, 41, 45, 263
Intercostal space, 36f, 38, 41
Intercostal veins, 41, 71f, 73, 74f, 85
Intercostobrachial nerve, 250f, 270f
Interfoveolar ligament, 90
Interlobular arteries, 133b
Intermaxillary process, face development from, 308–309, 308f
Intermediate femoral cutaneous nerve, 210f, 211f
Intermediolateral (lateral) horns, of spinal cord, 13
Intermesenteric plexus, 137, 152
Intermittent claudication, 220b
Intermuscular septum
  of arm, 267f
  of leg, 223f

Internal acoustic meatus, 297f
Internal auditory meatus, 297f, 299, 299f, 299t
Internal carotid artery, 300f, 311, 313f, 324f, 325, 331f, 337, 340f
Internal carotid nerve, 314, 353–354
Internal carotid nerve plexus, 341f
Internal iliac artery, 154–156, 155f, 204, 206f, 211f
Internal intercostal muscle, 39, 39f, 40f, 252f
Internal jugular vein, 312f, 323f, 324f, 325, 336f, 342f, 344
Internal laryngeal artery, 330f, 396f
Internal laryngeal nerve, 331f, 391f, 393, 395
Internal mammary artery, 333
Internal nasal nerve, 372f
Internal oblique muscle, of abdominal wall, 80f–82f, 81, 85, 86f
Internal pudendal artery, 154t, 155f, 156, 192–193, 192f, 193f
Internal pudendal vein, 159, 159f, 192, 193
Internal rectal venous plexus, 159, 159f
Internal spermatic fascia, 184f
Internal thoracic artery, 41, 66, 260f, 333
Internal thoracic vein, 41
Interosseous artery, 269f, 274f, 276f–279f
Interosseous border, of fibula, 222f
Interosseous fascia, 282
Interosseous membrane, 274f, 278f
Interosseous muscles
    of foot, 234t, 236–237, 236f, 240f
    of hand, 286, 286f, 287f
Interosseous nerve, 274f, 275t, 277, 277f, 288f
Interosseous recurrent artery, 279f
Interosseous talocalcaneal ligament, 230f
Interscalene triangle, 242, 244, 244f
Intersphincteric line (Hilton's white line), 157f, 158
Interspinous ligaments, of vertebral column, 29
Intertrochanteric crest, 198, 199f, 204f
Intertrochanteric line, 198, 199f, 204f
Intertubercular (bicipital) groove, 248, 248f
Intertubercular (transtubercular) line, 78, 78f
Intertubercular sulcus, of humerus, 249f
Interureteric crest, 167f
Interventricular artery, 55–56, 55f, 56f
Interventricular septum, 59f, 60, 64f, 65, 65f, 66f
Interventricular sulcus, 55
Intervertebral disks, 28–29
Intervertebral foramina, 24, 25f, 26f
Intestine. See Colon; Small intestine.
Intorsion, of eye, 351–353, 351f, 352f, 353t
Intraembryonic coelom, thoracic cavity development from, 43–44, 44f
Intramembranous bone formation, 247b
Intraperitoneal organs, 92–93, 94t
Intraventricular septum, 62f
Introitus, vaginal, 187, 187f
Inversion, of ankle joint, 221f, 229–230
Ischial spine, 142f, 143, 143f, 144f, 198f
Ischial tuberosity, 142f, 143, 179f, 180f, 198f
Ischioanal fossa, 185f, 189–190, 189b, 189f, 190f
Ischiocavernous muscle, 181f, 182, 182f, 186f, 187f
Ischiofemoral ligament, 201–202, 204f
Ischiopubic ramus, 143, 143f, 180f, 181f
Ischiorectal fossa, 181f
Ischium, 142f–145f, 143
Isthmus
    of fauces, 379
    of thyroid gland, 342f, 343
    of uterus, 173, 173f

J
Jejunal arcades, 106f
Jejunal artery, 106f, 111f
Jejunum, 106, 106f, 107t, 108, 108b, 108t, 126
Joint(s). See also specific joints.
    classification of, 6, 6t
    rib, 36f, 37, 37f
    shoulder region, 248–250, 248f, 249f
    vertebral, 28–29
    wrist, 281, 282f
Jugular foramen, 294f, 296f, 297f, 299, 299t
Jugular (superior) ganglion, 317, 339
Jugular (suprasternal) notch, 36f, 37, 38f, 299
Jugular vein, 54f, 67, 68f, 312f, 323f, 324f, 325, 328f, 336f, 339, 343–344
Jugular venous arch, 328f
Jugulodigastric node, 344
Jugulo-omohyoid nodes, 344
Juxtaglomerular cells, 135b

K
Kernig's sign, 31b, 397, 401
Kidney, 130–135
    blood supply to, 131f, 133, 133b, 134f
    calculi in, 398–399, 402
    cross-section of, 132f
    development of, 130, 134–135
    fascia of, 130–131, 131b
    function of, 130, 135b
    glomerular basement membrane of, 135b
    histology of, 135b
    innervation of, 133–134
    internal anatomy of, 130f, 131f, 133
    lateral surgical approach to, 133b
    left, 131, 132f, 133
    location of, 130, 130f
    lymphatic system of, 134
    morphology of, 130, 130f
    relationships of, 131, 131f, 132f, 133
    right, 131, 131f, 132f
    suprarenal gland on, 128f, 131, 131f, 134f, 135–136, 136t
    surface anatomy of, 130, 130f, 131f
    ureter attachment to, 130f, 134f, 135
Kiesselbach's area, 388
Klumpke's palsy, 245b
Knee joint
    blood supply to, 206f, 212f, 219–220, 219f
    bones of, 206, 208f
    innervation of, 204f, 217, 218f, 219, 219f
    ligaments of, 215–216, 215f–217f
    muscles of
        in anterior thigh compartment, 207–209, 209t, 210f
        in medial compartment, 210, 212f
        in posterior thigh compartment, 210, 211f, 213, 214f, 214t

L
Labia majora, 186–187, 186f, 187f
Labia minora, 185–186, 185f–187f
Labial artery, 186f, 300f, 307, 388
Labial nerve, 186f, 191, 193f
Labioscrotal folds, 187, 189f
Lacrimal artery, 356–357, 356f–358f
Lacrimal bone, 345, 346f, 347, 385f
Lacrimal crest, 346f, 347, 348f
Lacrimal gland, 349f, 350f, 354f, 356f, 357f
Lacrimal nerve, 307, 315, 315f, 349f, 355, 356f, 357f, 374f, 375, 387f
Lacrimal portion, of orbicularis oculi muscle, 303f, 304, 304f
Lacrimal sac, 348f, 349f
    fossa for, 346f, 347
Lacunar ligament, 83, 83f, 85
Lambdoid suture, 292f, 294f

Lamina cribrosa, 313f
Laminae
    of glomerular basement membrane, 135
    vertebral, 24–25, 25f
Laryngeal artery, 330f, 335f, 338, 393, 395, 396f
Laryngeal inlet, 389, 392, 395t
Laryngeal nerves, 68f, 330f, 331f, 332, 338, 339, 342f, 391f, 393, 393f, 395
Laryngeal vestibule, 393
Laryngopharynx, 388, 389
Larynx, 392–396
    blood supply to, 393, 395, 396f
    framework of, 392–393, 392f–394f
    innervation of, 393, 395, 395b, 395f
    muscles of, 393, 394f, 395t
Lateral antebrachial cutaneous nerve, 245, 264f, 271f, 283f
Lateral arcuate ligaments, 128f, 129–130
Lateral brachial cutaneous nerve, 270f
Lateral check ligament, 348, 348f
Lateral (fibular) collateral ligament, 208f, 215, 217f, 227f
Lateral compartment, of leg, 225, 226t, 227f
Lateral condyle
    of femur, 199f
    of tibia, 208f, 222f
Lateral cord, of brachial plexus, 243f, 244–245
Lateral cricoarytenoid muscle, 395t
Lateral cutaneous nerve of forearm, 265f, 268f, 271f
Lateral cutaneous nerve of thigh, 128f, 204f
Lateral dorsal cutaneous nerve, of foot, 237f
Lateral epicondyle
    of femur, 199f, 206
    of humerus, 262f
Lateral femoral circumflex artery, 205, 206f, 219–220, 219f
Lateral femoral cutaneous nerve, 136, 137, 137t, 207f, 210f, 211f
Lateral glossoepiglottic fold, 381
Lateral (intermediolateral) horns, of spinal cord, 13
Lateral lip, of femur, 199f, 205
Lateral malleolus, 220, 222f, 224f, 225f, 227f
Lateral meniscus, 215, 216f, 217f
Lateral nasal artery, 307
Lateral nodes, 140, 140t
Lateral palpebral artery, 356–357
Lateral palpebral ligament, 349f
Lateral pectoral nerve, 243f, 245, 250f, 253t, 259
Lateral plantar artery, 235f, 239, 239f
Lateral plantar nerve, 232f, 235f, 238–239, 238f, 239f
Lateral position, 1, 2f, 2t
Lateral pterygoid plate, 391f
Lateral rectus muscle, 348f–352f, 351, 354f, 356f–358f
Lateral region, of abdominal wall, 78, 78f
Lateral sacral artery, 154t, 155, 155f, 206f
Lateral sinus, groove for, 294f
Lateral supracondylar line, of femur, 206
Lateral sural cutaneous nerve, 224f, 238f
Lateral tarsal arteries, 240f
Lateral thoracic artery, 259, 260f
Lateral thoracic vein, 84f
Lateral thyrohyoid ligament, 392f
Latissimus dorsi muscle, 31, 32f, 253t, 254, 254f–256f, 265f
Latissimus dorsi tendon, 257f
Least splanchnic nerves, 74–75
Left anterior descending coronary artery, 54f
Left atrioventricular orifice, 59, 59f
Left atrium, 59
Left (main) coronary artery, 54f, 56, 56f

Left marginal artery, 54f, 55f
Left vagus nerve, 70, 71f
Left ventricle, 59–60, 59f, 60f
Leg, 220–231
    anterior compartment of, 225–226, 227t,
        228f
    blood supply to, 225f, 228f, 231
    bones of, 220, 222f, 223. *See also*
        individual bones.
    compartment syndrome in, 399, 402–403
    cross-section of, 223f
    definition of, 195, 196f, 220
    fascia of, 221f, 223, 223f
    innervation of, 228f, 230–231
    lateral compartment of, 225, 226t, 227f
    lymphatic system of, 231
    muscles of, 224–226, 224f, 225f, 226t, 227f,
        228f
    popliteal fossa of, 226, 228–229, 229f
    posterior compartment of, 224, 224f, 225f,
        226f
Lesser occipital nerve, 306f, 328f, 329,
        336f
Lesser omentum, 93f, 95, 99f, 100, 116f
Lesser palatine artery, 377, 377f
Lesser palatine canal, 371
Lesser palatine foramen, 370f, 371f, 376
Lesser palatine nerve, 372f, 373, 374f, 377,
        377f, 379
Lesser pelvis, versus greater pelvis, 144f,
        145–146
Lesser petrosal nerve, 298, 373
Lesser sac (omental bursa), 90–91, 92f, 93f,
        100–101, 102f
Lesser sciatic foramen, 146, 146t
Lesser splanchnic nerves, 74–75
Lesser trochanter, 198, 199f, 204f
Lesser tubercle, of humerus, 249f
Lesser wing, of sphenoid bone, 296, 298, 371,
        371f
Levator anguli oris muscle, 300f, 303t, 304
Levator ani muscles, 147f, 148f, 148t,
        149, 157f, 180f, 189–190, 189f, 190f,
        202f
Levator glandulae thyroidea muscle, 343
Levator labii superioris alaeque nasi muscle,
        300f, 303t, 304
Levator labii superioris muscle, 300f, 303t, 304
Levator palatini fold, 387f
Levator palpebrae muscle, 354f, 356f, 357f
Levator palpebrae superioris muscle, 348f,
        349f, 350–351, 350f, 357f, 358f
Levator scapulae muscle, 31, 32f, 253t, 254,
        255f, 256f, 327f
Levator veli palatini muscle, 378f, 378t, 379,
        379f, 391f
Ligament(s)
    of abdominal wall, 83, 83f, 83t
    of ankle joint, 229–230, 230f
    of bladder, 162, 162f
    of elbow, 262, 262f
    of foot, 232–233, 233f
    of gluteal region, 201–202, 204f
    of hand, 286, 286f
    of hip joint, 201–202, 204f
    of knee, 201f, 208f, 210f, 215–216,
        215f–217f
    of larynx, 392, 392f, 393, 394f
    of pelvis, 144f, 145f, 146
    peritoneal, 92, 92f, 150f, 151, 152f, 170f,
        173f, 174–175
    of shoulder, 248–250, 249f
    of uterus, 150f, 151, 170f, 173f, 174–175,
        175f
    of vagina, 176
    of vertebral column, 29

Ligament of Treitz, 105, 106b
Ligamentum arteriosum, 70, 71f
Ligamentum flavum, 29
Ligamentum nuchae, 29
Ligamentum teres
    of hip joint, 79, 202
    of liver, 101f, 114, 115f
Ligamentum transversum, 217f
Ligamentum venosum, 114
Limb(s). *See also* Lower limb; Upper limb;
        specific structures.
    development of, 195–197, 196b, 197f
Limb buds, 196, 197f
Line of gravity, in hip region, 204f
Linea alba, 80f–82f, 81, 83, 84f
Linea aspera, 199f, 205, 207
Lines
    of abdominal wall, 78, 78f
    of thoracic cavity, 43, 43f
Lingual artery, 330f, 335f, 338, 380f, 382,
        383
Lingual frenulum, 382
Lingual nerve, 374f, 380f, 383f, 384, 387f,
        389, 391, 396f
Lingual papillae, 380–381
Lingual tonsil, 381
Lingual vein, 338, 344, 380f, 382
Lingula, 48
Lip, 384f
    blood supply to, 307–308
    mucosa of, 376
    muscles of, 300, 304–305, 375
    skin of, 375
Lithotomy position, 178
Liver, 113–119
    biopsy of, 113–114
    blood supply to, 114, 117f, 118
    development of, 100
    extrahepatic duct of, 114, 117f, 118
    functional units of, 114
    innervation of, 107t, 119
    lobes of, 114, 115f, 116f
    location of, 113
    percussion of, 113–114
    peritoneal ligaments of, 114, 115f
    relationships of, 114, 115f–117f
    surface anatomy of, 113–114, 113f, 115f,
        116f
    veins of, 118–119, 118f
Lobar (secondary) bronchi, 48, 48f
Long buccal nerve, 307
Long ciliary artery, 357f, 359
Long ciliary nerve, 354f, 356, 357f
Long plantar ligament, 233, 233f
Long thoracic nerve, 243f, 244f, 245, 250f,
        253t, 258–259
Longissimus muscle, 33t
Longitudinal arch, 231–232, 232f
Longitudinal esophageal venous plexus, 72
Longitudinal ligaments, of vertebral column,
        29
Longitudinal muscle, 380f, 381–382
Lower limb, 195–240. *See also specific*
        structures.
    development of, 195–197, 196b, 197f
    fascia of, 195
    overview of, 195, 196f
    regions of, 195, 196f
Lower subscapular nerve, 259, 265f
Lower trunk, of brachial plexus, 242, 243f
Lumbar arteries, 138, 138t, 206f
Lumbar lymphatic trunk, 73, 140
Lumbar nodes, 139–140, 140t
Lumbar plexus, 136
Lumbar puncture, 31
Lumbar regions, of abdominal wall, 78, 78f

Lumbar spinal nerves, 136
Lumbar splanchnic nerves, 74–75, 98f,
        133–134, 137
Lumbar trunk, 172f
Lumbar veins, 73, 74f, 139, 139f
Lumbar vertebrae, 24f, 25f, 27
Lumbosacral nerves, 136
Lumbosacral plexus, 151, 217
Lumbosacral trunk, 128f, 155f, 202, 204f
Lumbrical muscles
    of lower limb, 234t, 235f, 236
    of upper limb, 285f, 286, 286f
Lunate, 270, 271f, 281, 282f
Lunate surface, of acetabulum, 197
Lung, 47–51
    blood supply to, 49
    bronchopulmonary segments of, 49
    collapsed, 45f
    development of, 44, 45f, 50–51, 50f
    diseases of, 49b
    external features of, 47–48, 47f
    histology of, 48b
    innervation of, 49–50
    internal features of, 48–49, 48f, 49t
    lymphatic system of, 50
    pleura covering. *See* Pleural cavity.
    right versus left, 47–48, 47f
    root of, 48
Lung buds, 50–51, 50f
Lymphatic system, 3–4
    of abdominal wall, 139–140, 140t
    of anal canal, 160–161, 160f
    of ankle joint, 231
    of breast, 39
    of colon, 112, 112f
    of epididymis, 166
    of face, 308
    of genital system, 177t
    of heart, 62
    of kidney, 134
    of knee joint, 207f, 220
    of leg, 231
    of lung, 50
    of mediastinum, 73–74
    of neck, 337f, 344–345
    of ovary, 171, 172f
    of perineum, 193
    of prostate gland, 169
    of rectum, 160–161, 160f
    of scalp, 308
    of submandibular triangle, 336, 337f
    of testis, 166
    of thigh, 207f, 220
    of thoracic wall, 41
    of thorax, 75
    of thymus, 67
    of uterus, 175

M
Male
    bladder of, 161–166, 162f, 165f
    pelvis of, 143f–146f, 146–147, 146t
    pseudohermaphroditism in, 170b
    rectal examination in, 161t
    urethra of, 163–164, 164f
    urogenital triangle of, urogenital diaphragm
        in, 179, 180f, 181, 181f
Male genital system, 166–170
    blood supply to, 168t
    development of, 169–170, 169f, 187–188,
        188f, 189t
    ductus deferens in, 155f, 162, 162f,
        166–167, 168t
    epididymis in, 166, 168t
    prostate gland in, 162, 162f, 167–169,
        168t

Male genital system (*cont'd*)
  seminal vesicle in, 162f, 167, 168t
  testis in. *See* Testis.
Malleolar artery, 240f
Malleolus, 220, 222f, 224f, 225f, 227f
Mamillary processes, vertebral, 27
Mammary artery, 333
Mammary gland (breast), 39, 41
Mandible, 292f, 293f, 302
Mandibular canal, 302
Mandibular nerve (V₃), 303t, 305, 305f, 307, 311, 358f, 375, 378, 379, 387f
  cavernous sinus and, 314–315
  function of, 317
Mandibular swellings, face development from, 308–309, 308f
Manubriosternal joint, 38f
Manubrium, 36f, 37–38, 38f
Marginal arcade, 357
Marginal artery, 54f, 55, 55f
  of Drummond, 111f, 112, 112f
Marginal mandibular nerve, 305, 305f
Marrow, 5
Masseter muscle, 300f, 327f
Mastoid canaliculus, 299t
Mastoid (posterolateral) fontanelle, 292, 294f
Mastoid foramen, 299t
Mastoid process, of temporal bone, 293f, 299
Maxilla, 292f, 293f, 302, 345, 346f, 347, 371
  frontal process of, 384f
  palatine process of, 377f, 387f
Maxillary artery, 308, 311, 331f, 338, 375, 388
Maxillary nerve (V₂), 305, 307, 311, 313f, 357f, 372–373, 372f, 374f, 387f
  branches of, 372f, 373, 374f
  cavernous sinus and, 314–315, 315f
Maxillary process, face development from, 308f, 309
Maxillary sinus, 346f, 386, 386t
Maxillary swellings, face development from, 308–309, 308f
Maxillary vein, 308, 312f
Meatus, 385f, 386
Meckel's (trigeminal) cave, 314–315
Medial antebrachial cutaneous nerve of the forearm, 250f, 270f, 271f
Medial arcuate ligament, 128f
Medial brachial cutaneous nerve of arm, 243f, 245, 250f, 263, 270f
Medial check ligament, 348, 348f
Medial circumflex artery, 218f
Medial (tibial) collateral ligament, 215, 215b, 217f
Medial compartment, of thigh, 209, 210f, 211, 212f, 213t
Medial concha, 385f
Medial condyle
  of femur, 199f
  of tibia, 222f
Medial cord, of brachial plexus, 243f, 244–245
Medial crus, 87
Medial cubital vein, 270
Medial epicondyle
  of femur, 206
  of humerus, 262f
Medial femoral circumflex artery, 205, 206f, 219–220, 219f
Medial intermuscular septum, 265f
Medial lip, of femur, 199f, 205
Medial malleolus, 220, 222f, 224f, 225f
Medial meniscus, 208f, 215, 217f
Medial palpebral artery, 357, 358
Medial palpebral ligament, 347, 349f

Medial pectoral nerve, 243f, 245, 250f, 253t, 259
Medial pharyngeal constrictor muscle, 379f, 390f
Medial plantar artery, 235f, 239, 239f
Medial plantar nerve, 232f, 235f, 238, 238f, 239f
Medial position, 1, 2f, 2t
Medial pterygoid muscle, 390f
Medial pterygoid plate, 370f, 385f
Medial rectus muscle, 348f, 350f, 351, 351f, 352f, 353, 357f
Medial supracondylar line, of femur, 206
Medial supracondylar ridge, of humerus, 262f
Medial sural cutaneous nerve, 223f, 224f, 238f
Medial tarsal arteries, 240f
Median arcuate ligament, 128f, 129–130
Median cricothyroid cartilage, 392f
Median cubital vein, 269, 270f, 271f
Median glossoepiglottic fold, 380f, 381
Median nerve, 243f, 245, 250f, 264f, 265f, 266, 271f, 274f, 275–276, 275t, 277f, 280f, 283f, 288–289, 289f
  in carpal tunnel, 279, 280, 281b
Median position, 1, 2t
Median sacral artery, 138t, 154, 154t
Median septum, of tongue, 380
Median thyrohyoid ligament, 392f
Median umbilical ligament, 152f, 162f
Mediastinal pleura, 44, 45f
Mediastinal surface, of lung, 47, 47f
Mediastinum
  anterior, 51, 54f
  heart in. *See* Heart.
  middle, 51, 51f
  midsagittal section of, 51f
  pericardium in, 51–53, 52f
  posterior, 70–75
  structures in, 51–53, 51f, 52f
  subdivisions of, 51
  superior, 51f, 65–70
Mediastinum testis, 166
Medulla
  of kidney, 130f, 133
  of suprarenal gland, 135, 136
Membranocranium, 292, 294f
Membranous urethra, 164, 164f, 167f, 181, 184f
Meningeal artery, 296, 310f, 311, 349f, 356f–358f
Meningeal layer, of dura mater, 309, 309f
Meningeal vein, 312, 313f
Meninges, 20
  cranial, 309–311, 309f, 310f
  spinal, 29–31, 29f–31f
Meningitis, 31, 31b, 397, 401
Meningoceles, 295b
Meniscus, of knee, 208f, 215, 216f, 217f
Menstrual cycle, 171b
Mental artery, 300f, 308, 331f
Mental foramen, 292f, 293f, 302, 302t
Mental nerve, 306f, 307, 375
Mentalis muscle, 300f, 303t, 304–305
Mesencephalic nucleus, 317–318
Mesenchyme, limb development from, 196
Mesenteric arteries, 99, 99f, 104f, 106, 106f, 111–112, 111f, 112f, 138t
  midgut development and, 122–123, 123f
Mesenteric ganglion, 98f, 113
Mesenteric plexus, 97
Mesenteric veins, 97, 104f, 108, 112, 118f
Mesentery, 92, 92f, 93f, 108
  liver development from, 99f, 100
  midgut development from, 122
Mesoappendix, 110, 110f

Mesocolon, 110
Mesoderm, 7–9, 7f, 8f
  diaphragm development from, 42, 42f
  peritoneum development from, 90
Mesogastrium, 99f
  liver development from, 100
  peritoneal ligament formation from, 101–102, 102f
  stomach development from, 95
Mesometrium, 175, 175f
Mesonephric duct, 165f, 166, 170, 170f, 178f, 189t
Mesonephros, 134, 165f
Mesosalpinx, 172f, 175, 175f
Mesovarium, 174, 175f
Metacarpal arteries, 288f, 290f
Metacarpal bones, 271f, 272
Metacarpal ligaments, 283f, 286f, 288f
Metacarpophalangeal joint, 282f
Metanephros, 134, 165f, 166
Metastasis, from breast cancer, 39, 41
Metatarsal arteries, 231, 232f, 239, 239f, 240f
Metatarsal bones, 220, 221f, 232f
Metopic (frontal) suture, 292, 294f
Mid-axillary line, 43, 43f
Midcarpal joint, 282f
Midclavicular line, 43, 43f, 46f
Middle cardiac vein, 55f, 57
Middle cerebral artery, 331f, 340f
Middle cervical ganglion, 330f, 340–341, 341f
Middle colic artery, 111f, 112f
Middle collateral artery, 269f, 279f
Middle concha, 386, 387f
Middle cranial fossa, 294f, 296, 296f–298f, 297t, 298, 299b
Middle meatus, 386, 387f
Middle meningeal artery, 296, 310f, 311, 356f, 357f, 358f
Middle meningeal vein, 313f
Middle palatine constrictor muscle, 378f, 380f
Middle pharyngeal constrictor muscle, 335f, 337, 389, 390t, 391f, 392t
Middle rectal artery, 154t, 155f, 156, 168t, 171f
Middle rectal vein, 118f, 159, 159f
Middle scalene muscle, 244f, 256f, 327, 327f, 330f
Middle supraclavicular nerve, 328f
Middle suprarenal artery, 134f
Middle thyroid vein, 342f, 343
Middle trunk, of brachial plexus, 242, 243f
Midgut
  arterial supply of, 99–100, 99f
  congenital abnormalities of, 125–126, 125f
  development of, 122–126
    fixation in, 123f, 124, 124f
    physiologic herniation in, 122, 123f
    physiologic reduction in, 122–123, 123f
Mid-inguinal lines, 78
Midline prelaryngeal (Delphian) node, 344
Midsagittal plane, 1
Midsternal line, 43
Mitral valve, 59, 59f, 60, 62, 63f
Modiolus, 304, 327f
Mons pubis, 186–187, 187f
Morphology, 2–3
Motor (efferent) neurons, 12, 12f, 17b
Motor root of the ciliary ganglion, 353, 354f, 357f
Mouth. *See* Oral cavity (mouth).
Mucoperiosteum, of palate, 376–377, 377f
Müllerian ducts, 169
Multifidus muscle, 33t
Multiple sclerosis, 12b
Multipolar neurons, 11

Muscle(s). *See also specific muscles.*
of abdominal wall
anterior, 80–85, 80f–84f
posterior, 127, 128f, 129t. *See also* Diaphragm.
of ankle joint, 224–226, 224f, 225f, 226t, 227f, 227t, 228f
of arm, 262–263, 264f, 266t
of auricle, 300f, 303t, 304
of back, 31–32, 32f, 33t
of bladder, 163
of elbow joint, 262–263, 264f, 266t
extraocular, 348–353, 349f–352f, 353t
of face, 300f, 303t, 304–305, 304f
fascia attached to, 5
of foot, 233, 233f, 234t, 235f–237f, 235t, 236
of forearm
extensor, 272f, 273–274, 273t, 274f, 275t
flexor, 266t, 272–273, 272f, 273t
of gluteal region, 198, 200, 200t, 202f, 203f, 204b
of hand, 282–286, 284f–288f, 284t, 285t
of hip joint, 198, 200, 200t, 202f, 203f
of larynx, 393, 394f, 395t
of leg, 224–226, 224f, 225f, 226t, 227f, 228f
of mouth, 300f, 301f, 303t, 304–305
of nose, 300f, 303t, 304
of orbit, 300f, 303t, 304, 348–353, 349f–352f, 353t
of palate, 377–379, 378f, 378t, 379f
of pelvis, 147–149, 147f, 148f, 148t
of penis, 182–183, 182f
of pharynx, 389, 390f, 390t, 391, 391f, 392f
of scalp, 295f, 300f, 301
of shoulder region
back, 253–254, 253f–255f, 253t
chest, 250–251, 251f, 252f, 253t
of thigh
in anterior compartment, 207–209, 209t, 210f
in medial compartment, 209, 210f, 211, 212f, 213t
in posterior compartment, 210, 211f, 213, 214f, 214t
of thorax, 38–39, 39f, 40f
of tongue, 380f, 381–382
types of, 5–6
of urogenital triangle, 179, 180f, 181–183
of wrist
extensor, 272f, 273–274, 273t, 274f, 275t
flexor, 266t, 272–273, 272f, 273t
Muscular branches, of cervical plexus, 328f, 329, 329t
Muscular fascia, of orbit, 348, 348f
Muscular interventricular septum, 64f, 65
Muscular triangle, of neck, 322f, 334t, 335f, 341–343, 342f, 342t
Musculocutaneous nerve, 243f, 245, 250f, 263, 264f, 265f, 266t, 267f, 269f
Musculophrenic artery, 41, 42, 85
Musculophrenic vein, 41, 85
Musculotendinous cuff, of shoulder, 257f, 258
Musculus uvulae muscle, 378t
Myelin, 11, 12b, 12f
Myenteric (Auerbach's) ganglion, 317
Mylohyoid cleft, 326, 382
Mylohyoid muscle, 323f, 327f, 333, 334t, 335f, 342f, 376f, 380f, 382, 391f
Mylohyoid nerve, 336, 387f
Mylohyoid raphe, 333
Myoblasts, back muscle development from, 32
Myocardial infarction, pain perception in, 17b

Myotome, 9, 9f, 21
back muscle development from, 32
vertebral development from, 27–28, 28f

N
Nares (nostrils), 384, 384f
Nasal aperture, 302
Nasal artery, 300f, 307, 358
Nasal bones, 292f, 302, 346f, 385f, 385f
Nasal branch, of olfactory nerve, 372f
Nasal cavity, 384–388
blood supply to, 387f, 388
bones of, 385–386, 385f
cartilages of, 384–385, 384f
innervation of, 386, 387f, 388
mucoperiosteum of, 386, 386t, 387f
pituitary access through, 389b
sinus openings in, 386, 386t, 387f
Nasal nerves, 306f, 307, 349f, 372f, 373
Nasal pit, face development from, 308, 308f
Nasal placodes, face development from, 308, 308f
Nasal process, face development from, 308, 308f
Nasal slit, 294f–296f
Nasal spine, 385f
Nasalis muscle, 300f, 303t, 304
Nasociliary nerve, 311, 315, 315f, 349f, 350, 354f, 355, 356f, 357f, 387f
Nasofrontal vein, 359
Nasolabial groove, 384f
Nasolacrimal canal, 347, 386
Nasolacrimal duct, 386
Nasopalatine nerve, 373, 377, 377f, 386, 388
Nasopharyngeal meatus, 387f
Nasopharynx, 388
Navicular bone, 220, 221f, 232f
Navicular fossa, 183, 183f, 187f
Neck
carotid sheath in, 324f, 325
cross-section of, 324f
definition of, 319
fascia of, 322–324, 323t, 324f, 325b, 325f
in visceral column, 321, 323f, 323t
of humerus, 248, 248f
infection of, spread of, 325b
larynx in, 392–396
lymphatic system of, 337f, 344–345
overview of, 319, 321, 322f, 322t
parotid space in, 322f, 334t, 342t, 365f, 366f, 368f, 369–370
triangles of, 325–343
anterior. *See* Anterior triangle, of neck.
carotid, 322f, 326f, 334t, 337–341
digastric (submandibular), 322f, 326f, 333, 334t, 335f, 336
muscular, 322f, 334t, 335f, 341–343, 342f, 342t
posterior. *See* Posterior triangle, of neck.
submental, 322f, 334t, 343
veins of, 343–344
vertebral column of, 322
visceral column of, 321–322, 323f, 341–343
Necrosis, avascular, 202b
Neonates
respiratory distress syndrome in, 50b
spinal cord of, 30–31
vertebral column of, 23
Nerve of Herring (carotid sinus nerve), 337
Nervous system, 4. *See also* Brain; Peripheral nervous system; Spinal cord.
of abdominal wall
anterior, 83–85, 84f
posterior, 128f, 136–137, 137t, 138t
of anal canal, 159
of ankle joint, 228f, 230–231

Nervous system (*cont'd*)
of arm, 263, 264f, 266, 267f
autonomic, 14–16
of back muscles, 32, 33t
of bladder, 163
of carotid triangle, 339–341, 341f
of cecum, 107t
of colon, 107t, 112–113
components of, 11
of diaphragm, 41–42
of duodenum, 105–106, 107t
of dura mater, 311
of epididymis, 166
of esophagus, 70, 72–73, 72t, 107t
of face, 295t, 303t, 305, 305f, 306f, 307
fibers of, 19, 19t
of foot, 238–239, 238f, 239f
of forearm, 275–278, 275t, 277f, 278f
of gallbladder, 107t, 120
of gastrointestinal tract, 107t
of genital system, 177t
of gluteal region, 200t, 202–204, 205f
of hand, 286–289, 288f, 289f
of heart, 60
of hip joint, 200t, 202–204, 205f
of ileum, 107t
of jejunum, 107t
of kidney, 133–134
of larynx, 393, 395, 395b, 395f
of leg, 228f, 230–231
of liver, 107t
of lung, 49–50
of nasal cavity, 386, 387f, 388
of orbit, 353–356, 354f, 355b, 356f, 357f
of ovary, 171
pain transmission in. *See* Pain.
of palate, 377, 377f, 379
of pancreas, 107t, 122
of pelvis, 150f, 151–152, 153f, 153t, 154
of pericardium, 53
of perineum, 191–193, 192f, 193f
of pharynx, 391–392, 391f
of pleura, 45–46
of prostate gland, 169
of pterygopalatine fossa, 372–373, 372f, 374f, 375
of scalp, 301
of shoulder region, 258–259, 258f, 259f
of spleen, 107t
of stomach, 97–99, 98f, 107t
of suprarenal gland, 136
of testis, 166
of thigh, 204f, 217, 218f, 219, 219f
of thymus, 67
tissue of, 12b
of tongue, 382
of trachea, 69
of upper limb, brachial plexus as, 241–246, 243f, 244f
of ureter, 135
of uterus, 175
of wrist, 275–278, 275t, 277f, 278f
Neural crest, 8, 9f, 19–21, 20f
Neural (occipital) triangle, 326, 327t
Neural tube, 8, 9f, 19–21, 20f
Neurocranium, 291
Neuroepithelial cells, 19–21, 20f
Neurons, 11, 11f, 12f
of autonomic nervous system, 14
development of, 19–21, 20f
fibers of, classification of, 19, 19t
first-order, 14
second-order, 14
of somatic nervous system, 14
Neurotransmitters, 11
Neurulation, 8, 9f

Nipple, 39
  in midclavicular line, 43, 43f
Nodes of Ranvier, 11, 12b, 12f
Nodose (inferior) ganglion, 319, 339
Nose. *See also* Nasal cavity.
  external, 384–385, 384f
  muscles of, 300f, 303t, 304
  septum of, 384, 384f, 385
Nostrils (nares), 384, 384f
Notochord, 7–8, 7f, 8f
Nucleus of Edinger-Westphal, 316
Nucleus pulposus, 28–29, 28f

O

Oblique arytenoid muscle, 395t, 396f
Oblique muscles
  of abdominal wall, 80–81, 80f–82f, 254, 254f
  of orbit, 348f–352f, 351–353, 354f, 356f, 358f
Oblique pericardial sinus, 52–53, 52f
Oblique vein (of Marshall), 55f, 56
Obstetrics, pelvic diameters in, 146f, 147
Obturator artery, 154t, 155f, 156, 206f, 211f
Obturator canal, 146, 146t, 147f
Obturator externus muscle, 202f, 210, 211f, 213t, 219f
Obturator fascia, 186f
Obturator foramen, 143, 143f
Obturator groove, of pubis, 142
Obturator internus fascia, 5, 153f
Obturator internus muscle, 147–148, 147f, 148f, 148t, 181f, 186f, 189–190, 189f, 190f, 200, 200t, 202f, 214f
Obturator internus tendon, 203f
Obturator membrane, 146, 186f
Obturator nerve, 128f, 136, 137, 137t, 153f, 155f, 156, 204f, 207f, 210, 210f, 211f, 213t, 217, 219, 219f
Occipital artery, 300f, 301, 302, 331f, 335f, 338
Occipital bone, 292f, 293f, 294f, 299
Occipital nerve, 300, 305f, 306f, 328f, 329, 336f
Occipital nodes, 344
Occipital sinus, 310f, 312
Occipital (neural) triangle, 326, 327t
Occipitalis muscle, 300, 300f, 303t
Occipitofrontalis (epicranius) muscle, 300, 303t
Oculomotor nerve (III), 313f, 316, 340f, 349f, 350f, 353, 357f, 358f
  cavernous sinus and, 314–315, 315f
Olecranon, 267f
Olecranon fossa, 261, 262f
Olecranon process, 261
Olfactory bulb, 372f, 387f
Olfactory foramina, 296
Olfactory nerve (I), 313f, 319, 372f, 386
Olfactory tract, 372f
Oligodendrocytes, 20
Omental (epiploic) appendices, 109, 109f
Omental bursa (lesser sac), 90–91, 92f, 93f, 100–101, 102f
Omental foramen, 91, 92f–94f
Omentum, 92f–94f, 95, 99f, 100–102, 101f, 116f, 124, 124f
Omohyoid muscle, 256f, 323f, 325, 326, 326f, 327f, 335f, 336f, 341
Omphalocele, 125, 125f
Ophthalmic artery, 301, 307–308, 311, 349f, 350, 354f, 356–357, 356f–358f
Ophthalmic nerve (V₁), 307, 313f, 349f, 355, 356, 358f, 372f, 374f, 375, 387f
  cavernous sinus and, 314–315, 315f
Ophthalmic vein, 308, 312f, 313f, 345, 349f, 359

Opponens digiti minimi muscle, 283, 285f, 285t, 286
Opponens pollicis muscle, 283, 284t, 285f
Opposition, 279, 280f, 281, 282f
Optic canal, 294f, 296f, 297f, 297t, 346f
Optic chiasm, 350f
Optic chiasmatic groove, 293, 294f
Optic chiasmatic sulcus, 297t
Optic foramen, 345
Optic nerve (II), 313f, 315f, 319, 345, 348f–350f, 353, 354f, 357f, 358f
Optic sheath, 348f
Oral cavity (mouth), 375–384. *See also* Lip.
  blood supply to, 382
  boundaries of, 375, 375t
  floor of (paralingual space), 326, 376f, 382–384, 383f
  muscles of, 300f, 301f, 303t, 304–305
  palate, 376–379, 377f–379f, 378t, 383f, 384
  paralingual (sublingual) space, 326, 376f, 382–384, 383f
  proper, 375–376, 375t, 376f
  tongue, 379–382, 380f, 381t
  tonsil, 378f, 379
  vestibule, 375–376, 376f
Orbicularis oculi muscle, 300f, 303t, 304, 304f, 348f
Orbicularis oris muscle, 300f, 304
Orbit, 291, 302, 345–359
  blood supply to, 356–359, 358f
  bones of, 345–347, 346f, 347t
  cross-section of, 348f
  fascia of, 347–348, 348f, 349f, 350
  innervation of, 353–356, 354f, 355b, 356f, 357f
  landmarks of, 347t
  movement of, 351, 351f, 352f
  muscles of, 300f, 303t, 304, 349f, 350–353, 350f, 352f
Orbital fissure, 297f, 297t, 298, 314, 345, 346f, 349f, 370f, 371f, 372
Orbital fossa, 296f
Orbital margin (aditus), 345
Orbital part
  of ethmoid bone, 295f
  of frontal bone, 293, 294f, 295f, 297f
  of orbicularis oculi muscle, 303t, 304, 304f
Orbital process, of palatine bone, 371f
Orbital septum, 347, 348f, 349f
Orbital strut, 345
Orbital tubercle, 345, 346f, 348f
  of the zygomatic bone, 346f, 348
Orbital walls, 345, 346f, 347, 351f
Oropharyngeal isthmus, 376
Oropharyngeal membrane, 308f, 309
Oropharynx, 388, 389
Osmotic pressure, 3b
Ostium secundum, 64, 64f
Otic ganglion, 317
Outer investing layer of deep fascia, 4f, 5
  of neck, 323, 323t, 324f
Ovarian artery, 138t, 154t, 156, 170f, 171–173, 171f, 173f, 177t
Ovarian fossa, 170
Ovarian ligament, 170, 170f, 175, 175f
Ovarian vein, 170f, 171, 171f, 177t
Ovary, 170–171, 171f, 177t
  descent of, 90
  development of, 169f, 171, 177–178, 178f
  nervous system of, 154, 177t
Oviducts (fallopian tubes), 171f, 172–173, 172f, 173b, 173f

P

Pacchionian (arachnoid) granulations, 309f, 311
Pachymeninx (dura mater), 309–311, 309f
Pain
  abdominal, 98–99, 98b
  in appendicitis, 110
  perception of, 17b
  referred, 17–18, 19f
    cardiac, 60–61, 61f
    from gastrointestinal tract, 107t
  in renal calculi, 398–399, 402
  in shingles, 397, 401
  visceral, 17–18, 19f
Palate, 376–379
  bone of, 385f
  cleft, 384b
  development of, 383f, 384
  hard, 376–377, 377f
  soft, 377–379, 378f, 378t, 379f
Palatine aponeurosis, 378
Palatine artery, 335f, 377, 377f, 396f
Palatine bone, 345, 346f, 347, 370f, 371, 371f, 372f, 376, 377f, 385, 385f
Palatine canal, 370f, 371, 376
Palatine constrictor muscle, 378f
Palatine folds, 376f, 377f
Palatine foramen, 370f, 371, 371f, 376, 377
Palatine glands, 377, 377f
Palatine groove, 371, 371f, 377f
Palatine nerve, 372f, 373, 374f, 377, 377f, 386, 391–392, 391f
Palatine raphe, 376f, 377, 377f
Palatine suture, 385f
Palatoglossal arch, 376, 376f, 379, 380f
Palatoglossus muscle, 378f, 378t, 380f, 381, 381t
Palatopharyngeal arch, 376f, 379, 380f, 387f
Palatopharyngeal fold, 379
Palatopharyngeal muscle, 378f, 378t, 379f
Palatopharyngeal sphincter (Passavant's ridge), 378f, 379, 389
Palatopharyngeus muscle, 379, 390t
Palatovaginal (pharyngeal) canal, 370f, 371, 371f
Palmar aponeurosis, 282, 283f
Palmar arch, 279f, 288f, 289, 290f
Palmar carpal arch, 290f
Palmar interosseous muscles, 286, 287f
Palmar metacarpal artery, 288f, 290f
Palmaris brevis muscle, 281, 283f
Palmaris longus muscle, 272, 272f, 275t
Palmaris longus tendon, 280f, 284f
Palpebral artery, 356–357, 358
Palpebral ligament, 347, 349f
Palpebral portion, of orbicularis oculi muscle, 303t, 304, 304f
Palsy, facial nerve, 400, 403
Pampiniform plexus, 171
Pancreas, 131
  bile duct in, 122
  blood supply to, 119f, 121
  development of, 100, 102–103, 103f
  innervation of, 107t
Pancreatic artery, 119f
Pancreatic bud, 100
Pancreatic duct (of Wirsung), 121
Pancreaticoduodenal arteries, 96f, 97f, 99, 105, 117f, 119f, 121, 122
Pancreaticoduodenal veins, 118f
Papilla of Vater, 104, 105f
Papillary muscles, 58, 58f, 59f
Para-aortic nodes, 75
Para-axial (somitic) mesoderm, 8–9, 9f
Paralingual (sublingual) space, 326, 376f, 382–384, 383f

Paralysis, of diaphragm, 42b
Paramesonephric ducts, 169, 169f, 178, 178f, 189t
Parametrium, 174
Paranasal sinuses, 385–386, 387f
Pararectal pouches, 151
Pararectal space, 150f
Pararenal fascia, 130, 132f
Parasagittal plane, 1, 2t
Parasternal line, 43
Parasternal nodes, 41, 75
Parasympathetic nervous system, 16, 18f, 19t
    of anal canal, 159
    of bladder, 163
    of colon, 113
    of duodenum, 105–106, 107t
    of pancreas, 122
    of pelvis, 154
    of perineum, 192
    of stomach, 97–99, 98f
    of ureter, 135
    of uterus, 175
Parathyroid glands, 343
Paratracheal nodes, 50
Paraurethral (Skene's) glands, 186, 187f
Paravesical space, 150f
Parietal bone, 292f, 293f, 294f, 299
Parietal emissary vein, 312
Parietal endopelvic fascia, 150
Parietal foramen, 292f
Parietal (somatic) mesoderm, 9
Parietal pericardium, 51–52, 52f, 54f
Parietal peritoneum, 90, 92f
Parietal pleura, 44–45, 45f
Parotid duct, 305f
Parotid gland, 300f, 305, 305f, 308, 336f
Parotid nodes, 308, 344
Passageways, of pelvis, 146, 146t
Passavant's ridge (palatopharyngeal sphincter), 378f, 379, 389
Patella, 206, 208f, 210f
Patellar ligament, 201f, 208f, 210f, 215, 215f–217f
Patellar retinaculum, 215
Patent ductus arteriosus, 65
Pecten of the pubis, 80, 81f, 142, 142f, 157f
Pectinate line, 157f, 158, 158t
Pectineal ligament, 83, 83f, 142
Pectineal line, 80, 81f, 142, 142f
Pectineus muscle, 208, 209t, 210, 210f, 212f, 218f, 219f
Pectoral nerve, 243f, 245, 250f, 253t, 259
Pectoralis major muscle, 250, 251f, 253t, 256f
Pectoralis minor muscle, 250–251, 251f, 253t
Pedicles, vertebral, 23–24, 25f
Pelvic diaphragm, 176
Pelvic floor, 147f
Pelvic inlet, 144f, 145, 179f
Pelvic outlet, 145–146, 146f
Pelvic splanchnic fibers, 16, 18f, 19t
Pelvic splanchnic nerves, 137, 152, 153f, 192, 205f, 317
Pelvis, 141–178
    versus abdomen, 141–142
    anorectal structures in. See Anal canal; Rectum.
    blood supply of, 154–156, 154t, 155f
    bones of, 142–145, 142f–145f, 197–198, 198f
    development of
        anorectal structures, 164–166, 165f
        bladder, 164–166, 165f
        female reproductive system, 177–178, 178f
        male reproductive system, 169–170, 169f, 170f

Pelvis (cont'd)
    diaphragms of, 147f, 148f, 148t, 149–150
    fascia of, 147f, 150f, 151, 152f
    genital system of. See Female genital system; Male genital system.
    greater, 144f, 145–146
    lesser, 144f, 145–146
    ligaments of, 144f, 145f, 146
    lower limb attachment to, 195, 196f
    muscles of, 147–149, 147f, 148f, 148t
    nervous system of, 150f, 151–152, 153f, 153t, 154
    organ prolapse in, 149b
    organization of, 145–149
    passageways of, 146, 146t
    sex dimorphisms in, 143f–146f, 146–147, 146t
    ureter in, 161, 162f
    urinary system of, 160f, 161–166, 162f, 164f
    urogenital hiatus in, 147f, 149–150
    wall of, versus abdominal wall, 142
Pelvis major (greater pelvis), versus lesser pelvis, 144f, 145–146
Penile (spongy) urethra, 164, 164f, 167f, 181–183, 182f–184f
Penis, 181–182, 182f
    deep artery of, 183f
    deep dorsal vein of, 152f
    dorsal nerve of, 180f, 191–192, 192f
    dorsal vein of, 183f
    erectile tissue of, 181–182, 182f
    fascia of, 184, 184f
    midsagittal section of, 183f
    muscles of, 182–183, 182f
    transverse section of, 183f
Peptic ulcer disease, 398, 402
Perforating femoral arteries, 219, 219f
Perianal space, 190f
Pericardiacophrenic artery, 42, 53
Pericardial cavity, 43–44, 44f, 52, 52f
Pericardiocentesis, 53b
Pericardium, 51–53, 54f
    arterial supply to, 53
    cavity of, 52
    development of, 52
    fibrous, 52, 52f
    innervation of, 53
    sinuses of, 52–53, 52f
Pericranium, 301, 309f
Perimuscular plexus, 159f
Perineal artery, 180f, 192f, 193, 193f
Perineal body (central tendon of perineum), 152f, 182f, 184f, 187f, 190f
Perineal flexure, of rectum, 156, 157f
Perineal ligament, 152f
Perineal membrane, 180f, 181f, 185f, 186f
Perineal muscles, 180f, 182f, 183, 184f, 190f
Perineal nerve, 180f, 191, 192f, 193f
Perineal space, deep, 186f
Perineum, 178–193
    anal triangle in, 178–179, 179f, 189–191, 189f, 190f
    boundaries of, 178–179, 179f, 180f
    definition of, 178
    development of, 187–188, 188f, 189t
    fascia of, 181f
    lymphatic system of, 160f, 172f, 193
    neurovascular bundles of, 191–193, 192f, 193f
        female superficial pouch in, 184–187, 185f–187f
        male superficial pouch in, 181–184, 181f–184f

Perineum (cont'd)
    urogenital triangle in
        urogenital diaphragm in, 179, 180f, 181, 181f
Perineurium, 12b
Periorbita, 347, 348f, 373
Periosteal (endosteal) layer, of dura mater, 309, 309f
Periosteum, 5
Peripheral arcade, 357
Peripheral nervous system. See also Autonomic nervous system.
    development of, 20f, 21
    overview of, 12, 12b, 12f
Perirenal fascia, 130, 132f
Peritoneal cavity, 90
    development of, 43–44, 100
    ovum release into, 172
Peritoneal ligaments, 92, 92f, 150f, 151, 152f, 170f, 173f, 174–175
    development of, 101–102, 102f
    of liver, 100, 114, 115f
Peritoneal reflections, 91–92
Peritoneum, 5, 82, 90–93, 92f, 93f, 94t
    development of, 90, 124
    innervation of, 85
    lesser sac of, 90–91, 92f, 93f, 101, 102f
    pouches of, 150f, 151, 152f
    on uterus, 174
Peroneal artery, 225f, 228t, 240f
Peroneal communicating nerve, 223f, 224f
Peroneal nerve, 203, 205f, 214f, 214t, 223f, 228f, 231, 237f
Peroneal retinaculum, 227f, 237f
Peroneus (fibularis) brevis muscle, 225, 227f, 228f, 235f
Peroneus (fibularis) brevis tendon, 228f
Peroneus (fibularis) longus muscle, 224f, 225, 225f, 227f, 228f
Peroneus (fibularis) tertius muscle, 226
Peroneus (fibularis) tertius tendon, 237f
Perpendicular plate, of palatine bone, 371f
Persistent truncus arteriosus, 65, 67f
Pes anserinus, 210, 213t
Petrocinoid ligament, 315
Petrosal artery, 298
Petrosal nerve, 298, 373, 375
    hiatus of, 297t
Petrosal sinus, 312f, 313f, 314, 390f
Petrosal sulcus, 296f
Petrous portion, of temporal bone, 296, 298, 298f, 299, 314
Petrous ridge, of temporal bone, 298
Phalanges, 221f, 223, 271f, 272
Pharyngeal arches, 319, 320f, 321t, 376f
Pharyngeal artery, 331f, 335f, 338, 379
Pharyngeal (palatovaginal) canal, 370f, 371, 371f
Pharyngeal constrictor muscles, 334t, 335f, 337, 378f, 379f, 389, 390f, 390t, 391f, 392t
Pharyngeal nerve, 372f, 373
Pharyngeal plexus, 339, 382, 391
Pharyngeal pouches, 319, 320f, 321t
Pharyngeal raphe, 389, 390f
Pharyngeal recess, 387f, 389
Pharyngeal vein, 344
Pharyngobasilar fascia, 391
Pharyngotympanic (auditory) tube, 298, 378f, 379f, 389
Pharynx, 389–392
    boundaries of, 388t
    divisions of, 388–389
    fascia of, 389
    innervation of, 391–392, 391f
    muscles of, 389, 390f, 390t, 391, 391f, 392t
Philtrum, 384f

Phrenic arteries, 42, 97f, 134f, 137–138, 138t
Phrenic nerve, 243f, 244f, 250f, 328f, 329, 330f, 331f
   to diaphragm, 41–42
   to esophagus, 71f
   to heart, 54f, 68f
   to pericardium, 53
   to pleural cavity, 45
Phrenic vein, 134f
Phrenicocolic ligament, 93f
Pia mater, 29f, 30, 30f, 309f, 311
Piriform aperture, 292f, 302
Piriform recess, 389, 396f
Piriformis muscle, 147–149, 147f, 148f, 148t, 200, 200t, 203f
Pisiform, 270, 272f, 282f
Pituitary gland, 311, 313f
   transsphenoidal surgical approach to, 389b
Planes, 1
   of abdominal wall, 78, 78f
   types of, 1, 2f, 2t
Plantar aponeurosis, 232–233, 232f
Plantar arteries, 235f, 239, 239f, 240f
Plantar digital arteries, 239f
Plantar digital nerves, 239f
Plantar interosseous muscles, 236–237
Plantar ligament, 230f, 233, 233f
Plantar metatarsal arteries, 232f, 239, 239f
Plantar muscles, 233, 233f, 233t, 235f–237f, 236–237
Plantar nerves, 232f, 235f, 238, 238f, 239, 239f
Plantarflexion, of ankle joint, 221f, 229
Plantaris muscle, 224f, 225, 226t
Plantaris tendon, 223f, 224f, 225
Platysma muscle, 300f, 305, 322
Pleural cavity, 44–47
   development of, 43–44, 44f
   features of, 44, 45f
   fluid removal from (thoracentesis), 45b, 47b
   neurovascular supply of, 45–47
   nomenclature of, 44–45, 45f
   parietal pleura in, 44–45, 45f
   pathology of, 47b
   recesses of, 45, 46f
   respiration and, 46–47
   visceral pleura in, 44–46, 45f
Pleural pressure, 46–47
Pleuropericardial folds, thoracic cavity development from, 44, 44f
Pleuroperitoneal folds, thoracic cavity development from, 44
Pleuroperitoneal membranes, diaphragm development from, 42, 42f
Plica fimbriata, 380f, 382
PMI (point of maximal impulse), 43b
Pneumocytes, 48b
Pneumothorax, in pleural cavity, 47b
Point of maximal impulse, 43b
Popliteal artery, 214f, 224f, 225f, 231
Popliteal fossa, 226, 228–229, 229f
Popliteal vein, 224f
Popliteus muscle, 223f, 225, 225f, 226t
Porta hepatis, 114, 116f
Portal hypertension, 159–160
Portocaval anastomosis, 159
Position, anatomic, 1–4, 2f, 2t, 3b, 3f
Posterior antebrachial cutaneous nerve, 267f, 268f, 270f, 271f
Posterior auricular artery, 300f, 302, 331f, 335f, 338
Posterior auricular muscles, 304
Posterior auricular nodes, 344
Posterior auricular vein, 308, 343
Posterior axillary line, 43, 43f

Posterior belly, of digastric muscle, 337
Posterior brachial cutaneous nerve, 267f, 268f
Posterior cerebral artery, 331f, 340f
Posterior ciliary artery, 358f
Posterior circumflex humeral artery, 268f, 271f
Posterior clinoid process, 296
Posterior communicating artery, 331f, 340f
Posterior compartment
   of arm, 263, 266t, 267f
   of leg, 224, 224f, 225f, 226t
   of thigh, 210, 211f, 213, 214f, 214t
Posterior cord, of brachial plexus, 243f, 244–245
Posterior cranial fossa, 294f, 297f, 298f, 299, 299t
Posterior cricoarytenoid ligament, 392f, 396f
Posterior cruciate ligament, 215–216, 215f–217f
Posterior cutaneous nerve of thigh, 193f, 204f
Posterior ethmoid groove, 295f
Posterior ethmoidal artery, 356f–358f, 357
Posterior ethmoidal foramen, 346f
Posterior ethmoidal nerve, 356, 356f, 357f
Posterior femoral cutaneous nerve, 186f, 191, 203, 203f, 205f
Posterior fontanelle, 292, 294f
Posterior gluteal line, 198, 198f
Posterior intermuscular septum, 223f
Posterior interosseous artery, 276f, 277f, 278, 279f
Posterior interosseous nerve, 275t, 277, 278f
Posterior interventricular artery, 55–56, 55f, 56f
Posterior lacrimal crest, 346f, 347, 348f
Posterior left ventricular vein, 55f
Posterior nasal spine, 385f
Posterior papillary muscle, 58, 58f, 59f
Posterior perforating arteries, of foot, 240f
Posterior position, 1, 2f, 2t
Posterior recess of the ischioanal fossa, 189, 190f
Posterior scalene muscle, 256f, 327, 327f
Posterior spinal artery, 332, 340f
Posterior superior alveolar canal, 293f
Posterior superior alveolar nerve, 387f
Posterior supraclavicular nerve, 328f
Posterior tibial artery, 225f, 231, 232f, 239, 239f
Posterior triangle, of neck, 325–333
   boundaries of, 325, 325t
   cervical plexus in, 253t, 327f, 328–329, 328f, 329t
   circulation in, 329, 330f, 331f, 332–333
   subdivisions of, 325–326, 327f, 327t
Posterior trunk, of brachial plexus, 244
Posterior vertebral artery, 332
Posteroinferior lateral nasal nerve, 386
Posterolateral (mastoid) fontanelle, 292, 294f
Posterosuperior lateral nasal nerve, 373, 386
Postganglionic (postsynaptic) neurons and fibers, 14–15, 15f, 16t, 17t, 169
   of diaphragm, 42
   of epididymis, 166
   of esophagus, 72–73
   of facial nerve, 373, 374f, 375
   of oral cavity, 383
   of palate, 379
   of pelvis, 151–152, 153f, 153t
   of stomach, 97–98
   of testis, 166
   of uterus, 175
Postsynaptic neurons and fibers. *See* Postganglionic (postsynaptic) neurons and fibers.
Pouch(es), peritoneal, 150f, 151, 152f

Pouch of Douglas (rectouterine pouch, cul-de-sac), 151, 152f, 156, 157f, 158, 170f, 174
Preaortic (prevertebral) ganglia, 16
Preaortic lymph nodes, 160f
Preaortic nodes, 75, 140, 140t
Preauricular nodes, 344
Precaval nodes, 160f
Preganglionic (presynaptic) neurons and fibers, 14–15, 15f, 16t, 17t
   of brachial plexus, 241
   of epididymis, 166
   of esophagus, 72–73
   of facial nerve, 373, 374f
   of heart, 61, 61f
   of ileum, 108
   of jejunum, 108
   of pelvis, 151–152, 153f, 153t
   of prostate, 169
   of stomach, 97
   of testis, 166
   of uterus, 175
Pregnancy
   cervical changes in, 173–174
   ectopic, 173b
Prepatellar bursa, 215f
Prepuce, 183f, 184
Presacral (Waldeyer's) fascia, 157, 190f
Presacral (superior hypogastric) plexus, 151–152
Presacral space, 190f
Presynaptic neurons and fibers. *See* Preganglionic (presynaptic) neurons and fibers.
Pretracheal layer, of neck fascia, 323–324, 324f
Pretracheal space, 324f, 325f
Prevertebral fascia, 324, 324f, 325f
Prevertebral (preaortic) ganglia, 16
Primitive atrium, 63, 63f
Primitive node, 7, 7f
Primitive pit, 7, 7f, 8f
Primitive sex cords, 169, 169f, 177–178
Primitive streak, 7, 7f, 8f
Primitive urogenital sinus, 189t
Primitive ventricle, 63, 63f
Princeps pollicis artery, 290f
Procerus muscle, 300f, 303t, 304, 304f
Processus vaginalis, 88, 88b, 89f, 90, 166
Profunda brachii artery, 265f
Profunda femoris artery, 219f
Pronation
   of elbow joint, 262, 263f
   of wrist, 270
Pronator quadratus muscle, 272f, 273, 274f, 275t, 277f, 285f
Pronator teres muscle, 271f, 272f, 273, 275t
Pronephros, 134
Proper digital arteries, 290f
Proper digital nerve, 284f, 287
Proper dorsal digital nerve, 237f
Proper hepatic artery, 93f, 114, 119f
Proper palmar digital artery, 283f
Proper plantar digital nerve, 232f, 239f
Proprioception, 12, 317–318, 318t
Prostate gland, 162, 162f, 167–170, 167f, 168t, 169b
Prostatic fascia, 150
Prostatic plexus of veins, 168
Prostatic sheath, 168
Prostatic urethra, 163–164, 164f, 168
Prostatic utricle, 152f, 167f
Prostatic venous plexus, 163, 168
Pseudoglandular phase, of lung development, 50
Pseudohermaphroditism, male, 170b

Pseudounipolar neurons, 11
Psoas major muscle, 128f, 129, 129t, 208, 209t, 211f
Psoas minor muscle, 129, 208, 209t
Psoas sign, 209b
Pterygoid canal, 297t, 370f, 371, 371f
    artery of, 375
    nerve of (vidian nerve), 373, 374f
Pterygoid hamulus, 377f
Pterygoid muscle, 379f
Pterygoid plate, 370f, 385f, 391f
Pterygoid plexus, 308, 312f, 359
Pterygoid process, of sphenoid bone, 370, 370f, 371f
Pterygoideus hamulus, 379f
Pterygomandibular raphe, 304, 378f
Pterygomandibular space, 335f
Pterygomaxillary fissure, 370f, 372
Pterygopalatine fossa, 370–375, 371, 371f, 372, 372f
    blood supply to, 368f, 375
    bones of, 360–362, 370f–372f
    neurovascular bundles of, 372–373, 372f, 374f, 375
    passageways of, 370–371, 370f
Pterygopalatine (sphenopalatine) ganglion, 316, 354f, 372f, 373, 374f, 375, 379, 387f
Pterygopalatine nerve, 372f, 373
Pubic crest, 142, 144f
Pubic rami, 142
Pubic symphysis, 142, 144f, 179f
Pubic tubercle, 142, 144f, 145f, 179f
Pubis, 79–80, 81f, 142, 142f–145f
Pubocervical ligament, 150f, 175
Pubococcygeus muscle, 147f, 148f, 148t, 149
Pubofemoral ligament, 201, 204f
Puboprostatic ligament, 150, 152f, 162, 162f
Puborectalis muscle, 147f, 148f, 148t, 149, 156, 191
Pubovesical ligament, 150, 152f, 157f
Pudendal artery, 154t, 155f, 192–193, 192f, 193f, 210f, 212f
Pudendal (Alcock's) canal, 189f, 191
Pudendal nerve, 191–192, 192f, 193f, 204f, 205f
Pudendal veins, 159, 159f, 192, 193
Pulmonary artery(ies), 48–49, 48f, 58–59, 58f, 59f, 69f
Pulmonary edema, 49b
Pulmonary embolism, 49b
Pulmonary ligament, 44, 47f
Pulmonary plexuses, 49–50
Pulmonary trunk, development of, 66f
Pulmonary valve, 58–59, 58f, 60f, 62, 63f
Pulmonary veins, 49, 55f
Purkinje fibers, 61b, 62, 62f
Pus, in pleural cavity (pyothorax), 47b
Pylorus, 94f, 95
Pyothorax, 47b
Pyramidal lobe, of thyroid gland, 342f, 343
Pyramidal process, of palatine bone, 370f, 371, 371f
Pyramidalis muscle, 80f, 81f, 82

Q
Quadrangular membrane, 393, 393f
Quadrangular space, of shoulder, 258, 258f
Quadrants, of abdominal wall, 78, 78f, 79t
Quadrate lamina, 393
Quadrate lobe, of liver, 114, 116f
Quadrate tubercle, of femur, 198, 199f
Quadratus femoris muscle, 200, 200t, 203f
Quadratus lumborum muscle, 128f, 129, 129t
Quadratus plantae muscle, 233, 234t, 235f, 239f

Quadriceps femoris muscle, 207–208, 208f, 209t
Quadriceps femoris tendon, 208f, 215f

R
Radial artery, 269f, 277f, 278–279, 279f, 284f, 288f, 289, 290f
Radial collateral artery, 269f, 279f
Radial collateral ligament, 262
Radial fossa, 261
Radial groove, 248, 248f
Radial nerve, 243f, 250f, 263, 265f, 266, 266t, 267f, 268f, 271f, 275t, 276–277, 278f, 279f, 289, 290f
Radial notch, 262, 262f, 263f
Radial recurrent artery, 269f, 279f
Radial tuberosity, 261, 261f
Radialis indicis artery, 288f, 290f
Radiocarpal joint, 282f
Radius
    distal, 270, 271f
    proximal, 261, 261f
Rami communicantes, 14–15, 15f
Raynaud's syndrome, 289b
Recesses, of pleural cavity, 45, 46f
Rectal arteries, 111f, 112, 112f, 154t, 155f, 156, 168t, 171f, 192f, 193, 203f
Rectal fascia, 150, 150f, 157f, 162f, 190f
Rectal folds, 157
Rectal nerves, 191, 193f, 203f
Rectal plexus, 159f
Rectal veins, 118f, 159, 159f, 192f, 193
Rectal venous plexus, 159f
Rectouterine pouch (pouch of Douglas, cul-de-sac), 151, 152f, 156, 157f, 158, 170f, 174
Rectouterine space, 150f
Rectovesical ligament, 162
Rectovesical pouch, 151, 152f, 158
Rectovesical septum (Denonvilliers' fascia), 151, 158, 162, 167, 168, 190f
Rectum, 156–158, 157f
    digital examination of, 161, 161t
    fascia of, 157–158, 157f
    lymphatic system of, 160–161, 160f
    prolapse of, 149b, 151
    relationships of, 161, 161t
Rectus abdominis muscle, 80f, 81, 81f, 84f, 85
Rectus femoris muscle, 201f, 209t, 210f, 211f, 218f
Rectus muscles, of orbit, 348–351, 348f, 350f, 353, 354f, 356f–358f
Rectus sheath, 80f–82f, 82–83, 252f
Recurrent articular nerve, 238f
Recurrent interosseous artery, 269f
Recurrent lacrimal artery, 357
Recurrent laryngeal nerve, 332, 339, 395, 396f
Recurrent meningeal artery, 349f, 358f
Recurrent meningeal nerve, 311
Recurrent tentorial nerve, 311
Recurrent thyroid nerve, 391f
Recurrent vagus nerve, 330f
Reference lines, of thoracic cavity, 43, 43f
Referred pain, 17–18, 19f
    cardiac, 60–61, 61f
    from gastrointestinal tract, 107t
Reflections
    in pericardial cavity, 52–53, 52f
    peritoneal, 91–92
        near bladder, 162
        near uterus, 174
    in pleural cavity, 44, 45f
Reflex, cremaster, 88
Relationships, 3

Renal artery, 97f, 130, 130f, 132f, 133, 133b, 134f, 138t
Renal fascia, 130–131, 131b, 132f
Renal vein, 73, 74f, 104f, 130, 130f, 132f, 134, 139, 139f
Renin, 135b
Reproductive system. See Female genital system; Male genital system.
Respiration, pleural cavity function in, 46–47
Respiratory distress syndrome, 50b
Rete cords, 169f
Rete ovarii, 169f
Rete testis, 169f
Retina, central artery of, 358
Retinaculum
    of ankle, 221f, 224, 224f
    of patella, 208f
Retroflexion, of uterus, 174, 174f
Retromammary space, 39
Retromandibular vein, 308, 343
Retroperitoneal organs, 93, 94t, 110
Retropharyngeal nodes, 344
Retropharyngeal space, 325b
Retropubic space, 150f, 162f
Retroversion, of uterus, 174, 174f
Retrovisceral space, 325b, 325f
Rhomboid muscles, 31, 32f
Rhomboideus major muscle, 253t, 254, 255f, 258f
Rhomboideus minor muscle, 253t, 254, 255f, 258f
Rib(s), 35–37, 36f, 37f
    articulations of, 37, 37f
    classification of, 36f, 37
    development of, 27–28
    elevation of, diaphragm function in, 41
    parts of, 36–37, 36f
    unique features of, 37
Rib cage, 35–38, 36f–38f, 46f, 79
Right aortic sinus, 59f
Right atrium, 54f, 57
Right border, of heart, 53
Right coronary artery, 54f–56f, 55–56
Right marginal artery, 55, 56f
Right sigmoid sinus, 312f
Right vagus nerve, 70, 71f
Right ventricle, 58, 58f
Rima glottidis, 393, 395t
Rima vestibuli, 393
Risorius muscle, 300f, 303t
Roof, of orbit, 345, 347
Root(s)
    of brachial plexus, 242, 243f, 245
    of penis, 182, 182f
Rostral position, 1, 2t
Rotation
    in midgut development, 122–126, 123f–125f
    of shoulder, 246, 246f
    of stomach, 100–101, 101f
Rotator cuff muscles, 255, 257f, 258
Rotatores muscle, 33t
Round ligament, 88, 90
    of liver, 115f, 118f
    of uterus, 87, 170f, 175f

S
Sacral artery, 134f, 138t, 154, 154t, 155, 155f, 206f
Sacral crest, 145
Sacral flexure, of rectum, 156, 157f
Sacral foramina, 143f
Sacral hiatus, 27, 27f, 145
Sacral nerve, 202
Sacral nodes, 172f

Sacral plexus, 153f, 202–203, 204f, 205f
Sacral promontory, 127, 128f, 143f, 144f, 145
Sacral splanchnic nerves, 152, 153f
Sacral vertebrae, 24f, 27, 27f
Sacrococcygeal teratoma, 7b
Sacrogenital folds, 151
Sacroiliac joint, 144–145, 144f
Sacrospinous ligament, 144f, 146, 179f, 192f, 202f
Sacrotuberous ligament, 144f, 146, 179f, 180f, 202f, 203f, 214f
Sacrovesical ligament, 151
Sacrum, 143f, 144f, 145
Sagittal plane, 1, 2f, 2t
Sagittal sinus, 312, 312b, 312f
Sagittal suture, 292f, 294f
Salivatory nucleus, 316, 317, 374f
Salpingopharyngeal fold, 387f, 389
Salpingopharyngeus muscle, 378f, 379, 389
Salpinx (fallopian tube), 171f–173f, 172–173
Saphenous nerve, 207f, 211f, 212f, 216–217, 218f, 223f, 228t
Saphenous opening, in fascia lata, 205, 207f
Saphenous vein, 207f, 210f, 212f, 223f, 224f, 228t
Sartorius muscle, 207–208, 207f, 209t, 210f–212f, 213t, 218f, 224f
Scalene muscle, 244f, 256f, 326–328, 326f, 327b, 327f, 330f
Scalene triangle, 242, 244, 244f
Scalene tubercle, 37
Scalp, 299–302, 300f, 301f
Scaphoid, 270, 271f, 281, 282f
Scapula, 246–248, 247f
   winged deformity of, 259, 259f
Scapular artery, 330f, 332–333
Scapular ligament, 249f, 258f
Scapular line, 43
Scapular nerve, 243f, 244f, 245, 250f, 253t, 258–259, 258f
Scapular spine, 247, 247f
Scarpa's fascia, 79, 87, 184f
Sciatic foramen, 144f, 146, 146t
Sciatic nerve, 128f, 202f, 203f, 204, 204f, 213t, 214f, 214t, 219, 226, 228, 238f
Sciatic notches, 142f, 143
Sclerotome, 9, 9f
   nervous system development from, 21
   vertebral development from, 27–28, 28f
Scoliosis, 25b
Scrotal artery, 192f
Scrotal nerves, 191
Scrotum, 183–184, 184f
   development of, 187–188, 188f
   layers of, 87–88, 88t
Secondary (lobar) bronchi, 48, 48f
Sections, 1
Segmental bronchi, 48, 48f
Sella tunica, 294f
Sella turcica, 296, 296f, 298
Semicircular (arcuate) line, 80f, 81f, 83
Semilunar line, 81f
Semimembranosus muscle, 203f, 211, 213t, 214f, 214t, 224f
Semimembranosus tendon, 225f
Seminal hillock (colliculus seminalis, verumontanum), 168
Seminal vesicle, 162f, 167, 167f, 168t
Semispinalis muscle, 33t
Semitendinosus muscle, 203f, 210, 211, 213t, 214f, 214t, 224f
Sensory (afferent) neurons, 11f, 12
   morphology of, 17b
   visceral, 16
Sensory root of the ciliary ganglion, 341f, 354f, 357f

Septal arteries, 388
Septal internal nasal nerves, 386
Septal papillary muscle, 58, 58f
Septomarginal trabecula, 58, 58f
Septum primum, 64, 64f
Septum secundum, 64f
Septum transversum
   diaphragm development from, 42, 42f
   liver development from, 100, 101f
Serous cavity, 4f, 5
Serratus anterior muscle, 251, 251f, 252f, 253, 256f
Serratus muscles, 31, 32f, 80f
Serratus posterior muscle, 258f
Sesamoid bones, 220, 221f, 233f
Sex dimorphisms, of pelvis, 143f–146f, 146–147, 146t
Shaft, rib, 36–37, 36f
Shingles, 397, 401
Short ciliary artery, 358–359
Short ciliary nerve, 341f, 354f, 357f
Short plantar ligament, 233, 233f
Short saphenous vein, 224f
Shoulder region, 246–261
   axilla in, 250, 250f
   blood supply to, 259, 260f, 261
   bones of, 246–248, 246f–248f
   definition of, 242f
   innervation of, 258–259, 258f, 259f
   joints of, 248–250, 248f, 249f
   movement of, 246, 246f
   muscles of
      back, 253–254, 253f–255f, 253t
      chest, 250–251, 251f, 252f, 253t
      intrinsic, 254–255, 255f–258f, 256t, 258
   separation in, 399–400, 403
Sibson's fascia, 44–45
Sigmoid arteries, 111f, 112, 112f
Sigmoid dural sinus, 299
Sigmoid sinus, 312f, 313f, 314, 390f
   groove for, 294f, 297f
Sigmoid veins, 118f
Sinoatrial node, 57, 61–62, 62f
Sinovaginal bulbs, 178
Sinus venarum (sinus of the venae cavae), 57
Sinus venosus, 63, 63f, 64f
Sites of reflection. See Reflections.
Skeletal muscle, 6
Skeletal system, 5. See also Bone(s); Joint(s); specific bones and joints.
Skene's (paraurethral) glands, 186, 187f
Skin, 4, 4f
   of abdominal wall, 79
   of scalp, 299
Skull, 291–299
   anterior cranial fossa in, 293–296, 294f–296f, 295t, 296b
   development of, 292, 294f
   middle cranial fossa in, 294f, 296, 296f–298f, 297t, 298, 299b
   morphology of, 291–292
   posterior cranial fossa in, 294f, 297f, 298f, 299, 299t
Sliding inguinal hernia, 90b
Small cardiac vein, 54f, 55f
Small intestine
   development of, 122–126, 123f–125f
   duodenum of, 102f, 103–105, 104f, 105f
   ileum of, 106, 106f, 107t, 108, 108t
   jejunum of, 106, 106f, 107t, 108, 108t
Smooth muscle, 5–6
Soft palate, 377–379, 378f, 378t, 379f
Soleal line, 220, 222f
Soleus muscle, 213t, 223f–225f, 224–225, 226t, 227f, 228t
Somatic (parietal) mesoderm, 9

Somatic nervous system, 12
   versus autonomic nervous system, 14
Somitic (para-axial) mesoderm, 8–9, 9f
Somitomeres, 8–9
Spasms, of scalene muscles, 327b
Special visceral efferent and afferent fibers, in cranial nerves, 316–317, 318t, 319
Spermatic cord, 87–88, 88t, 91f, 166
Spermatic fascia, 81f, 86f, 87, 89f, 91f, 184f
Sphenoethmoid recess, 385f, 386, 386t, 387f
Sphenoid bone, 293, 293f, 294f, 296, 298, 298f, 299, 345, 346f, 370–371, 370f, 371f
Sphenoid process, of palatine bone, 371, 371f
Sphenoid sinus, 298f, 315f, 386t
Sphenoidal (anterolateral) fontanelle, 292, 294f
Sphenoidal jugum, 294f, 296
Sphenoidal sinus, 385, 385f, 387f
Sphenopalatine artery, 388
Sphenopalatine foramen, 370f, 371, 385f, 386
Sphenopalatine notch, 370f, 371, 371f
Sphenopalatine (pterygopalatine) nucleus, 316
Sphenoparietal sinus, 312f, 313f
Sphincter of Oddi, 122
Sphincter urethrae muscle, 181
Sphincter urethrovaginalis muscle, 180f, 181
Sphincter vesicae, 163
Spigelian hernia, 90b
Spinal accessory nerve (XI), 244f, 250f, 253t, 313f, 317, 318, 338f, 339
Spinal artery, 332, 340f
Spinal cord
   development of, 19–21, 20f, 30–31
   function of, 13–14
   preganglionic fibers in, 17t
   structure of, 13–14, 13f
Spinal meninges, 29–30, 29f–31f
Spinal nerves, 12, 13f, 14
   development of, 32
   lumbar, 136
   to pelvis, 151
   to pericardium, 53
Spinal tap, 31
Spinalis muscles, 33t
Spinoglenoid (great scapular) notch, 247, 247f
Spinotransverse muscles, 33t
Spiral ganglion, 319
Spiral valve (of Heister), 119
Splanchnic nerves, 15–16, 15f, 16t
   to colon, 113
   to duodenum, 105–106, 107t
   to heart, 71f
   to ileum, 108
   to jejunum, 108
   to kidney, 133–134
   lumbar, 74–75, 98f, 133–134, 137
   pelvic, 137, 152, 153f, 192, 205f, 317
   sacral, 152, 153f
   to stomach, 97, 98f
Spleen, 107t, 119f, 120–121, 120f
Splenic artery, 93f, 96f, 97f, 101–102, 117f, 119f, 120–121
Splenic flexure, 103f
Splenic vein, 97, 112, 118f, 121
Splenius capitis muscle, 33t
Splenius cervicalis muscle, 33t
Splenorenal ligament, 92f, 93f, 95, 99f, 101–102, 101f, 102f, 120
Spondylolisthesis, 26b
Spongy (penile) urethra, 164, 164f, 167f, 181–183, 182f–184f
Spring (calcaneonavicular) ligament, 230f, 232–233, 233f
Squamous portion
   of frontal bone, 295, 295f, 302
   of temporal bone, 293f, 296, 298

Stellate (cervicothoracic) ganglion, 241–242, 340–341, 341f
Sternal angle, 36f, 38, 38f, 46f
Sternal end, of clavicle, 246, 246f
Sternoclavicular joint, 248, 249f
Sternoclavicular ligament, 249f
Sternocleidomastoid muscle, 244f, 250f, 300f, 319, 321, 322f–324f, 322t, 325, 326f, 326t
Sternocostal surface, 53, 54f
Sternocostal triangle, 128f, 129
Sternohyoid muscle, 323f, 327f, 335f, 336f, 341
Sternothyroid muscle, 323f, 327f, 341, 342f
Sternum, 37–38, 38f
Stomach, 94–102
   blood supply to, 96–97, 96f, 97f, 99–100, 99f
   development of, 95, 99–101, 99f, 101f
   innervation of, 97–99, 98f, 107t
   pain in, 98b
   parts of, 94–95, 94f, 95f
   peptic ulcer disease of, 398, 402
   relationships of, 95–96, 95f
   rotation of, 100–101, 101f
   tube in, 96b
Stones, kidney, 398–399, 402
Straight arteries, 106, 106f
Straight sinus, 310f, 312, 312f, 313f
Strap (infrahyoid) muscles, 324, 324f, 325f, 341–342
Styloglossus muscle, 335f, 380f, 381, 381t, 389, 391, 391f
Stylohyoid ligament, 391f
Stylohyoid muscle, 323f, 327f, 334t, 335f, 336, 342f, 379f, 390f
Stylohyoideus muscle, 380f
Styloid process
   of fibula, 208f
   of radius, 270, 271f, 288f
   of skull, 293f
   of ulna, 270, 271f, 288f
Stylomandibular ligament, 323, 335f
Stylomastoid foramen, 305
Stylopharyngeus muscle, 335f, 378f–380f, 390f, 390t, 391f
Subacromial bursa, 258
Subarachnoid space, 29, 29f, 309f, 311
Subclavian arteries, 68, 68f, 69f, 71f, 250f, 259, 260f, 261, 326, 329, 330f, 331f, 332
Subclavian artery impression, 47f
Subclavian nerve, 245, 259
Subclavian (vascular) triangle, 326, 327t
Subclavian vein, 54f, 68f, 250f, 326–327, 333
Subclavius muscle, 251, 253t
Subcoracoid bursa, 257f
Subcostal muscles, 39
Subcostal nerve, 41, 128f, 129, 207f, 210f
Subcostal plane, 78, 78f
Subcostal vein, 74f
Subdeltoid bursa, 257f
Subdural hematoma, 312b
Subdural space, 29
Sublingual caruncle, 382
Sublingual duct of Bartholin, 383
Sublingual fold, 380f
Sublingual gland, 374f, 376f, 380f, 383, 383f
Sublingual plica, 383
Sublingual (paralingual) space, 326, 376f, 382–384, 383f
Submandibular (Wharton's) duct, 336, 382, 383f
Submandibular ganglion, 316–317, 374f, 384, 387f

Submandibular gland, 323f, 335f, 336, 336f, 374f, 376f, 382–383, 383f
Submandibular nodes, 344
Submandibular space, 336, 382
Submandibular (digastric) triangle, 322f, 326f, 333, 334t, 335f, 336
Submaxillary space, 382
Submental nodes, 343, 344
Submental triangle, 322f, 334t, 343
Subscapular artery, 260f
Subscapular fossa, 246, 247f
Subscapular nerve, 245, 250f, 256t, 259, 265f
Subscapularis muscle, 252f, 255, 256t, 257f, 258, 264f, 265f
Subscapularis tendon, 257f
Subserous (extraserous, extraperitoneal) fascia, 4f, 5, 82, 83, 86f, 87, 130, 150–151
Sulcus limitans, 20f, 21
Sulcus terminalis, 380, 380f
Superciliary ridge, 346f
Superficial branches, of cervical plexus, 328–329, 328f, 329t
Superficial cardiac plexus, 60
Superficial cervical artery, 330f, 333
Superficial circumflex femoral artery, 210f
Superficial circumflex iliac artery, 84f, 85, 206f, 207f
Superficial circumflex iliac vein, 84f, 207f
Superficial epigastric artery, 84f, 207f, 210f, 212f
Superficial fascia, 4–5, 4f
   of abdominal wall, 79
   of neck, 322
   of scrotum, 183–184, 184f
Superficial fibular nerve, 228t, 238f
Superficial inguinal ring, 86f, 87
Superficial middle cerebral vein, 313f
Superficial palmar arch, 279f, 289, 290f
Superficial peroneal nerve, 223f, 228f, 231
Superficial peroneal retinaculum, 224f
Superficial petrosal artery, 298
Superficial position, 1, 2t
Superficial postanal space, 190f
Superficial pouch
   female, 184–187, 185f–187f
   male, 181–184, 181f–184f
Superficial radial artery, 284f
Superficial radial nerve, 276–277
Superficial temporal artery, 300f, 301–302, 301f, 305f, 338
Superficial temporal vein, 308
Superficial transverse metacarpal ligaments, 283f
Superficial transverse perineal muscles, 182f, 183, 184f, 190f
Superior auricular muscles, 304
Superior cervical ganglion, 340–341, 341f, 374f
Superior collateral artery, 265f
Superior concha, 386, 387f
Superior duodenal flexure, 104
Superior epigastric artery, 41, 84f, 85
Superior epigastric vein, 85
Superior extensor retinaculum, 227f
Superior (jugular) ganglion, 317, 339
Superior gemellus muscle, 200, 200t, 202f, 203f, 214f
Superior gluteal artery, 154t, 155, 202f, 203f, 204, 205, 206f, 211f
Superior gluteal nerve, 151, 202f, 203, 204f, 205f
Superior hypogastric plexus, 137, 151–152, 153f, 153t, 175
Superior intercostal vein, 74f

Superior labial artery, 300f, 307
Superior laryngeal artery, 330f, 331f, 335f, 338, 393, 396f
Superior laryngeal nerve, 338, 339, 342f, 391f, 393, 396b
Superior longitudinal muscle, 380f, 381
Superior meatus, 385f, 386
Superior mesenteric artery, 99, 99f, 104f, 106, 106f, 111, 111f, 112f, 138t
   midgut development and, 122–123, 123f
Superior mesenteric vein, 104f, 108, 112, 118f
Superior nuchal line, 293f
Superior oblique muscle, 349f–352f, 351–353, 352t, 356f–358f
Superior ophthalmic vein, 308, 345, 349f, 359
Superior orbital fissure, 297f, 297t, 298, 314, 345, 346f, 371f
Superior orbital fossa, 296f
Superior orbital margin, 345
Superior palatine constrictor muscle, 378f, 380f
Superior peroneal retinaculum, 227f
Superior petrosal sinus, 312f, 313f, 314, 390f
Superior pharyngeal constrictor muscle, 334t, 335f, 337, 379, 379f, 389, 390f, 390t, 391f, 392t
Superior phrenic artery, 42
Superior position, 1, 2f, 2t
Superior rectal artery, 111f, 112, 112f
Superior rectus muscle, 350f, 351, 351f, 352f, 353, 353t, 354f, 356f–358f
Superior sagittal sinus, 310f, 312, 312b, 312f
Superior salivatory nucleus, 316, 374f
Superior subscapular nerve, 243f
Superior tarsus (Muller's) muscle, 348f, 349f, 350–351
Superior temporal line, 292f, 293f
Superior thoracic aperture, 38
Superior thyroid artery, 300f, 330f, 331f, 335f, 337–338, 342f, 343
Superior thyroid vein, 342f, 343
Superior trunk, of brachial plexus, 242, 243f
Superior ulnar collateral artery, 266, 269f, 279f
Superior vena cava, 54f, 57, 57f, 67–68, 68f, 71f
Superior vena cava impression, 47f
Superior vesical artery, 155f
Superolateral aspect, of cavernous sinus, 310
Supination
   of elbow joint, 262, 263f
   of wrist, 270
Supinator crest, 262f
Supinator muscle, 274, 274f, 275t, 276f, 277f, 278f, 279f
Supracilary arch, of frontal bone, 295f, 302
Supraclavicular nerve, 306f, 328f, 329
Supraclavicular nodes, 344
Supracondylar lines, of femur, 206
Supracrestal plane, 78f
Supraduodenal vein, 118f
Supraglenoid fossa, 247f
Supraglenoid tubercle, 248
Supraorbital artery, 300f, 307–308, 356f, 357, 358f
Supraorbital foramen, 302, 302t
Supraorbital nerve, 300, 307, 306f, 349f, 356f, 387f
Supraorbital notch, 292f, 295f, 302, 345, 346f
Supraorbital vein, 359
Suprapatellar bursa, 208f, 215f
Suprapubic (hypogastric) region, 78–79, 78f
Suprarenal artery, 134f, 136, 138t
Suprarenal gland, 128f, 131, 131f, 134f, 135–136, 136t
Suprarenal vein, 134f, 136, 136t

Suprascapular artery, 244f, 259, 260f, 261, 330f, 331f, 332
Suprascapular nerve, 243f, 244f, 245, 250f, 256t, 259, 332
Suprascapular notch, 247f, 248
Supraspinatus artery, 258f
Supraspinatus muscle, 255, 256t, 257f, 258, 258f
Supraspinatus nerve, 258f
Supraspinatus tendon, 258
Supraspinous fossa, 247
Supraspinous ligaments, of vertebral column, 29
Suprasternal notch, 36f, 37, 38f
Suprasternal space of Burns, 323
Supratrochlear artery, 300f, 307, 358, 358f
Supratrochlear nerve, 300, 306f, 307, 349f, 356f, 387f
Supraventricular crest, 58
Supreme genicular artery, 218f
Supreme intercostal artery, 41
Supreme intercostal vein, 74f
Supreme thoracic artery, 259, 260f
Sural cutaneous nerve, 223f, 224f, 238f
Sural nerve, 228–229, 238f
Surfactant deficiency, 50b
Surgical neck, of humerus, 248, 248f
Suspensory ligament (of Lockwood), 348
Suspensory ligament of the ovary, 170, 170f, 178f
Suspensory ligament of the thyroid gland (suspensory ligament of Berry), 342
Suspensory ligaments (of Cooper) of the breast, 39
Sustenaculum tali, 220, 221f, 230f
Sutures, in bones, 6t, 292, 292f, 294f
Sweat glands, 4
Sympathetic nervous system, 14–15, 15f, 16t, 17t, 19t
  of anal canal, 159
  of bladder, 163
  of brachial plexus, 241
  of cecum, 107t
  of colon, 107t, 113
  of duodenum, 105–106, 107t
  of epididymis, 166
  of esophagus, 107t
  of gallbladder, 107t
  of gastrointestinal tract, 107t
  of ileum, 107t
  of jejunum, 107t
  of kidney, 133–134
  of liver, 107t
  of pancreas, 107t, 122
  of pelvis, 151–152, 153f, 153t
  of spleen, 107t
  of stomach, 97–99, 98f, 107t
  of ureter, 135
  of uterus, 175
Sympathetic trunk, 14, 71f, 74–75, 129, 330f, 331f, 340, 341f
Symphysis, 6t
Synapses, 11, 13, 15–16
Synarthrodial joints, 6, 6t
Synchondrosis, 6t
Syndesmosis, 6t

T
Teniae coli, 109, 109f, 110f
Talocalcaneal ligament, 230f
Talofibular ligament, 230f
Talus, 220, 221f, 232f
Tarsal arteries, 240f
Tarsal bones, 220, 221f
Tarsometatarsal ligament, 230f, 233f
Taste buds, 381

Tegmen tympani, 298
Temporal artery, 300f, 301–302, 301f, 305f, 338, 358
Temporal bone, 293f, 294f, 298, 298f, 299, 314
Temporal fossa, 359–360, 359f
Temporal nerve, 303t, 305
Temporal vein, 305f, 308
Temporalis muscle, 300f, 304f, 356f
Tenon's capsule, 347–348
Tensor fasciae latae muscles, 198, 200, 200t, 201f, 210f, 211f, 218f
Tensor veli palatini muscle, 377–378, 378f, 378t, 379f
Tentorial nerve, 311
Tentorial notch, 310
Tentorium cerebelli, 298, 310, 310f, 312, 312f
Teratoma, sacrococcygeal, 7b
Teres major muscle, 252f, 255f–258f, 256t, 258, 265f, 268f
Teres major tendon, 257f
Teres minor muscle, 255, 256t, 256t, 257f, 258, 267f, 268f
Teres minor tendon, 257f
Terminal cutaneous rami to foot, 238f
Terminal line, of pelvis, 144
Terminal phase, of lung development, 50–51
Terminology, 1–4, 2f, 2t, 3b, 3f
Testicular artery, 138f, 148f, 166, 168t
Testicular veins, 166
Testis, 162f, 166, 168t
  cancer of, 399, 402
  descent of, 88, 89f
  development of, 169–170, 169f, 170f
  undescended, 90b
Testis-determining factor, 169
Tetralogy of Fallot, 65, 67f
Thebesian veins, 57
Thenar muscles, 282–283, 284f, 285f
Thigh, 205–220
  adductor canal in, 216–217, 218f
  anterior compartment of, 207–209, 209t, 210f
  blood supply to, 206f, 212f, 219–220, 219f
  bones of, 199f, 205–206, 208f
  definition of, 195, 196f, 205
  fascia of, 205, 207f
  femoral sheath in, 216, 218f
  femoral triangle of, 212f, 216
  innervation of, 204f, 217, 218f, 219, 219f
  medial compartment of, 209, 210f, 211, 212f, 213t
  muscles of
    in anterior compartment, 207–209, 209t, 210f
    in medial compartment, 209, 210f, 211, 212f, 213t
    in posterior compartment, 210, 211f, 213, 214f, 214t
  posterior compartment of, 210, 211f, 213, 214f, 214t
  superficial fascia of, 186f
Third occipital nerve, 306f
Thoracentesis, 45b, 47b
Thoracic apertures, 38
Thoracic artery, 41, 66, 68f, 259, 260f, 333
Thoracic duct, 73–74
Thoracic ganglion, 330f
Thoracic nerve, 243f, 244f, 245, 250f, 253t, 258–259
Thoracic spinal nerves, 42, 83–84, 244
Thoracic vein, 41, 84f
Thoracic vertebrae, 24f, 27
Thoracis muscle, 33t
Thoracoabdominal nerves, 84–85, 84f
Thoracoabdominal outflow, 16

Thoracoacromial artery, 259, 260f
Thoracodorsal artery, 258f, 260f
Thoracodorsal nerve, 243f, 250f, 253t, 259
Thoracoepigastric vein, 84f, 85
Thoracolumbar fascia, 256f
Thoracolumbar outflow, 14
Thorax. *See also* Heart; Mediastinum; *specific structures.*
  cavity of, 43–51
    development of, 43–44, 44f
    lung in, 47–51, 47f, 48f, 49t, 50f
    pleural cavity as, 44–47, 45f–47f
    reference lines of, 43, 43f
  diaphragm in, 41–43, 42f
  point of maximal impulse on, 43b
  shape of, 35–36
  surface anatomy of, 43, 43f
  wall of, 35–41
    bones of, 35–38, 36f–38f. *See also* Rib(s).
    breast in, 39, 41
    inferior thoracic aperture of, 38
    muscles of, 38–39, 39f, 40f, 250–251, 251f, 252f, 253t
    neurovascular structures of, 40f, 41
    superior thoracic aperture of, 38
Thumb, movement of, 281, 282f
Thymus, 66–67
Thyroarytenoid muscle, 394f, 395t
Thyrocervical trunk, 259, 260f, 330f, 332
Thyroepiglottic ligament, 392f, 393f
Thyroepiglottic muscle, 395t
Thyrohyoid ligament, 323f, 392f
Thyrohyoid membrane, 391f–394f
Thyrohyoid muscle, 323f, 327f, 329, 337, 341, 342f
Thyroid artery, 66, 300f, 330f, 332, 335f, 337–338, 342f, 396f
Thyroid cartilage, 322, 323f, 342f, 343, 391f, 392–393, 392f, 394f, 396f
Thyroid gland, 323f, 327f, 342–343, 342f
Thyroid membrane, 392
Thyroid nerve, 391f
Thyroid notch, 392
Thyroid vein, 68f, 342f, 343
Thyroidea ima, 343
Tibia, 206, 208f, 220, 222f
Tibial artery, 225f, 228f, 231, 232f, 239, 239f, 240f
Tibial (medial) collateral ligament, 215, 215f, 217f
Tibial ligament, 208f
Tibial nerve, 203, 204, 205f, 214f, 223f–225f, 226t, 228, 230–231, 238, 238f
Tibial plateau, 206
Tibial tuberosity, 208f, 217f, 222f
Tibialis anterior muscle, 223f, 226, 227f, 227t, 240f
Tibialis anterior tendon, 237f
Tibialis posterior muscle, 213t, 223f, 225, 225f, 226t, 235f
Tibialis posterior tendon, 236f
Tibiofibular ligament, 230f
Tongue, 379–382, 380f, 381t
Tonsil
  lingual, 380f, 381
  palatine, 378f, 379, 380f
  pharyngeal, 389
Tonsillar artery, 335f, 379, 396f
Tonsillar nerve, 377
Torus tubarius, 387f
Trabecular carneae, 58, 58f, 59f
Trachea, 48, 48f, 69, 70–71
Tracheal cartilage, 392f
Tracheal impression, 47f
Tracheal nodes, 41
Tracheobronchial nodes, 50

Tracheoesophageal groove, 343
Transesophageal echocardiography, 72b
Transposition of the great vessels, 65, 67f
Transpyloric plane, 78, 78f
Transsphenoidal surgical approach, to pituitary gland, 389b
Transtubercular (intertubercular) line, 78, 78f
Transversalis fascia, 5, 80f, 81f, 82, 84f, 86f, 87, 90, 91f, 129–130, 184f
Transverse arch, 231–232, 232f
Transverse arytenoid muscle, 395t
Transverse cervical artery, 244f, 258f, 259, 260f, 330f, 332–333
Transverse cervical (cardinal) ligament, 150f, 151, 156, 175
Transverse cervical nerve, 328f, 329, 336f
Transverse cruciate ligament, 237f
Transverse facial artery, 300f, 331f
Transverse fascia, 283f
Transverse mesocolon, 124, 124f
Transverse metacarpal ligament, 288f
Transverse muscle, 380f, 381
Transverse palatine suture, 385f
Transverse part, of nasalis muscle, 304
Transverse pericardial sinus, 52, 52f
Transverse perineal ligament, 152f, 181
Transverse plane, 1, 2f, 2t
Transverse processes, vertebral, 24–25, 25, 25f
Transverse rectal folds, 157
Transverse scapular ligament, 258f
Transverse sinus, 297f, 310f, 312f, 313f, 314
Transversospinal muscles, 32, 33t
Transversus abdominis muscle, 80f–82f, 81, 85, 86f
Transversus thoracis muscle, 39, 40f
Trapezium, 271f, 272, 282f
Trapezius muscle, 31–32, 32f, 244f, 253–254, 253t, 254f–256f, 319, 320f, 321, 322f, 322t, 326f, 326t, 327f
Trapezoid, 271f, 272, 282f
Trapezoid ligament, 249, 249f
Trapezoid tubercle, of clavicle, 246, 246f
Trendelenburg test, 200, 203f
Triangles, of neck. See Neck, triangles of.
Triangular ligaments, 114, 116f
Triangular space, of shoulder, 258, 258f
Triceps brachii muscle, 257f, 258f, 263, 266t, 267f, 268f, 272f
Triceps surae, 225
Tricuspid valve, 58, 58f, 60f, 62, 63f
Trigeminal (Meckel's) cave, 314–315
Trigeminal ganglion, 313f, 314, 315f, 318, 357f, 358f
Trigeminal impression, 298
Trigeminal nerve, 305, 311, 315, 387f
Trigone muscle, of bladder, 163
Trilaminar embryo, 6–7, 6f–8f
Triquetrum, 270, 271f, 282f
Trochanter, 198, 199f, 204f
Trochlea, 261, 261f, 263f, 358f
Trochlea tali, 220, 221f
Trochlear fossa, 346f
Trochlear nerve (IV), 313f, 316, 353–355, 356f–358f
  cavernous sinus and, 314–315, 315f
Trochlear notch, 261, 262f, 263f
True conjugate, of pelvis, 146f, 147
True (lesser) pelvis, versus greater pelvis, 144f, 145–146
True ribs, 37
True vocal cords, 393
Truncoaortic sac, 63, 63f
Truncoconal ridges, 65
Truncus arteriosus, 63, 63f, 66f, 68
  persistent, 65, 67f

Trunk(s), of brachial plexus, 242, 243f, 244–245, 244f
Trunk wall, organization of, 4–6, 4f, 5b, 6t
Tubercle, rib, 36, 36f, 37
Tuberculum sellae, 296f, 311
Tumor(s). See also Cancer.
  breast, 39, 41
Tunica albuginea, 166, 169f, 171, 182, 183f, 184f
Tunica vaginalis, 88, 166
Tympanic artery, 298

U
Ulna
  distal, 270, 271f
  proximal, 261–262, 261f
Ulnar artery, 266, 269f, 271f, 277f, 278–279, 279f, 289, 290f
Ulnar collateral artery, 264f, 266, 267f, 269f, 279f
Ulnar collateral ligament, 262
Ulnar nerve, 243f, 245, 250f, 264f, 265f, 266, 267f, 268f, 274f, 276, 279f, 283f, 286–287, 288f
Ulnar recurrent arteries, 269f, 279f
Ulnar tuberosity, 261–262, 261f
Umbilical artery, 154t, 155f, 156
Umbilical ligaments, 79, 152f, 162f
Umbilical region, 78, 78f
Umbilical vein, 114, 118f
Umbilicus, 79
Uncinate process, 385f, 386, 387f
Unhappy triad, in knee injury, 215b
Upper limb, 241–290. See also specific structures.
  development of, 195–197, 196b, 197f
  overview of, 241, 242f
  regions of, 241, 242f
Upper subscapular nerve, 250f, 259, 265f
Upper trunk, of brachial plexus, 242, 243f, 244, 245
Urachus, 165, 165f
Ureter
  abdominal, 130f, 134f, 135
  development of, 134
  pelvic, 153f, 161, 162f
Ureteric arteries, 134f
Ureteric bud, 165f
Urethra, 163–164
  bladder orifice for, 163
  external orifice of, 180f, 185f, 187f
Urethral artery, 180f
Urethral crest, 168
Urethral sphincter, 148t
Urethrovaginal sphincter, 148t, 149
Urinary system. See specific components, eg, Bladder; Kidney.
Urogenital diaphragm, 147f, 148f, 162f, 167f, 179, 180f, 181, 181f
Urogenital folds, 187–188, 189t
Urogenital hiatus, 147f, 149–150, 179, 180f, 181
Urogenital sinus, 164–165, 165f, 178f, 188f, 189t
Urogenital triangle
  urogenital diaphragm in, 179, 180f, 181, 181f
  superficial pouch in
    female, 184–187, 185f–187f
    male, 181–184, 181f–184f
Urorectal fold, 164
Urorectal septum, 164, 165f
Uterine artery, 154t, 156, 171–173, 171f, 173f, 175, 175f, 177t
Uterine (fallopian) tubes, 171f–173f, 172–173
Uterine vein, 175, 175f, 177t
Uterine venous plexus, 177t
Uterosacral fold, 170f

Uterosacral ligament, 150f, 151, 170f, 175, 176
Uterovaginal canal, 178, 178f
Uterovesical ligament, 150f
Uterus, 173–176
  blood supply of, 171f, 175, 177t
  development of, 177–178, 178f
  fibroids of, 174b
  innervation of, 175, 177t
  ligaments of, 150f, 151, 170f, 173f, 174–175, 175f
  lymphatic system of, 172f, 175, 177t
  peritoneal covering of, 174
  position of, 173–174, 174f
  prolapse of, 151, 174
  relationships of, 175–176, 176f
Uvula, 376f, 377

V
Vagal trunks, 97, 98f, 105–106, 107t
Vagina, 176–177, 176f, 177t, 186f
  cervix in, 173–174, 173f, 174f, 176, 177t
  development of, 177–178, 178f
  prolapse of, 149b, 151
  urogenital diaphragm penetration by, 181
Vaginal artery, 154t, 156, 171f
Vaginal vestibule, 185, 185f, 186f
Vagus nerve (X)
  branches of, 339
  in carotid sheath, 325
  to colon, 113
  to dura mater, 311, 313f
  to esophagus, 70, 71f
  function of, 317, 318, 319
  to heart, 54f, 61, 68f
  to ileum, 108
  to jejunum, 108
  to larynx, 393
  to lung, 49–50
  in neck, 330f
  to palate, 379
  to stomach, 97–99, 98f
Vallate (circumvallate) papillae, 380f, 381, 396f
Valleculae epiglotticae, 380f, 381, 394f
Valves of Houston (transverse rectal folds), 157, 157f
Varicella-zoster virus infection, 397, 401
Vas deferens, 153f
Vasa recta, 133f
Vascular (subclavian) triangle, 326, 327t
Vastus intermedius muscle, 207–208, 209t, 218f
Vastus lateralis muscle, 201f, 203f, 207, 209t, 211f, 218f
Vastus medialis muscle, 209t, 210f, 211f, 213t, 218f
Vein(s), 3, 3f
  of abdominal wall, 84f, 85
  of anal canal, 159–160, 159f
  of arm, 269, 270f
  of bladder, 160f, 163
  of colon, 112
  of face, 308
  of kidney, 133
  of mediastinum, 67–68, 68f
  of neck, 343–344
  of ovary, 177t
  of pelvis, 156
  of stomach, 97
  of thoracic wall, 40f, 41
  of thymus, 66
  of uterine tubes, 177t
  of uterus, 177t
  of vagina, 176, 177t
Vena cava. See Inferior vena cava; Superior vena cava.
Venae cordis minimae, 57

Venous sinuses, dural. *See* Dural venous sinuses.
Ventral horns, of spinal cord, 13, 13f
Ventral mesentery, liver development from, 100, 101f
Ventral mesogastrium
  liver development from, 100
  stomach development from, 95
Ventral position, 1, 2f, 2t
Ventral ramus, of spinal cord, 13f, 14
Ventricle
  development of, 62–65, 63f–66f, 65t
  left, 59–60, 59f, 60f
  primitive, 63, 63f
  right, 58, 58f
Ventricular septum, 59f, 60, 62f, 64f, 65, 65f, 66f
Ventricular vein, 55f
Venules, 3, 3f
Vermilion border, 384f
Vertebrae and vertebral column, 23–30
  cervical, 24f, 25–27, 26f
  coccygeal, 24f, 145
  curvature of, 23, 24f, 25b
  development of, 27–28, 28f
  joints of, 28–29
  ligaments of, 79
  lumbar, 24f, 25f, 27
  neonatal, 23
  parts of, 23–25, 24f–26f
  rib attachment to, 36, 36f, 37
  sacral, 24f, 27, 27f, 145
  thoracic, 24f, 27
  in thoracic apertures, 38
Vertebral artery, 69f, 311, 331f, 332, 340f
Vertebral column, of neck, 322
Vertebral vein, 332
Vertebral venous system (Batson's plexus), 163, 168, 309
Vertical muscle, 380f, 382
Verumontanum (seminal hillock, colliculus seminalis), 168
Vesical arteries, 154t, 155f, 156, 167f, 168, 168t

Vesical venous plexus, 163
Vesicocervical space, 157f
Vesicouterine fossa, 157f
Vesicouterine ligament, 162
Vesicouterine pouch, 151, 152f
Vesicouterine space, 150f
Vestibular fold, 393, 394f
Vestibular ganglion, 319
Vestibular (Bartholin's) glands, 186, 186f, 187f
Vestibular ligament, 393, 393f
Vestibule
  oral cavity, 375–376, 376f
  vaginal, 185, 185f, 186f
Vestibulocochlear nerve (VIII), 313f, 319
Vidian nerve (nerve of pterygoid canal), 373, 374f
Visceral afferent neurons, 16
Visceral column, of neck, 321–322, 323f, 341–343
Visceral endopelvic fascia, 150
Visceral lateral mesoderm, 9
Visceral nerves. *See* Splanchnic nerves.
Visceral pain, 17–18, 19f
Visceral pericardium, 51–52, 52f
Visceral peritoneum, 90, 92, 92f
Visceral pleura, 44–46, 45f
Visceral surface, of spleen, 120, 120f
Viscerocranium, 291
Vocal folds (cords), 388f, 393, 394f, 395t, 396f
Vocal ligament, 393f
Vocalis muscle, 395t
Volvulus, 125f, 126
Vomer, 385
Vorticose vein, 359
Vulva, 184–187

W
Waldeyer's (presacral) fascia, 157, 190f
Waldeyer's lymphatic ring, 381
Wharton's (submandibular) duct, 336, 382
White matter, 11, 13, 13f
White ramus communicans, 14, 15f
Whitnall's (orbital) tubule, 345

Winged scapula, 259, 259f
Wings, of sphenoid bone, 296, 298, 371, 371f
Wrist
  anatomic snuffbox at, 281, 281f
  bones of, 270, 271f, 272, 281, 282f
  carpal tunnel in, 279, 280f, 281b
  cross-section of, 280f
  innervation of, 275–278, 275t, 277f, 278f
  joints of, 281, 282f
  movement of, 270
  muscles of
    extensor, 272f, 273–274, 273t, 274f, 275t
    flexor, 266t, 272–273, 272f, 273t

X
Xiphisternal joint, 38f
Xiphoid process, 36f, 38

Y
Yolk sac, 6, 6f

Z
Zone of polarizing activity, in limb development, 196
Zygapophyseal joints, 29
Zygomatic arch, 293f
Zygomatic artery, 357
Zygomatic bone, 292f, 293f, 302, 345, 346f
Zygomatic nerve, 303t, 305, 305f, 349f, 354f, 372f, 373
Zygomatic process, 292f, 293f, 295f, 302
Zygomaticofacial foramen, 293f, 302, 302t, 345, 346f, 373
Zygomaticofacial nerve, 306f, 307, 349f, 373, 374f
Zygomaticomaxillary suture, 346f
Zygomatico-orbital artery, 300f
Zygomatico-orbital foramen, 345
Zygomaticotemporal foramen, 302, 302t, 345, 373
Zygomaticotemporal nerve, 306f, 307, 349f, 355, 373, 374f
Zygomaticus major muscle, 300f, 303t, 304
Zygomaticus minor muscle, 300f